Tumor Necrosis Factors

IMMUNOLOGY SERIES

1. Mechanisms in Allergy: Reagin-Mediated Hypersensitivity
   Edited by Lawrence Goodfriend, Alec Sehon and Robert P. Orange
2. Immunopathology: Methods and Techniques
   Edited by Theodore P. Zacharia and Sidney S. Breese, Jr.
3. Immunity and Cancer in Man: An Introduction
   Edited by Arnold E. Reif
4. *Bordetella pertussis:* Immunological and Other Biological Activities
   J.J. Munoz and R.K. Bergman
5. The Lymphocyte: Structure and Function (in two parts)
   Edited by John J. Marchalonis
6. Immunology of Receptors
   Edited by B. Cinader
7. Immediate Hypersensitivity: Modern Concepts and Development
   Edited by Michael K. Bach
8. Theoretical Immunology
   Edited by George I. Bell, Alan S. Perelson, and George H. Pimbley, Jr.
9. Immunodiagnosis of Cancer (in two parts)
   Edited by Ronald B. Herberman and K. Robert McIntire
10. Immunologically Mediated Renal Diseases: Criteria for Diagnosis and Treatment
    Edited by Robert T. McCluskey and Giuseppe A. Andres
11. Clinical Immunotherapy
    Edited by Albert F. LoBuglio
12. Mechanisms of Immunity to Virus-Induced Tumors
    Edited by John W. Blasecki
13. Manual of Macrophage Methodology: Collection, Characterization, and Function
    Edited by Herbert B. Herscowitz, Howard T. Holden, Joseph A. Bellanti, and Abdul Ghaffar
14. Suppressor Cells in Human Disease
    Edited by James S. Goodwin
15. Immunological Aspects of Aging
    Edited by Diego Segre and Lester Smith
16. Cellular and Molecular Mechanisms of Immunologic Tolerance
    Edited by Tomáš Hraba and Milan Hašek

17. Immune Regulation: Evolution and Biological Significance
Edited by Laurens N. Ruben and M. Eric Gershwin

18. Tumor Immunity in Prognosis: The Role of Mononuclear Cell Infiltration
Edited by Stephen Haskill

19. Immunopharmacology and the Regulation of Leukocyte Function
Edited by David R. Webb

20. Pathogenesis and Immunology of Treponemal Infection
Edited by Ronald F. Schell and Daniel M. Musher

21. Macrophage-Mediated Antibody-Dependent Cellular Cytotoxicity
Edited by Hillel S. Koren

22. Molecular Immunology: A Textbook
Edited by M. Zouhair Atassi, Carel J. van Oss, and Darryl R. Absolom

23. Monoclonal Antibodies and Cancer
Edited by George L. Wright, Jr.

24. Stress, Immunity, and Aging
Edited by Edwin L. Cooper

25. Immune Modulation Agents and Their Mechanisms
Edited by Richard L. Fenichel and Michael A. Chirigos

26. Mononuclear Phagocyte Biology
Edited by Alvin Volkman

27. The Lactoperoxidase System: Chemistry and Biological Significance
Edited by Kenneth M. Pruitt and Jorma O. Tenovuo

28. Introduction to Medical Immunology
Edited by Gabriel Virella, Jean-Michel Goust, H. Hugh Fudenberg, and Christian C. Patrick

29. Handbook of Food Allergies
Edited by James C. Breneman

30. Human Hybridomas: Diagnostic and Therapeutic Applications
Edited by Anthony J. Strelkauskas

31. Aging and the Immune Response: Cellular and Humoral Aspects
Edited by Edmond A. Goidl

32. Complications of Organ Transplantation
Edited by Luis H. Toledo-Pereyra

33. Monoclonal Antibody Production Techniques and Applications
Edited by Lawrence B. Schook

34. Fundamentals of Receptor Molecular Biology
Donald F. H. Wallach

35. Recombinant Lymphokines and Their Receptors
Edited by Steven Gillis

36. Immunology of the Male Reproductive Organs
Edited by Pierluigi E. Bigazzi

37. The Lymphocyte: Structure and Function
Edited by John J. Marchalonis

38. Differentiation Antigens in Lymphohemopoietic Tissues
Edited by Masayuki Miyasaka and Zdenek Trnka

39. Cancer Diagnosis In Vitro Using Monoclonal Antibodies
Edited by Herbert Z. Kupchik

40. Biological Response Modifiers and Cancer Therapy
Edited by J. W. Chiao

41. Cellular Oncogene Activation
Edited by George Klein

42. Interferon and Nonviral Pathogens
Edited by Gerald I. Byrne and Jenifer Turco

43. Human Immunogenetics: Basic Principles and Clinical Relevance
Edited by Stephen D. Litwin, with David W. Scott, Lorraine Flaherty, Ralph A. Reisfeld, and Donald M. Marcus

44. AIDS: Pathogenesis and Treatment
Edited by Jay A. Levy

45. Cell Surface Antigen Thy-1: Immunology, Neurology, and Therapeutic Applications
Edited by Arnold E. Reif and Michael Schlesinger

46. Immune Mechanisms in Cutaneous Disease
Edited by David A. Norris

47. Immunology of Fungal Diseases
Edited by Edouard Kurstak

48. Adoptive Cellular Immunotherapy of Cancer
Edited by Henry C. Stevenson

49. Colony-Stimulating Factors: Molecular and Cellular Biology
Edited by T. Michael Dexter, John M. Garland, and Nydia G. Testa

50. Introduction to Medical Immunology, Second Edition
Edited by Gabriel Virella, Jean-Michel Goust, and H. Hugh Fudenberg

51. Tumor Suppressor Genes
Edited by George Klein

52. Organ-Specific Autoimmunity
Edited by Pierluigi E. Bigazzi, Georg Wick, and Konrad Wicher

53. Immunodiagnosis of Cancer: Second Edition
Edited by Ronald B. Herberman and Donald W. Mercer

54. Systemic Autoimmunity
Edited by Pierluigi E. Bigazzi and Morris Reichlin

55. Molecular Immunobiology of Self-Reactivity
Edited by Constantin A. Bona and Azad K. Kaushik

56. Tumor Necrosis Factors: Structure, Function, and Mechanism of Action
Edited by Bharat B. Aggarwal and Jan Vilček

Tumor Necrosis Factors

Structure, Function, and Mechanism of Action

edited by

Bharat B. Aggarwal

University of Texas M.D. Anderson Cancer Center
Houston, Texas

Jan Vilček

New York University Medical Center
New York, New York

Marcel Dekker, Inc. New York • Basel • Hong Kong

ISBN 0-8247-8554-1

This book is printed on acid-free paper

Marcel Dekker, Inc.
270 Madison Avenue, New York, New York, 10016

Current Printing (last digit):
10 9 8 7 6 5 4 3 2 1

PRINTED IN THE UNITED STATES OF AMERICA

Series Introduction

Science, it can be said, moves not as steady stream but in fits and starts. A vivid impression of this is obtained as one reviews the history of the tumor necrosis factor (TNF). At the very dawn of immunology, an astute surgeon, Dr. Cooley, observed that in some of his cancer patients the tumor seemed to melt away if they had a concurrent infection. He hit upon the idea of administering a "vaccine"—"Cooley's toxins"—consisting of killed bacteria. He claimed some beneficial results, but without formal clinical trials and without experimental bases his case reports had little impact on the flow of immunological research.

It was only later, when it became possible to conduct the research described in this volume, that Dr. Cooley's observation was confirmed and the tumor necrosis factor became a reality. Why such a long delay? Advances in scientific thinking require new experimental tools and new conceptual scaffolding, but it was not until the 1970s that these necessary elements were in place and scientists could return to some of the lingering questions of the past. Investigations on TNF and similar factors have proceeded with dazzling speed during the past decade. Factors have been isolated, characterized, cloned, sequenced, and named, putting the unexplained and unexplainable observations of the past on a solid molecular basis.

This latest addition to the Immunology Series exemplifies the extraordinary contributions molecular science is making to the flow of immunological knowledge.

Noel R. Rose

Preface

The field of tumor necrosis factor (TNF) research evolved from several independent sources. As most readers will recall, TNF owes its name to the work of Lloyd Old and his colleagues at the Memorial Sloan-Kettering Cancer Center in New York, published in 1975, showing that tumor necrotizing activity in the sera of bacillus Calmette-Guérin-sensitized mice injected with endotoxin was due to an endotoxin-induced host factor, which they christened TNF. The work of Old's group was preceded by investigations carried out over the span of several decades, demonstrating that injection of tumor-bearing animals with crude bacterial filtrates or, more recently, with purified preparations of bacterial lipopolysaccharide can lead to a hemorrhagic necrosis of well-vascularized tumors. The most important contribution of Old's group was to show conclusively that hemorrhagic necrosis was mediated by a host-derived factor. They also showed that TNF had a direct inhibitory effect on some tumor cells in culture and correctly proposed that macrophages were the major source of TNF.

The second chapter in the history of TNF research began with the discovery of lymphotoxin, a factor independently described by two groups of investigators in the late 1960s, before the first publications on TNF. Nancy Ruddle and Byron Waksman described a factor released from T-lymphocytes in the presence of specific antigen. This factor was later shown to be identical to a cytotoxic factor described by Gale (Mori) Granger and coworkers, which they had called "lymphotoxin." At about the same time, other groups, including Werner Rosenau's, described cytotoxic proteins made by lymphocytes that were probably identical to lymphotoxin. For many years lymphotoxin and TNF had been studied by separate groups of investigators, and despite some obvious similarities in their actions (both TNF and lymphotoxin were known to be cytotoxic for certain tumor cell lines) there was no clear evidence that the two proteins were closely related. Until 1984, that is, when Bharat Aggarwal (then at Genentech in South San Francisco) and coworkers purified both the lymphotoxin and TNF proteins, demonstrated a significant degree of sequence homology between these two molecules, and went on to show that they share a common receptor. These accomplishments were rapidly followed by the elucidation of the relatedness of the lymphotoxin and TNF genes by David Goeddel, Pat Gray and their colleagues at Genentech.

The beginning of the third major chapter in the history of TNF can be traced to the completely independent studies in the early 1980s by Anthony Cerami and coworkers at New York's Rockefeller University, who analyzed a hypertriglyceridemic state and wasting in rabbits infected with *Trypanosoma brucei*. (To readers unfamiliar with Manhattan's topography it is worth pointing out that Old's laboratory at Sloan-Kettering and Cerami's lab at Rockefeller were but a stone's throw apart.) In 1985, Bruce Beutler, Cerami, and coworkers isolated a macrophage-derived, endotoxin-inducible factor capable of suppressing the enzyme lipoprotein lipase. The protein factor was termed "cachectin" because of its presumed role in the genesis of cachexia. To everybody's surprise, the amino-terminal sequence of murine cachectin was found to be highly homologous to the sequence of human TNF as determined some months earlier by Aggarwal, Goeddel, and coworkers at Genentech. Cachectin and TNF turned out to be one and the same, "two sides of the same biological coin," as Beutler and Cerami put it. The rest is history—recorded in this volume.

The purification and cloning of TNF proteins and genes were followed by a veritable information explosion. Up to 1984 there had been fewer than one hundred studies published in this field in the span of approximately ten years. Within the last five years over five thousand publications have dealt with TNF. Although in 1985 TNF was still viewed by most investigators as a selective antitumor agent, the many chapters in this volume devoted to TNF's pleiotropic activities admirably illustrate the numerous newly discovered functions of TNF in the host defenses, inflammation, pathogenesis, regulation of gene expression, differentiation, etc. (An irreverent graduate student recently observed that TNF stands for "too numerous functions.")

Even though there have been many review articles written on TNF, and proceedings of several international conferences on TNF, no in-depth treatise on the subject has been published until now. This volume is the first to provide a thorough and critical evaluation of the TNF field. Considering the extremely rapid development in this field, no book can be completely up to date. However, efforts have been made by all the authors, who include many pioneers in TNF research, to provide as much current information as possible. It is our hope that this book will serve well both the newcomers and the veterans of the field of TNF and cytokine research.

We wish to thank many people whose hard work made possible the successful completion of this project. We are most grateful to all the authors for devoting the time and enormous effort necessary for the timely completion of their chapters. We apologize to them for being so much "on their backs" during the final months before the completion of the manuscript. In the end, it seems, the joint effort has paid off. Our secretaries Ilene Toder and Barbara Nash were most helpful during the entire process of the preparation of this volume. We also wish to express our appreciation to the staff of Marcel Dekker, Inc., and especially to Connie Casella, the Production Editor of this volume, whose devotion to this project helped to shorten the publication time.

Bharat B. Aggarwal
Jan Vilček

Contents

Part II: Receptors and Mechanism of Action of TNFs

Part III: Biological Actions of TNFs

Contributors

Bharat B. Aggarwal The University of Texas M. D. Anderson Cancer Center, Houston, Texas

Corrado Baglioni Albany Medical College and State University of New York at Albany, Albany, New York

Frances R. Balkwill Biological Therapies Laboratory, Imperial Cancer Research Fund, London, England

Benjamin Bonavida UCLA School of Medicine and the Jonsson Comprehensive Cancer Center, University of California, Los Angeles, California

L. F. Bonewald The University of Texas Health Science Center at San Antonio, San Antonio, Texas

Anthony Cerami Rockefeller University, New York, New York

I. A. Clark Zoology Department and John Curtin School of Medical Research, Australian National University, Canberra, Australia

W. B. Cowden Zoology Department and John Curtin School of Medical Research, Australian National University, Canberra, Australia

Jean-Michel Dayer University Hospital, Geneva, Switzerland

Stephan Deutsch University of Wisconsin, Madison, Wisconsin

Sarah J. Fashena Yale University School of Medicine, New Haven, Connecticut

W. Fiers State University, Ghent, Belgium

Georges E. Grau University of Geneva, Geneva, Switzerland

Edward A. Havell Trudeau Institute, Inc., Saranac Lake, New York

E. Y. Jones University of Oxford, Oxford, England

Martin Krönke Max-Planck-Society, Göttingen, Germany

Donald W. Kufe Dana Farber Cancer Institute, Boston, Massachussetts

Hansruedi Loetscher F. Hoffmann-LaRoche Ltd., Basel, Switzerland

Saleem T. A. Malik Biological Therapies Laboratory, Imperial Cancer Research Fund, London, England

G. R. Mundy The University of Texas Health Science Center at San Antonio, San Antonio, Texas

Ruth Neta Armed Forces Radiobiology Research Institute, Bethesda, Maryland

Naoto Oku Setsunan University, Hirakata, Osaka, Japan

Joost J. Oppenheim National Cancer Institute, Frederick, Maryland

Vito J. Palombella Harvard University, Cambridge, Massachusetts

Nina L. Paul Yale University School of Medicine, New Haven, Connecticut

Klaus Pfizenmaier Max-Planck-Society, Göttingen, Germany

Pierre-François Piguet University of Geneva, Geneva, Switzerland

G. D. Roodman The University of Texas Health Science Center at San Antonio, San Antonio, Texas

Michael Rosenblum University of Texas M. D. Anderson Cancer Center, Houston, Texas

Jay L. Rothstein The Wistar Institute, Philadelphia, Pennsylvania

Berish Y. Rubin Fordham University, Bronx, New York

Nancy H. Ruddle Yale University School of Medicine, New Haven, Connecticut

M. Sabatini The University of Texas Health Science Center at San Antonio, San Antonio, Texas

Sam Saks Xoma Corporation, Berkeley, California

Thomas J. Sayers Program Resources, Inc./DynCorp, Frederick, Maryland

Peter Scheurich Max-Planck-Society, Göttingen, Germany

Hans Schreiber The University of Chicago, Chicago, Illinois

Stefan Schütze Max-Planck-Society, Göttingen, Germany

Philippe Seckinger University Hospital, Geneva, Switzerland

Richard A. Smith Albany Medical College and State University of New York at Albany, Albany, New York

David R. Spriggs University of Wisconsin, Madison, Wisconsin

D. I. Stuart University of Oxford, Oxford, England

Kevin J. Tracey New York Hospital-Cornell University Medical Center, New York, New York

Giorgio Trinchieri The Wistar Institute, Philadelphia, Pennsylvania

Masafumi Tsujimoto Suntory Institute for Biomedical Research, Mishima, Osaka, Japan

Regina L. Turetskaya Institute of Molecular Biology, USSR Academy of Science, Moscow, USSR, and Yale University School of Medicine, New Haven, Connecticut

Pierre Vassalli University of Geneva, Geneva, Switzerland

Jan Vilček New York University Medical Center, New York, New York

N. P. C. Walker BASF A. G., Ludwigshafen, Germany

T. Yoneda The University of Texas Health Science Center at San Antonio, San Antonio, Texas

I

PROTEIN AND GENE STRUCTURE OF TNF-α AND TNF-β

1

Genomic Structure, Induction, and Production of TNF-α

DAVID R. SPRIGGS and STEPHAN DEUTSCH
University of Wisconsin, Madison, Wisconsin

DONALD W. KUFE
Dana Farber Cancer Institute, Boston, Massachussetts

I. THE TNF GENE: CHROMOSOMAL LOCATION AND STRUCTURAL FEATURES

The tumor necrosis factor (TNF) α gene and its regulation have been a major focus of research since the TNF protein was first identified (Carswell et al., 1975). Because of its promise for anticancer therapy, it was one of the first recombinant proteins to be prepared for clinical trials. To better understand the production and action of TNF in vivo, attention has been directed to its chromosomal location, the structure of the gene, and the nature of surrounding regulatory sequences.

A. Chromosomal Location

Certain disease states may be associated with inappropriate production of TNF, a mediator of the inflammatory response. Knowledge of the chromosomal location of the TNF gene aids in the understanding of the pathophysiology of TNF within a genetic context. In early mapping studies, Southern blot analysis of human–murine somatic cell hybrids using a TNF cDNA probe localized the TNF genes to a portion of chromosome 6 flanking the centromere, between 6p23 and 6p12. This includes the region containing the major histocompatibility complex, on the proximal end of the short arm, 6p21.1-6p21.3 (Nedwin et al., 1985; Strominger, 1986). More recently, chromosome walking with overlapping cosmid clones found the TNF genes to be 210 kb from the HLA-B locus of the class I gene family, more proximal to the

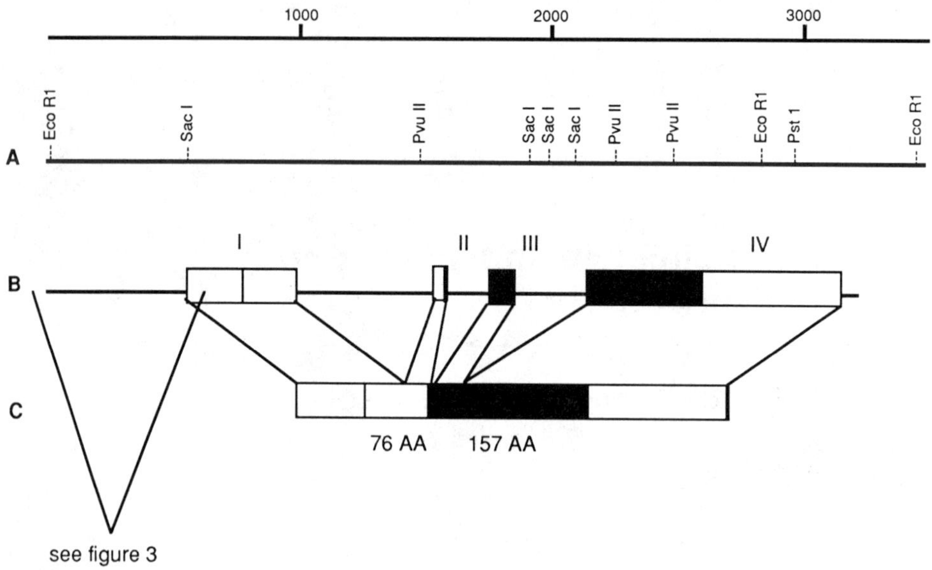

Figure 1 Schematic of the TNF-α gene: (a) restriction map; (b) arrangement of exons; (c) mature mRNA. The regions corresponding to the 76-residue propeptide and the 157-residue mature protein are indicated. (From Nedwin et al., 1985, Fig. 2.)

centromere, toward the distal end of the class III loci (Spies et al., 1989). In the mouse, the chromosomal context of the TNF gene is very similar. The murine TNF genes are located within the mouse MHC on chromosome 17, approximately 70 kb proximal to the H2-D locus, the murine equivalent of HLA-B (Muller et al., 1987). The juxtaposition of TNF among the MHC suggests interesting possibilities for the relationship between the recognition and effector components of the immune system, as well as the role of the TNF locus in inflammatory disease.

B. Organization of the TNF Gene

1. Coding Structure

Molecular cloning of the TNF-α gene from genomic libraries has permitted detailed structural analysis by different groups of investigators (Marmenout et al., 1985; Nedwin et al., 1985; Shirai et al., 1985; Wang et al., 1985). The TNF coding regions consist of four exons arranged over approximately 3 kb of DNA (see Figs. 1 and 2).More than 80% of the sequence contributing to mature TNF is encoded in the fourth exon, while exons I and II contain almost entirely leader peptide sequence. The TNF amino acid sequence is conserved between species, with 79% homology between humans and mice and greater than 70% homology between humans and rabbits (Ito et al., 1986; Marmenout et al., 1985). Two cysteine residues are highly conserved in all three species (Goeddel et al., 1986). The region corresponding to residues 114 to 130 is most highly conserved, suggesting that a functionally important structure is encoded there. The high levels of sequence conservation are consistent with the lack of species specificity in response to TNF administration. There are also highly conserved sequence regions in the 5′ and 3′ flanking regions that are potentially associated with gene regulation (see below).

2. *Transcriptional Control Elements*

Knowledge of the structural elements involved in the control of TNF gene activity is essential to the understanding of the function and regulation of TNF. The approximately 1000 base pairs of the TNF gene's 5′ flanking region contains a number of important regulatory elements that affect TNFs transcription in response to various stimuli. The basic promotor region is defined by the Goldberg–Hogness (TATA box) sequence, located approximately 20 bp upstream from the transcription site and about 200 bp from the translation start codon. A GC box/SP-1 binding site is about 20 bp farther upstream and inverted in orientation (Ito et al., 1986; Marmenout et al., 1985; Shakhov et al., 1990). Elements that may provide more specific control of TNF transcription are found farther upstream.

Jongeneel and co-workers have identified some of the 5′ control sites associated with induction by lipopolysaccharide (LPS) (Jongeneel et al., 1989). Having searched the 5′ flanking sequences of rabbit, mouse, and human TNF genes for regulatory sites, they determined that the 200 bp flanking the transcription start site is highly conserved, implying that important control elements reside there, including but not limited to the TATA and GC boxes. Furthermore, upstream of the mouse TNF gene they identified sequences similar to the κB enhancers of immunoglobulin genes, located 480 and 820 bp upstream from the TATA box (see Fig. 3). At positions 230 bp and 650 bp 5′ to TATA are two other sequences resembling the "cytokine-1" motif of the IL-2, IL-3, G-CSF, and GM-CSF promotors ["κB (CK-1)" in Fig. 2], believed to be a variant of the κB enhancer. Enhancers of the latter type were conserved in all three species. Also, a decanucleotide resembling the "Y-box" of MHC class II promotors is located 240 bp upstream from TATA. When the 5′ flanking region of the murine TNF gene was linked to the chloramphenicol acetyltransferase (CAT) gene and transfected into bone marrow-derived macrophages, induction of CAT activity by LPS was observed. Sequential deletions of portion s of the 5′ flanking region diminished the LPS response when fewer than two of the κB enhancer-like sequences were present. Inducibility was further reduced when the Y-box sequence was deleted. In addition, LPS induction was conferred by attachment of copies of the central κB enhancer-like sequence to the heterologous thymidine kinase promotor in a CAT gene construct. A second set of experiments demonstrated the induction of nuclear factors in LPS-activated macrophages, which bound specifically to DNA fragments containing the κB en-

```
101  ATCCTGTCTGGAAGTTAGAAGGAAACAGACCACAGACCTGGTCCCCAAAAGAAATGGAGGCAATAGGTTTTGAGGGGCATGGGGACGGGGTTCAGCCTCC  200
201  AGGGTCCTACACACAAATCAGTCAGTGGCCCAGAAGACCCCCCTCGGAATCGGAGCAGGGAGGATGGGGAGTGTGAGGGGTATCCTTGATGCTTGTGTGT  300
301  CCCCAACTTTCCAAATCCCCGCCCCCGCGATGGAGAAGAAACCGAGACAGAAGGTGCAGGGCCCACTACCGCTTCCTCCAGATGAGCTCATGGGTTTCTC  400
401  CACCAAGGAAGTTTTCCGCTGGTTGAATGATTCTTTCCCCGCCCTCCTCTCGCCCCAGGGACATATAAAGGCAGTTGTTGGCACACCCAGCCAGCAGACG  500
501  CTCCCTCAGCAAGGACAGCAGAGGACCAGCTAAGAGGGAGAGAAGCAACTACAGACCCCCCCTGAAAACAACCCTCAGACGCCACATCCCCTGACAAGCT  600
601  GCCAGGCAGGTTCTCTTCCTCTCACATACTGACCCACGGCTCCACCCTCTCTCCCCTGGAAAGGACACCATGAGCACTGAAAGCATGATCCGGGACGTGG  700
                                         T
                                                                        MetSerThrGluSerMetIleArgAspValG
701  AGCTGGCCGAGGAGGCGCTCCCCAAGAAGACAGGGGGGCCCCAGGGCTCCAGGCGGTGCTTGTTCCTCAGCCTCTTCTCCTTCCTGATCGTGGCAGGCGC  800
     luLeuAlaGluGluAlaLeuProLysLysThrGlyGlyProGlnGlySerArgArgCysLeuPheLeuSerLeuPheSerPheLeuIleValAlaGlyAl
801  CACCACGCTCTTCTGCCTGCTGCACTTTGGAGTGATCGGCCCCCAGAGGGAAGAGGTGAGTGCCTGGCCAGCCTTCATCCACTCTCCCACCCAAGGGGAA  900
     aThrThrLeuPheCysLeuLeuHisPheGlyValIleGlyProGlnArgGluGlu
901  ATGGAGACGCAAGAGAGGGAGAGAGATGGGATGGCTGAAAGATGTGCGCTGATAGGGAGGGATGGAGAGAAAAAAACGTGGAGAAAGACGGGGATGCAGA  1000
       ΔA                                                                       A                     C
1001 AAGAGATGTGGCAAGAGATGGGGAAGAGAGAGAGAGAAAGATGGAGAGACAGGATGTCTGGCACATGGAAGGTGCTCACTAAGTGTGTATGGAGTGAATG  1100
1101 AATGAATGAATGAATGAACAAGCAGATATATAAATAAGATATGGAGACAGATGTGGGGTGTGAGAAGAGAGATGGGGGAAGAAACAAGTGATATGAATAA  1200
1201 AGATGGTGAGACAGAAAGAGCGGGAAATATGACAGCTAAGGAGAGAGATGGGGGAGATAAGGAGAGAAGAAGATAGGGTGTCTGGCACACAGAAGACACT  1300
1301 CAGGGAAAGAGCTGTTGAATGCCTGGAAGGTGAATACACAGATGAATGGAGAGAGAAAACCAGACACCTCAGGGCTAAGAGCGCAGGCCAGACAGGCAGC  1400
1401 CAGCTGTTCCTCCTTTAAGGGTGACTCCCTCGATGTTAACCATTCTCCTTCTCCCCAACAGTTCCCCAGGGACCTCTCTCTAATCAGCCCTCTGGCCCAG  1500
                                                                                PheProArgAspLeuSerLeuIleSerProLeuAlaGln
1501 GCAGTCAGTAAGTGTCTCCAAACCTCTTTCCTAATTCTGGGTTTGGGTTTGGGGGTAGGGTTAGTACCGGTATGGAAGCAGTGGGGGAAATTTAAAGTTT  1600
     AlaValA
1601 TGGTCTTGGGGGAGGATGGATGGAGGTGAAAGTAGGGGGGTATTTTCTAGGAAGTTTAAGGGTCTCAGCTTTTTCTTTTCTCTCTCCTCTTCAGGATCAT  1700
                                                                                                 rgSerS
1701 CTTCTCGAACCCCGAGTGACAAGCCTGTAGCCCATGTTGTAGGTAAGAGCTCTGAGGATGTGTCTTGGAACTTGGAGGGCTAGGATTTGGGGATTGAAGC  1800
     erSerArgThrProSerAspLysProValAlaHisValValA
1801 CCGGCTGATGGTAGGCAGAACTTGGAGACAATGTGAGAAGGACTCGCTGAGCTCAAGGGAAGGGTGGAGGAACAGCACAGGCCTTAGTGGGATACTCAGA  1900
1901 ACGTCATGGCCAGGTGGGATGTGGGATGACAGACACAGAGGACACGGAACCGGATGTGGGGTGGGCAGAGCTCGAGGGCCAGGATGTGGAGAGTGAACCGA  2000
2001 CATGGCCACACTGACTCTCCTCTCCCTCTCTCCCTCCCTCCAGCAAACCCTCAAGCTGAGGGGCAGCTCCAGTGGCTGAACCGCCGGGCCAATGCCCTCC  2100
                                                  laAsnProGlnAlaGluGlyGlnLeuGlnTrpLeuAsnArgArgAlaAsnAlaLeuL
2101 TGGCCAATGGCGTGGAGCTGAGAGATAACCAGCTGGTGGTGCCATCAGAGGGCCTGTACCTCATCTACTCCCAGGTCCTCTTCAAGGGCCAAGGCTGCCC  2200
     euAlaAsnGlyValGluLeuArgAspAsnGlnLeuValValProSerGluGlyLeuTyrLeuIleTyrSerGlnValLeuPheLysGlyGlnGlyCysPr
2201 CTCCACCCATGTGCTCCTCACCCACACCATCAGCCGCATCGCCGTCTCCTACCAGACCAAGGTCAACCTCCTCTCTGCCATCAAGAGCCCCTGCCAGAGG  2300
     oSerThrHisValLeuLeuThrHisThrIleSerArgIleAlaValSerTyrGlnThrLysValAsnLeuLeuSerAlaIleLysSerProCysGlnArg
2301 GAGACCCCAGAGGGGGCTGAGGCCAAGCCCTGGTATGAGCCCATCTATCTGGGAGGGGTCTTCCAGCTGGAGAAGGGTGACCGACTCAGCGCTGAGATCA  2400
     GluThrProGluGlyAlaGluAlaLysProTrpTyrGluProIleTyrLeuGlyGlyValPheGlnLeuGluLysGlyAspArgLeuSerAlaGluIleA
2401 ATCGGCCCGACTATCTCGACTTTGCCGAGTCTGGGCAGGTCTACTTTGGGATCATTGCCCTGTGAGGAGGACGAACATCCAACCTTCCCAAACGCCTCCC  2500
     snArgProAspTyrLeuAspPheAlaGluSerGlyGlnValTyrPheGlyIleIleAlaLeuEnd
2501 CTGCCCCAATCCCTTTATTACCCCCTCCTTCAGACACCCTCAACCTCTTCTGGCTCAAAAAGAGAATTGGGGGCTTAGGGTCGGAACCCAAGCTTAGAAC  2600
2601 TTTAAGCAACAAGACCACCACTTCGAAACCTGGGATTCAGGAATGTGTGGCCTGCACAGTGAAGTGCTGGCAACCACTAAGAATTC  2686
```

(A)

Figure 2 Nucleotide sequence of the human TNF-α gene (A) with deduced amino acid sequence (B). (From Marmenout et al., 1985, Fig. 3.)

```
HUMAN  (-76) MET SER THR GLU SER MET ILE ARG ASP VAL GLU LEU ALA GLU GLU ALA LEU PRO LYS
MOUSE        MET SER THR GLU SER MET ILE ARG ASP VAL GLU LEU ALA GLU GLU ALA LEU PRO GLN
                                   (-70)                                     (-60)

LYS THR GLY GLY PRO GLN GLY SER ARG ARG CYS LEU PHE LEU SER LEU PHE SER PHE LEU ILE VAL ALA GLY ALA THR THR LEU PHE CYS
LYS MET GLY GLY PHE GLN ASN SER ARG ARG CYS LEU CYS LEU SER LEU PHE SER PHE LEU LEU VAL ALA GLY ALA THR THR LEU PHE CYS
                        (-50)                         (-40)                                        (-30)

LEU LEU HIS PHE GLY VAL ILE GLY PRO GLN ARG  -  GLU GLU PHE PRO ARG ASP LEU SER LEU ILE SER PRO LEU ALA GLN ALA  -   - ↓
LEU LEU ASN PHE GLY VAL ILE GLY PRO GLN ARG ASP GLU LYS PHE PRO ASN GLY LEU PRO LEU ILE SER SER MET ALA GLN THR LEU THR
                (-20)                                           (-10)

(1)                                 (10)                                (20)                                (30)
VAL ARG SER SER SER ARG THR PRO SER ASP LYS PRO VAL ALA HIS VAL VAL ALA ASN PRO GLN ALA GLU GLY GLN LEU GLN TRP LEU ASN
LEU ARG SER SER SER GLN ASN SER SER ASP LYS PRO VAL ALA HIS VAL VAL ALA ASN HIS GLN VAL GLU GLU GLN LEU GLU TRP LEU SER

                                   (40)                                (50)                                (60)
ARG ARG ALA ASN ALA LEU LEU ALA ASN GLY VAL GLU LEU ARG ASP ASN GLN LEU VAL VAL PRO SER GLU GLY LEU TYR LEU ILE TYR SER
GLN ARG ALA ASN ALA LEU LEU ALA ASN GLY MET ASP LEU LYS ASP ASN GLN LEU VAL VAL PRO ALA ASP GLY LEU TYR LEU VAL TYR SER

                                   (70)                                (80)                                (90)
GLN VAL LEU PHE LYS GLY GLN GLY CYS PRO SER THR HIS VAL LEU LEU THR HIS THR ILE SER ARG ILE ALA VAL SER TYR GLN THR LYS
GLN VAL LEU PHE LYS GLY GLN GLY CYS PRO ASP TYR  -  VAL LEU LEU THR HIS THR VAL SER ARG PHE ALA ILE SER TYR GLN GLU LYS

                                   (100)                               (110)                               (120)
VAL ASN LEU LEU SER ALA ILE LYS SER PRO CYS GLN ARG GLU THR PRO GLU GLY ALA GLU ALA LYS PRO TRP TYR GLU PRO ILE TYR LEU
VAL ASN LEU LEU SER ALA VAL LYS SER PRO CYS PRO LYS ASP THR PRO GLU GLY ALA GLU LEU LYS PRO TRP TYR GLU PRO ILE TYR LEU

                                   (130)                               (140)                               (150)
GLY GLY VAL PHE GLN LEU GLU LYS GLY ASP ARG LEU SER ALA GLU ILE ASN ARG PRO ASP TYR LEU ASP PHE ALA GLU SER GLY GLN VAL
GLY GLY VAL PHE GLN LEU GLU LYS GLY ASP GLN LEU SER ALA GLU VAL ASN LEU PRO LYS TYR LEU ASP PHE ALA GLU SER GLY GLN VAL

                        (157)
TYR PHE GLY ILE ILE ALA LEU
TYR PHE GLY VAL ILE ALA LEU
```

(B)

Figure 2 (Continued)

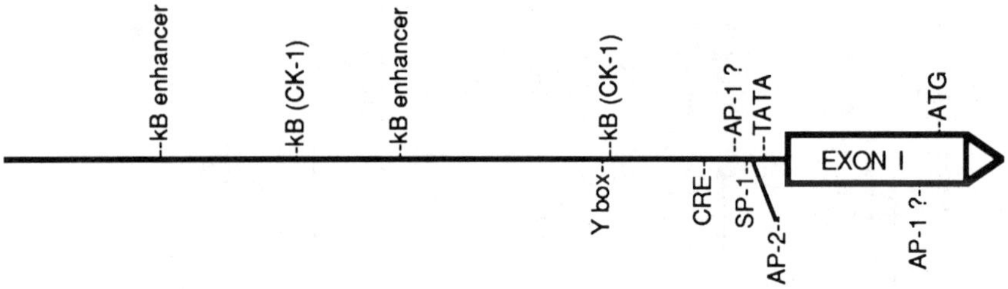

Figure 3 The 5′ flanking region of the TNF gene. This figure corresponds to an enlargement of the left end of Fig. 1B, showing the relative positions of regulatory sites identified by homology to known motifs or through reporter gene and gel binding analyses. κB enhancer: Igκ chain κB enhancer homolog. κB (CK-1): Cytokine-1-type κB enhancer variant homolog. Y box: homolog of a MHC class II promoter element. CRE: Cyclic AMP- responsive element. AP-1: C-jun/AP-1 binding site homolog. SP-1: GC box/SP-1 binding site. AP-2: AP-2 binding site. TATA: TATAAA box. ATG: Translation start site. (Adapted from Shakhov et al., 1990, Fig. 1.)

hancer-like or Y-box sequences in gel retardation assays. These results strongly suggest that these features participate in the induction of TNF by LPS in the mouse (Shakhov et al., 1990).

TNF protein also acts as an autocrine inducer of TNF expression (see below). In human leukemia cells, TNF induced protein kinase C–independent activation of nuclear factor kB (Meichle et al., 1990). In other studies, TNF-induced expression of mouse MHC class I genes was dependent on the presence of two imperfect palindromic repeats. TNF treatment induced an NF-κB-like activity that displaced two constituitive transcription factors, AP2 and KBF1 (Israel et al., 1990). A NF-κB-like factor is also involved in the transcriptional activation of the inflammatory cytokine IL-6 and TNF stimulation (Shimizu et al., 1990).

Other putative regulatory sites are indicated by studying the sequence adjoining the TATA box. Approximately 80 bp 5′ to the TATA box is an eight-nucleotide palindrome almost identical to a sequence found in the cyclic AMP–responsive element (CRE) of the somatostatin gene promoter (Economou et al., 1989; Montminy et al., 1986). It differs in that the central dinucleotide is inverted (CG versus GC). This sequence is usually associated with cyclic AMP–induced genes; however, TNF transcription is inhibited by agents that elevate cyclic AMP levels (see below). An inhibitory effect by a cyclic AMP–activated factor that recognizes this CRE-like sequence remains an interesting possibility.

The induction of TNF by phorbol esters (see below) can be associated with 5′ flanking sequences. A sequence very similar to the c-jun/AP-1 binding site consensus sequence, a seven-nucleotide motif associated with the promotors of phorbol ester-inducible genes, is located between the TATA box and the translation start site, but its functional relevance in that location is unclear. However, a somewhat less homologous, though possibly functional sequence resembling the AP-1 binding site occurs 40 bp upstream from the TATA box, a position observed in other systems (Angel et al., 1987). In this location it may be participating in TNF induction by phorbol esters.

Other phorbol ester-responsive elements are indicated by experimental data. Krönke and co-workers, using CAT gene constructs and gel retardation assays analogous to those of Jongeneel and co-workers, identified a region 90 to 165 bp 5′ of the TATA box that appears to contain a TPA-responsive element (Hensel et al., 1989). Economou and co-workers found that TPA induction is associated with a region within 95 bp 5′ to the transcription start site, using deletion analysis of the human 5′ flanking region linked to the reporter gene luciferase. Their examination of the 5′ flanking sequence also identified a binding site for the phorbol ester-responsive transcription factor AP-2, directly 5′ to the TATA box, in addition to the putative AP-1 site 40 bp farther upstream (Economou et al., 1989).

The NF-κB protein may also be involved in TPA-induced expression of TNF. An inactive form of NF-κB is present in all cell types and may be activated by exposure to TPA (Sen and Baltimore, 1986). This activation appears to occur through protein kinase C-mediated phosphorylation of the NF-κB inhibitor, IkB (Ghosh and Baltimore, 1990).

3. 3′ Sequences and Posttranscriptional Regulation

A conserved sequence element in the 3′ untranslated region affects the posttranscriptional regulation of TNF gene expression. Beutler and co-workers identified an octanucleotide, TTATTTAT, in the 3′ untranslated regions of human and murine TNF and the genes of several other cytokines (Caput et al., 1986). The presence of this sequence is associated with both the accelerated degradation of mRNA and interference with translation (Kruys et al., 1989; Shaw and Kamin, 1986; Wilson and Treisman, 1988). Beutler and co-workers have demonstrated that mouse macrophages contain a ribonuclease that selectively degrades mRNA possessing this sequence, and have recently shown that addition of TTATTTAT-containing sequences to CAT gene constructs confers a negative response to endotoxin that is mediated at the translational level (Beutler et al., 1988; Han et al., 1990).

II. REGULATION OF TNF GENE EXPRESSION

The production of TNF-α is tightly regulated in a tissue-specific manner. Transcription, translation, and secretion/release all appear to be controlled in a multiple-step process. The production of TNF by cells of the monocyte/macrophage lineage has been studied most extensively, but TNF expression by nonhematopoietic cells may also be important in certain disease states.

A. Leukocyte Production of TNF

A variety of stimuli have been observed to induce the production of TNF by monocytes and macrophages. A list of agents that have been reported to induce production of TNF in vitro is shown in Table 1. This list includes bacterial products such as LPS, a variety of cytokines, membrane active agents, nitrites, γ-irradiation, and phorbol esters. The mechanisms by which these diverse stimuli induce TNF expression is not known. In vivo, the situation is even less clear. TNF has been implicated in the pathophysiology of many disease states, but the signals that initiate TNF production in these diseases remain unknown. The relationship of TNF to the pathophysiology of disease is discussed elsewhere in this volume.

1. Inducers of TNF: LPS

Lipopolysaccharide (LPS) is the best known inducer of tumor necrosis factor. However, the molecular mechanisms responsible for the induction of TNF expression in monocytes are not well understood. In monocytes, regulation of TNF transcription appears to be an important control mechanism for TNF expression. LPS stimulation of monocytes has been the most extensively studied model of TNF production. The production of TNF by monocytes is generally associated with activation. However, basal TNF gene transcription has been observed in some systems. Thioglycollate-elicited peritoneal macrophages from C3H/HeN mice have detectable levels of TNF transcription but no measurable TNF protein production (Beut-

Table 1 Partial List of Stimuli Known to Induce TNF Production In Vitro

Lipopolysaccharide
Bacterial extracts
Synthetic lipid A
Phorbol esters
Cytokines
Tumor necrosis factor
Interleukin-1
GM-CSF
"Cytotoxicity triggering factor"
Interleukin-2
Other stimuli
DMSO and nonpolar solvents
Gamma-irradiation
Free oxygen radicals
Peroxidases
FC receptor cross-linking

ler et al., 1986). This basal level of TNF transcription is increased more than threefold by stimulation with 10 ng/mL of LPS. In C3H/HeJ mutant mice, this concentration of LPS does not induce detectable levels of TNF transcripts. However, 1000 ng/mL of LPS induces TNF mRNA production in both the C3H/HeJ endotoxin-resistant strain and the wild-type C3H/HeN strain. Dexamethasone (1μM) decreases the basal transcription of TNF and inhibits the LPS-induced increase of TNF mRNA.

The activation of monocytes by LPS may involve a number of signal transduction pathways, including phospholipase C, phospholipase A_2, protein kinase C, calcium flux, and cyclic nucleotides. In murine macrophages, the PKC inhibitors H-7 and retinal both decrease TNF mRNA levels after exposure to 10 μg/mL LPS. The protein kinase C inhibitors are effective even 2 hr after the addition of LPS. The cyclic nucleotide inhibitor HA 1004 has no inhibitory effect. In contrast, inhibitors of calmodulin-dependent kinase (W7, calmidazolium, and trifluorperazine) do not alter the induction of TNF transcripts. The role of calcium in LPS-mediated macrophage activation has also been examined by other investigators. Calcium ionophore (A23187) actives monocytes to produce soluble cytotoxin, which is probably identical with TNF (Drysdale et al., 1983). However, in studies of starch-elicited mouse monocytes, LPS does not induce ^{45}Ca uptake, and depletion of extracellular calcium does not abrogate LPS-induced cytotoxin production (Drysdale et al., 1987). However, chelators of intracellular calcium decrease monocyte activation. Thus it appears that calcium-dependent processes are required for LPS-mediated TNF production but that extracellular calcium fluxes are not induced by LPS.

A brief exposure to LPS is not sufficient to induce significant TNF production. LPS induction of TNF requires continued presence of LPS during the entire induction/secretion process (Gifford and Lohmann, 1986). The effect of LPS is markedly enhanced by pretreatment with γ-interferon (IFN-γ). Treatment with IFN-γ alone does not result in significant TNF secretion by mouse or human monocytes. However, treatment with both IFN-γ and LPS has a synergistic effect on TNF production, especially for very low concentrations of LPS (1 to 10 ng/mL) (Gifford and Lohmann, 1987). Reactive oxygen species result in similar enhancement of LPS-induced release of TNF. The presence of 40 μM H_2O_2 or 5 mM $NaIO_4$ markedly enhances the release of TNF from mouse monocytes following stimulation with a suboptimal concentration of LPS (Chaundhri and Clark, 1989).

In studies of HL-60 cells, induction of TNF transcripts by LPS is associated with phospholipase A_2 activity (Mohri et al., 1990). LPS significantly increases membrane-bound phospholipase A_2 activity after as little as 5 min of exposure time (see Table 2). In contrast, no alterations in protein kinase C activity are observed. Inhibitors of phospholipase A_2 significantly decrease the levels of TNF mRNA induced by LPS (Fig. 4A). Mellitin, a potent direct activator of phospholipase A_2, induces TNF gene expression, and this effect is also inhibited by pretreatment with

Table 2 Effects of LPS on Substrate-specific Membrane-Bound Phospholipase A_2 in HL-60 Cells[a]

Substrate	Phospholipase A_2 activity (pmol/mg protein/h)			
		+LPS		
	Control	5 min	10 min	15 min
1-Stearoyl-2-arachidonyl PC	278 ± 14	321 ± 13	361 ± 20	280 ± 14
1,2-Dipalmitoyl PC	125 ± 6	155 ± 91	58 ± 13	145 ± 11

Source: Mohri et al., 1990, Table 1.

[a]Cells were exposed to 250 ng/mL of LPS for up to 15 min. The membrane fraction was collected and phospholipase A_2 activity measured against the substrates indicated. $*p < 0.05$; $** p < 0.01$.

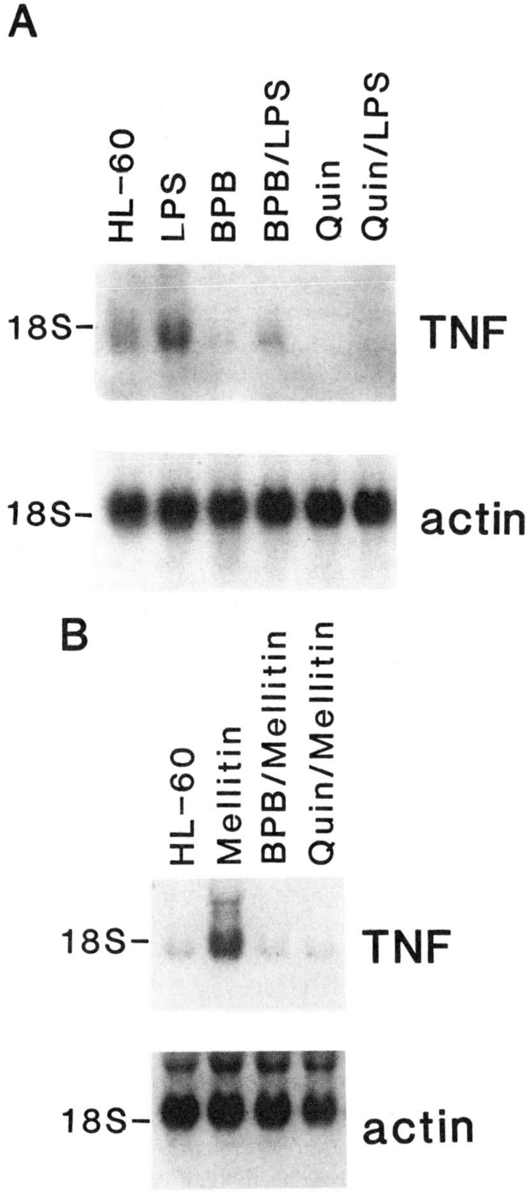

Figure 4 (A) Effect of bromophenacylbromide (BPD) and quinacrine on LPS-induced TNF mRNA levels. HL-60 cells were treated with 250 ng/mL LPS for 1 h. Cells were preincubated with 10 μM BPD or 50 mM quinacrine for 30 min. Total cellular RNA (20 μg/lane) was then hybridized to the labeled actin or TNF probes. (B) Cells were preincubated with 10 μM BPB or 50 μM quinacrine for 30 min and then exposed to 5 μg/mL mellitin. (From Mohri et al., 1990, Fig. 3.)

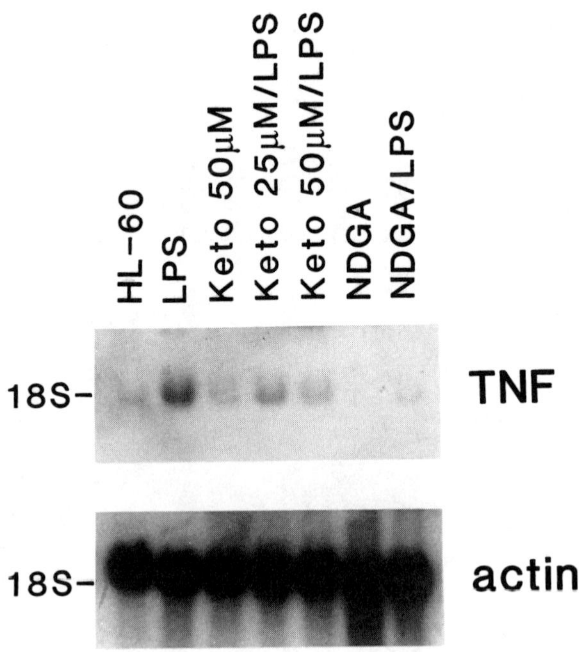

Figure 5 Effects of lipoxygenase inhibitors [ketoconazole and nordihydroguaiaretic acid (NDGA)] on LPS-induced TNF expression in HL-60 cells. Cells were pretreated with NDGA (10 μM) or the indicated concentrations of ketoconazole for 30 min followed by LPS (250 ng/mL) for 60 min. The RNA was collected and analyzed by Northern blotting. Total RNA was hybridized to the \$32P-labeled TNF or actin cDNA. (From Mohri et al., 1990, Fig. 4.)

BPB (Fig. 4B). These findings suggested that eicosanoid production is associated with induction of TNF expression and prompted further studies of arachidonic acid metabolism. Indomethacin, an inhibitor of cyclooxygenase activity, has no effect on TNF mRNA levels following LPS stimulation. However, inhibitors of lipoxygenase activity (nordihydroguaiaretic acid and ketoconazole) inhibit TNF gene expression, implying that leukotrienes or other lipoxygenase metabolites may be involved in TNF induction (Fig. 5).

In studies comparing the regulation of IL-1 and TNF secretion, it appeared that LPS induction of these two mediators differs significantly. Following LPS stimulation, the amount of TNF protein released is regulated primarily by a more prolonged period of increased transcription and by increased translation (Burchett et al., 1988). In contrast, IL-1 secretion after LPS exposure is regulated primarily through posttranscriptional regulation of IL-1 α and β mRNA species. No significant alterations of IL-1 translation have been observed.

2. Inducers of TNF: Phorbol Esters

Another group of inducers of TNF are the phorbol esters. In vitro, 12-O-tetradecanoylphorbol-13-acetate (TPA) induces production of tumor necrosis factor mRNA by human monocytes in as little as 3 hr. Maximal levels of TNF transcripts are observed after 12 h (Sariban et al., 1988). This induction of TNF mRNA is accompanied by the secretion of bioactive TNF into the cell culture supernatant. The protein synthesis inhibitor cycloheximide has no effect on basal levels of TNF mRNA, but following TPA exposure, cycloheximide increases TNF mRNA levels 50-fold. The regulation of TNF expression following TPA stimulation appears to involve both transcriptional and posttranscriptional mechanisms. In transcriptional run on assays, the TNF gene is transcriptionally inactive in unstimulated human monocytes. TNF gene transcription is increased after 20 min of exposure to TPA (Fig. 6A). An additional 12-fold enhancement of TNF gene transcription is observed when cycloheximide is added to activated monocytes (Fig. 6B). When the transcription inhibitor actinomycin D is added to activated monocytes, a 90% decrease in TNF mRNA levels is observed in 1 hr, implying an intracellular half-life of <20 min. In contrast, the combination of cycloheximide and actinomycin D does not appreciably decrease the level of TNF transcripts in activated monocytes. These observations suggest that in normal human monocytes, TNF mRNA levels are regulated transcriptionally and degraded by a labile protein.

The mechanism by which TPA activates TNF transcription is not known. While phorbol esters are well known to active protein kinase C, these agents also stimulate arachidonic acid metabolism (Castagna et al., 1982). After 30 min of TPA exposure, HL-60 cells demonstrate a significant increase in arachidonic acid release, which persists for up to 6 H. As in human monocytes, TPA stimulation of HL-60 cells increases TNF mRNA levels through transcriptional activation (Horiguchi et al., 1989). This TPA-induced increase in TNF transcripts is blocked by preincubation with the inhibitors of phospholipase A_2, BPB, and quinacrine (Quin) (Fig. 7). Indomethacin, an inhibitor of cyclooxygenase activity, has no effect on TNF transcripts, but the lipoxygenase inhibitor ketoconazole also blocks TNF induction. Furthermore, the lipoxygenase metabolite leukotriene B_4 (LTB_4) increases TNF mRNA levels (Fig. 8). In these studies, TPA induces a 50% increase in membrane-bound protein kinase C activity, and this effect is not affected by the inhibitors BPB or ketoconazole. H7, an inhibitor of protein kinase C action, also prevented TNF mRNA increases induced by TPA. Other activators of protein kinase C, such as bryostatin 1, also induced TNF gene expression in HL-60 cells (Stone et al., 1988). From these studies it appears that phospholipase A_2 occupies a key role in the induction of TNF by TPA. In some cases this effect may be mediated through activa-

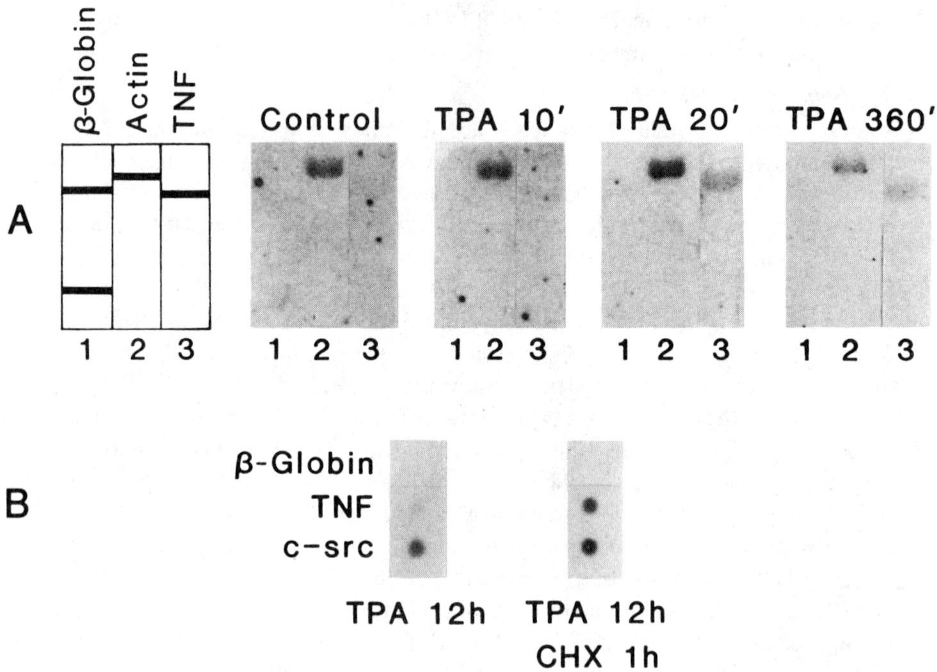

Figure 6 Analysis of TNF gene transcription in resting TPA-activated and cycloheximide (CHX)-monocytes, (A) Five micrograms of linearized β-globin, TNF, and actin plasmid DNA were electrophoresed and transferred to nitrocellulose paper by Southern blotting. The filters were hybridized to similar amounts of ^{32}P-labeled nuclear RNA. (B) Five micrograms of linearized β-globin, TNF, and c-src plasmid DNA were spotted on nitrocellulose hybridized to ^{32}P-labeled nuclear RNA isolated from monocytes exposed to TPA for 12 h, with or without 1 h or cycloheximide. (From Sariban et al., 1988, Fig. 4.)

tion of protein kinase C. As discussed above, TPA is an activator of NF-κB via protein kinase C, and NF-κB has been shown to regulate TNF transcription.

3. Inducers of TNF: Cytokines

a. GM-CSF. The colony-stimulating factor, GM-CSF, also induces TNF gene expression. In studies of U937 human myelomonocytic leukemia cells, 2500 pg/mL of recombinant human GM-CSF induced increased TNF mRNA levels after 2 h (Cannistra et al., 1987). Peak transcript levels were seen after 6 h and persisted for up to 24 h of continued exposure. Similar effects were observed after GM-CSF treatment of T-lymphocyte-depleted peripheral mononuclear cells. These alterations are accompanied by increased secretion of an inhibitory TNF-like molecule,

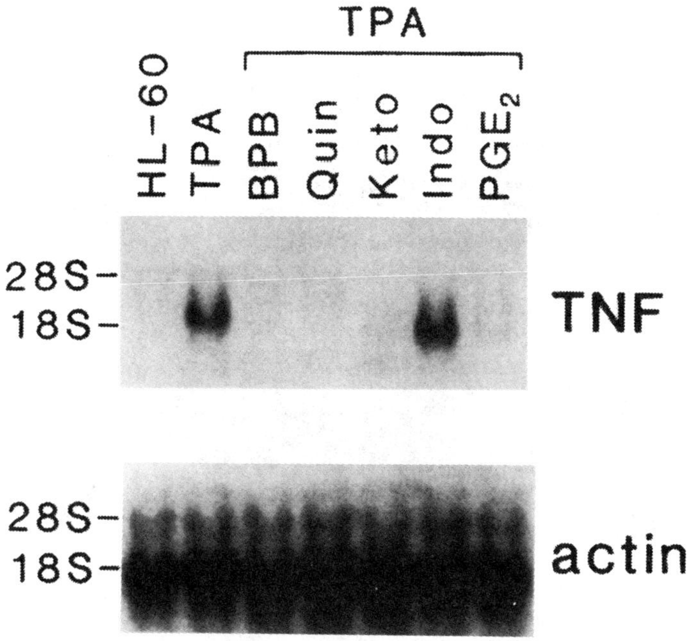

Figure 7 Effect of BPB, quinacrine, ketoconazole, indomethacin, and PGE_2 on induction of TNF mRNA. HL-60 cells were treated with 8 n*M* TPA for 3 h. Cells were also preincubated with 10 μM BPB, 100 μM quinacrine, 100 μM ketoconazole, 10 μM indomethacin, or 1 μM PGE_2 for 30 min before addition of TPA. (From Horiguchi et al., 1989, Fig. 8.)

which could be inhibited by anti-TNF antibody. GM-CSF also enhances TNF release by monocytes stimulated with either TPA or LPS.

b. TNF. TNF induces its own expression at both the RNA and protein levels in HL-60 cells (Hensel et al., 1987). TNF transcripts are induced 15–30 min after stimulation with TNF. This effect is associated with an increase in the rate of TNF transcription (Spriggs et al., 1990). Postreceptor events associated with the autoinduction of TNF expression have also been examined in HL-60 cells. Following TNF stimulation, there is no detectable alteration in phospholipase C activity as measured by inositol phosphate generation or release of choline metabolites. TNF increases the release of arachidonic acid metabolites and this effect is associated with a 40% increase in phospholipase A_2 activity. The release of arachidonic acid metabolites and induction of TNF gene expression are blocked by inhibitors of phospholipase A_2. The autoinduction of TNF mRNA is also blocked by inhibitors of lipoxygenase, while the cyclo-oxygenase inhibitor indomethacin has no detectable effect. Furthermore, TNF transcripts are induced by metabolites of the

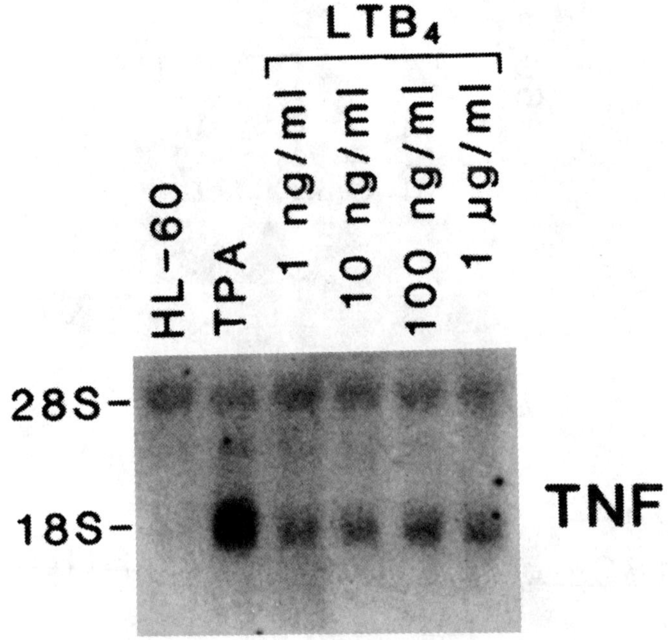

Figure 8 Effects of TPA and LTB_4 on TNF mRNA levels. HL-60 cells were treated with 8 n*M* TPA or various concentration of LTB_4 for 3 h. Total cellular RNA was then hybridized with the ^{32}P-labeled TNF cDNA. (From Horiguchi et al., 1989, Fig. 9.)

5-lipoxygenase pathway, 5-hydroperoxyeicosatetraenoic acid and leukotriene B_4 (Fig. 9). Leukotriene B_4 increases transcription of TNF in transcriptional run on assays (unpublished observation). These findings suggest that phospholipase A_2 and 5-lipoxygenase activity are involved in the transcriptional activation of TNF gene expression associated with TNF stimulation of HL-60 cells.

c. IL-1. Both IL-1 and TNF are potent activators of immune effector cells, including T-cells, NK cells, PMNs, and monocytes (Dinarello, 1984). In studies of monocyte toxicity, IL-1 induces increased monocyte cytotoxic activity, which is neutralized by anti-TNF antibody (Philip and Epstein, 1986). TNF and IL-1 are frequently induced by the same stimuli and appear to have regulatory mechanisms that are similar but not identical.

d. IFN. γ-Interferon (IFN-γ) has been reported to be synergistic with TNF in many of its actions. Some workers have reported that IFN-γ increases TNF gene transcription (Collart et al., 1986). Exposure of mouse or human monocyte /macrophages to IFN-γ is not associated with measurable TNF secretion (Gifford and

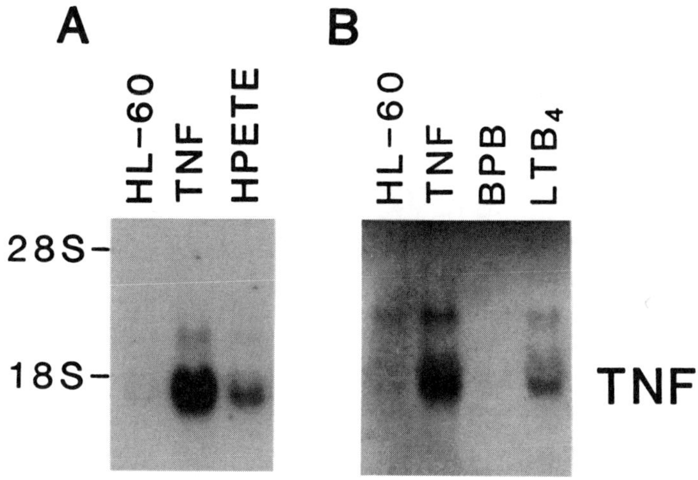

Figure 9 Effect of (A) 5-hydroperoxyeicosatetraenoic acid (HPETE) (1 μM) and (B) leukotriene B_4 and (LTB_4) (1 μM) on TNF mRNA levels in HL-60 cells. Cells were exposed to the indicated eicosanoids for 30 min.

Lohmann, 1987; Hart et al., 1989). However, IFN-γ appears to be a potent enhancer of TNF production in response to other stimuli. When mouse peritoneal monocytes are exposed to 20 μ/mL of IFN-γ, no detectable TNF production is observed. However, when IFN-γ primed mice are exposed to LPS, there is a marked enhancement in the TNF mRNA levels compared to that with LPS alone (Fig. 10). IFN-γ priming also markedly increases the sensitivity to LPS stimulation (Koerner et al., 1987).

4. Inducers of TNF: Other Stimuli

Induction of TNF transcripts by polar solvents has been described. In U937 human myelomoncytic leukemia cells, 1.5% DMSO induces TNF mRNA after 12–24 h (Fig. 11). This increase in TNF transcripts is related to the appearance of the mature monocyte phenotype, including nonspecific esterase staining and monocyte surface antigen expression (Mac 1). As is the case for LPS and TPA induction, the increase in TNF expression is paralleled by an increase in phospholipase A_2 activity (Fig. 12). Pretreatment with dexamethasone prevents the increase in phospholipase A_2 activity and prevents the DMSO-induced increase in TNF transcripts. This inhibition of TNF gene expression is associated with failure to express a mature monocytic phenotype. Similar results have been observed with other polar solvents (S. Bernstein, personal communication).

Ionizing radiation also appears to enhance TNF production. In studies using X-rays, 5 of 13 human sarcoma cell lines examined could be induced to secrete TNF

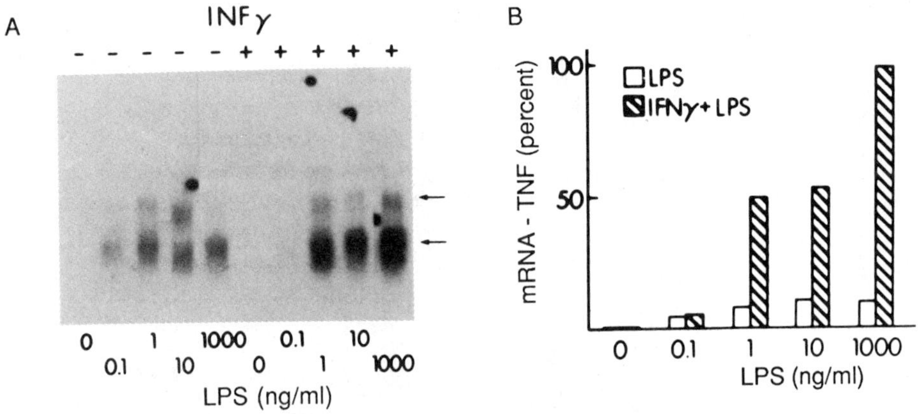

Figure 10 Effect of IFN-γ on induction of TNF mRNA by LPS (A). Macrophage cultures were treated for 5 h with the indicated concentrations of LPS in the absence (-) or presence (+) of 20 U/mL IFN-γ. The total RNA was then examined for TNF sequences. Arrows mark the 18S and 28S ribosomal RNA. (B) To quantify the relative expression, the autoradiographs were analyzed by densitometry and standardized to the maximum value observed in the experiment. (From Koerner et al., 1987, Fig. 2.)

into the cell structure supernatant following 500 cGy (Table 3) (Hallahan et al., 1989). Two normal human fibroblast lines and four human squamous cell carcinoma cell lines do not produce measurable amounts of TNF after radiation. When the TNF producing lines are examined, some heterogeneity is observed. In two of the five lines (STSAR-13 and -48), TNF transcripts are present in unirradiated controls. Exposure to 500 cGy significantly increases TNF transcripts by 3 to 6 h in each of the TNF producing lines. These findings imply that some posttranscriptional mechanisms may also be active in certain cell types.

Oxygen free-radical species also induce the production of TNF. As shown in Table 4, thioglycollate-induced mouse macrophages secrete significant amounts of TNF into the cell culture supernatant after exposure to a variety of peroxidases (Lefkowitz et al., 1989). The TNF-inducing effect appears to be maximal after 6 h, but the effect of horseradish peroxidase also induces TNF secretion by resident peritoneal macrophages. In other studies of mouse peritoneal macrophages, $NaIO_4$ and H_2O_2 both increase TNF production following stimulation with LPS, while the free-radical scavengers butylated hydroxyanisole and butylated hydroxytoluene decrease production (Chaudhri and Clark, 1989).

A variety of other stimuli have been reported to induce TNF production by leukocytes, including Fc receptor cross-linking, interleukin-2, and a lymphokine provisionally referred to as *cytotoxicity triggering factor* (Debets et al., 1988;

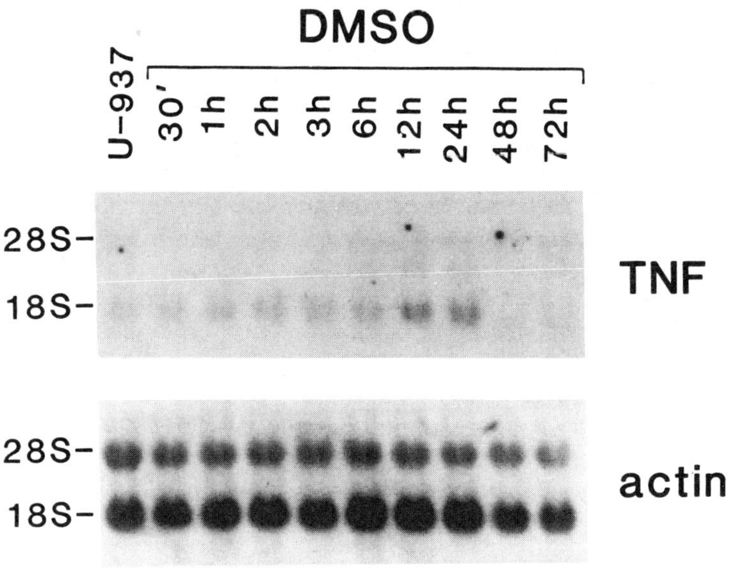

Figure 11 Effect of DMSO on TNF gene expression. U937 cells were exposed to 1.5% DMSO for the times indicated. Total RNA was hybridized to the ^{32}P-labeled TNF or actin cDNA. (From Nakamura et al., 1990, Fig. 4).

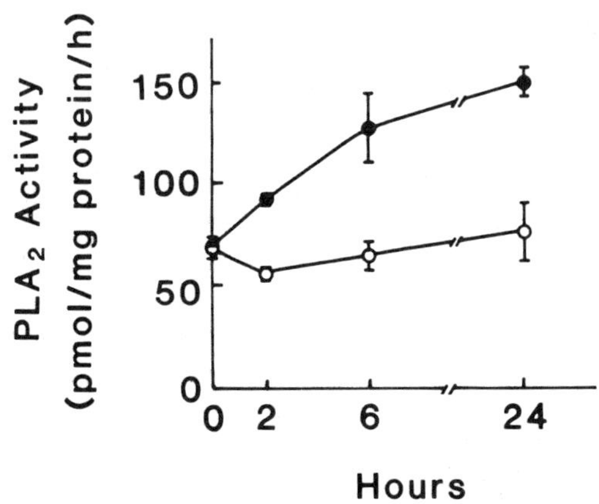

Figure 12 Effects of DMSO and dexamethasone on phospholipase A_2 activity in U937 cells. U937 cells were treated with 1.5% DMSO (●) or 1.5% DMSO amd dexamethasone 4 μM (○) for the times indicated. The results are presented as the mean ± standard deviation. (From Nakamura et al., 1990, Fig. 5.)

Table 3 Production of TNF in Human Sarcoma Cell Lines[a]

Cell line	Origin	TNF produced (U/mL)	
		Control	X-ray treated
STSAR-5	Malignant fibrous histiocytoma	0.4	>2.0
STSAR-13	Liposarcoma	0.0	0.34
STSAR-33	Ewing sarcoma	0.17	>2.0
STSAR-43	Osteosarcoma	0.41	1.3
STSAR-48	Neurofibrosarcoma	0.28	0.43

Source: Hallahan et al., 1989, Table 1.
[a]TNF levels were measured in confluent (control) and irradiated confluent cell cultures by ELISA.

Table 4 Induction of TNF Protein in Thioglycollate-Induced Macrophages by Peroxidases

Inducer	Concentration	TNF (U/mL)
HRP	0.88 μ*M*	80. ± 10.77
	17.70	1850. ± 30.18
LPO	1.77 μ*M*	120. ± 37.0
	17.70	1740. ± 30.9
MyPO	0.16 μ*M*	80. ± 10.7
LPS	10.ng/mL	20. ± 4.0

Source: Lefkowitz et al., 1989, Table 1.

Kornbluth et al., 1988). Bacterial extracts, synthetic lipids related to LPS, and other microbial stimuli have also been implicated as inducers of TNF production.

B. Inhibitors of TNF Production

1. Prostaglandin E_2

Regardless of the inducing stimulus for TNF production, certain mechanisms appear to participate in the subsequent down-regulation of TNF expression and secretion. TNF stimulation of fibroblasts and monocytes results in increased production of the arachidonic acid metabolite prostaglandin E_2 (PGE_2) (Bachwich et al., 1986; Dayer et al., 1985). In murine macrophages stimulated by LPS, 0.1 μM PGE_2 is sufficient to decrease TNF transcript levels by 50% (Fig. 13) (Kunkel et al., 1988). In nuclear run on transcription assays this effect is mediated, at least in part, by a marked decrease in TNF transcription. PGE_2 appears to act through a cell surface receptor coupled to adenyl cyclase by a G-protein. This cell surface receptor may be desensitized by prolonged exposure to PGE_2. The amount of TNF secreted by mouse monocytes following LPS exposure is decreased 16-fold by concurrent treatment with 1 μM PGE_2. However, when the monocytes are preincubated with 0.1 μM PGE_2 for 4 h, TNF secretion is decreased slightly, but addition of 1 μM PGE_2 has no further attenuating effect (Spengler et al., 1989b). Similarly, pretreatment with PGE_2 attenuates the ability of PGE_2 to decrease LPS-stimulated TNF mRNA levels. The effect of cyclo-oxygenase inhibitors is also complex. When indomethacin is added simultaneously with LPS, the production of TNF is enhanced. However, pretreatment of the monocytes with indomethacin decreases the production of TNF and sensitized the monocytes to the inhibitory effects of exogenous PGE_2.

2. cAMP

The inhibitory effects of PGE_2 appear to be mediated through cAMP. Direct manipulation of cAMP levels has also been reported to alter TNF expression. The cell permeant cAMP analogs dibutryl cyclic AMP and 8-bromo cyclic AMP both decrease TNF production in LPS-stimulated monocytes (Katakami et al., 1988; Spengler et al., 1989a). This inhibition of TNF production is observed at both the mRNA and protein levels. Forskolin and cholera toxin, activators of adenyl cyclase, also increase cAMP levels and decrease production of TNF. In related studies, a variety of phosphodiesterase inhibitors decrease TNF production in mouse macrophages (Strieter et al., 1988). Pentoxyfylline (2.5×10^{-5} M), isobutylmethylxanthine (5×10^{-5} M), and theophylline (1×10^{-4} M) all decrease LPS-induced secretion of TNF by more than 50%. This effect is associated with decreased accumulation of TNF mRNA following TNF stimulation.

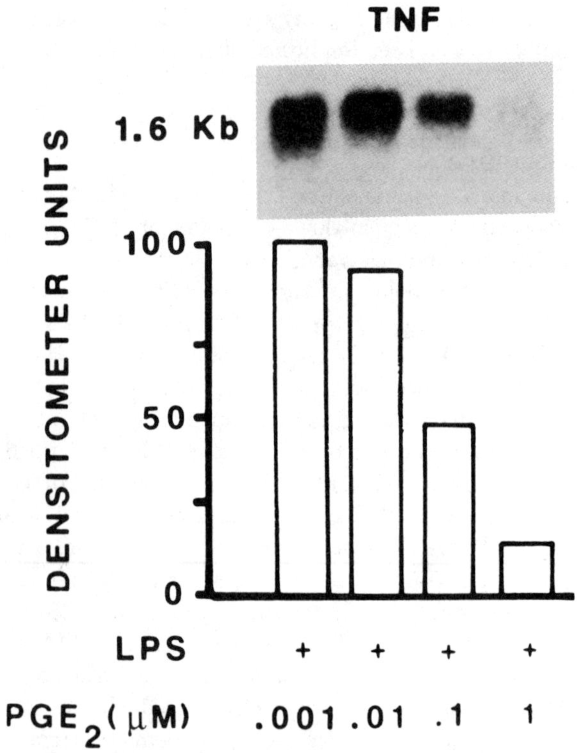

Figure 13 Northern blot analysis of the dose-dependent suppression of LPS-induced TNF mRNA accumulation by graded doses of PGE_2. Graded doses of PGE_2 were added concomitantly with 1 μg/mL LPS and 90 min later samples collected for total RNA isolation. TNF expression was decreased 50% by 0.1 μM PGE_2 and more than 90% by 1 μM PGE_2. (From Kunkel et al., 1988, Fig. 2.)

C. Inhibitors of Secretion

The regulation of TNF secretion remains unclear. As noted above, investigators have identified a cytokine that may specifically stimulate secretion of previously formed TNF. It appears that TNF is initially synthesized as a 26-kDa membrane-associated protein (Kriegler et al., 1988). This 26-kDa protein is cytotoxic only when associated with membrane components as microsomes. This protein is cleaved to form the secreted 17-kDa TNF protein. The regulation of cleavage and the mechanism of secretion are not known. However, the serine protease inhibitor *p*-toluenesulfonyl-l-arginine decreases LPS-stimulated TNF secretion by 47%

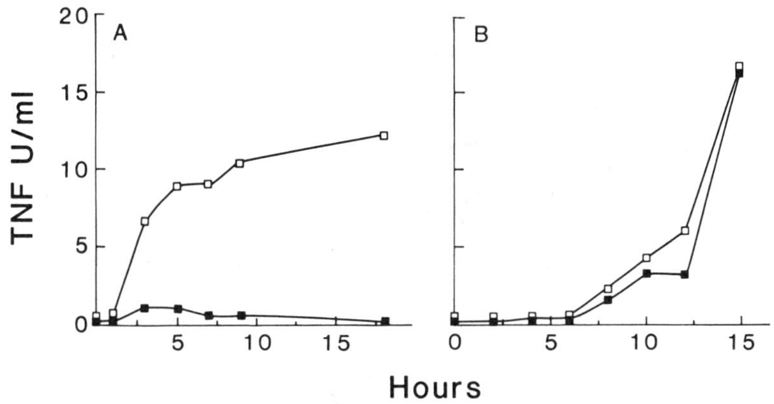

Figure 14 Effects of botulinum toxin type D on secretion of TNF from LPS- and TPA-stimulated human monocytes. The cells (2×10^6 per 0.5 mL) were treated with 50 n*M* LPS (A) or 33 n*M* (B) for the times indicated. Control cells (□) were compared to monocytes preincubated for 15 h with 2 μg of botulinum toxin type D per milliliter (■). (From Imamura et al., 1989, Fig. 1.)

without significantly altering IL-1 secretion (Scuderi, 1989). Recently, studies of RAW 264.7 cells demonstrated a partially processed precursor that is not cytotoxic to L929 cells (Cseh and Beutler, 1989). This alternative cleavage site has been mapped to a scission site 10 amino acids before the amino terminal of the mature 17-kDa protein.

In some secretory cells, exocytotic secretion is regulated by a distinct guanine nucleotide binding protein (G-protein) (Burgoyne, 1987; Goud et al., 1988). Type D botulinum toxin specifically ADP ribosylates an M_r 21,000 protein in bovine adrenal cell membranes (Ohashi and Narumiya, 1987). In normal human monocytes, botulinum D toxin markedly inhibits the secretion of TNF into the cell supernatant following LPS stimulation but not following TPA stimulation (Fig. 14) (Imamura et al., 1989). This effect is not associated with decreased TNF gene expression at the mRNA level. LPS-induced TNF mRNA levels are unchanged by treatment with LPS and botulinum D toxin. Moreover, when cell lysates are examined for TNF protein, the botulinum D toxin-pretreated monocytes have more immunoreactive TNF protein. This inhibitory effect on TNF release following LPS appears to be dependent on a G-protein. When botulinum-pretreated monocytes are treated with the GTP analog GTP-γ-S, a partial reversal of the secretory block is observed. As was observed in adrenal cell membranes, treatment with botulinum D toxin results in ADP-ribosylation of an M_r 21,000 protein.

In summary, intracellular TNF protein trafficking is not well understood. Additional studies are needed to delineate the processes related to TNF translation, processing, and release.

D. TNF Secretion by Nonmyeloid Cells

Initially, TNF was thought to be exclusively a monokine. However, it is now clear that many tissues have the capacity to express TNF, either constituitively or in response to stimuli. In studies of normal tissue, TNF mRNA was present in organ homogenates from spleen, liver, and kidney (Tovey et al., 1988). The expression of TNF was closely correlated to the cellular levels of IL-1α, IL-1β, and IL-6 mRNA. These findings suggest that TNF may act in consort with other cytokines to control growth and function in normal tissues. Both TNF mRNA and TNF protein have been identified in cultured human diploid fibroblasts (Niitsu et al., 1988a).

TNF production has also been observed in cells of the central nervous system. LPS-induced expression of TNF mRNA and cytotoxic protein is detectable in cultured rat astrocytes after exposures of 1 h (Chung and Benveniste, 1990; Lieberman et al., 1989). This LPS-induced secretion of TNF is enhanced by pretreatment with IFN-γ or IL-1β, although neither cytokine induces significant TNF production alone (Chung and Benveniste, 1990). TNF expression is also induced by exposure of the astrocytes to a neurotropic paramyxovirus, Newcastle disease virus (NDV) (Lieberman et al., 1989). This increase in TNF mRNA levels occurs with 3 h of exposure and is associated with release of TNF protein into the supernatant.

Cultured human tumor cells also produce TNF in vitro. In studies of 14 human epithelial tumor cells, 3 or 14 cell lines examined had detectable levels of TNF mRNA by Northern blot analysis (Fig. 15A) (Spriggs et al., 1988). If the cells are pretreated with cycloheximide, Northern blot analysis demonstrates TNF transcripts in 12 of 14 lines, suggesting regulation by a labile inhibitory protein (Fig. 15B). This expression of TNF is not correlated with the number of TNF cell surface receptors. These observations have been confirmed by other investigators (Krönke et al., 1988; Niitsu et al., 1988b). Not all of the cells that have detectable TNF mRNA secrete TNF protein into the supernatant. Immunoprecipitation studies have demonstrated immunoreactive protein in the cell culture supernatant of one ovarian carcinoma line (Spriggs et al., 1988). The cell culture supernatant from some tumor cell cultures is cytotoxic for L929 cells (Krönke et al., 1988). Additional cell culture lines have membrane-bound TNF and can be induced to secrete bioactive TNF into the cell culture supernatant by treatment with TPA.

TNF acts as a stimulus for autocrine production of TNF in epithelial tumor cells. Human carcinoma cells exposed to TNF also produce TNF mRNA and TNF protein (Niitsu et al., 1988a; Spriggs et al., 1987). Prolonged in vitro exposure of carcinoma cells to increasing concentrations of TNF produces stable TNF resistance (Rubin et al., 1986; Spriggs et al., 1987). In these cell lines, there is induction of

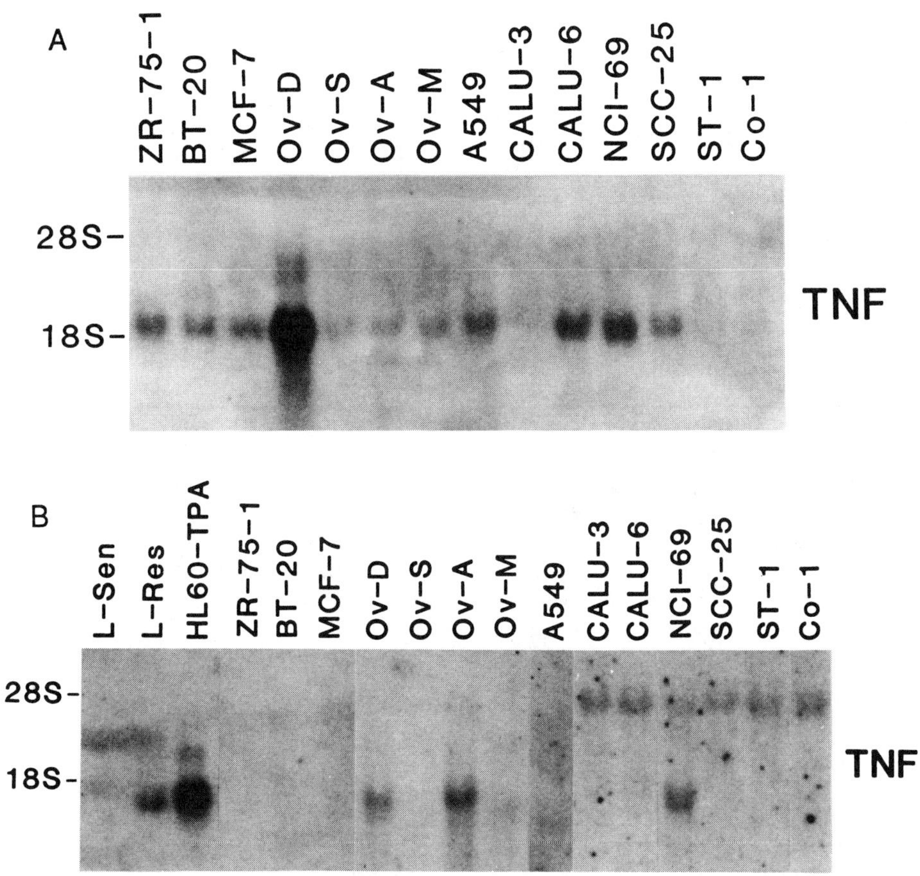

Figure 15 Levels of TNF in tumor cell culture. (A) Total RNA was purified and hybridized to the ^{32}P-labeled TNF probe. (B) The same cell lines were treated with 10 μg/mL cycloheximide prior to collection of the RNA. (From Spriggs et al., 1988, Figs. 2 and 3.)

TNF MRNA following TNF exposure, and the resistant sublines show a marked increase in the levels of TNF mRNA present (Fig. 16). These resistant sublines also secrete bioactive TNF into the cell culture supernatant (Fig. 17). The production of TNF by tumor cells is of particular interest because murine studies suggest that TNF secreting tumors produce a wasting syndrome similar to the cachexia observed in cancer patients (Oliff et al., 1987).

The expression of TNF by tumor cells in vivo remains a controversial area. In a study of 10 patients with colorectal carcinoma, Northern blot analysis of tumor homogenates has shown detectable TNF mRNA. However, the TNF mRNA ap-

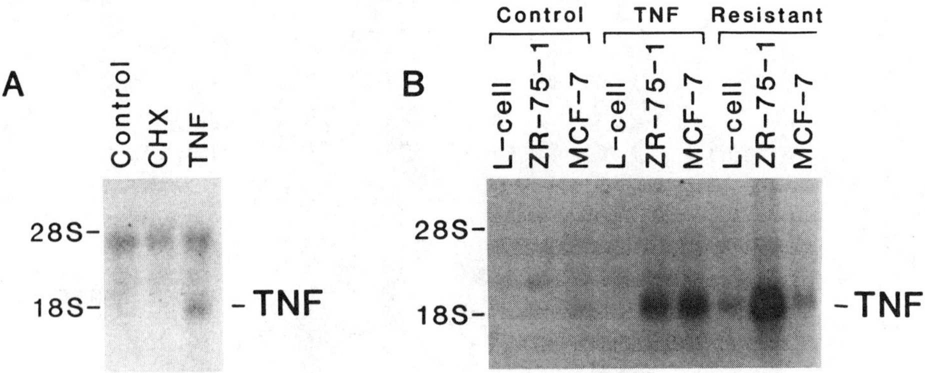

Figure 16 Effect of cycloheximide and TNF on TNF mRNA levels in ZR-75-1 human breast carcinoma cells. (B) Effect of acute and chronic exposure to TNF on TNF mRNA levels in cell culture of ZR-75-1, MCF-7, and L-cells (L929 cells). In both panels, the control cells were untreated. Cells were treated for 60 min with 1 μg/mL cycloheximide in the CHX lane. The TNF lanes were prepared from cell cultures exposed to TNF (0.45 μg/mL) for 3 h. The "resistant" lanes in panel B were prepared from stable resistant sublines, prepared by chronic exposure to increasing concentrations of TNF.

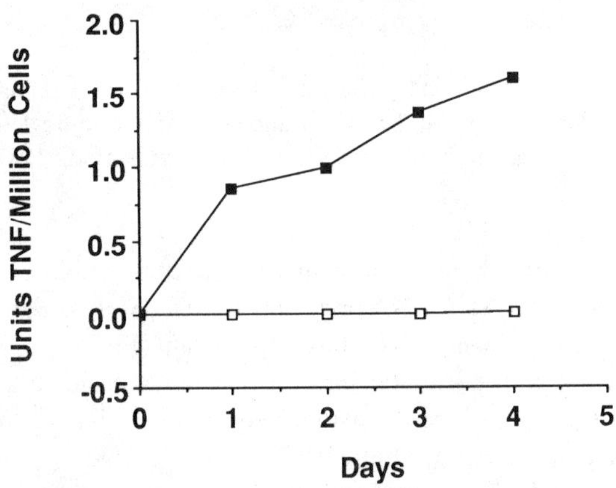

Figure 17 Production of bioactive TNF into cell culture supernatant by wild-type ZR-75-1 cells (□) and TNF-resistant ZR-75-1 cells (■).

pears to be localized in infiltrating mononuclear cells and is not present in the tumor cells as detected by in situ hybridization (Beissert et al., 1989). This may not be the case for all tumor types. In analogous studies of ovarian carcinoma, we have observed TNF protein by immunoperoxidase staining in the epithelial tumor cells. In situ hybridization techniques indicated that TNF mRNA was present in ovarian tumor cells of some but not all tumor biopsies examined.

III. SUMMARY

The TNF gene is located in close proximity to the HLA-B locus in both humans and mouse. TNF has a high degree of sequence observation across species, and this is reflected in its relatively high cross-species activity. The 5′ flanking region of the TNF gene contains multiple potential regulatory sites, including consensus sequences for the AP-1 and AP-2 sites, the cAMP-responsive element, and sequences similar to the κB sequences found in immunoglobulin and cytokine regulatory elements. This sequence has been demonstrated to be responsive to LPS and TNF stimulation. The 3′ untranslated region contains a sequence element affecting posttranslational control of TNF through mRNA stability and translation efficiency. The functional importance and interactions of these regulatory elements remain undefined.

TNF is widely expressed in granulocytes, macrophages, fibroblasts, and epithelial cells. Induction of TNF can occur through a variety of stimuli, including LPS, TPA, cytokines, calcium flux, and oxygen free-radical mechanisms. A common pathway for these diverse agents remains unknown. In human monocytes, the regulation of TNF expression is regulated at both transcriptional and posttranscriptional levels. Experimental evidence suggests that phospholipase A_2 and the lipoxygenase pathway may be central in the process of TNF induction in leukocytes. Down-regulation of TNF expression is better understood. The inhibition of expression appears to result from high levels of cAMP, frequently induced through the action of PGE_2. TNF secretion is separately regulated and may involve the action of G binding proteins.

REFERENCES

Angel, P., Imagawa, M., Chiu, R., Stein, B., Imbra, R. J., Rahmsdorf, H. J., Jonal, C., Herlich, P., and Karin, M. (1987). Phorbol ester inducible genes contain a common cis element recognized by TPA modulated trans acting factor, *Cell*, *49*: 729.

Bachwich, P. R., Chensue, S. W., Larrick, J. W., and Kunkel, S. L. (1986). Tumor necrosis factor stimulates interleukin-1 and prostaglandin E_2 production in resting macrophages, *Biochem. Biophys. Res. Commun.*, *136*: 94.

Beissert, S., Bergholz, M., Waase, I., Lepsien, G., Schauer, A., Pfizenmaier, K., and Kronke, M. (1989). Regulation of tumor necrosis factor gene expression in colorectal adenocarcinoma: in vivo analysis by in situ hybridization, *Proc. Natl. Acad. Sci. USA*, *86*: 5064.

Beutler, B., Krochin, N., Milsark, I. W., Luedke, C., and Cerami, A. (1986). Control of cachectin (tumor necrosis factor) synthesis: mechanisms of endotoxin resistance, *Science*, *232*: 977.

Beutler, B., Thompson, P., Keyes, J., Hagerty, K., and Crawford, D. (1988). Assay of a ribonuclease that preferentially hydrolyses mRNAs containing cytokine-derived UA-rich instability sequences, *Biochem. Biophys. Res. Commun.*, *152*: 973.

Burchett, S. K., Weaver, W. M., Westall, J. A., Larsen, A., Kronheim, S., and Wilson, C. B. (1988). Regulation of tumor necrosis factor/cachectin and IL-1 secretion in human mononuclear phagocytes, *J. Immunol.*, *140*: 3473.

Burgoyne, R. D. (1987). Control of exocytosis, *Nature*, *328*: 112.

Cannistra, S. A., Rambaldi, A., Spriggs, D. R., Herrmann, F., Kufe, D., and Griffin, J. D. (1987). Human granulocyte-macrophage colony-stimulating factor induces expression of the tumor necrosis factor gene by the U937 cell line and by normal human monocytes, *J. Clin. Invest.*, *79*: 1720.

Caput, D., Beutler, B., Hartog, K., Thayer, R., Brown, S. S., and Cerami, A. (1986). Identification of a common nucleotide sequence in the 3′-untranslated region of mRNA molecules specifying inflammatory mediators, *Proc. Natl. Acad. Sci. USA*, *83*: 1670.

Carswell, E. A., Old, L. J., Kassel, R. L., Green, S., Fiore, N., and Williamson, B. (1975). An endotoxin induced serum factor which causes necrosis of tumors, *Proc. Natl. Acad. Sci. USA*, *72*: 3666.

Castagna, M., Takai, Y., Kaibuchi, K., Sano, Kikkawa, V., and Nishizuka, Y. (1982). Direct activation of calcium activated phospholipid dependent protein kinase by tumour promoting phorbol esters, *J. Biol. Chem.*, *257*: 7847.

Chaudhri, G., and Clark, I. A. (1989). Reactive oxygen species facilitate the in vitro and in vivo lipopolysaccharide-induced release of tumor necrosis factor, *J. Immunol.*, *143*: 1290.

Chung, I. Y., and Benveniste, E. N. (1990). Tumor necrosis factor production by astrocytes, *J. Immunol.*, *144*: 2999.

Collart, M. A., Belin, D., Vassalli, J. D., de Kossodo. S., and Vassalli, P. (1986). Gamma interferon enhances macrophage transcription of the tumor necrosis factor/cachectin, interleukin 1, and urokinase genes, which are controlled by short-lived repressors, *J. Exp. Med.*, *164*: 2113.

Cseh, K., and Beutler, B. (1989). Alternative cleavage of the cachectin/tumor necrosis factor propeptide results in a larger, inactive form of secreted protein, *J. Biol. Chem.*, *264*: 16256.

Dayer, J. M., Beutler, B., and Cerami, A. (1985). Cachectin/tumor necrosis factor stimulates collagenase and prostaglandin E_2 production by human synovial cells and dermal fibroblasts, *J. Exp. Med.*, *162*: 2163.

Debets, J. M., Van, d. L. C. J., Dieteren, I. E., Leeuwenberg, J. F., and Buurman, W. A. (1988). FC-receptor cross-linking induces rapid secretion of tumor necrosis factor (cachectin) by human peripheral blood monocytes, *J. Immunol.*, *141*: 1197.

Debets, I. M., Van, d. L. C. J., Dieteren, I. E., Leeuwenberg, J. F., and Buurman, W. A. (1989). Fc-receptors regulate secretion of tumor necrosis factor by human monocytes, *Transplant. Proc.*

Dinarello, C. A. (1984). Interleukin 1 and the pathogenesis of the acute phase response, *N. Engl. J. Med.*, *311*: 1413.

Drysdale, B., Zacharchuk, C. M., and Shin, H. S. (1983). Mechanism of macrophage-mediated cytotoxicity: production of a soluble cytotoxic factor, *J. Immunol.*, *131*: 1315.

Drysdale, B. E., Yapundich, R. A., Shin, M. L., and Shin, H. S. (1987). Lipopolysaccharide-mediated macrophage activation: the role of calcium in the generation of tumoricidal activity, *J. Immunol.*, *138*: 951.

Economou, J. S., Rhoades, K., Essner, R., McBride, W. H., Gasson, J. C., and Morton, D. L. (1989). Genetic analysis of the human tumor necrosis factor alpha/cachectin promotor region in a macrophage cell line, *J. Exp. Med.*, *170*: 321.

Ghosh, S., and Baltimore, D. (1990). Activation in vitro of NF-kB by phosphorylation of its inhibitor IkB, *Nature*, *344*: 678.

Gifford, G. E., and Lohmann, M. M. L. (1986). Requirement for the continual presence of lipopolysaccharide for production of tumor necrosis factor by thioglycollate-induced peritoneal murine macrophages, *Int. J. Cancer*, *38*: 135.

Gifford, G. E., and Lohmann, M. M. L. (1987). Gamma interferon priming of mouse and human macrophages for induction of tumor necrosis factor production by bacterial lipopolysaccharide, *J. Natl. Cancer Inst.*, *78*: 121.

Goeddel, D. V., Aggarwal, B. B., Gray, P. W., Leung, D. W., Nedwin, G. E., Palladino, M. A., Patton, J. S., Pennica, D., Shepard, H. M., Sugarman, B. J., et al. (1986). Tumor necrosis factors: gene structure and biological activities, *Cold Spring Harbor Symp. Quant. Biol.*, *1*: 597.

Goud, B., Salminen, N. C., Walworth, N. C., and Novick, P. J. (1988). A GTP binding protein required for secretion rapidly associates with secretory vesicles and the plasma membrane in yeast, *Cell*, *53*: 753.

Hallahan, D. E., Spriggs, D. R., Beckett, M. A., Kufe, D. W., and Weichselbaum, R. R. (1989). Increased tumor necrosis mRNA after cellular exposure to ionizing radiation, *Proc. Natl. Acad. Sci. USA*, *86*: 10104.

Han, J., Brown, T., and Beutler, B. (1990). Endotoxin-responsive sequences control cachectin/tumor necrosis factor biosynthesis at the translational level, *J. Exp. Med.*, *171*: 465.

Hart, P. H., Whitty, G. A., Piccoli, D. S., and Hamilton, J. A. (1989). Control by IFN-gamma and PGE2 of TNF alpha and IL-1 production by human monocytes, *Immunology*, *66*: 376.

Hensel, G., Mannel, D. N., Pfizenmaier, K., and Krönke, M. (1987). Autocrine stimulation of TNF-alpha mRNA expression in HL-60 cells, *Lymphokine REs.*, *6*: 119.

Hensel, G., Meichle, A., Pfizenmaier, K., and Krönke, M. (1989). PMA-responsive 5′ flanking sequences of the human TNF gene, *Lymphokine Res.*, *8*: 347.

Horiguchi, J., Spriggs, D., Imamura, K., Stone, R., Luebbers, R., and Kufe, D. (1989). Role of arachidonic acid metabolism in transcriptional induction of tumor necrosis factor gene expression by phorbol ester, *Mol. Cell. Biol.*, *9*: 252.

Imamura, K., Ohno, T., Spriggs, D. R., and DW, K. (1989). Effects of botulinum type D toxin on secretion of tumor necrosis factor from human monocytes, *Mol. Cell. Biol.*, *9*: 2239.

Israel, A., Le Bail, O., Hatat, D., et al. (1990). TNF stimulates expression of mouse MHC class I genes by inducing an NFkB-like enhance binding activity which displaces constituitive factors, *EMBO J.*, *8*: 3793.

Ito, H., Shirai, T., Yamamoto, S., Akira, M., Kawahara, S., Todd, C. W., and Wallace, R. B. (1986). Molecular cloning of the gene encoding rabbit tumor necrosis factor, *DNA*, *5*: 157.

Jongeneel, C. V., Shakhov, A. N., Nedospasov, S. A., and Cerottini, J. C. (1989). Molecular control of tissue-specific expression at the mouse TNF locus, *Eur. J. Immunol.*, *19*: 549.

Katakami, Y., Nakao, Y., Koizumi, T., Katakami, N., Ogawa, R., and Fujita, T. (1988). Regulation of tumor necrosis factor production by mouse peritoneal macrophages: the role of cellular cyclic AMP, *Immunology*, *64*: 719.

Koerner, T. J., Adams, D. O., and Hamilton, T. A. (1987). Regulation of tumor necrosis factor (TNF) expression: interferon-gamma enhances the accumulation of mRNA for TNF induced by lipopolysaccha ride in murine in peritoneal macrophages, *Cell. Immunol.*, *109*: 437.

Kornbluth, R. S., Gregory, S. A., and Edgington, T. S. (1988). Initial characterization of a lymphokine pathway for the immunologic induction of tumor necrosis factor-alpha release from human peripheral blood mononuclear cells, *J. Immunol.*, *141*: 2006.

Kriegler, M., Perez, C., DeFay, K., Albert, I., and Lu, S. D. (1988). A novel form of TNF/cachectin is a cell surface cytotoxic transmembrane protein; ramifications for the complex physiology of TNF, *Cell*, *53*: 45.

Krönke, M., Hensel, G., Schluter, C., Scheurich, P., Schutze, S., and Pfizenmaier, K. (1988). Tumor necrosis factor and lymphotoxin gene expression in human tumor cell lines, *Cancer Res.*, *48*: 5417.

Kruys, V., Marinx, O., Shaw, G., Deschamps, J., and Huez, G. (1989). Translational blockade imposed by cytokine derived UA rich sequences, *Science*, *245*: 852.

Kunkel, S. L., Spengler, M., May, M. A., Spengler, R., Larrick, J., and Remick, D. (1988). Prostaglandin E_2 regulates macrophage-derived tumor necrosis factor gene expression, *J. Biol. Chem.*, *263*: 5380.

Lefkowitz, D. L., Mone, J., Mills, K., Hsieh, T. C.,and Lefkowitz, S. S. (1989). Peroxidases enhance macrophage-mediated cytoxicity via induction of tumor necrosis factor, *Proc. Soc. Exp. Biol. Med.*, *190*: 144.

Lieberman, A. P., Pitha, P. M., Shin, H. S., and Shin, M. L. (1989). Production of tumor necrosis factor and other cytokines by astrocytes stimulated with lipopolysaccharide or a neurotropic virus, *Proc. Natl. Acad. Sci. USA*, *86*: 6348.

Marmenout, A., Fransen, L., Tavernier, J., Van, d. H. J., Tizard, R., Kawashima, E., Shaw, A., Johnson, M. J., Semon, D., Muller, R., et al. (1985). Molecular cloning and expression of human tumor necrosis factor and comparison with mouse tumor necrosis factor, *Eur. J. Biochem.*, *152*: 515.

Meichle, A., Schutze, S., Hensel, G., Brunsing, D., and Krönke, M. (1990). Protein kinase C independent activation of nuclear factor κB by tumor necrosis factor, *J. Biol. Chem.*, *265*: 8339.

Mohri, M., Spriggs, D. R., and Kufe, D. (1990). Effects of lipopolysaccharide on phospholipase A_2 activity and tumor necrosis factor expression in HL-60 cells, *J. Immunol.*, *144*: 2678.

Montminy, M. R., Sevarino, K. A., Wagner, J. A., and Mandel, G. (1986). Identification of a cyclic AMP responsive element with the rat somatostatin gene, *Proc. Natl. Acad. Sci. USA*, *83*: 6682.

Muller, U., Jongeneel, C. V., Nedoospasov, S. A., Lindahl, K. F., and Steinmetz, M. (1987). Tumour necrosis factor and lymphotoxin genes map close to H-2D in the mouse major histocompatibility complex, *Nature*, *325*: 265.

Nakamura, T., Kharbanda, S., Spriggs, D., and Kufe, D. (1990). Effects of dexamethasone on induction of monocytic differentiation in human U-937 cells by dimethylsulfoxide, *J. Cell. Phys.*, *142*: 261.

Nedwin, G. E., Naylor, S. L., Sakaguchi, A. Y., Smith, D., Jarrett, N. J., Pennica, D., Goeddel, D. V., and Gray, P. W. (1985). Human lymphotoxin and tumor necrosis factor genes: structure, homology and chromosomal localization, *Nucleic Acids Res.*, *13*: 6361.

Niitsu, Y., Watanabe, N., Neda, H., Yamauchi, N., Maeda, M., Sone, H., and Kuriyama, H. (1988a). Induction of synthesis of tumor necrosis factor in human and murine cell lines by exogenous recombinant human tumor necrosis factor, *Cancer Res.*, *48*: 5407.

Niitsu, Y., Watanabe, N., Umeno, H., Sone, H., Neda, H., Yamauchi, N., Maeda, M., and Urushizaki, I. (1988b). Synergistic effects of recombinant human tumor necrosis factor and hyperthermia on in vitro cytotoxicity and artificial metastasis, *Cancer Res.*, *48*: 654.

Ohashi, Y., and Narumiya, S. (1987). ADP ribosylation of a M_r 21,000 membrane protein by type D botulinum toxin, *J. Biol. Chem.*, *262*: 1430.

Oliff, A., Defeo, J. D., Boyer, M., Martinez, D., Kiefer, D., Vuocolo, G., Wolfe, A., and Socher, S. H. (1987). Tumors secreting human TNF/cachectin induce cachexia in mice, *Cell*, *50*: 555.

Philip, R., and Epstein, L. B. (1986). Tumour necrosis factor as immunomodulator and mediator of monocyte cytotoxicity induced by itself, gamma-interferon and interleukin-1, *Nature*, *323*: 86.

Rubin, B. Y., Anderson, S. L., Sullivan, S. A., Williamson, B. D., Carswell, E. A., and Old, L. J. (1986). Nonhematopoietic cells selected for resistance to tumor necrosis factor produce tumor necrosis factor, *J. Exp. Med.*, *164*: 1350.

Sariban, E., Imamura, K., Luebbers, R., and Kufe, D. (1988). Transcriptional and posttranscriptional regulation of tumor necrosis factor gene expression in human monocytes, *J. Clin. Invest.*, *81*: 1506.

Scuderi, P. (1989). Suppression of human leukocyte tumor necrosis factor secretion by the serine protease inhibitor *p*-toluenesulfonyl-L-arginine methyl ester (TAME), *J. Immunonol.*, *143*: 168.

Sen, R., and Baltimore, D. (1986). Inducibility of a immunoglobulin enhancer-binding protein by a post translational mechanism, *Cell*, *47*: 921.

Shakhov, A. N., Collart, M. A., Vassalli, P., Nedospasov, S. A., and Jongeneel, C. V. (1990). Kappa B-type enhancers are involved in lipopolysaccharide-mediated transcriptional activation of the tumor necrosis factor alpha gene in primary macrophates, *J. Exp. Med.*, *171*: 35.

Shaw, G., and Kamin, R. (1986). A conserved AU sequence from the 3′ untranslated region of GM-Csf mRNA mediates selective mRNA degradation, *Cell*, *456*: 659.

Shimuzu, H., Mitomo, K., Watanabe, T., Okamoto, S., and Yamamoto, K. (1990). Involvement of a NF-κB-like transcription factor in the activation of the interleukin 6 gene by inflammatory lymphokines, *Mol. Cell. Biol.*, *10*: 561.

Shirai, T., Yamaguchi, H., Ito, H., Todd, C. W., and Wallace, R. B. (1985). Cloning and expression in *Escherichia coli* of the gene for human tumour necrosis factor, *Nature, 313*: 803.

Spengler, R. N., Spengler, M. L., Lincoln, P., Remick, D. G., Strieter, R. M., and Kunkel, S. L. (1989a). Dynamics of dibutyryl cyclic AMP- and prostaglandin E_2-mediated suppression of lipopolysaccharide-induced tumor necrosis factor alpha gene expression, *Infect. Immun.*, *57*: 2837.

Spengler, R. N., Spengler, M. L., Strieter, R. M., Remick, D. G., Larrick, J. W., and Kunkel, S. L. (1989b). Modulation of tumor necrosis factor-alpha gene expression: desensitization of prostaglandin E_2-induced suppression, *J. Immunol.*, *142*: 4346.

Spies, T., Blanck, G., Bresnahan, M., Sands, J., and Strominger, J. L. (1989). A new cluster of genes within the human major histocompatibility complex, *Science*, *243*: 214.

Spriggs, D., Imamura, K., Rodriguez, C., Horiguchi, J., and Kufe, D. W. (1987). Induction of tumor necrosis factor expression and resistance in a human breast tumor cell line, *Proc. Natl. Acad. Sci. USA*, *84*: 6563.

Spriggs, D. R., Imamura, K., Rodriguez, C., Sariban, E., and Kufe, D. W. (1988). Tumor necrosis factor expression in human epithelial tumor cell lines, *J. Clin. Invest.*, *81*: 455.

Spriggs, D. R., Sherman, M. L., Imamura, K., Mohri, M., Rodriguez, C., Robbins, G., and Kufe, D. W. (1990). Phospholipase A_2 activation and the auto induction of TNF gene expression by TNF, *Cancer Res.*, *50*: 7101..

Stone, R. M., Sariban, E., Pettit, G. R., and Kufe, D. W. (1988). Bryostatin 1 activates protein kinase C and induces monocytic differentiation of HL-60 cells, *Blood*, *72*: 208.

Streiter, R. M., Remick, D. G., Ward, P. A., Spengler, R. N., Lynch, J. P., III, Larrick, J., and Kunkel, S. L. (1988). Cellular and molecular regulation of tumor necrosis factor-alpha production by pentoxyifylline, *Biochem. Biophys. Res. Commun.*, *155*: 1230.

Strominger, J. L. (1986). Human major histocompatibility complex genes: class I antigens and tumor necrosis factors, *Cold Spring Harbor Symp. Quant. Biol.*, *1*: 63.

Tovey, M. G., Content, J., Gresser, I., Gugenheim, J., Blanchard, B., Guymarho, J., Poupart, P., Gigou, M., Shaw, A., and Fiers, W. (1988). Genes for IFN-beta-2 (IL-6), tumor necrosis factor, and IL-1 are expressed at high levels in the organs of normal individuals, *J. Immunol.*, *141*: 3106.

Wang, A. M., Creasey, A. A., Ladner, M. B., Lin, L. S., Strickler, J., Van, A. J. N., Yamamoto, R., and Mark, D. F. (1985). Molecular cloning of the complementary DNA for human tumor necrosis factor, *Science*, *228*: 149.

Wilson, T., and Treisman, R. (1988). Removal of poly(A) and consequent degradation of c-fos mRNA facilitated by 3′ AU rich sequences, *Nature*, *336*: 396.

2

Genomic Structure, Induction, and Production of TNF-β

REGINA L. TURETSKAYA
Institute of Molecular Biology, USSR Academy of Science, Moscow, USSR; Yale University School of Medicine, New Haven, Connecticut

SARAH J. FASHENA
Yale University, New Haven, Connecticut

NINA L. PAUL and NANCY H. RUDDLE
Yale University School of Medicine, New Haven, Connecticut

1. INTRODUCTION

Tumor necrosis factor β (TNF-β), the first of the TNFs to be described, was discovered almost simultaneously by Ruddle and Waksman (1968c), who called it *cytotoxic factor*, and by Granger and Williams (1968), who called it *lymphotoxin* (LT). The latter name indicated both the cell of the origin and one activity of the material. The factor was produced by lymphocytes and was toxic to syngeneic embryo fibroblasts or L929 cells, and is now known to be a glycoprotein of 25 kDa (Aggarwal et al., 1983, 1985b). The realization that lymphotoxin and tumor necrosis factor are 35% homologous (Li et al., 1987) and share some activities, including killing L929 cells, inducing necrosis of the Meth A sarcoma in vivo (Gray et al., 1984), and activating polymorphonuclear leukocytes (Shalaby et al., 1985), prompted a change in the name of lymphotoxin to TNF-β and tumor necrosis factor to TNF-α. This nomenclature will be used throughout the remainder of this chapter.

TNF-α and TNF-β appear to be members of a duplicated gene family because their genes are tightly linked within the MHC and show similar organization, and the encoded proteins share many biologic activities, including competition for the same cell surface receptor (Aggarwal et al., 1985a). Nevertheless, important differences do exist between TNF-α and TNF-β, both at the level of protein sequence and function and with regard to gene regulation. Functionally, TNF-α appears to be more potent than TNF-β in some assays (Browning and Ribolini, 1989). There are also distinct differences in the mode of secretion, in that TNF-α can either be secreted or displayed as a membrane protein, utilizing its unusually long leader sequence (Kriegler et al., 1988), whereas TNF-β has a more conventional signal peptide and is a secretory protein. There are also similarities and differences in the nature of cells producing TNF-α and TNF-β. TNF-α was originally described as a macrophage product (reviewed in Beutler and Cerami, 1989); TNF-β was originally described as a T-cell product (reviewed in Paul and Ruddle, 1988). In fact, many cells, including primary T cells (Sung et al., 1988), T-cell clones (Sheehan et al., 1989), B-cell lines (Laskov et al., 1990), astrocytes (Lieberman et al., 1989), and lymphokine-activated killer cells (Chambers et al., 1991), can be induced to make both TNF-α and TNF-β. Even in those cases in which the same cell can be induced to make TNF-α and TNF-β, the intracellular signaling pathways may be different. For example, TNF-α is induced from astrocytes by lipopolysaccharide (LPS) and Newcastle disease virus, and TNF-β is induced from those cells only by Newcastle disease virus (Lieberman et al., 1989). Furthermore, in the study of Lieberman et al. (1989), the kinetics of TNF-α and TNF-β mRNA accumulation also differed. Such observations, and the fact that TNF-α is the only TNF made by LPS-activated macrophages and TNF-β is the predominant TNF secreted by human T-cell leukemia virus type I (HTLV-I)-infected T-cell lines (Tschachler et al., 1989; Krönke et al., 1988; Paul et al., 1990) indicates that there are important induction signal-specific and cell-specific differences in the expression of these two proteins.

It is crucial to understand the molecular basis of regulation of TNF-α and TNF-β, because these molecules play important roles in defense and in the pathogenesis of disease. These roles, particularly those of TNF-β, were reviewed by Paul and Ruddle (1988), and an expanded update is included in Chapter 18 of the present volume. Briefly, TNF-β has been implicated as a mediator of cytolytic T-cell (CTL) killing (Ruddle and Schmid, 1987) and defense against virus-infected cells (Aderka et al., 1985), *Chlamydia* infections (Byne and Kreuger, 1985), and tumors (Gray et al., 1984). TNF-β appears to be produced by HIV-infected T cells (Ratner et al., 1987), and it has been suggested that along with TNF-α, it could contribute to the pathogenesis of AIDS (Ruddle, 1986). Its production by HTLV-I-infected T lymphomas implicates it in the hypercalcemia and tropical spastic paraparesis associated with infection by that virus. Our recent demonstration that production of TNF-β by myelin basic protein-specific T-cell clones correlates with their ability to transfer experimental allergic encephalomyelitis (Powell et al., 1990), and that anti-TNF-α/TNF-β monoclonal antibody inhibits transfer of the disease (Ruddle et al., 1990), further implicates TNF-β in the pathogenesis of autoimmune disease. Insight into signals that induce TNF-β production will allow definition of responsive elements in TNF-β expression at the level of gene transcription, mRNA stability, translation, and secretion. This, in turn, may provide insight into the role of TNF-β in health and disease and direct development of treatments to regulate TNF-β expression and activity.

II. INDUCTION OF TNF-β: CELLS AND CONDITIONS

A. TNF-β Production by Normal T Cells and T-Cell Clones

1. Induction of TNF-β from CD4+ T Cells by Antigen in Association with Class II Gene Products

The original description of antigen-specific induction of cytotoxic factors involved an analysis of lymph node cells from rats immunized with tubercle bacilli (Ruddle and Waksman, 1967), ovalbumin, bovine gamma globulin, or haptenated proteins (Ruddle and Waksman, 1968a,b). These studies demonstrated that lymph node cells from immunized rats produce a cytotoxic factor when reexposed in vitro to the original immunizing antigen. They established the antigen specificity of the phenomenon and revealed that the cytotoxic activity was a property of cells involved in "cellular" rather than "humoral" immunity. It is now understood that these cells were probably producing both TNF-α and TNF-β. Later studies with mouse lymphocytes demonstrated that T cells produced TNF-β in response to reexposure to antigen following immunization with soluble proteins in complete Freund's adjuvant (Ruddle, 1978, 1979), and the predominant TNF-β producing cell was identified as an Lyt-1, $CD4^+$ cell (Eardley et al., 1980). The CD4 phenotype and class II restriction of T cells activated by soluble protein antigen was established definitively with murine T-cell clones (Conta et al., 1983, 1985). Once a panel of murine $CD4^+$ T-cell clones had been analyzed, it became apparent that not all clones were alike with regard to the amount of TNF-β that they produced. These differences were noted by Tite et el. (1985), who also established that a T-cell clone's ability to kill target cells was directly correlated with the titer of cytotoxic factors that it produced. These results were extended by Mosmann et al. (1986), who demonstrated that one T-cell subset (TH1) generally produced IL-2, IFN-γ, and TNF-β and TNF-α, whereas the other CD4 subset (TH2) produced IL-4 and little or no TNF-α or β. The definition of these subsets by their functional capabilities as inflammatory (TH1) or regulatory (TH2) T cells has been established by Bottomly and her colleagues (Kim et al., 1985). Although many exceptions to this classification have been noted (Wong et al., 1988), variations in the ability of various cells to produce TNF-β and IL-4 suggest differential regulation of cytokine gene expression in T-cell subsets. Molecular characterization of TNF-β gene regulation will provide interesting information regarding T-cell subset differential gene expression patterns.

2. *Induction of TNF-β from CD8+ T cells in Response to Antigen in Association with Class I Gene Products*

TNF-β is produced by most CD8+ T cells after antigenic stimulation. This has been noted in cells from animals undergoing graft rejection which were exposed to allogeneic antigens or contract sensitizers. Conta et al. (1985) and Schmid et al. (1985) established the molecular requirements for activation of CD8+ cells to produce TNF-β. T-cell clones were established from cells of mice skin-painted with picryl chloride. These CD8+ T cells were class I restricted and TNP-specific in their proliferation, cytokine production, and CTL activity against haptenated target cells. They produced variable amounts of IFN-γ and IL-2 and all produced TNF-β. A wide variety of CD8+ clones that produce both TNF-α and TNF-β after activation with antigen have been described, indicating that this is a common, though not invariant (Jongeneel et al., 1988) characteristic of CD8+ cytotoxic T cells. These observations, those of Tite et al. (1985), and the fact that TNF-β and TNF-α can induce target cell DNA fragmentation (Schmid et al., 1986, 1987; Dealtry et al., 1987), a characteristic of CTL killing, prompted Ruddle and Schmid (1987) to suggest that these cytokines play a pivotal role in cytotoxicity. Unrelated factors such as perforin (Podack et al., 1985) and the serine proteases (Lobe et al., 1986) also contribute to this phenomenon. Other factors that may be related to TNF-β but have not been as thoroughly characterized, such as leukolexin (Liu et al., 1987), have also been suggested as cytotoxic mediators.

3. *Induction of TNF-β by Nonspecific Mitogens and Activation Through the T-Cell Receptor*

There have been many studies describing TNF-β production by T cells activated by nonspecific mitogens, including phytohemagglutinin (PHA), phorbol myristate acetate(PMA), PMA and PHA, or concanavalin A (Con A). Most have been reviewed by Paul and Ruddle (1988). These studies do not clearly establish the signaling structure, but those using PMA do suggest an involvement of protein kinase C. Studies designed to analyze signaling through the T-cell receptor have utilized antibodies to the T-cell receptor isotype or CD3; most have used T-cell clones or T-cell hybridomas. The results shown in Fig. 1 are typical of such studies. They show a dot blot of RNA obtained from three T-cell clones after activation with plate-bound antibodies to the T-cell receptor. They clearly demonstrate that such anti-isotype or anticlonotypic antibodies can induce TNF-β mRNA accumulation. The fact that such antibodies are most effective when presented on a matrix suggests that cross-linking of the T-cell receptor is necessary for activation. These studies are further substantiated by those of Sung et al. (1988) and Thompson et al. (1989), which indicate that antibodies to CD3 are most effective in activation of TNF-β when bound to plates, on other cells, or when added together with an antibody to another T-cell surface molecule, such as CD28.

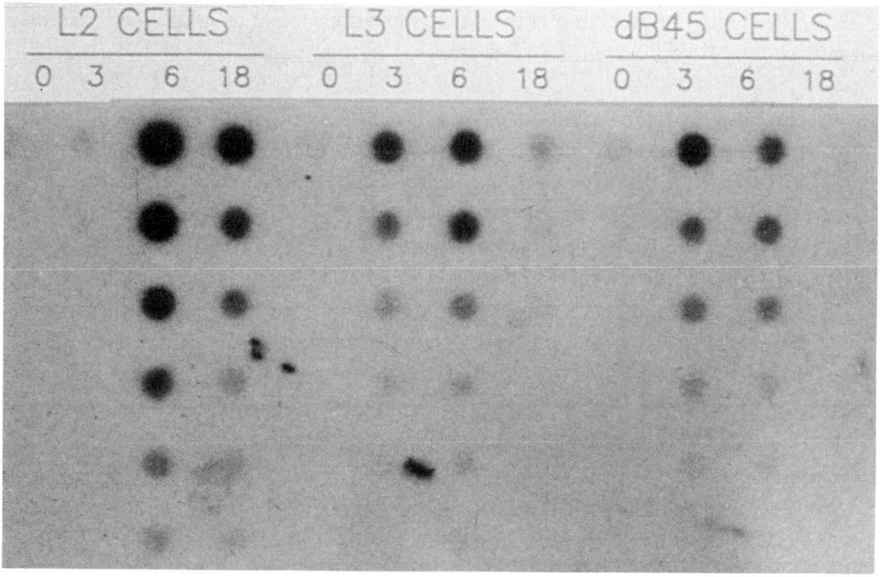

Figure 1 Production of TNF-β mRNA by cloned T cells stimulated with immobilized anticlonotypic mAb 384.5 or antiisotypic mAb F23.1 ThL2 cells and CTL dB45 cells were stimulated with mAb 384.5 for the indicated times after which the cells were harvested and their RNA spotted in twofold dilutions. Dot blots were performed with the TNF-β cDNA probe. (This experiment was performed by K. McGrath, K. C. Herold, D. M. Lancki, F. Fitch, and N. H. Ruddle.)

B. TNF-β Production by T Lymphomas

Transformed human T-cell lines are valuable reagents for the analysis of TNF-β production. Human T-cell lines can be roughly divided into three classes: those that constitutively produce high levels of TNF-β protein, those that can be induced to produce high levels of TNF-β, and those that do not produce TNF-β protein. The cell lines that constitutively produce high levels of TNF-β are HTLV-I infected. We and others have shown that HTLV-I-infected T cells produce high levels of TNF-β mRNA and protein (Hinuma et al., 1985; Kobayashi et al., 1984; Ratner et al., 1987; Krönke et al., 1988; Tschachler et al., 1989; Paul et al., 1990). The constitutive production of TNF-β mRNA in a T-cell clone after HTLV-I infection (Tschachler et al., 1989) suggests a direct role of that virus in TNF-β induction. The production of TNF-β mRNA and protein in the C-81-66a cell line, which expresses some but not all HTLV-I proteins (Tschachler et al., 1989; Paul et al., 1990), indicates that the entire replicating HTLV-I virus is not necessary to activate TNF-β production. TNF-β production by HTLV-I-infected cell lines implicates a role for

TNF-β in HTLV-I-associated clinical manifestations, such as adult T-cell leukemia-associated hypercalcemia and tropical spastic paraparesis-associated demyelination.

Noninfected human T lymphomas can also produce TNF-β. The phorbol ester PMA is commonly used to increase TNF-β mRNA and protein production in T-cell lines (Krönke et al., 1988; Sung et al., 1988). The HUT-78 cell line constitutively produces low levels of TNF-β mRNA and protein that increase after PMA stimulation (Krönke et al., 1988; Steffen et al., 1988). We have activated TNF-β production in the H9 subline of HUT-78 by using the T-cell mitogen PHA (Paul et al., 1990). Mitogen and phorbol ester were both required for maximal production of TNF-β from a TNF-β-producing hybridoma II-23 (Ware et al., 1986). Anti-CD3 (coupled to Sepharose) stimulation of the T-cell receptor complex also induced TNF-β production from this hybridoma, albeit to lower levels. We have found that anti-CD3 (adhered to a plastic dish) stimulates the production of high levels of TNF-β by H9 cells (Paul et al., 1990).

A third type of human T-cell line includes Jurkat and CEM cells. These cells can be stimulated with phorbol ester or antibody to CD3 to produce IL-2 but do not produce detectable TNF-β protein. However, they may produce increased levels of TNF-β mRNA after PMA stimulation (Sung et al., 1988).

In contrast with human T lymphomas, there have been very few reports of TNF-β production from murine T lymphomas, despite the fact that several T-cell clones can be induced to produce high levels. One murine hybridoma, 24/G1, does produce both TNF-α and TNF-β RNA and protein, but the levels are low compared to those obtained with clones (Sheehan et al., 1989). Other frequently studied murine T lymphomas such as EL-4, BW 5147, and YAC-1 cannot be induced to produce TNF-β or TNF-α (Sheehan et al., 1989; Fashena et al., 1990).

C. TNF-β Production by Normal B Cells

TNF-β production was originally considered an exclusive property of activated T cells. However, several investigators have determined that some B cells produce TNF-β mRNA and protein. Bersani and co-workers (1987) showed that normal human tonsillar B lymphoblasts stimulated with *Staphylococcus aureus* Cowan I (SAC) for 72 h and purified by positive selection for the B-cell surface marker B1 produce cytotoxic activity, measured as lysis of actinomycin D- treated WEHI 164 sarcoma cells. This cell line is routinely used to evaluate levels of TNF-β- and TNF-α-mediated killing, although, like L929, it does not distinguish between the two cytokines. Sung et al. (1989) examined the production of TNF-β by primary human purified tonsillar B cells activated by a variety of agents, including PMA, SAC, B-cell growth factor, or anti-μ antibodies, alone and in combination. They concluded that tonsillar B cells require two concurrent activation signals, one supplied by PMA and the other provided by either SAC or anti-μ to induce maximum

TNF-β mRNA accumulation. They also demonstrated that the supernatants from activated tonsillar B cells contain TNF-β cytotoxic activity that is largely neutralized by TNF-β-specific antibodies. These data clearly establish that human B cells can be activated to produce TNF-β. Thus far there have been no reports of antigen-specific induction of TNF-β from human or murine B cells under conditions similar to the antigen-specific induction of TNF-β from T cells. There has been one suggestion by Welsh et al. (1986) that virus-specific killer B cells may use TNF-β as an effector molecule.

D. TNF-β Production by Human B Lymphomas

Many Epstein-Barr virus (EBV)–infected human B-cell lines make TNF-β and related molecules. The human B cell line RPM1-1788 was the source of material for the original sequencing of TNF-β. It secretes TNF-β constitutively and can be induced 10- to 20-fold upon PMA induction (Aggarwal et al., 1983, 1985b). Bersani et al. (1987) demonstrated that a constitutive cytotoxic activity derived from EBV-transformed B-cell lines is inhibited by antibodies specific for TNF-β but unaffected by anti-TNF-α antibodies. In a similar study, Sung et al. (1989) showed that activation with PMA causes an increase in TNF-β mRNA and protein secretion in a variety of EBV-transformed B-cell lines. Cytotoxic factors derived from the supernatants of these activated cell lines are neutralized by anti-TNF-β antibodies. The kinetics of TNF-β mRNA accumulation are different from those of tonsillar B cells induced in a similar manner, in that TNF-β mRNA production peaked at 8 h rather than 48 h. Another study showed that K160b, an EBV-transformed B-lymphoblast lymphoblastoid line produces a cytotoxic lymphokine similar but not identical to either TNF-β or TNF-α (Yamanaka and Karpas, 1989; see below). Several additional studies indicated that EBV-transformed human B-cell lines produce cytotoxic activity before (Rubin et al., 1985) and after (Williamson et al., 1983) PMA induction. This suggests that viral transformation may supply one of the two signals required for B-cell activation, thereby facilitating TNF-β induction.

The role of EBV transformation in activation of TNF-β mRNA and protein production by these B-cell lines is unclear. The virus may indirectly or directly activate the TNF-β gene transcriptionally and/or posttranscriptionally. Alternatively, EBV may preferentially infect a particular lineage of B cells capable of producing TNF-β, or it may infect cells during a developmental stage in which the TNF-β gene is constitutively expressed. TNF-β production by these cells may therefore be a consequence of EBV infection and/or EBV may immortalize a TNF-β expressing B cell and freeze its cellular gene expression patterns. A role for direct viral activation is suggested by the studies cited above implicating HTLV-I induction of TNF-β and those of Wong and Goeddel (1986) in which several viruses could induce TNF-β mRNA from peripheral blood leukocytes.

Some EBV negative B lymphoblastoid lines also produce TNF-β. The human lymphoblastoid B-cell line RPM1-6410t and its subclones constitutively secrete factors that kill L929 cells and provide autocrine growth factor activity. Upon activation, the cells are induced to increase TNF-β transcript and protein levels. These cells also accumulate TNF-α mRNA but do not secrete TNF-α. The growth-promoting and cytotoxic effects of cell supernatants are neutralized by anti-TNF-β but not anti-TNF-α antibodies, thereby demonstrating that the factor is TNF-β (Seregina et al., 1989). Additionally, a tumor cell line established directly from a patient with myeloma spontaneously produces TNF-β mRNA and cytotoxic and osteoclast activating activity (Garrett et al., 1987). Anti-TNF-β antibodies inhibited the cytotoxic activity and most of the in vitro bone resorbing activity observed in supernatants derived from this line. This study suggests that TNF-β, which is also an osteoclast-activating factor (Bertolini et al., 1986), may play a role in osteolytic bone lesions and hypercalcemia associated with multiple myeloma.

E. TNF-β Production by Murine B Lymphomas

Some transformed murine B cells also produce TNF-β. Laskov et al. (1990) reported that TNF-β is produced by murine tumor cells of the B-cell lineage. Their data suggest that TNF-β expression varies during B-cell development in that it is expressed early and is repressed as B cells mature. They base their hypothesis on the finding that three Abelson virus transformed pre-B-cell lines (PD, 2M-3, and L12) and three B-cell lymphomas (M12, X16, and L10A) constitutively produce cytotoxic activity that is neutralized by anti-TNF antibodies that neutralize TNF-α and TNF-β. TNF activity from these cells is not further induced by PMA or LPS. They also analyze TNF expression by Northern analysis of RNA derived from the B cell lines. The data show that TNF-α and TNF-β mRNAs are present in the three Abelson transformed pre-B-cell lines (PD, 2M-3, and L12) and in one Abelson virus negative lymphoma (M12). TNF-β seems to be under more stringent regulation, as its mRNA is absent in some B-cell lymphomas in which TNF-α mRNA is found. The B cell myelomas 4T00.1 and P3X63Ag8.653 are negative for cytotoxic activity and TNF-β and TNF-α mRNA.

We have extended the studies of Laskov et al. (1990) to include additional murine pre-B-cell lines. The pre-B-cell hybridoma (15-79-2) and five Abelson virus transformed pre-B-cell lines (PD31, 1-8, 38B9, 22D6P) and ABE 8.1/2 were examined for TNF-β mRNA expression. Two of the Abelson virus positive lines (38B9 and 22D6P) were negative for TNF-β mRNA (S. Fashena and N. Ruddle, in preparation). These results indicate that Abelson virus transformation alone is not sufficient for TNF-β mRNA expression, although this phenomenon may be due in part to varying *abl* oncogene expression levels in the different lines. The pre-B hybridoma 15-79-2, which is the product of a fusion between fetal liver cells and the myeloma P3X63.Ag8, was negative for TNF-β mRNA. The repression of

TNF-β mRNA may have been mediated by a trans-acting negative regulatory protein contributed by the myeloma component of the hybridoma. TNF-β expression in the pre-B Abelson transformed cells may be a function in part of virus infection as noted above (Wong and Goeddel, 1986) and/or developmental stage. These questions are similar to those raised in the case of EBV transformed cells. Careful analysis of the contribution of individual viral gene products, cellular activation signals, and TNF-β gene responsive elements will provide the answers to these queries.

In summary, TNF-β mRNA and protein can be produced by a variety of normal and malignant human and murine B cells. Determination of the physiological role of TNF-β production by B cells will be an important avenue of research. TNF-β is known to act as a costimulator of growth of normal B cells (Kashiwa et al., 1987; Kehrl et al., 1987). TNF-β also functions as an autocrine growth factor for malignant B cells (Seregina et al., 1989) and aberrantly high levels of TNF-β production observed in transformed B-cell lines may be associated with immunopathology. Alternatively, TNF-β expression could play an important role in B-cell development through its pleiotropic effects as both a growth and cytotoxic factor. B-cell-derived TNF-β production could account for cytotoxic activity in certain microenvironments that are enriched for B cells. It could contribute to apoptotic suicide by developing B cells and thus play a role in the elimination of autoreactive cells or B cells with nonproductive immunoglobulin gene rearrangements.

III. TNF-β GENE ORGANIZATION AND REGULATION

A. TNF-β Genomic Structure

TNF-β is encoded by a single gene in human (Goeddel et al., 1986; Nedospasov et al., 1985, 1986b), murine (Nedospasov et al., 1986a; Ruddle et al., 1987), bovine (Goeddel et al., 1986) and rabbit (Nedospasov et al., 1988; Shakhov et al., 1990b) genomes. Both the TNF-β and TNF-α genes are approximately 3 kbp in size and are split by three introns (Fig. 2) (Goeddel et al., 1986; Gray et al., 1987, Shakhov et al., 1990b). In all species analyzed, the TNF-β and TNF-α genes are tightly linked in a tandem array. The TNF-β gene is always 5′ to the TNF-α gene and the genes are transcribed in the same direction (Fig. 2). The TNF-α and TNF-β proteins are approximately 35% homologous in human and mouse (Gray et al., 1984; Li et al., 1987) with the greatest homology in the carboxyl-terminal amino acids. This is due to the highly (56%) homologous fourth exons which encode the carboxyl-terminal amino acids. Similarities in gene organization, linkage relationships, and their common biological properties suggest that the TNF-α and TNF-β genes are evolutionarily related and probably are the result of gene duplication. Divergence of the genes has resulted in sequence changes and in differential regulation.

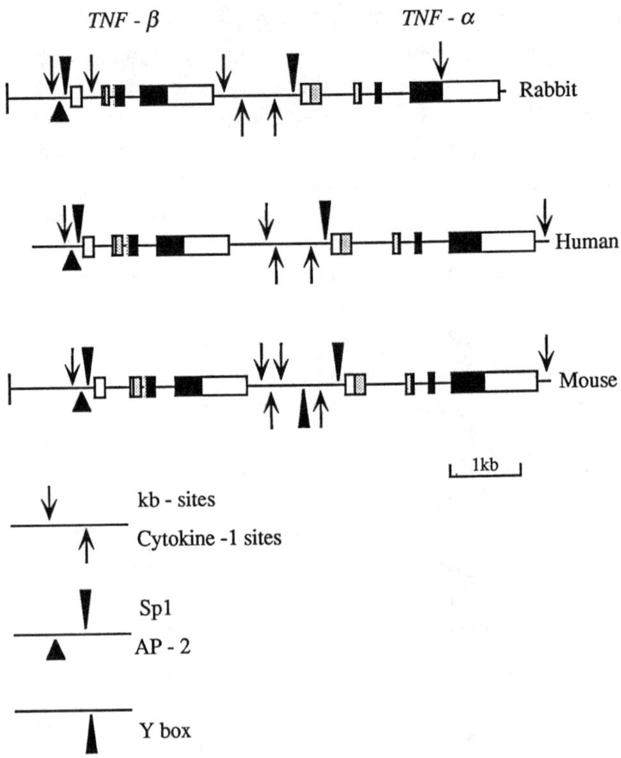

Figure 2 Schematic comparison of the TNF loci of rabbit, human, and mouse with putative transcriptional elements. (Alignment courtesy of Dmitry Kuprash.)

The complete nucleotide sequences of the TNF-β locus of human, murine, and rabbit genomes have been determined (Nedospasov et al., 1986a;b; Semon et al., 1987, Gray et al., 1987; Gardner et al., 1987; Ito et al., 1986; Shakhov et al., 1990b). A comparison of the gene sequences and organization in Fig. 2 depicts conserved exon structure and provides information regarding putative regulatory elements. The gene organization and the identification of coding regions were derived from the original sequencing of the human TNF-β protein (Aggarwal et al., 1985b) and the cloning of the human (Gray et al., 1984) and murine (Li et al., 1987) TNF-β cDNAs.

B. TNF-β Gene Regulatory Elements

Upon alignment of the human, rabbit, and mouse TNF-β genes, extensive similarities are seen. The most complete homology among the three species in the 5′ region is in the 300 bases upstream of the putative transcription initiation sites (Shakhov et al., 1990a,b; Fashena et al., 1990; Paul et al., 1990). Our laboratory has carried out primer extension and RNase protection analysis of murine TNF-β mRNA derived from anti-CD3-activated T-cell clones and PD and PD31 pre-B cells and identified two functional cap sites within 15 bases of each other (Fashena et al., 1990). The numbering of the sequences used throughout the remainder of this chapter is based on the predominantly used CAGG cap site (Fig. 3). In the three species analyzed, within 110 bp upstream of theTATA box are an consensus site transcription factor SP1 and a near consensus site for AP-2.

κB enhancers have also been detected in the upstream regions of several cytokine and cytokine receptor genes (for a review, see Lenardo and Baltimore, 1989) and have been implicated in the transcriptional activation of many of these genes. We have identified several NF-κB-like sites in the TNF-β genes of human, mouse, and rabbit. The human upstream NF-κB-like sequence, which is identical to the murine sequence, forms a complex after incubation with nuclear extracts from a variety of cells (PHA/PMA-activated Jurkat, C81-66-45, MT-2) which are known to contain active NF-κB (Paul et al., 1990). This site has also been determined to be a functional element in TNF-β gene transcription (Paul et al., 1990; see below). The upstream NF-κB site by itself is not responsible for the tissue-specific induction of TNF-β expression. Additional enhancer sequences are being identified in other regions of the TNF-β and neighboring TNF-α genes. It is possible that these other enhancer sequences cooperate with the already identified 5′ NF-κB site to provide inducible activation of the TNF-β gene. An additional κB sequence is located 3′ to the TNF-β gene in all species analyzed (Fig. 2). This sequence, which is upstream of the TNF-α gene, binds weakly to NF-κB protein (Collart et al., 1990). It does not appear to be a crucial element in LPS induction of TNF-α production (Shakhov et al., 1990a). Its activity as a transcriptional enhancer of the TNF-β gene has not been experimentally considered at this time, nor has that of an additional κB sequence in rabbit intron 1. This sequence is not seen in murine or human TNF-β genes. There is no information available on rabbit TNF-β expressions. Additional sequences upstream of the murine TNF-β gene have been identified after comparison of the 5′ flanking regions of the genes coding for several cytokines and cytokine receptor. It is of interest that there are similarities among these TNF-β 5′ sequences and some of the other genes that are also expressed by the TH1 cell subset, perhaps reflecting common sites for DNA binding factors and the possibility of coordinate regulation. A region of homology (22 of 25 bp) is shared by the TNF-β and IL-2 receptor upstream sequences. A short TNF-β sequence is present in IL-2 and IFN-γ 5′ flanking regions (9 and 7 bp, respectively).

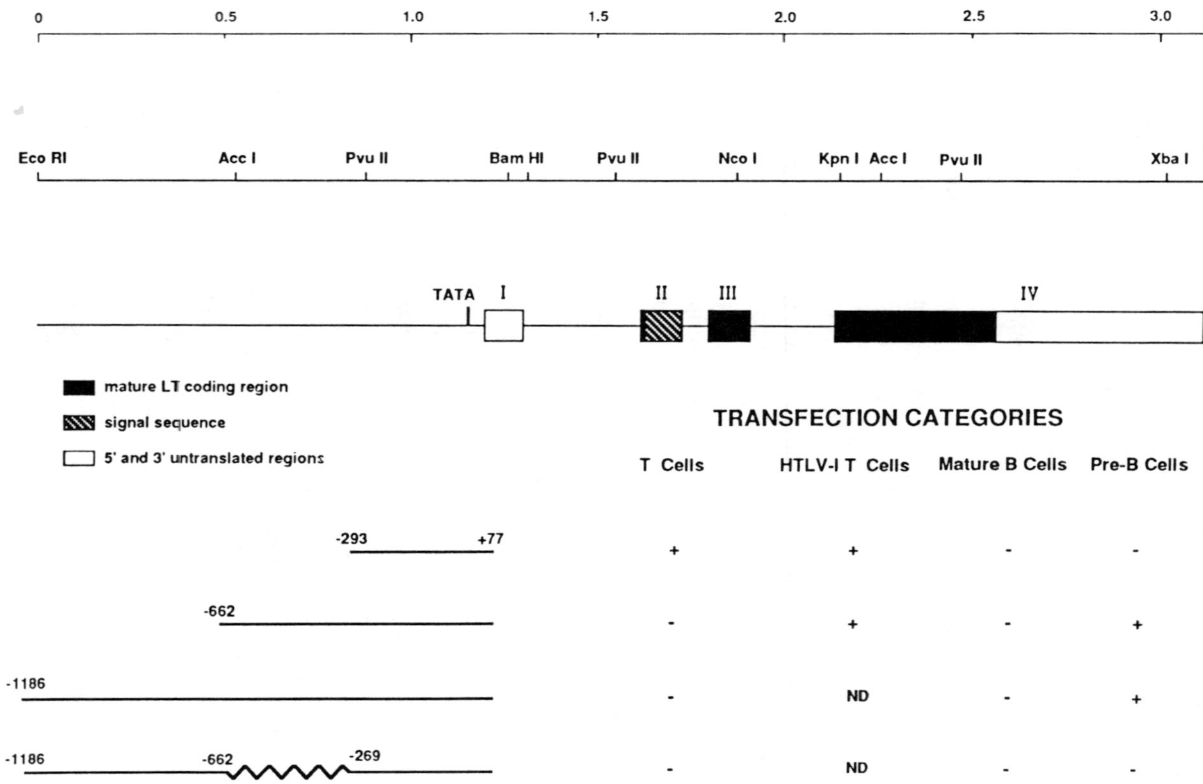

Figure 3 Murine TNF-β gene and its regulatory elements defined by transfection analysis. T cells include EL-4, YAC-1, and H9; HTLV-I T cells include MT-2; mature B cells include A20 and P3 × 63 · .Ag.8; pre-B cells include PD and PD31 cells. [Data are summarized from Fashena et al. (1990), Paul et al. (1990), and Fashena and Ruddle (in preparation).]

In addition, a 7 bp sequence was found in the TNF-β, IFN-γ, IL-3, GM-CSF, and IL-2 receptor genes (Gardner et al., 1987). Additional sequences found in the upstream region of the TNF-β gene include a 178 bp segment (-762 to-584) that is 93% homologous to the mouse B1 (Alu-like) repeat. One perfect and two nearly perfect matches to the heat-shock consensus sequence (C--GAA--TTC--G) (Pelham, 1985; Bienz, 1985) were also found in the TNF-β 5′ flanking regions (Fashena et al., 1990).

C. Functional TNF-β Regulatory Elements Identified by Transfection Studies

As noted above, we have identified by RNase protection and primer extension the predominantly used cap sites that are components of the endogenous TNF-β gene promoter in activated T-cell clones and murine PD and PD31 pre-B cells. To isolate and analyze the role of 5′ regulatory elements in TNF-β, a nested series of 5′ deletion mutants were linked to the bacterial gene-encoding chloramphenicol acetyl transferase (CAT) using the vector system of Gorman et al. (1982). These constructs depicted in Fig. 3 were transfected into a variety of cells and analyzed to determine the ability of the inserted 5′ fragments to drive CAT expression (Fashena et al., 1990).

The smallest fragment (-293 to +77 in relation to the cap site) exhibits promoter activity, which drives CAT expression in transfected murine fibroblasts, the murine T lymphomas EL-4 and YAC-1, and the human T-cell lymphomas MT-2 and H9. This fragment includes the TATA box, cap site, an inverted Sp1 binding site, a putative AP-2 site, and the 5′-κB-like consensus sequence noted above. Larger 5′ fragments (-662 to +77), (-1186 to +77), and [-1186 to +77 (Δ-662/-269)], which include additional 5′ sequences, exhibit no promoter activity in transfected murine fibroblasts and human and murine T cells. These data, summarized in Fig. 3, suggest that at least one upstream negative regulatory element (NRE) exists that can inhibit TNF-β promoter activity. It is not possible to overcome the negative regulation of the larger constructs in these transfection systems by cellular activation. However, this negative regulation is overcome in MT-2, an HTLV-I-infected cell line that makes high levels of TNF-β constitutively (Paul et al., 1990). It was concluded that the mechanism inhibiting the expression of the endogenous TNF-β gene in many cells may be similar to that which suppresses the CAT gene under the control of 5′ regulatory sequences. We predict from our data that these NREs may prevent endogenous TNF-β expression prior to activation signals, thereby controlling the expression of this potent biological modifier. TNF-β production in some cell systems may therefore, be the result of derepression rather than activation. NREs have been demonstrated to control the expression of a variety of other eukaryotic genes, including the human cytokine

IFN-α and IFN-β genes (Goodbourn et al., 1986; Boss and Strominger, 1986; Zinn and Maniatis, 1986; Kuhl et al., 1987).

The functional promoter fragment and the larger 5′ fragments do not drive CAT expression in transfected mature murine B cells. These data imply that regulatory factors required for TNF-β gene promoter activity are absent and/or that inhibitory proteins are present in these mature B cells. These findings are of particular interest because they indicate that the TNF-β gene promoter can be regulated at several levels. In addition to the control exerted by upstream NREs in some systems, the promoter itself is differentially regulated in other systems.

The TNF-β 5′ deletion mutants were differentially regulated within the context of LT-producing murine pre-B cells. The promoter fragment (−293 to +77) did not function in transfected PD and PD31 cells. Interestingly, the larger fragments (-662 to +77 and -1186 to +77) exhibit significant promoter activity. These data suggest that these larger 5′ fragments contained enhancer elements that were responsive to the pre-B, Abelson infected environment. Deletion of a 393-bp region (-662 to -269) abolished the enhancer activity, implying that the essential elements were located within this region. We are currently investigating this enhancer region in greater detail (S.J. Fashena, R. Reeves, and N.H. Ruddle, submitted).

We have analyzed the function of the 5′ NF-*k*B in TNF-β transcription in transfection experiments by mutating the *k*B site of the smallest functional TNF-β promoter fragment. The basal TNF-β promoter which contains the mutated κB site that inhibits formation of the NF-κB specific complex (see above), is not able to drive CAT activity when transfected into H9 and MT-2 T-cell lines (Paul et al., 1990). These data indicate that this upstream NF-κB site is necessary for TNF-β promoter activity in these particular cell lines.

D. Posttranscriptional Regulation

TNF-β production is regulated posttranscriptionally as well as transcriptionally. Though, in general, in activated T cells the extent of mRNA accumulation correlates with the amount of secreted TNF-β biologic activity, mRNA accumulation may be due to a combination of transcriptional activation and stabilization of TNF-β mRNA. Support for this suggestion comes from nuclear run on assays with activated T-cell clones and lymphomas in our laboratory (T. Sarr, R. L. Turetskaya, and N. H. Ruddle, in preparation) and those of Jongeneel et al. (1989) indicating that the rate of transcription of TNF-β mRNA in T-cell clones after activation is enhanced but remains rather low. This suggests that induction may stabilize mRNA. Many cytokine mRNA transcripts have short half lives that are increased in the presence of cycloheximide. This is true for TNF-β in T as well as pre-B cells (K. McGrath and N. H. Ruddle, unpublished; S. J. Fashena and N. H. Ruddle, in preparation). It has been suggested that a TTATTTAT motif found in the 3′ region of human and murine TNF-β genes and several other cytokine and proto-oncogenes (Caput et al., 1986) confers instability (Shaw and Kamen, 1986).

As mentioned previously, anti-CD3 and anti-CD28 antibodies synergize to activate TNF-β mRNA accumulation (Thompson et al., 1989). It has been demonstrated that anti-CD28 selectively increases the half-life of cytokine mRNAs (Lindsten et al., 1989), suggesting a possible mechanism of TNF-β activation through the CD28 signaling pathway.

An additional mechanism for regulation of cytokine expression exists at the level of translation of accumulated mRNA. Han et al. (1990) have recently demonstrated the importance of this mechanism in LPS induction of TNF-α secretion and have identified elements in the 3′ end of that gene that are responsible for the enhanced translatability of such mRNA after activation. The 3′ region of the TNF-β gene has not yet been analyzed in this regard. Additional posttranslational modifications such as glycosylation may also contribute to TNF-β regulation.

E. Summary of Regulation As It Relates to Induction

In Section II we summarized conditions that result in activation of TNF-β production. These include activation through the T-cell receptor through T-cell accessory molecules such as CD3 or CD28, by EBV or HTLV-I infection, by B-cell-specific signals, and in pre-B and B lymphomas. In this section we investigate elements of the gene that may respond to such signals. We have identified the transcription initiation site in T cells and pre-B cells. The 5′ NF-κB is identified as an HTLV-I-responsive element. An element that functions as an NRE for T cells has been identified, as has a positive regulatory element for pre-B cells. Posttranscriptional regulation is suggested by properties of the mRNA; it is likely that this mechanism plays a role in anti-CD28 activation and may be a property of the 3′ untranslated region of the gene. Those sequences on the TNF-β gene that are responsive to stimulation through the T cell receptor have not been identified. They await additional analysis of intronic sequences and transfections in antigen specific T-cell clones.

IV. CHROMOSOMAL POSITION OF THE TNF-β GENE AND ITS RELATIONSHIP TO THE MHC

The genes encoding TNF-α and TNF-β are tightly linked to each other, separated by approximately 1 kb and located on murine chromosome 17 (Nedospasov et al., 1986a, Ruddle et al., 1987; Gardner et al., 1987) and human chromosome 6 (Nedwin et al., 1985a,b). The TNF gene complex is tightly linked to the MHC in both species (Spies et al., 1986; Carroll et al., 1987; Müller et al., 1987) and is in fact located within it. The TNF genes are centromeric to murine H-2-D and human HLA-B between the class I and class III gene clusters. The distance between the

TNF locus and H-2-D cluster in mice is 70 kb; the distance to HLA-B in humans is 220 kb (Müller et al., 1987; Carroll et al., 1987). In both cases the TNF genes and class I genes are transcribed in opposite directions. A 435 kb human MHC region has been characterized that includes the genes encoding TNF-β, TNF-α, a series of HLA-B-associated transcripts (BAT) (Spies et al., 1989a), and a heat shock protein (Spies et al., 1989b).

Population studies suggest that some HLA-B and DR alleles are associated with certain types of heritable immune disorders, although the role of MHC antigens in these autoimmune diseases in unclear. It has been suggested that MHC genes could be markers for closely linked genes, rather than causative genes (Jacob et al., 1990; Spies et al., 1989a). It is possible that the MHC linkage of some diseases is a reflection of the activity of the TNF genes. Evidence for this possibility is provided by a correlation in the levels of TNF-α production with certain H-2 haplotypes (Jacob and McDevitt, 1988) and in their association with an autoimmune phenotype. Two alleles of the human TNF-β gene have been described (Partanen and Koskimies, 1988), and one is associated with diabetes (Pociot et al., 1990).

Polymorphism in the structure of TNF-α and TNF-β genes at the level of restriction fragment length polymorphism has also been reported (Müller et al., 1987; Gardner et al., 1987; Jacob and McDevitt, 1988; Richter et al., 1989). Recently, a polymorphic microsatellite sequence between the mouse TNF-β and TNF-α genes has been described which is unique to NZW mice. The MHC allele of this locus correlates with development of lupus-like glomerulonephritis and might serve as a convenient marker for TNF polymorphism (Jongeneel et al., 1990). This particular microsatellite is absent from the homologous position in human and rabbit genes (Nedospasov et al., 1986b; Shakhov et al., 1990b). A complex polymorphic sequence has been detected in the human gene 4 kb upstream of the TNF-β gene (Nedospasov, Udalova, Kuprash, Turetskaya, submitted) in a region where structural differences between the two alleles were previously noted (Nedospasov et al., 1986b). Analysis of polymorphism at this locus may provide new insight into the role of TNF-α and TNF-β genes in hereditary immune diseases.

V. PROTEIN PRODUCTS OF THE TNF-β GENE

A predominant species of TNF-β, a 25 kDa glycoprotein, and a smaller 20 kDA species were derived from a human B lymphoblastoid cell line RPM1 1788 (Aggarwal et al., 1983, 1985b; Gray et al., 1984). The smaller of the two TNF-β species lacks the 23 amino-terminal residues. Despite the amino-terminal differences, both forms are cytotoxic for L929 cells. Recombinant human and murine TNF-β kill L929 cells, indicating that glycosylation is not necessary for cytotoxic activity. Recombinant human and murine TNF-β translated in vitro are usually detected in

```
                                                                            1
HUMAN      -34 M T P P E R L F L P R V C G T T L H L L L L G L L L V L L - P G A Q G L P G V G L T P S A A Q T A R Q
BOVINE     -33 M T P P G R L Y L L R V C S T P P - L L L L G L L L A L P - L E A Q G L R G I G L T P S A A Q P A H Q
RABBIT     -26 M T P P G R L Y L P - - - - - - - - - L L L G L L L A P P P P G A Q G L P G A E F P P S A A R N A Q Q
MURINE     -33 M T L L G R L H L L R V L G T P P V F - L L G L L L A L P - L G A Q G L S G V R F - - S A A R T A H P
CONSENSUS      M T       R L   L           T           L L G L L L             A Q G L   G           S A A     A

HUMAN       17 H P K M H L A H S T L K P A A H L I G D P S K Q N S L L W R A N T D R A F L Q D G F S L S N N S L L
BOVINE      17 Q L P T P F T R G T L K P A A H L V G D P S T Q D S L R W R A N T D R A F L R H G F S L S N N S L L
RABBIT      17 R L Q K H F G H S T L K P A A H L V G D P S A Q D S L R W R A N T D R A F L R H G F S L S N N S L L
MURINE      15 L P Q K H L T H G I L K P A A H L V G Y P S K Q N S L L W R A S T D R A F L Q D G F S L S N N S L L
CONSENSUS                          L K P A A H L   G   P S   Q   S L   W R A   T D R A F L     G F S L S N N S L L

HUMAN       67 V P T S G I Y F V Y S Q V V F S G K A Y S P K A T S S P L Y L A H E V Q L F S S Q Y P F H V P L L S
BOVINE      67 V P T S G L Y F V Y S Q V V F S G R G C F P R A T P T P L Y L A H E V Q L F S P Q Y P F H V P L L S
RABBIT      67 V P S S G L Y F V Y S Q V V F S G E G C S P K A V P T P L Y L A H E V Q L F S S Q Y S F H V P L L S
MURINE      65 I P T S G L Y F V Y S Q V V F S G E S C S P R A I P T P I Y L A H E V Q L F S S Q Y P F H V P L L S
CONSENSUS        P   S G   Y F V Y S Q V V F S G         P   A       P   Y L A H E V Q L F S   Q Y   F H V P L L S

HUMAN      117 S Q K M V Y P G L Q E P W L H S M Y H G A A F Q L T Q G D Q L S T H T D G I P H L V L S P S T V F F
BOVINE     117 A Q K S V C P G P Q G P W V R S V Y Q G A V F L L T R G D Q L S T H T D G I S H L L L S P S S V F F
RABBIT     117 A Q K S V C P G P Q G P W V R S V Y Q G A V F L L T Q G D Q L S T H T D G I A H L L L S P S S V F F
MURINE     115 A Q K S V Y P G L Q G P W V R S M Y Q G A V F L L S K G D Q L S T H T D G I S H L H F S P S S V F F
CONSENSUS        Q K   V   P G   Q   P W     S   Y   G A   F   L     G D Q L S T H T D G I   H L     S P S   V F F

HUMAN      167 G A F A L 171
BOVINE     167 G A F A L 171
RABBIT     167 G A F A L 171
MURINE     165 G A F A L 169
CONSENSUS      G A F A L
```

Figure 4 Comparative amino acid sequence of of human, bovine, rabbit, and mouse TNF-*β*s. [A summary of data obtained from Goeddel et al. (1986), Ito et al. (1986), Li et al. (1987), and Shakhov et al. (1990b).]

Western blots as two bands of 18 and 34 kDa (Li et al., 1987); the high-molecular-weight species is presumably an oligomeric form of the protein.

On the basis of the sequence derived from human TNF-*β* protein and human and murine TNF-*β* cDNA cloning, the coding sequence of the genes and the putative amino acid sequence of the proteins have been identified. The rabbit and bovine protein sequences are derived from genomic clones and still must be confirmed by direct analysis. TNF-*β* protein are highly conserved among mammalian species (Fig. 4) (Goeddel et al., 1986; Gray et al., 1984; Li et al., 1987; Ito et al., 1986; Shakhov et al., 1990b). The cDNAs code for polypeptides of 205 amino acids (human), 204 amino acids (cow), 197 amino acids (rabbit), and 202 amino acids (mouse). There is some divergence in the length and sequences in the N-terminal signal of 34 residues (human), 33 residues (cow and mouse), or 26 residues (rabbit).

As noted above, the first 23 amino acids do not appear to be essential for function, and this region is not particularly conserved among the four species. However, the remainder of the molecule is quite similar with 106 of 148 amino acids (72%) identical in all four species. As indicated in Fig. 4, when one considers residues that are identical in three of the four species, rather than all four, the homology is even more striking. One interesting difference is the presence of a cysteine residue conserved in mouse (residue 84), cow (residue 86), and rabbit (residue 86), which is a tyrosine in human. This cysteine is also conserved between murine TNF-β and TNF-α (Li et al., 1987). A second cysteine that is found only in TNF-α may facilitate intra-and intermolecular disulfide bonding.

It is possible that additional high molecular weight forms of TNF-β exist, and there are several reports of cytotoxic proteins with unusual neutralization properties. As noted above, Yamanaka and Karpas (1989) described a cytotoxic protein secreted by a human lymphoblastoid line K160b which has an N-terminal amino acid sequence identical to that of human TNF-β. Its cytotoxic activity, however, is not neutralized by antibodies raised against recombinant TNF-β. Green et al. (1985) also described heterogeneous cytotoxic lymphokines that were only partially neutralized by antibodies to TNF-β. Yamamoto et al. (1986) described a high molecular weight cytotoxic factor produced by human lymphoid cells that was only partially neutralized by antibodies to TNF-β. Complete neutralization was achieved by a mixture of antibodies to TNF-α and TNF-β. Liu et al. (1987) also described a high-molecular-weight factor produced by T lymphocytes termed leukalexin which was antigenically related to TNF-β and TNF-α. Although Northern blot analysis with TNF-α and TNF-β probes did not reveal specific TNF mRNAs, the possibility remains that this cytotoxin is encoded by the TNF locus.

There are several nonmutually exclusive explanations for the novel forms of TNF-β that have been described. It is likely that TNF-β forms oligomers and that such multimeric forms are less easily neutralized by antibodies. Many of the samples undoubtedly contain TNF-α, and simultaneous addition of both anti-TNF-β and anti-TNF-α antibodies might achieve neutralization. TNF-β/TNF-α oligomers may also exist. Unusual posttranslational modifications of TNF-β might occur in some cells resulting in changes in antigenicity, or alternatively spliced forms of TNF-β mRNA might give rise to different carboxyl-termini.

The TNF-α and TNF-β genes are very tightly linked and high molecular weight mRNAs have been seen that hybridize with both TNF-β and TNF-α cDNAs (Ruddle et al., 1990). These data suggest that transcripts arise that result from transcriptional read-through of the entire locus and subsequent alternative splicing. Even more intriguing is the discovery of a short open reading frame in the 3′ untranslated region of the fourth exon of the human, mouse, and rabbit TNF-β genes

```
Human     CCC TCG ATG AAG CCC AAT AAA CCT CTT TTC TCT GAA ATG CTG TCT GCT
          Pro Ser Met Lys Pro Asn Lys Pro Leu Phe Ser Glu Met Leu Ser Ala

           *   *       *                               *
Mouse     CCA TCT GTG AAA CCC AAT AAA CCT CTT TTC TCT GAG ATT CTG TCT GCT
          Pro Ser Val Lys Pro Asn Lys Pro Leu Phe Ser GLu Ile Leu Ser Ala

           *   *       *                               *
Rabbit    CCC TCA GTG AAG CCC AAT AAA CCT CTT TTC TCT GAA GTG CTG TCT GCT
          Pro Ser Val Lys Pro Asn Lys Pro Leu Phe Ser Glu Val Leu Ser Ala
```

Figure 5 Putative additional carboxyl-terminal amino acid residues of TNF-β derived from the exon 4, 3′ untranslated region. (Data from Shakhov et al., 1990b.)

(Shakhov et al., 1990b). The potential 16-residue peptide encoded by this sequence is conserved among the three species analyzed (Fig. 5; Shakhov et al., 1990b). It is possible that TNF-β mRNA could be alternatively spliced to give rise to this form.

ACKNOWLEDGMENTS

This work was supported by NIH CA-16885, CA-47878 T32 AI-07019, and a fellowship from the International Union Against Cancer (RLT). We thank Dr. Sergei Nedospasov for his interest, comments, and prepublication results and Dmitry Kuprash for schematic alignments of TNF loci. We are grateful to Frances Larvey for expert manuscript preparation.

REFERENCES

Aderka, D., Novick, D., Hahn, T., Fischer, D. G., and Wallach, D. (1985). Increase of vulnerability to lymphotoxin in cells infected by vesicular stomatitis virus and its further augmentation by interferon, *Cell. Immunol.*, *92*: 918.

Aggarwal, B. B., Moffat, B., and Harkins, R. N. (1983). Purification and characterization of lymphotoxin from human lymphoblastoid cell line 1788, *Interleukins, Lymphokines, and Cytokines* (J. J. Oppenheim and S. Cohen, eds.), Academic Press, New York, p. 521.

Aggarwal, B. B., Eessalu, T. E., and Hass, P. E. (1985a). Characterization of receptors for human tumor necrosis factor and their regulation by interferon, *Nature*, *318*: 665.

Aggarwal, B. B., Henzel, W. J., Moffat, B., Kohr, W. J., and Harkins, R. N. (1985b). Primary structure of human lymphotoxin derived from 1788 lymphoblastoid cell line, *J. Biol. Chem.*, *260*: 2334.

Bersani, L., Colotta, F., Peri, G., and Mantovani, A. (1987). Cytotoxic effector function of B lymphoblasts, *J. Immunol.*, *139*: 645.

Bertolini, D. R., Nedwin, G. E., Bringman, T. S., Smith, D. D., and Mundy, T. R. (1986). Stimulation of bone resorption and inhibition of bone formation in vitro by human tumor necrosis factor, *Nature*, *319*: 516.

Beutler, B., and Cerami, A. (1989). The biology of cachectin/TNF a primary mediator of the host response, *Annu. Rev. Immunol.*, *7*: 625.

Bienz, M. (1985). Transient and developmental activation of heat-shock genes. *Trends Biochem.*, *10*: 157.

Boss, J. M., and Strominger, J. L. (1986). Regulation of a transfected human class II major histocompatibility complex gene in human fibroblasts, *Proc. Natl. Acad. USA*, *83*: 9139.

Browning, J., and Ribolini, A. (1989). Studies on the differing effects of tumor necrosis factor and lymphotoxin on the growth of several human tumor lines, *J. Immunol.*, *143*: 1859.

Byne, G. I., and Kreuger, D. A. (1985). In vitro expression of factor-mediated cytotoxic activity generated during immune response to Chlamydia in the mouse, *J. Immunol.*, *134*: 4189.

Caput, D., Beutler, B., Hartog, K., Thayer, R., Brown-Shimer, S., and Cerami, A. (1986). Identification of a common nucleotide sequence in the 3′-untranslated region of mRNA molecules specifying inflammatory mediators, *Proc. Natl. Acad. Sci USA*, *83*: 1670.

Carrol, M. C., Katzman, P., Alicot, E. M., Koller, B. H., Geraghty, D. E., Orr, H. T., Strominger, J. L., and Spies, T. (1987). Linkage map of the human major histocompatibility complex including the tumor necrosis factor genes, *Proc. Natl. Acad. Sci. USA*, *84*: 8535.

Chambers, W. H., Vujanovic, N. L., Olszowy, M. W., Ruddle, N. H., Herberman, R. B., and Hiserodt, J. C. (1991). Cytokine production by lymphokine activated killer (LAK) cells. I. Secretion of tumor necrosis factors, in preparation.

Collart, M. A., Baeuerle, P. A., and Vassalli, P. (1990). Regulation of TNF-α transcription in macrophages: involvement of four DNA κB-like motifs and of constitutive and inducible forms of NF-κB, *Mol. Cell. Biol.*, *10*: 1498.

Conta, B. S., Powell, M. B., and Ruddle, N. H. (1983). Production of lymphotoxin, IFN-γ and IFN-α, β by murine T-cell lines and clones, *J. Immunol.*, *130*: 2231.

Conta, B. S., Powell, M. B., and Ruddle, N. H. (1985). Activation of Lyt-1+ and Lyt-2$^+$ T-cell cloned lines: stimulation of proliferation, lymphokine production, and self-destruction, *J. Immunol.*, *134*: 2185

Dealtry, G. B., Naylor, M. S., Fiers, W., and Balkwill, F. R. (1987). DNA fragmentation and cytotoxicity caused by tumor necrosis factor is enhanced by interferon-γ, *Eur. J. Immunol.*, *17*: 689.

Eardley, D. D., Shen, F. W., Gershon, R. K., and Ruddle, N. H. (1980). Lymphotoxin production by subsets of cells, *J. Immunol.*, *124*: 1199.

Fashena, S. J., Tang, W.-L., Sarr, T., and Ruddle, N. H. (1990). The murine lymphotoxin gene promoter: characterization and negative regulation, *J. Immunol.*, *145*: 177.

Gardner, S. M., Mock, B. A., Hilgers, J., Huppi, K. E., and Roeder, W. D. (1987). Mouse lymphotoxin and tumor necrosis factor: structural analysis of the cloned genes, physical linkage, and chromosomal postition, *J. Immunol.*, *139*: 476.

Garrett, I. R., Durie, B. G. M., Nedwin, G. E., Gillespie, A., Bringman, T., Sabatini, M., Bertolini, D. R., and Mundy, G. R. (1987). Production of lymphotoxin, a bone-resorbing cytokine, by cultured human myeloma cells, *N. Engl. J. Med.*, *317*: 526.

Goeddel, D. V., Aggarwal, B. B., Gray, P. W., Leung, D. W., Nedwin, G. E., Palladino, M. A., Patton, J. S., Pennica, D., Shepard, H. M., Sugarman, B. J., and Wong, G. H. W. (1986). Tumor necrosis factor: gene structure and biological activities, *Cold Spring Harbor Symp. Quant. Biol.*, *51*: 597.

Goodbourn, S., Burstein, H., and Maniatis, T. (1986). The human β-interferon gene enhancer is under negative control, *Cell*, *45*: 601.

Gorman, G. M., Moffat, L. F., and Howard, B. F. (1982). Recombinant genomes which express chloramphenicol acetyltransferase in mammalian cells, *Mol. Cell. Biol.*, *2*: 1044.

Granger, G. A., and Williams, T. W. (1968). Lymphocyte cytotoxicity in vitro: activation and release of a cytotoxic factor, *Nature*, *218*: 1253.

Gray, P. W., Aggarwal, B. B., Benton, C. V., Bringman, T. S., Henzel, W. J., Jarrett, J. A., Leung, D. W., Moffat, B., Ng, P., Svedersky, L. P., Palladino, M. A., and Nedwin, G. E. (1984). Cloning and expression of cDNA for human lymphotoxin, a lymphokine with tumor necrosis activity, *Nature*, *312*: 721.

Gray, P. W., Chen , E., Li, C.-B., Tang, W.-L., and Ruddle, N. H. (1987). The murine tumor necrosis factor-beta (lymphotoxin) gene sequence, *Nucleic Acids Res.*, *15*: 3937.

Green, L. M., Stern, M. L., Haviland, D. L., Mills, B. J.,and Ware, C. F. (1985). Cytotoxic lymphokines produced by cloned human cytotoxic T lymphocytes. I. Cytotoxins produced by antigen-specific and natural killer-like CTL are dissimilar to classical lymphotoxins, *J. Immunol.*, *135*: 4034.

Han, J., Brown, T., and Beutler, B. (1990). Endotoxin-responsive sequences control cachectin/tumor necrosis factor biosynthesis at the translational level, *J. Exp. Med.*, *171*: 465.

Hinuma, S., Naruo, K.-I., Tsukamoto, K., Sugamura, K., and Hiuma, Y. (1985). Production of cytotoxic factors in human T-cell lines transformed by a human retrovirus, *Biochem. Biophys. Res. Commun.*, *130*: 1051.

Ito, H., Shiraui, T., Yamamoto, S., Akira, M., Kawahara, S., Todd, C. W., and Wallace, R. B. (1986). Molecular cloning of the gene encoding rabbit tumor necrosis factor, *DNA*, *5*: 157.

Jacob, C. O., and McDevitt, H. O. (1988). Tumor necrosis factor-α in murine autoimmune "lupus" nephritis, *Nature*, *331*: 356.

Jacob, C. O., Fronek, Z., Lewis, G. D., Koo, M., Hansen, J. A., and McDevitt, H. O. (1990). Heritable major histocompatibility complex class II-associated differences in production of tumor necrosis factor α: relevance to genetic predisposition to systemic lupus erythematosus, *Proc. Natl. Acad. Sci. USA*, *87*: 1233.

Jongeneel, C. V., Nedospasov, S. A., Plaetinck, G., Naquet, P., and Cerottini, J. C. (1988). Expression of the tumor necrosis factor locus is not necessary for the cytolytic activity of T lymphocytes, *J. Immunol.*, *140*: 1916.

Jongeneel, C. V., Shakhov, A. N., Nedospasov, S. A., and Cerottini, J.-C. (1989). Molecular control of tissue-specific expression at the mouse TNF locus, *Eur. J. Immunol.*, *19*: 549.

Jongeneel, C. V., Acha-Orbea, H., and Blankenstein, T. (1990). A polymorphic microsatellite in the tumor necrosis factor α promoter identifies an allele unique to the NZW strain, *J. Exp. Med.*, *171*: 2141.

Kashiwa, H., Wright, S. C., and Bonavida, B. (1987). Regulation of B cell maturation and differentiation. I. Suppression of pokeweed mitogen-induced B cell differentiation by tumor necrosis factor (TNF), *J. Immunol.*, *138*: 1383.

Kehrl, J. H., Alvarez-Mon, M., Delsing, G. A., and Fauci, A. S. (1987). Lymphotoxin is an important T-cell-derived growth factor for human B cells, *Science*, *238*: 1144.

Kim, J., Woods, A., Becker-Dubb, E., and Bottomly, K.(1985). Distinct functional phenotypes of cloned Ia-restricted helper T cells, *J. Exp. Med.*, *162*: 188.

Kobayashi, Y., Asado, M., and Osawa, T. (1984). Mechanism of phorbol myristate-acetate-induced lymphotoxin production by a human T-cell hybridoma, *J. Biochem.*, *95*: 1775.

Kriegler, M., Perez, C., DeFay, K., Albert, I., and Lu, S. D. (1988). A novel form of TNF/cachectin is a cell surface cytotoxic transmembrane protein: ramifications for the complex physiology of TNF, *Cell*, *53*: 45.

Krönke, M., Hensel, G., Schluter, C., Scheurich, P., Schutze, S., and Pfizenmaier, K. (1988). Tumor necrosis factor and lymphotoxin gene expression in human tumor cell lines, *Cancer Res.*, *48*: 5417.

Kuhl, D., de la Fuenta, J., Chaturvedi, M., Parimoo, S., Ryals, J., Meyer, F., and Weissmann, C. (1987). Reversible silencing of enhancers by sequences derived from the human IFN-α-promoter, *Cell*, *50*: 1057.

Laskov, R., Lancz, G., Ruddle, N. H., McGrath, K. M., Spector, S., Klein, T., Djeu, J. Y., and Friedman, H. (1990). Production of tumor necrosis factor (TNF-α) and lymphotoxin (TNF-β) by murine pre-B and B-cell lymphomas, *J. Immunol.*, *144*: 3424.

Lenardo, M. J., and Baltimore, D. (1989). NF-κB: a pleiotropic mediator of inducible and tissue-specific gene control, *Cell*, *58*: 227.

Li, C.-B., Gray, P., P.-F., McGrath, K. M., Ruddle, F. H., and Ruddle, N. H. (1987). Cloning and expression of murine lymphotoxin cDNA, *J. Immunol.*, *138*: 4496.

Lieberman, A. P., Pitha, P., Shin, H. S., and Shin, M. L. (1989). Production of tumor necrosis factor and other cytokines by astrocytes stimulated with lipopolysaccharide or a neurotropic virus, *Proc. Natl. Acad. Sci. USA*, *86*: 6348.

Lindsten, T., June, C. H., Ledbetter, J. A., Stella, G., and Thompson. C. P. (1989). Regulation of lymphokine messenger RNA stability by surface-mediated T-cell activation pathway, *Science*, *244*: 339.

Liu, C.-C., Steffen, M., King, F., and Young, J. D.-E. (1987). Identification, isolation, and characterization of a novel cytotoxin in murine cytolytic lymphocytes, *Cell*, *51*: 393.

Lobe, G. C. G., Finley, B. B., Paranchyck, W., Paetkau, V. H., and Bleakley, R. C. (1986). Novel serine proteases encoded by two cytotoxic T lymphocyte-specific genes, *Science*, *232*: 858.

Mosmann, T., Cherwinski, H., Bond, M. W., Giedlin, M. A., and Coffman, R. L. (1986). Two types of murine helper T-cell clone. I. Definition according to profiles of lymphokine activities and secreted proteins, *J. Immunol.*, *136*: 2348.

Müller, U., Jongeneel, C. V., Nedospasov, S. A., Fisher-Lindahl, K., and Steinmetz, M. (1987). Tumor necrosis factor and lymphotoxin genes map close to H-2D in the mouse major histocompatibility complex, *Nature*, *325*: 265.

Nedospasov, S. A., Shakhov, A. N., Turetskaya, R. L., Mett, V. A., Georgiev, G. P., Korobko, V. G. (1985). Molecular cloning of human tumore necrosis factor gene: tandem arrangement of TNF-alpha and TNF-beta genes in short segment of human genome, Dokl. *Acad. Nauk SSSR, 285*: 1487 (in Russian).

Nedospasov, S. A., Hirt, B., Shakhov, A. N., Dobrynin, V. N., Kawashima, E., Accolla, R. S., and Jongeneel, C. V. (1986a). The genes for tumor necrosis factor (TNF-alpha) and lymphotoxin (TNF-beta) are tandemly arranged on chromosome 17 of the mouse, *Nucleic Acids Res.*, *14*: 7713.

Nedospasov, S. A., Shakhov, A. N., Turetskaya, R. L., Mett, V. A., Azizov, M. M., Georgiev, G. P., Korobko, V. G., Dobrynin, V. N., Filippov, S. A., Bystrov, N. S., Boldyreva, E. F., Chuvpilo, S. A., Chumakov, A. M., Shingarova, L. N., and Ovchinnikov, Y. A.

(1986b). Tandem arrangement of genes coding for tumor necrosis factor (TNF-alpha) and lymphotoxin (TNF-beta) in the human genome, *Cold Spring Harbor Symp. Quant. Biol.*, *51*: 611.

Nedospasov, S. A., Turetskaya, R. L., and Shakhov, A. N. (1988). Cloning and characterization of the rabbit lymphotoxin (TNF-beta) gene and its tight linkage to the gene coding for tumor necrosis factor, *Nucleic Acids Res.*, *16*: 3112.

Nedwin, G. E., Jarrett-Nedwin, J., Smith, D. H., Naylor, S. L., Sakaguchi, A. Y., Goeddel, D. V., and Gray, P. W. (1985a). Structure and chromosomal localization of the human lymphotoxin gene, *J. Cell. Biochem.*, *29*: 171.

Nedwin, G. E., Naylor, S. L., Sakaguchi, A. Y., Smith, D. H., Jarrett-Nedwin, J., Pennica, D., Goeddel, D. V., and Gray, P. W. (1985b). Human lymphotoxin and tumor necrosis factor genes: structure, homology and chromosomal localization, *Nucleic Acids Res.*, *13*: 6361.

Partanen, J., and Koskimies, S. (1988). Low degree DNA polymorphism in the HLA-linked lymphotoxin (tumor necrosis factor β) gene, *Scand. J. Immunol.*, *28*: 313.

Paul, N., and Ruddle, N. H. (1988). Lymphotoxin, *Annu. Rev. Immunol.*, *6*: 407.

Paul, N. L., Lenardo, M. J., Novak, K. D., Sarr, T., Tang, W.-L., and Ruddle, N. H. (1990). Lymphotoxin activation by human T-cell leukemia virus type I infected cell lines: role for NK-κB, *J. Virol.*, *64*: 5412.

Pelham, H. (1985). Activation of heat-shock genes in eukaryotes, *Trends Gen et.*, *1*: 31.

Pociot, F., Molvig, J., Wogensen, L., Worsaee, H. Dalboge, H. Baek, L. and Nerup, J. (1990). A tumor necrosis factor beta gene polymorphism in relation to monokine secretion and insulin dependent diabetes mellitus, *Scand. J. Immunol.*, *32*: 297–311.

Podack, E. R., Young, J.-D.-E., and Cohn, Z, (1985). Isolation and biochemical and functional characterization of perforin-1 from cytolytic T-cells granules, *Proc. Natl. Acad. Sci. USA*, *82*: 8629.

Powell, M. B., Mitchell, D., Lederman, J., Buchmeier, S., Zamvil, S. S., Graham, M., Ruddle, N. H., and Steinman, L. (1990). Lymphotoxin production by myelin basic protein specific clones correlates with encephalitogenicity, *Int. Immunol.*, 2: 539 .

Ratner, L., Polmar, S. H., Paul, N., and Ruddle, N. (1987). Cytotoxic factors secreted by cells infected by human immunodeficiency virus type I, *AIDS Res. Hum. Retroviruses*, *3*: 147.

Richter, G., Qin, Z., Diamanstein, T., and Blankenstein, T. (1989). Analysis of restriction fragment length polymorphism in lymphokine genes of normal and autoimmune mice, *J. Exp. Med.*, *170*: 1439.

Rubin, B. Y., Anderson, S. L., Sullivan, S. A., Williamson, B. D., Carswell, E. A., and Old, L. J. (1985). Purification and characterization of a human tumor necrosis factor from the LukII cell line, *Proc. Natl. Acad. Sci. USA*, *82*: 6637.

Ruddle, N. H. (1978). Delayed hypersensitivity to soluble antigens in mice. I. Analysis in vivo, *Int. Arch. Allergy Appl. Immunol.*, *58*: 560.

Ruddle, N. H. (1979). Delayed hypersensitivity to soluble antigens in mice. II. Analysis in vitro, *Int. Arch. Allergy Appl. Immunol.*, *58*: 44.

Ruddle, N. H., and Schmid, D. S. (1987). The role of lymphotoxin in T-cell mediated cytotoxicity, *Ann. Inst. Pasteur Immunol.*, *138*: 314.

Ruddle, N. H. (1986). Lymphotoxin production in AIDS. *Immunol. Today*, *7*: 8.

Ruddle, N. H., and Waksman, B. H. (1967). Cytotoxic effect of lymphocyte-antigen interaction in delayed hypersensitivity, *Science*, *157*: 1060.

Ruddle, N. H., and Waksman, B. H. (1968a). Cytotoxicity mediated by soluble antigen and lymphocytes in delayed hypersensitivity. I. Characterization of the phenomenon, *J. Exp. Med., 128*: 1237.

Ruddle, N. H., and Waksman, B. H. (1968b). Cytotoxicity mediated by soluble antigen and lymphocytes in delayed hypersensitivity. II. Correlation of the in vitro response with skin reactivity, *J. Exp. Med., 128*: 1255.

Ruddle, N. H., and Waksman, B. H. (1968c). Cytotoxicity mediated by soluble antigen and lymphocytes in delayed hypersensitivity. III. Analysis of mechanism, *J. Exp. Med., 128*: 1267.

Ruddle, N. H., Li, C.-B., Tang, W.-L., Gray, P., and McGrath, K. M. (1987). Lymphotoxin: cloning, regulation and mechanism of killing, *Tumor Necrosis Factor and Related Cytotoxins*, Ciba Foundation Symposium 131, (G. Bock and J. Marsh, eds.), Wiley, Chichester, England, p.64.

Ruddle, N. H., Bergman, C., McGrath, K. M., Lingenheld, E. G., Grunnet, M. L., Padula, S. J., and Clark, R. B. (1990). An antibody to lymphotoxin and tumor necrosis factor prevents transfer of experimental allergic encephalomyelitis, *J. Exp. Med.*, 172*: 1193* .

Schmid, D. S., Powell, M. B., Mahoney, K. A., and Ruddle, N. H. (1985). A comparison of lysis mediated by Lyt 2^+ TNP-specific cytotoxic T lymphocyte (CTL) lines with that mediated by rapidly internalized lymphotoxin-containing supernatant fluids: evidence for a role of soluble mediators in CTL-mediated killing, *Cell. Immunol., 93*: 68.

Schmid, D. S., Tite, J. P., and Ruddle, N. H. (1986). DNA fragmentation: manifestation of target cell destruction mediated by cytotoxic T-cell lines, lymphotoxin-secreting helper T-cell clones, and cell-free lymphotoxin containing supernatants, *Proc. Natl. Acad. Sci. USA, 83*: 1881.

Schmid, D. S., McGrath, K. M., Hornung, R. L., Paul, N., and Ruddle, N. H. (1987). Target cell DNA fragmentation is mediated by lymphotoxin and tumor necrosis factor, *Lymphokine Res., 6*: 195.

Semon, D., Kawashima, E., Jongeneel, C. V., Shakhov, A. N., and Nedospasov, S. A. (1987). Nucleotide sequence of the murine TNF locus, including the TNF-α (tumor necrosis factor) and TNF-β (lymphotoxin) genes, *Nucleic Acids Res., 15*: 9083.

Seregina, T. M., Mekshenkov, M. I., Turetskaya, R. L., and Nedospasov, S. A. (1989). An autocrine growth factor constitutively produced by a human lymphoblastoid B-cell line is serologically related to lymphotoxin (TNF-β), *Mol. Immunol., 26*: 339.

Shakhov, A. N., Collart, M. A., Vassalli, P., Nedospasov, S. A., and Jongeneel, C. V. (1990a). κB-type enhancers are involved in LPS-mediated transcriptional activation of the tumor necrosis factor-α gene in primary macrophages, *J. Exp. Med., 171*: 35.

Shakhov, A. N., Kuprash, D. V., Azizov, M. M., Jongeneel, C. V., and Nedospasov, S.A. (1990b). Structural analysis of the rabbit TNF locus, containing the genes encoding TNF-β (lymphotoxin) and TNF-α (tumor necrosis factor), *Gene, 95*: 215.

Shalaby, M. R., Aggarwal, B. B., Rinderknecht, E., Svedersky, L. P., Finkle, B. S., and Palladino, M. A. (1985). Activation of human polymorphonuclear leukocyte functions by interferon-α and tumor necrosis factors, *J. Immunol., 135*: 2069.

Shaw, G., and Kamen, R. (1986). A conserved AU sequence from the 3′ untranslated region of GM-CSF mediated selective mRNA degradation, *Cell, 46*: 659.

Sheehan, K. C. F., Ruddle, N. H., and Schreiber, R. D. (1989). Generation and characterization of hamster monoclonal antibodies that neutralize murine tumor necrosis factors, *J. Immunol.*, *142*: 3884.

Spies, T., Morton, C. C., Nedospasov, S. A., Fiers, W., Pious, D., and Strominger, J. L. (1986). Genes for the tumor necrosis factors alpha and beta are linked to the human major histocompatibility complex, *Proc. Natl. Acad. Sci. USA*, *83*: 8699.

Spies, T., Blanck, G., Bresnahan, M., Sands, J., and Strominger, J. L. (1989a). A new cluster of genes within the human major histocompatibility complex, *Science*, *243*: 214.

Spies, T., Bresnahan, M., and Strominger, J. L. (1989b). Human major histocompatibility complex contains a minimum of 19 genes between the complement cluster and HLA-B, *Proc. Natl. Acad. Sci. USA*, *86*: 8955.

Steffen, M., Ottmann, O. G., and Moore, M. A. S. (1988). Simultaneous production of tumor necrosis factor-a and lymphotoxin by normal T cells after induction with IL-2 and anti-T3. *J. Immunol.*, *140*: 2621.

Sung, S.-S., Bjorndahl, J., Wang, C. Y., Kao, H. T., and Fu, S. M. (1988). Production of tumor necrosis factor/cachectin by human T-cell lines and peripheral blood T lymphocytes stimulated by phorbol myristate acetate and anti-CD3 antibody, *J. Exp. Med.*, *167*: 937.

Sung, S.-S. J., Jung, L. K. L., Walters, J. A., Jeffes, E. W. B., Granger, G. A., and Fu, S. M. (1989). Production of lymphotoxin by isolated human tonsillar B lymphocytes and B lymphocyte cell lines, *J. Clin. Invest.*, *84*: 236.

Thompson, C. B., Lindsten, T., Ledbetter, J. A., Kunkel, S. L., Young, H. A., Emerson, S. G., Leiden, J. M., and June, C. H. (1989). CD28 activation pathway regulates the production of multiple T-cell derived lymphokines/cytokines, *Proc. Natl. Acad. Sci. USA*, *86*: 1333.

Tite, J. P., Powell, M. B., and Ruddle, N. H. (1985). Protein-antigen specific Ia-restricted cytolytic T cells: analysis of frequency, target cell susceptibility, and mechanism of cytolysis, *J. Immunol.*, *135*: 25.

Tschachler, E., Robert-Gurroff, M., Gallo, R. C., and Reitz,M. S. (1989). Human T-lymphotropic virus I-infected T cells constitutively express lymphotoxin in vitro, *Blood*, *73*: 194.

Ware, C.-F., Green, L. M., Reade, J., Stern, M. L., and Berger, A. E. (1986). Human T-cell hybridomas producing cytotoxic lymphokines: induction of lymphotoxin release and killer cell activity by anti CD3 monoclonal antibody or lectins and phorbol ester, *Lymphokine Res.* *5*: 313.

Welsh, R. M., Haspel, M. V., Parker, D. C., and Holmes, K. V. (1986). Natural cytotoxicity against mouse hepatitis virus-infected cells. II. A cytotoxic effector cell with B lymphocyte phenotype, *J. Immunol.*, *136*: 1454.

Williamson, B. D., Carswell, E. A., Rubin, B. Y., Prendergast, J. S., and Old, L. J. (1983). Human tumor necrosis factor produced by human B-cell lines: synergistic cytotoxic interaction with human interferon, *Proc. Natl. Acad. Sci USA*, *80*: 5397.

Wong, G. H. W., and Goeddel, D. V. (1986). Tumor necrosis factors α and β inhibit virus replication and synergize with interferons, *Nature*, *323*: 819.

Wong, R. L., Ruddle, N. H., Padula, S. J., Lingenheld, E. G., Bergman, C. M., Rugen, R. V., Epstein, D. I., and Clark, R. B. (1988). Subtypes of helper cells: non-inflammatory type 1 helper T cells, *J. Immunol.* *141*: 3329.

Yamamoto, R. S., Ware, C. F., and Granger, G. A. (1986). The human LT system. XI. Identification of LT and "TNF-like" forms from stimulated natural killers, specific and nonspecific cytotoxic human T cells in vitro, *J. Immunol.*, *137*: 1878.

Yamanaka, H. I., and Karpas, A. (1989). Identity of human B-cell line cytotoxic lymphokine with tumor necrosis factor-type β, *Proc. Natl. Acad. Sci. USA*, *86*: 1343.

Zinn, K., and Maniatis, T. (1986). Detection of factors that interact with the human β-interferon regulatory region in vivo by DNase I footprinting, *Cell*, *45*: 611.

3

Comparative Analysis of the Structure and Function of TNF-α and TNF-β

BHARAT B. AGGARWAL
The University of Texas M.D. Anderson Cancer Center, Houston, Texas

I. INTRODUCTION

We know now that the antiproliferative factor produced primarily by activated macrophages is called tumor necrosis factor α (TNF-α), whereas that produced by activated lymphocytes is called TNF-β (previously called lymphotoxin; see Aiyer and Aggarwal, 1988; Goeddel et al., 1986). Extensive research during the last few years demonstrated that TNF-α is produced not only by macrophages but by several other cell types, including natural killer cells, certain B-lymphoblastoid cells, T-lymphocytes, mast cells, astrocytes, Kupffer's cells, granulosa cells, and smooth muscle cells (Table 1). Even certain tumor cells, such as breast and ovarian tumors, have been shown to produce TNF-α. The production of TNF-β, however, seems to be restricted to lymphocytes, although a recent report (Garrett et al., 1987) indicates that myeloma cells may also be a source of this cytokine.

The induction of TNF-α and TNF-β by cells is regulated differently. TNF-α production is controlled by a wide variety of agents, including gram-negative bacteria, viruses, protozoa, mitogens, various cytokines, tumor cells, and phorbol esters. Little is known about the induction of TNF-β. Agents that induce TNF-α do not necessarily cause the synthesis of TNF-β (Cuturi et al., 1987). Lipopolysaccharides, for instance, induce the synthesis of TNF-α without any effect on TNF-β induction, whereas phorbol esters and certain other mitogens induce both cytokines

Table 1 Sources, Inducers, and Suppressors of TNF-α and TNF-β Production

TNF-α	TNF-β (LT)
Sources	
Monocytes	Lymphocytes
Lymphocytes	Myeloma cells
Natural killer cells	
Endothelial cells	
Mast cells	
Glial cells	
Astrocytes	
Kupffer cells	
Granulosa cells	
Smooth muscle cells	
Inducers	
Endotoxin	Mitogens
Poly I:C	Phorbol ester
Mitogens	Poly I:C
Virus	Interleukin-2
Parasites	OKT-3
Protozoa	
Tumor cells	
Granulocyte-macrophage colony-stimulating factor	
Interleukin-1	
Interleukin-2	
Interferons	
Phorbol esters	
Ionophores	
Indomethacin	
Silica	
Suppressors	
Cyclosporin A	Cyclosporin A
Transforming growth factor β	
Dexamethasone	
Prostaglandin E_2	
Cyclic nucleotides	
Platelet-activating factor receptor antagonists	
Lipooxygenase inhibitors	
Interleukin-4	
Interleukin-6	

(Sung et al., 1988, 1989; Steffen et al., 1988). The production of TNF-β is downregulated by various agents (Espevik et al., 1987; Dubois et al., 1989; Hamilton, 1989; Renz et al., 1988), among them cyclosporin A, which is known to suppress the production of TNF-β as well (Espevik et al., 1987). Whether other agents also reduce TNF-β production is not known.

The focus of this chapter is on the physicochemical properties of TNF-α and TNF-β. Various structural and functional similarities and differences of these cytokines will be reviewed here, and, wherever possible, the known differences of TNFs among species will also be discussed.

II. PURIFICATION OF TNFs

TNF-α was first isolated to homogeneity from the conditioned media of a phorbol ester-treated human promyelomonocytic cell line, HL-60; TNF-β was isolated from the human B-lymphoblastoid cell line RPMI-1788 (Aggarwal et al., 1984; Aggarwal and Kohr, 1985; Aggarwal, 1985). The purification scheme for TNF-α consisted of controlled pore glass chromatography (CPG), diethylaminoethyl (DEAE) ion-exchange chromatography, mono Q-fast protein liquid chromatography (FPLC), and reversed phase high-performance liquid chromatography (HPLC). Isolation of TNF-α from the serum-free conditioned media of an HL-60 cell line was also reported by another group (Lin and Yamamoto, 1987), who used two sequential steps of DEAE sepharose chromatography followed by hydrophobic interaction chromatography on a TSK Phenyl 5PW column. The isolation scheme for TNF-β involved CPG and DEAE ion-exchange chromatography, followed by lentil lectin chromatography (Aggarwal et al., 1984; Aggarwal, 1985; Aggarwal et al., 1985b). Both TNF-α and TNF-β bind to CPG, and the fact that their binding may be reversed by ethylene glycol suggests that both are hydrophobic proteins. These cytokines also bind to DEAE resin at low salt concentrations, a binding that can be reversed by about 0.1 M NaCl, indicating that they are acidic proteins with a similar isoelectric point. In contrast to TNF-α, TNF-β binds to lentil lectin, and this binding may be reversed by α-methylmannoside, indicating that it is a glycoprotein. TNF-α has also been isolated from human peripheral-blood mononuclear cells by immunoaffinity chromatography (Hahn et al., 1985). A form of TNF distinct from TNF-α and TNF-β was reported to have been purified from the human B-lymphoblastoid cell line LuK II and designated LuK II TNF (Rubin et al., 1985). The latter was isolated by CPG, lentil lectin Sepharose, and procion red agarose chromatography. The amino terminal sequence analysis of Luk II TNF subsequently showed it to be identical to TNF-β (Cerletti et al., 1987).

TNF-α has been purified to homogeneity from several other species. Murine macrophage cell lines RAW 264.7 and J774.1, and sera from endotoxin-treated mice, rabbits, and guinea pigs have been used as the source of this cytokine (Beutler et al., 1985; Haranaka et al., 1985, 1986; Kull and Cuatrecasas, 1984; Abe et al.,

1985; Tamatani et al., 1989; Adams et al., 1987). Unlike human TNF-α, murine TNF-α is a glycoprotein. TNF-β has not yet been isolated from species other than humans.

III. PHYSICOCHEMICAL PROPERTIES

Under native conditions of gel filtration, human TNF-α and TNF-β display an apparent molecular size of about 45 and 65 kDa, respectively (Aggarwal et al., 1984; 1985c). A molecular weight of 17,000 for TNF-α and 25,000 for TNF-β is determined, however, under denaturing conditions on sodium dodecyl sulfate polyacrylamide gel electrophoresis (SDS-PAGE). These observations suggest that both cytokines exhibit a molecular weight approximately equivalent to that of a trimer under nondenaturing conditions. In addition to gel filtration results, ultracentrifugation and crystallographic studies have confirmed the trimeric nature of TNF-α (Davis et al., 1987; Narhi and Arakawa, 1987; Arakawa and Yphantis, 1987; Wingfield et al., 1987; Lewit-Bentley et al., 1988; Jones et al., 1989; Eck and Sprang, 1989; Eck et al., 1988; Smith and Baglioni, 1987). TNF-α from all other species exists as an oligomeric structure under native conditions (Table 2). That the self-association of human TNF-α cannot be reversed by the presence of reducing agents, as determined by both gel filtration and ultracentrifugation studies, suggests the lack of involvement of cysteine residues (Davis et al., 1987; Narachi et al., 1987). Oligomerization of both cytokines seems to depend on protein concentration, and both can be dissociated into monomeric form by lowering the pH or by the presence of chaotropic agents, thereby indicating that both hydrophobic and electrostatic interactions are responsible for trimer formation (Smith and Baglioni, 1987). X-ray crystallographic studies indicate that human TNF-α is a trimeric structure arranged in antiparallel β-sheet form (Jones et al., 1989; Eck and Sprang, 1989).

Molecular heterogeneity in human TNF-β was suggested when two different forms of this cytokine with molecular weights of 20 and 25 kDa were isolated by SDS-PAGE (Aggarwal et al., 1985b). The two forms differ in amino terminal sequence by 23 amino acid residues. Even greater heterogeneity was demonstrated for LuK II TNF, which exhibited molecular sizes of 80, 70, 43, 25, 23, 21, and 19 kDa on SDS-PAGE. These forms seemed to be related according to peptide mapping, immunoblotting methods, and amino terminal sequence analysis (Rubin et al., 1985; Cerletti et al., 1987).

Both forms of human TNF have an isoelectric point between pH 5 and 6 (Aggarwal et al., 1984, 1985c). Since human TNF-β is a glycoprotein, removal of the carbohydrate moiety enhances its basicity but lowers its solubility (Hains and Aggarwal, 1989) without significantly affecting its biological activity. The isoelectric point of TNFs from other species is also in the acidic range similar to that of human TNF (Table 2).

Table 2 Characteristics of TNFs Isolated from Various Species

	Human		Murine		Rabbit		Guinea pig	
	TNF-α	TNF-β	TNF-α	TNF-β	TNF-α	TNF-β	TNF-α	TNF-β
Source	HL-60 PBMC	RMPI-1788 LUK II	RAW-264.7 J-774.1 Serum	—	Serum	—	Serum	—
Molecular weight (kDa)								
Gel filtration	45	65	39	—	34	—	45	—
SDS-PAGE	17	25	16–18	—	18	—	18	—
Isoelectric point	5.6	5.8	3.9–4.7	—	5.0	—	5.2	—
Carbohydrates	No	Yes	Yes	Yes	—	—	—	—
Protease sensitivity	Sensitive	Resistant	Sensitive	—	—	—	—	—
Cysteine residues	2	None	2	1	2	—	—	—
Amino acid length	157	171	156	169	156	—	—	—
Amino terminal	VAL	LEU	LEU	LEU	SER	—	SER	—
Amino acid length	157	171	156	169	156	—	—	—

TNF-α and TNF-β differ remarkably in their sensitivity to proteases. Treatment of TNF-β with as much as 10% (w/w) of trypsin, chymotrypsin, or *Staphylococcus aureas* V8 protease does not affect its biological activity (Aggarwal et al., 1984, 1985b). Yet, of the potentially nine trypsin sites in the TNF-β structure, only one site (i.e., arginine residue at position 89) is susceptible to the enzyme trypsin, and the cleavage at this site is not sufficient to abolish biological activity. The reason why other trypsin sites in TNF-β are not susceptible to the enzyme is not understood. The presence of proline residue next to the basic residue is known to be resistant to trypsin, but TNF-β contains only one such bond, at position 28. The resistance of TNF-β to chymotrypsin and V8 protease also remains unexplained.

In contrast, TNF-α is highly susceptible to trypsin, chymotrypsin, and V8 protease (Aggarwal et al., 1985c), and its biological activity is sensitive to all of them. In TNF-α, trypsin cleaves after all arginine and lysine residues. There are two arginine residues next to each other, at positions 31 and 32 in TNF-α. This region of TNF-α is highly susceptible to porteolytic attack, which then results in loss of all biological activity (Aggarwal et al., unpublished data). The biological instability on storage leads to a reduction of molecular weight of TNF-α from 17 to 14 kDa by SDS-PAGE. This is due to a cleavage at the two adjacent arginine residues. The difference in sensitivity of the two cytokines to various proteases suggests that compared with TNF-α, TNF-β is a tightly packed structure. In the case of TNF-β, this structural difference may hinder the access of various proteases to certain amino acid residues. Further support for this hypothesis comes from experiments showing high sensitivity of TNF-β to acidic conditions and various organic solvents. Treatment with these agents may unfold the protein that leads to its denaturation, and it is possible that this treatment makes TNF-β susceptible to cleavage by proteases. By themselves, these unfolding agents destroy the biological activity of TNF-β. In contrast, TNF-α is relatively stable under these conditions. TNF-α contains one disulfide bridge, whereas TNF-β has no cysteine residue. The presence of disulfide bridges is usually believed to offer rigidity to proteins. Despite this, TNF-β seems to be more stable to protease and temperature. The presence of carbohydrates also makes a protein more soluble. The presence or absence of carbohydrates in TNF-β does not alter its susceptibility to protease, pH, or organic solvents, but its solubility in aqueous solvents is dramatically affected by the absence of carbohydrates (Hains and Aggarwal, 1989).

IV. TNF PRIMARY STRUCTURE

The amino acid sequences of human TNF-α and TNF-β, determined from the purified protein (Aggarwal et al., 1985b,c), are shown in Fig. 1. These two primary structures are identical to that predicted from the nucleotide sequence (Pennica et al., 1984; Gray et al., 1984; Marmenout et al., 1985). TNF-α and TNF-β are 157

TNF-α																			VAL
TNF-β	NH_2	LEU	PRO	GLY	VAL	GLY	LEU	THR	PRO	SER	ALA	ALA	GLN	THR	ALA	ARG	GLN	HIS	PRO
											10								
									10										20
TNF-α	ARG	SER	SER	SER	ARG	THR	PRO	SER	ASP	LYS	PRO	VAL	ALA	HIS	VAL	VAL	ALA	ASN	PRO
TNF-β	LYS	MET	HIS	LEU	ALA	HIS	SER	THR	LEU	<u>LYS</u>*	<u>PRO</u>	ALA	<u>ALA</u>	<u>HIS</u>	LEU	ILE	GLY	ASP	<u>PRO</u>
		20													30				
										30									
TNF-α	GLN	ALA	GLU	GLY	GLN	LEU	GLN	TRP	LEU	ASN	ARG	ARG	ALA	ASN	ALA	LEU	LEU	ALA	ASN
TNF-β	SER	LYS	GLN	ASN	SER	<u>LEU</u>	LEU	<u>TRP</u>	ARG	ALA	ASN	THR	ASP	ARG	<u>ALA</u>	PHE	<u>LEU</u>	GLN	ASP
			40										50						
	40										50								
TNF-α	GLY	VAL	GLU	LEU	ARG	ASP	ASN	GLN	LEU	VAL	VAL	PRO	SER	GLU	GLY	LEU	TYR	LEU	ILE
TNF-β	<u>GLY</u>	PHE	SER	<u>LEU</u>	SER	ASN	<u>ASN</u>	SER	<u>LEU</u>	LEU	<u>VAL</u>	<u>PRO</u>	THR	SER	<u>GLY</u>	ILE	<u>TYR</u>	PHE	VAL
				60										70					
		60										70							
TNF-α	TYR	SER	GLN	VAL	LEU	PHE	LYS	GLY	GLN	GLY	CYS	PRO	SER	THR	HIS	VAL	LEU	LEU	THR
TNF-β	<u>TYR</u>	<u>SER</u>	<u>GLN</u>	<u>VAL</u>	VAL	<u>PHE</u>	SER	<u>GLY</u>	LYS	ALA	TYR	SER	PRO	LYS	ALA	THR	SER	SER	PRO
					80											90			
			80										90						
TNF-α	HIS	THR	ILE	SER	ARG	ILE	ALA	VAL	SER	TYR	GLN	THR	LYS	VAL	ASN	LEU	LEU	SER	ALA
TNF-β	LEU	TYR	LEU	ALA	HIS	GLU	VAL	GLN	LEU	PHE	SER	SER	GLN	TYR	PRO	PHE	HIS	VAL	PRO
						100										110			
				100										110					
TNF-α	ILE	LYS	SER	PRO	CYS	GLN	ARG	GLU	THR	PRO	GLU	GLY	ALA	GLU	ALA	LYS	PRO	TRP	TYR
TNF-β	LEU	LEU	<u>SER</u>	SER	GLN	LYS	MET	VAL	TYR	<u>PRO</u>	GLY	LEU	GLN	<u>GLU</u>	----	----	<u>PRO</u>	<u>TRP</u>	LEU
							120												130
					120										130				
TNF-α	GLU	PRO	ILE	TYR	LEU	GLY	GLY	VAL	PHE	GLN	LEU	GLU	LYS	GLY	ASP	ARG	LEU	SER	ALA
TNF-β	HIS	SER	MET	<u>TYR</u>	HIS	<u>GLY</u>	ALA	ALA	<u>PHE</u>	<u>GLN</u>	<u>LEU</u>	THR	GLN	<u>GLY</u>	<u>ASP</u>	GLN	<u>LEU</u>	<u>SER</u>	THR
										140									140
						140										150			
TNF-α	GLU	ILE	ASN	ARG	PRO	ASP	TYR	LEU	ASP	PHE	ALA	GLU	SER	GLY	GLN	VAL	TYR	PHE	GLY
TNF-β	HIS	THR	ASP	GLY	ILE	PRO	HIS	<u>LEU</u>	VAL	LEU	SER	PRO	<u>SER</u>	THR	----	<u>VAL</u>	PHE	<u>PHE</u>	<u>GLY</u>
	150										160								
TNF-α	ILE	ILE	ALA	LEU	--COOH														
TNF-β	ALA	PHE	<u>ALA</u>	<u>LEU</u>	--COOH														
			170																

Figure 1 Comparative amino acid sequences of TNF-α and TNF-β. Underscores designate areas of homology.

and 171 amino acid proteins in length, respectively. A variation in the amino terminal sequence of TNF-α has been reported (Wang et al., 1985). Since no complementary DNA corresponding to these alternate structures has been found, however, the heterogeneity observed at the amino terminal of TNF-α may be the result of experimental error. The primary structure of TNF-α shows a significant homology with that of TNF-β (Aggarwal et al., 1985c; Pennica et al., 1984); the two cytokines are 31% identical and 51% homologous. An amino terminal extension of 14 amino acids in TNF-β seems to be absent in TNF-α, but a form of TNF-β lacking this amino terminal extension has also been isolated from human B-lymphoblastoid cell line RPMI-1788 (Aggarwal et al., 1984). The absence of 23 amino acid residues from TNF-β's amino terminal seems not to affect its biological activity, and, in fact, after deletion of 24 amino acid residues from the cytokines amino terminal, a threefold increase in its biological activity has been reported (Hillen et al., 1989). In both TNF-α and TNF-β, the number and position of tryptophan residues are well conserved. Despite several similarities, the two cytokines have interesting structural differences. TNF-α, for instance, contains two cysteine residues at positions 69 and 101, while TNF-β totally lacks cysteine residues. Instead, TNF-β has tyrosine residues at the two positions. TNF-β contains three methionine residues, whereas TNF-α contains none. In contrast to TNF-α, TNF-β is a glycoprotein with one N-linked glycosylation site at position 63 and several O-linked carbohydrate attachment sites, probably at the amino terminal extension. The TNF-β protein contains nine histidine residues; TNF-α has only three. Isolation from both natural and recombinant sources of a truncated form of TNF-β with cleavage at the histidine residue (Aggarwal et al., 1985b; Hains and Aggarwal, 1989), suggesting that the histidine residues in TNF-β's amino terminal region are highly susceptible to proteolytic cleavage.

The gene for TNF-α and TNF-β is each approximately 3 kb in size, contains three introns, and both genes are very closely linked on human chromosome 6 in the major histocompatibility complex region (Spies et al., 1986; Müller et al., 1987). TNF-α and TNF-β have signal sequences of 76 and 34 amino acid residues, respectively (Pennica et al., 1984; Gray et al., 1984), unusually long signal sequences whose importance is not known. In the case of TNF-α, a cell membrane-bound form of the protein with a molecular weight of 26 kDa (instead of 17 kDa for the secreted form) has been demonstrated (Kriegler et al., 1988), which suggested that the signal sequence acts as a membrane-anchoring domain of TNF-α. The membrane-bound form of TNF-α is believed to be active and responsible for cell-mediated cytotoxicity for monocytes (Philip and Epstein, 1986). However, whether the soluble form of TNF-α with a molecular weight of 26 kDa is biologically active is not known. Interestingly, the propeptide of murine TNF-α with additional 10 amino acid residues at the amino terminal has been shown to be biologically inactive (Cseh and Beutler, 1989). No information is available about either the soluble precursor form or the membrane-bound form of TNF-β.

V. BIOLOGICAL EFFECTS

TNF-α was originally defined as possibly a macrophage-derived soluble mediator that causes hemorrhagic necrosis of methylcholanthrene-transformed sarcoma in mice (Carswell et al., 1975). Subsequently, an identical activity was also assigned to TNF-β (Gray et al., 1984. Both proteins were isolated based on in vitro L-929 cytolytic assay (Aggarwal et al., 1984, 1985b,c; Aggarwal and Kohr, 1985; Aggarwal, 1985). They could be distinguished in this assay only by the antibody neutralization assay (Aggarwal et al., 1985c). No cross-neutralization among different antibodies against TNF-α and TNF-β has been reported (Bringman and Aggarwal, 1987).

Once enough of the TNFs became available through recombinant DNA technology, they were soon found to be highly pleiotropic proteins (Aiyer and Aggarwal, 1988; Goeddel et al., 1986). In most systems, TNF-β was found to exhibit activities similar as TNF-α, which is not surprising, since both of these cytokines were shown to have a common cell surface receptor (Aggarwal et al., 1985a; Stauber and Aggarwal, 1989). Although on most cell types the binding of TNF-α can be displaced by TNF-β, and vice versa, these cytokines differ qualitatively and quantitatively in their biological responses (Table 3) (Locksley et al., 1985; Seregina et al., 1989; Oster et al., 1987; Desch et al., 1990; Canalis, 1987; Koeffler et al., 1987; Kramer et al., 1986; Beran et al., 1987; Buck et al., 1990; Holt et al., 1989; Stemme et al., 1990; Browning and Ribolini, 1989). TNF-α was shown, for instance, to interact with endothelial cells, causing the production of interleukin-1, whereas TNF-β was found minimally active in this system (Locksley et al., 1985). For the production of macrophage colony-stimulating factor from macrophages, TNF-α was found to be highly potent, and TNF-β totally lacked this activity (Oster et al., 1987). Furthermore, TNF-β acted as an antagonist to the effects of TNF-α in macrophages, which suggested that these cytokines bind to a similar receptor, but their signal transduction mechanisms differ (Oster et al., 1987). Similar differences in the effects of TNF-α and TNF-β have been reported in other cell systems, including fibroblasts, B-lymphocytes, neutrophils, and osteoblasts (Koeffler et al., 1987; Kramer et al., 1986; Beran et al., 1987; Buck et al., 1990; Holt et al., 1989). The growth of B lymphocytes is stimulated by TNF-β, whereas TNF-α seems to have no effect (Seregina et al., 1989). Differences have also been found in cytotoxic effects of these two cytokines on wide variety of tumor cells (Kramer et al., 1986; Beran et al., 1987; Browning and Ribolini, 1989).

Unlike interferons, TNF-α and TNF-β are not in general considered to be species-specific. However, differences in the biological activity of TNF-α have been

Table 3 Differences in Biological effects of TNF-α and TNF-β

Target (response)	TNF-α	TNF-β	Reference
1. Endothelial cells (production of interleukin-1)	+++	+	Locksley et al., 1985
2. Myeloid cells (KBM-5) (clonogenic survival)	+++	–	Beran et al., 1987
3. Fibroblasts (production of macrophage colony-stimulating factor)	+++	+	Koeffler et al., 1987
4. Macrophages (production of macrophage colony-stimulating factor)	+++	–	Oster et al., 1987
5. Neutrophils (activation of neutrophils)	++	+	Desch et al., 1990; Kapp et al., 1989
6. Osteoblasts (proliferation, release of Ca^{+2} collagen degradation)	++	+	Canalis, 1987
7. Vascular smooth muscle cells (interferon-γ-dependent expression of human lymphocyte antigen-DR)	++	–	Stemme et al., 1990
8. Firing rate of central nervous system sympathetic–efferent nerves to intracapsular brown adipose tissues	↓↓	↑↑	Holt et al., 1989
Rectal temperature	↓↓	↑↑	Holt et al., 1989
9. Lung lymph and plasma levels of β-keto PGF$^1\alpha$	++	–	Kreil et al., 1989
Systemic vasodilation and hypotension	++	–	Kreil et al., 1989
10. B lymphocytes (growth factor)	–	++	Seregina et al., 1989; Buck et al., 1990
11. T-cell hybridoma (MHC-I expression)	++	–	Andrews et al., 1990

noted in certain systems of different species (Kramer et al., 1988; Brouckaert et al., 1986; Talmadge et al., 1988; Rice et al., 1990; Smith et al., 1986; Fransen et al., 1986; Zentella et al., 1989; Ranges et al., 1988, 1989; Ehrke et al., 1988). For instance, murine TNF-α induces the proliferation of murine thymocytes in the presence of comitogenic stimulus, whereas human TNF-α has no effect on murine thymocytes (Ranges et al., 1988; Ehrke et al., 1988). Furthermore, in the thymocyte system, the human TNF-α was found to antagonize the proliferative effects of murine TNF-α (Ranges et al., 1988). The proliferation of murine T-cell line CT6 was also induced by murine but not human TNF-α; the latter also failed to compete for binding of murine TNF-α on the CT6 cell line (Ranges et al., 1989). Species-related differences in TNF-α activities were also noticed on murine 3T3 cells. In rapidly dividing 3T3 cells, murine TNF was cytotoxic, whereas human TNF had no effect on these cells (Palombella and Vilček, 1989). Species preference rather than species specificity has also been shown for several other cell types in vitro (Smith et al., 1986; Fransen et al., 1986) and in vivo (Kramer et al., 1988; Brouckaert et al., 1986; Talmadge et al., 1988; Zentella et al., 1989).

Recently, when a TNF-α binding protein was isolated from the urine of healthy persons and of cancer patients (Peetre et al., 1988; Olsson et al., 1989; Seckinger et al., 1989; Engelmann et al., 1989a); this protein was found to bind to TNF-α with much higher affinity than TNF-β. Because antibodies against this binding protein can immunoprecipitate TNF-α cross-linked to the cell surface receptor, and because this antibody exhibits TNF-like activity, the suggestion was made that this binding protein may be a shedded form of the TNF-α receptor (Engelmann et al., 1989b). A difference in the binding affinities of TNF-α and TNF-β was also observed for their receptors on various cell types (Locksley et al., 1985; Browning and Ribolini, 1989; Andrews et al., 1990). Solubilized cell membranes derived from human cervical carcinoma ME-180 cells and from placenta bind to TNF-α, but its binding can be displaced only by TNF-α and not TNF-β (Aiyer and Aggarwal, 1990). Two different cDNAs of receptors for TNF have recently been isolated using recombinant DNA methods (see Chapter 8 in the present volume). The receptor structure showed a complete sequence homology to the TNF binding proteins isolated from serum and urine samples. Both of these receptor cDNAs when expressed bind TNF-α and TNF-β with equal affinities. Four distinct areas of primary sequence conservation, including 11-18, 48-64, 119-133, and 152-157 (TNF numbering), have been identified between TNF-α and TNF-β (Tavernier et al., 1989), and these regions also show a high degree of homology among various species. They may be important for receptor interaction. The mechanism by which this receptor transduces a wide variety of signals is not yet understood.

VI. CONCLUSIONS

TNF-α and TNF-β are genetically, structurally, and functionally related cytokines. Perhaps this relationship is similar to that observed previously with other peptide hormones, such as that between luteinizing hormone and human chorionic gonadotropin, platelet growth factors AA and BB, acidic and basic fibroblast growth factor, interleukin-1 α and interleukin-1 β, interferon-α and interferon-β, transforming growth factors β_1 and β_2, interleukin-3 and granulocyte–macrophage colony-stimulating factor, transforming growth factor α, and epidermal growth factor. The precise reason for this kind of redundancy in related cytokines is not known. Since TNF-β is known to be produced only by lymphocytes, whereas TNF-α is secreted by a wide variety of cell types and the two are regulated differently but bind to the same cell-surface receptor, it is possible that these two cytokines are meant to play both agonist and antagonist roles, depending on physiological situations.

ACKNOWLEDGMENT

I thank all my co-workers for their contribution to some of the research described here, and I am grateful to Barbara Nash for her help in preparing the manuscript. This research was conducted, in part, by the Clayton Foundation for Research and was supported, in part, by new program development funds from the University of Texas M.D. Anderson Cancer Center.

REFERENCES

Abe, S., Gatanaga, T., Yamazaki, M., Soma, G., and Muzuno, D. (1985). Purification of rabbit tumor necrosis factor, *FEBS Lett.*, *180*: 203.

Adams, B., Regenass, U., and Cerletti, N. (1987). An efficient method for the purification of tumor necrosis factor from rabbit serum, *Lymphokine Res.*, *6*: 203.

Aggarwal, B. B. (1985). Human lympohotoxin, *Methods of Enzymology*: *Immunochemical Techniques*, Vol. 116 (G. DiSabato, ed.), Academic Press, New York, p. 441.

Aggarwal, B. B., and Kohr, W. H. (1985). Human tumor necrosis factor, *Methods of Enzymology*: *Immunochemical Techniques*, Vol. 116 (G. DiSabato, ed.), Academic Press, New York, p. 448.

Aggarwal, B. B., Moffat, B., and Harkins, R. N. (1984). Human lymphotoxin: production by a lymphoblastoid cell line, purification and initial characterization, *J. Biol. Chem.*, *259*: 686.

Aggarwal, B. B., Eessalu, T. E., and Hass, P. E. (1985a). Characterization of receptors for human tumour necrosis factor and their regulation by gamma-interferon, *Nature*, *318*: 665.

Aggarwal, B. B., Henzel, W. J., Moffat, B., Kohr, W. J., and Harkins, R. N. (1985b). Primary structure of human lymphotoxin derived from 1788 lymphoblastoid cell line, *J. Biol. Chem.*, *260*: 2334.

Aggarwal, B. B., Kohr, W. J., Hass, P. E., Moffat, B., Spencer, S. A., Henzel, W. J., Bringman, T. S., Nedwin, G. E., Goeddel, D. V., and Harkins, R. N. (1985c). Human tumor necrosis factor: production, purification, and characterization, *J. Biol. Chem.*, *260*: 2345.

Aiyer, R. A., and Aggarwal, B. B. (1988). Tumor necrosis factors, *CRC Handbook on Cytolytic Lymphocytes and Complement: Effectors of the Immune System* (E. R. Podack, ed.), CRC Press, Boca Raton, Fla., p. 105.

Aiyer, R. A., and Aggarwal, B. B. (1990). Characterization of receptors for recombinant human tumor necrosis factor-α from human placental membranes, *Lymphokine Res.*, *9*: 333.

Andrews, J. A., Berger, A. E., and Ware, C. F. (1990). Characterization of the receptor for human necrosis factor (TNF) and lymphotoxin (LT) on human T lymphocytes, *J. Immunol.*, *144*: 2582.

Arakawa, T., and Yphantis, D. A. (1987). Molecular weight of recombinant human tumor necrosis factor-α, *J. Biol. Chem.*, *262*: 7484.

Beran, M., Anderson, B. S., Kelleher, P., Whalen, K., McCredie, K., and Gutterman, G. (1987). Diversity of the effect of recombinant tumor necrosis factor-α and -β on human myelogenous leukemia cell lines, *Blood*, *69*: 721-726.

Beutler, B., Mahoney, J., Le Trang, N., Pekala, P., and Cerami, A. (1985). Purification of cachectin, a lipoprotein lipase-suppressing hormone secreted by endotoxin-induced raw 264.7 cells, *J. Exp. Med.*, *161*: 984.

Bringman, T. S., and Aggarwal, B. B. (1987). Monoclonal antibodies to human tumor necrosis factors alpha and beta: application for affinity purification, immunoassays and as structural probes, *Hybridoma*, *6*: 489.

Brouckaert, P. G. G., Leroux-Roels, G. G., Guisez, Y., Tavernier, J., and Fiers, W. (1986). In vivo anti-tumour activity of recombinant human and murine TNF, alone and in combination with murine IFN-γ, on a syngeneic murine melanoma, *Int. J. Cancer*, *38*: 763.

Browning, J., and Ribolini, A. (1989). Studies on the differing effects of tumor necrosis factor and lymphotoxin on the growth of several human tumor lines, *J. Immunol.*, *143*: 1859.

Buck, C., Digel, W., Shöninger, W., Stepanic, M., Raghavachar, A., Heimpel, H., and Porzsolt, E. (1990). Tumor necrosis factor-α but not lymphotoxin stimulates growth of cells in hairy cell leukemia, *Leukemia*, *4*: 431.

Canalis, E., (1987). Effect of tumor necrosis factor on bone resorption in vitro, *Endocrinology*, *121*: 1596.

Carswell, E. A., Old, L. J., Kassel, R. L., Green, S., Fiore, N., and Williamson, B. (1975). An endotoxin-induced serum factor that causes necrosis of tumors, *Proc. Natl. Acad. Sci. USA*, *72*: 3666.

Cerletti, N., Knecht, R., Chang, J.-Y., and Regenass, U. (1987). Lymphotoxin from the human lymphoblastoid cell line LUK II: isolation and characterization and N-terminal sequence deterioration, *5th International Workshop on Molecular Basis of Lymphokine Action*, Clearwater, Fla., Abstract 1452A.

Cseh, K., and Beutler, B. (1989). Alternative cleavage of the cachectin/tumor necrosis factor propeptide results in a larger, inactive form of secreted protein, *J. Biol. Chem.*, *264*: 16256.

Cuturi, M. C., Murphy, M., Costa-Giomi, M. P., Weinmann, R., Perussia, B., and Trinchieri, G. (1987). Independent regulation of tumor necrosis factor and lymphotoxin production by human peripheral blood lymphocytes, *J. Exp. Med.*, *165*: 1581.

Davis, J. M., Narachi, M. A., Alton, N. K., and Arakawa, T. (1987). Structure of human tumor necrosis factor α derived from recombinant DNA, *Biochemistry*, *26*: 1322.

Desch, C. E., Dobrina, A., Aggarwal, B. B., and Harlan, J. M. (1990). Tumor necrosis factor-alpha exhibits greater proinflammatory activity than lymphotoxin in vitro, *Blood*, *75*: 2030.

Dubois, C., Bissonnette, E., and Rola-Pleszczynski, M. (1989). Platelet activating factor (PAF) enhances tumor necrosis factor production by alveolar macrophates, *J. Immunol.*, *143*: 964.

Eck, M. J., and Sprang, S. R. (1989). The structure of tumor necrosis factor-α at s.6 Åresolution: implications for receptor binding, *J. Biol. Chem.*, *264*: 17595.

Eck, M. J., Beutler, B., Kuo, G., Merryweather, J. P., and Sprang, S. R. (1988). Crystallization of trimeric recombinant human tumor necrosis factor (cachectin), *J. Biol. Chem.*, *263*: 12816.

Ehrke, M. J., Ho, R. L. X., and Hori, K. (1988). Species-specific TNF induction of thymocyte proliferation , *Cancer Immunol. Immunother.*, *27*: 103.

Engelmann, H., Aderka, D., Rubinstein, M., Rotman, D., and Wallack, D. (1989a). A tumor necrosis factor-binding protein purified to homogeneity from human urine protects cells from tumor necrosis factor toxicity, J. Biol. Chem., *264*: 11974.

Engelmann, G. Holtman, H., Brakebusch, C., Shemer Avni, Y., Sarov, I., Nophar, Y., and Wallach, D. (1989b). Soluble forms of the TNF receptors, purified from human urine inhibit TNF effects: antibodies against the soluble receptors induce TNF-like effects, *Cytokine*, *1*: 148A.

Espevik, T., Figari, I. S., Shalaby, M. R., Lackides, G. A., Lewis, G. D., Shepard, H. M., and Palladino, M. A., Jr. (1987). Inhibition of cytokine production by cyclosporin A and transforming growth factor β, *J. Exp. Med.*, *166*: 571.

Fransen, L., Ruysschaert, M.-R., Van der Heyden, J., and Fiers, W. (1986). Recombinant tumor necrosis factor: species specificity for a variety of human and murine transformed cell lines, *Cell. Immunol.*, *100*: 360.

Garrett, I. R., Durie, B. G. M., Nedwin, G. E., Gillespie, A., Bringman, T., Sabatini, M., Bertolini, D. R., and Mundy, G. R. (1987). Production of lymphotoxin, a bone-resorbing cytokine, by cultured human myeloma cells, *N. Engl. J. Med.*, *317*: 526.

Goeddel, D. V., Aggarwal, B. B., Gray, P. W., Leung, D. W., Nedwin, G. E., Palladino, M. A., Patton, J. S., Pennica, D., Shepard, H. M., Sugarman, B. J., and Wong, G. H. W. (1986). Tumor necrosis factors: gene structure and biological activities, *Cole Spring Harbor Symp. Quant. Biol.*, *51*: 597.

Gray, P. W., Aggarwal, B. B., Benton, C. V., Bringman, T. S., Henzel, W. J., Jarrett, J. A., Leung, D. W., Moffat, B., Ng, P., Svedersky, L. P., Palladino, M. A., and Nedwin, G. A. (1984). Cloning and expression of the cDNA for human lymphotoxin: lymphokine with tumor necrosis activity, *Nature*: *312*: 721.

Hahn, T., Toker, L., Budilovsky, S., Aderka, D., Eshhar, Z., and Wallach, D. (1985). Use of monoclonal antibodies to a human cytotoxin for its isolation and for examining the self-induction of resistance to this protein, *Proc. Natl. Acad. Sci. USA*, *82*: 3814.

Hains, J. M., and Aggarwal, B. B. (1989). Characterization of recombinant human lymphotoxin (TNF-β) produced by a mammalian cell line, *Arch. Biochem. Biophys.*, *274*: 417.

Hamilton, J. A. (1989). Potential antiinflammatory effects of interleukin 4: suppression of human monocyte tumor necrosis factor alpha, interleukin 1 and prostaglandin E2, *Proc. Natl. Acad. Sci. USA*, *86*: 3803.

Haranaka, K., Satomi, N., Sakurai, A., and Nariuchi, H. (1985). Purification and partial amino acid sequence of rabbit tumor necrosis factor, *Int. J. Cancer*, *36*: 395.

Haranaka, K., Carswell, E. A., Williamson, B. D., Prendergast, J. S., Satomi, N., and Old, L. J. (1986). Purification, characterization, and antitumor activity of nonrecombinant mouse tumor necrosis factor, *Proc. Natl. Acad. Sci. USA*, *83*: 3949.

Hillen, H., Keilhauer, G., Daum, L., Kluge, M., Emling, F., Moller, A., Schlick, E., and Schollmeier, K. (1989). Lymphotoxin muteins and their biological activities, *2nd International Conference on Tumor Necrosis Factor and Related Cytokines*, Napa, Calif., Abstract WA-354.

Holt, S. J., Grimble, R. F., and York, D. a. (1989). Tumor necrosis factor-α and lymphotoxin have opposite effects on sympathetic efferent nerves to brown adipose tissue by direct action in the central nervous system, *Brain Res.*, *497*: 183.

Jones, E. Y., Stuart, D. I., and Walker, N. P. C. (1989). Structure of tumour necrosis factor, *Nature*, *338*: 225.

Kapp, A., Zeck-Kapp, G., and Blohm, D. (1989). Human tumor necrosis factor is a potent activator of the oxidative metabolism in human polymorphonuclear neutrophilic granulocytes: comparison with human lymphotoxin, *J. Invest. Dermatol.*, *92*: 348.

Koeffler, H. P., Gasson, J., Ranyard, J., Souza, L., Shapard, M., and Munker, R. (1987). Recombinant human TNF-a stimulates production of granulocyte colony stimulating factor, *Blood*, *70*: 55.

Kramer, S. M., Carver, M. E., and Apperson, S. M. (1986). Comparison of TNF-α and TNF-β cytolytic biological activities in a serum free bioassay, *Lymphokine Res.*, *5*: S139.

Kramer, S. M., Aggarwal, B. B., Eessalu, T. E., McCabe, S. M., Figari, I. S., Ferraiolo, B. L, and Palladino, M. A. (1988). Characterization of the in vitro and in vivo species preference of human and murine tumor necrosis factor-α, *Cancer Res.*, *48*: 920.

Kreil, E. A., Green, E., Fitzgibbon, C., Robinson, D. R., and Zapol, W. M. (1989). Effects of recombinant human tumor necrosis factor alpha, lylmphotoxin, and *Escherichia coli* lipopolysaccharide on hemodynamics, lung microvascular permeability, and eicosanoid synthesis in anesthetized sheep, *Circ. Res.*, *65*: 502.

Kull, F. C., and Cuatrecasas, P. (1984). Necrosin: purification and properties of a cytotoxin derived from a murine macrophage-like cell line, *Proc. Natl. Acad. Sci. USA*, *81*: 7932.

Lewit-Bentley, A., Fourme, R., Kahn, R., Prangé, T., Vachette, P., Tavernier, J., Hauquier, g., and Fiers, W. (1988). Structure of tumour necrosis factor by x-ray solution scattering and preliminary studies by single crystal x-ray diffraction, *J. Mol. Biol.*, *199*: 389.

Lin, L. S., and Yamamoto, R. (1987). Purification of recombinant human interleukin 1β produced from yeast, *Protein Purification, Micro to Macro* (R. Burgess, ed.), UCLA Symposia on Molecular and Cellular Biology, New Series, alan R. Liss, New York, vol. 168, p. 401.

Locksley, R. M., Heinzel, F. B., Shepard, H. M., Agosti, J., Eessalu, T. E., Aggarwal, B. B., and Harlan, J. M. (1985). Tumor necrosis factor-α and -β differ in their capacities to generate interleukin-1 release from human endothelial cells, *J. Immunol., 139*: 1891.

Marmenout, A., Fransen, L., Tavernier, J., Van Der Heyden, J., Tizard, R., Kawashima, E., Shaw, A., Johnson, M.-J., Semon, D., Müller, R., Ruysschaert, M.-R., Van Vliet, A., and Fiers, W. (1985). Molecular cloning and expression of human tumor necrosis factor and comparison with mouse tumor necrosis factor, *Eur. J. Biochem., 152*: 515.

Müller, U., Jongeneel, C. V., Nedospasov, S. A., Lindahl, K. F., and Steinmetz, M. (1987). Tumour necrosis factor and lymphotoxin genes map close to H-2D in the mouse major histocompatibility complex, *Nature, 325*: 265.

Narachi, M. A., Davis, J. M., Hsu, Y.-R., and Arakawa, T. (1987). Role of single disulfide in recombinant human tumor necrosis factor-α, *J. Biol. Chem., 262*: 13107.

Narhi, L. O., and Arakawa, T. (1987). Dissociation of recombinant tumor necrosis factor α studied by gel permeation chromatography, *Biochem. Biophys. Res. Commun., 147*: 740.

Nedwin, G. E., Naylor, S. L., Sakaguchi, A. Y., Smith, D., Jarrett-Nedwin, J., Pennica, D., Goeddel, D. V., and Gray, P. W. (1985). Human lymphotoxin and tumor necrosis factor genes: structure, homology and chromosomal localization, *Nucleic Acids Res., 13*: 6361.

Olsson, I., Lantz, M., Nilsson, E., Peetre, C., Thysell, H., Grubb, A., and Adolph, G. (1989). Isolation and characterization of a tumor necrosis factor binding protein from urine, *Eur. J. Haematol., 42*: 270.

Oster, W., Lindemann, A., Horn, S., Mertelsmann, R., and Herrmann, F. (1987). Tumor necrosis factor-α and not TNF-β induces secretion of colony-stimulating factor for macrophages (CSF-1) by human monocytes, *Blood, 70*: 1700.

Palombella, V. J., and Vilček, J. (1989). Mitogenic and cytotoxic actions of tumor necrosis factor in BALB/c 3T3 cells: role of phospholipase activation, *J. Biol. Chem., 264*: 18128.

Peetre, C., Thysell, H., Grubb, A., and Olsson, I. (1988). A tumor necrosis factor binding protein is present in human biological fluids, *Eur. J. Haematol., 41*: 414.

Pennica, D., Nedwin, G. E., Hayflick, J. F., Seeburg, P. H., Palladino, M. A., Kohr, W. J., Aggarwal, B. B., and Goeddel, D. V. (1984). Human tumor necrosis factor: precursor structure, expression and homology to lymphotoxin, *Nature, 312*: 724.

Philip, R., and Epstein, L. B. (1986). Tumour necrosis factor as immunomodulator and mediator of monocyte cytotoxicity induced by itself, γ-interferon and interleukin-1, *Nature, 323*: 86.

Ranges, G. E., Zlotnik, A., Espevik, T., Dinarello, C. A., Cerami, A., and Palladino, M. A., Jr. (1988). Tumor necrosis factor α/cachectin is a growth factor for thymocytes: synergistic interactions with other cytokines, *J. Exp. Med., 167*: 1472.

Ranges, G. E., Bombara, M. P., Aiyer, R. A., Rice, G. G., and Palladino, M. A., Jr. (1989). Tumor necrosis factor-α as a proliferative signal for an IL-2 dependent T cell line: strict species specificity of action, *J. Immunol., 142*: 1203.

Renz, H., Gong, J.-H., Schmidt, A., Nain, M., and Gesma, D. (1988). Release of tumor necrosis factor-α from macrophages: enhancement and suppression are dose-dependently regulated by prostaglandin E_2 and cyclic nucleotides, *J. Immunol., 141*: 2388.

Rice, G. C., Kramer, S. M., Figari, I. S., Ranges, G. E., and Palladino, M. A. (1990). Tumor necrosis factor-alpha: a species-specific cytokine? *Tumor Necrosis Factor: Structure, Mechanism of Action, Role in Disease and Therapy* (B. Bonavida and G. Granger, eds.), S. Karger, Basel, pp. 87–93.

Rubin, B. Y., Anderson, S. L., Sullivan, S. A., Williamson, B. D., Carswell, E. A., and Old, L. J. (1985). Purification and characterization of a human tumor necrosis factor from the LuK II cell line, *Proc. Natl. Acad. Sci. USA*, *82*: 6637.

Seckinger, P., Isaaz, S., and Dayer, J.-M. (1989). Purification and biologic characterization of a specific tumor necrosis factor-α inhibitor, *J. Biol. Chem.*, *264*: 11966.

Seregina, T. M., Mekshenkov, M. I., Turetskaya, R. L., and Nedospasov, S. A. (1989). An autocrine growth factor constitutively produced by a human lymphoblastoid B-cell line is serologically related to lymphotoxin (TNF-β), *Mol. Immunol.*, *26*: 339.

Smith, R. A., and Baglioni, C. (1987). The active form of tumor necrosis factor is a trimer, *J. Biol. Chem.*, *262*: 6951.

Smith, R. A., Kirstein, M., Fiers, W., and Baglioni, C. (1986). Species specificity of human and murine tumor necrosis factor, *J. Biol. Chem.*, *261*: 14871.

Spies, T., Morton, C. C., Nedospasov, S. A., Fiers, W., Pious, D., and Strominger, J. L. (1986). Genes for the tumor necrosis factors α and β are linked to the human major histocompatibility complex, *Proc. Natl. Acad. Sci. USA*, *83*: 8699.

Stauber, G. B., and Aggarwal, B. B. (1989). Characterization and affinity cross linking of receptors for human recombinant lymphotoxin (TNF-β) on a human histiocytic lymphoma cell line U937, *J. Biol. Chem.*, *264*: 3573.

Steffen, M., Ottmann, O. G., and Moore, M. A. S. (1988). Simultaneous production of tumor necrosis factor-α and lymphotoxin by normal T cells after induction with IL-2 and anti-T3, *J. Immunol.*, *140*: 2621.

Stemme, S., Fager, G., and Hansson, G. K. (1990). MHC class II antigen expression in human vascular smooth muscle cells is induced by interferon-gamma and modulated by tumour necrosis factor and lymphotoxin, *Immunology*, *69*: 243.

Sung, S.-S. J., Bjorndahl, J. M., Wang, C. Y., Kao, H. T., and Fu, S. M. (1988). Production of tumor necrosis factor/cachectin by human T cell lines and periopheral blood T lymphocytes stimulated by phorbol myristate acetate and anti-CD3 antibody, *J. Exp. Med.*, *167*: 937.

Sung, S.-S. J., Jung, L. K. L., Walters, J. A., Jeffes, E. W. B., III, Granger, G. A., and Fu, S. M. (1989). Production of lymphotoxin by isolated human tonsillar B lymphocytes and B lymphocyte cell lines, *J. Clin. Invest.*, *84*: 236.

Talmadge, J. E., Phillips, H., Schneider, M., Rowe, T., and Pennington, R. (1988). Immunomodulatory properties of recombinant murine and murine tumor necrosis factor, *Cancer Res.*, *48*: 544.

Tamatani, T., Kimura, S., Hashimoto, T., and Onozaki, K. (1989). Purification of guinea pig tumor necrosis factor (TNF): comparison of its antiproliferative and differentative activities for myeloid leukemic cell lines with those of recombinant human TNF, *J. Biochem.*, *105*: 55.

Tavernier, J., van Ostade, X., Hauquier, G., Prange, T., Lasters, I., de Maeyer, M., Lewit-Bentley, A., and Fourme, R. (1989). Conserved residues of tumour necrosis factor and lymphotoxin constitute the framework of the trimeric structure, *FEBS Lett.*, *257*: 315.

Wang, A. M., Creasey, A. A., Ladner, M. B., Lin, L. S., Strickler, J., Van Arsdell, J. N., Yamamoto, R., and Mark, D. F. (1985). Molecular cloning of the complementary DNA for human tumor necrosis factor, *Science*, *228*: 149.

Wingfield, P., Pain, R. H., and Craig, S. (1987). Tumour necrosis factor is a compact trimer, *FEBS Lett.*, *211*: 179.

Zentella, A., Davatelis, G., and Cerami, A. (1989). Species specificity of cachectin/TNF, *2nd International Conference on Tumor Necrosis Factor and Related Cytokines, UCLA Symp.*, *41*: 216.

4

Precursor Structures and Structure-Function Analysis of TNF and Lymphotoxin

W. FIERS
State University, Ghent, Belgium

I. INTRODUCTION

Conditions for the synthesis of lymphotoxin (now also called TNF-β) were first described by Ruddle and Waksman (1967), and for in vivo production of TNF in experimental animals by Carswell et al. (1975). By the identification of producer cell lines, by the establishment of appropriate induction protocols, and by the development of sensitive and reproducible assays (Ruff and Gifford, 1981), the foundation was laid for the subsequent cloning of the respective genes. Aggarwal and co-workers (1984) purified human lymphotoxin from appropriately induced lymphoblastoid RPMI 1788 cells, and by microsequencing Aggarwal et al. (1985) could derive the almost complete amino acid sequence. On the basis of this information, oligonucleotide probes were made which allowed the cloning of the human lymphotoxin gene, and from its nucleotide sequence, the complete primary structure of the human lymphotoxin precursor polypeptide was deduced (Gray et al., 1984).

Human TNF was purified from induced HL-60 cells, and on the basis of the resulting structural information, probes could be derived that allowed cloning of the human TNF gene (Pennica et al., 1984; Wang et al., 1985). Other groups used serum from BCG/ lipopolysaccharide-treated rabbits as a source from which to purify rabbit TNF; on the basis of this structural information, oligonucleotide probes could be used for heterologous hybridization resulting in the cloning of the human (Marmenout et al., 1985; Shirai et al., 1985) and the murine TNF gene (Fransen et al., 1985; Pennica et al., 1985). Kull and Cuatrecasas (1984) described the purification of a factor, which they named necrosin, from the supernatant of a stimulated murine macrophage cell line; this factor was undoubtedly identical to murine TNF. Cachectin was a protein purified by Beutler et al. (1985) from the supernatant of a mouse macrophage-type cell line on the basis of its suppression of lipoprotein lipase activity; the N-terminal amino acid sequence revealed that this protein was in fact TNF.

II. PRESEQUENCE OF TNF

The lymphotoxin messenger RNA codes for the mature lymphotoxin preceded by a 34-amino-acid signal sequence (Gray et al., 1984). Undoubtedly, the prepolypeptide is secreted and processed as most other extracellular glycoproteins. But remarkably, the mature human TNF is preceded by a 76-amino-acid-long presequence (Fig. 1). A comparison between the sequences of different mammalian species reveals that the amino acid conservation is almost as high in the preregion as in the mature TNF, suggesting that the former must exert an important biological function (Table 1). There are especially two segments of very high sequence conservation, namely the N-terminal -76 to -63 (we only use the human numbering) and the region -44 to -26. The hydrophilicity plot reveals that the latter segment is fairly hydrophobic and presumably plays a role in the membrane insertion of the prepolypeptide. This transmembrane domain is interrupted by two threonine residues and one serine residue. Moreover, the segment is preceded in all species, except bovine, by two basic residues, which is often a mechanism for preventing further transmembrane migration and for anchoring the polypeptide. If such a mechanism is correct, the residues -76 to - 50 may constitute an intracellular domain of the TNF-producing cells, but so far there is neither evidence nor hints for its putative function. The region between residue -14 to -1 is the most variable and may constitute a stem from which the mature TNF is cleaved off before position 1.

That the presequence could not be considered an ordinary signal sequence was already evident from the fact that the TNF mRNA, when added to a translation mixture supplemented with dog pancreas microsomes, could be translated to a full-length precursor form (26 kDa) but was not further processed under conditions where "classical" signal sequences are readily clipped off (Müller et al., 1986). Nevertheless, the release of mature TNF by cleavage before amino acid 1 is not a property restricted to macrophages, as mature TNF (17 kDa) can be produced by many other cell types. However, Müller et al. (1986) found that transformed Chinese hamster ovary cells also produce substantial amounts of polypeptides with intermediate length (e.g., 20 and 18.5 kDa, the latter possibly being a doublet). Whether these represented intermediates in the processing or products of an alter-

	-76					-70										-60										
MAN	Met	Ser	Thr	Glu	Ser	Met	Ile	Arg	Asp	Val	Glu	Leu	Ala	Glu	Glu	Ala	Leu	Pro	Lys	Lys	Thr	Gly	Gly	Pro	Gln	Gly
PIG																										
COW	Met	Ser	Thr	Lys	Ser	Met	Ile	Arg	Asp	Val	Glu	Leu	Ala	Glu	Glu	Val	Leu	Ser	Glu	Lys	Ala	Gly	Gly	Pro	Gln	-
RABBIT	Met	Ser	Thr	Glu	Ser	Met	Ile	Arg	Asp	Val	Glu	Leu	Ala	Glu	Gly	Pro	Leu	Pro	Lys	Lys	Ala	Gly	Gly	Pro	Gln	Gly
RAT	Met	Ser	Thr	Glu	Ser	Met	Ile	Arg	Asp	Val	Glu	Leu	Ala	Glu	Glu	Ala	Leu	Pro	Lys	Lys	Met	Gly	Gly	Leu	Gln	Asn
MOUSE	Met	Ser	Thr	Glu	Ser	Met	Ile	Arg	Asp	Val	Glu	Leu	Ala	Glu	Glu	Ala	Leu	Pro	Gln	Lys	Met	Gly	Gly	Phe	Gln	Asn

	-50										-40										-30										-20		
MAN	Ser	Arg	Arg	Cys	Leu	Phe	Leu	Ser	Leu	Phe	Ser	Phe	Leu	Ile	Val	Ala	Gly	Ala	Thr	Thr	Leu	Phe	Cys	Leu	Leu	His	Phe	Gly	Val	Ile	Gly	Pro	Gln	Arg	Glu
PIG																		Ala	Thr	Thr	Leu	Phe	Cys	Leu	Leu	His	Phe	Glu	Val	Ile	Gly	Pro	Gln	Lys	Glu
COW	Ser	Arg	Ser	Cys	Leu	Cys	Leu	Ser	Leu	Phe	Ser	Phe	Leu	Leu	Val	Ala	Gly	Ala	Thr	Thr	Leu	Phe	Cys	Leu	Leu	His	Phe	Gly	Val	Ile	Gly	Pro	Gln	Arg	Glu
RABBIT	Ser	Lys	Arg	Cys	Leu	Cys	Leu	Ser	Leu	Phe	Ser	Phe	Leu	Leu	Val	Ala	Gly	Ala	Thr	Thr	Leu	Phe	Cys	Leu	Leu	His	Phe	Arg	Val	Ile	Gly	Pro	Gln	Glu	Glu
RAT	Ser	Arg	Arg	Cys	Leu	Cys	Leu	Ser	Leu	Phe	Ser	Phe	Leu	Leu	Val	Ala	Gly	Ala	Thr	Thr	Leu	Phe	Cys	Leu	Leu	Asn	Phe	Gly	Val	Ile	Gly	Pro	Asn	Lys	Glu
MOUSE	Ser	Arg	Arg	Ser	Leu	Cys	Leu	Ser	Leu	Phe	Ser	Phe	Leu	Leu	Val	Ala	Gly	Ala	Thr	Thr	Leu	Phe	Cys	Leu	Leu	Asn	Phe	Gly	Val	Ile	Gly	Pro	Gln	Arg	Asp

							-10										↓ 1									10						
MAN	Glu	Phe	-	Pro	Arg	Asp	Leu	Ser	Leu	Ile	Ser	Pro	Leu	Ala	Gln	Ala	-	-	VAL	ARG	SER	SER	SER	ARG	THR	PRO	SER	ASP	LYS	PRO	VAL	ALA	HIS	VAL	VAL
PIG	Glu	Phe	-	Pro	Ala	Gly	Pro	Leu	Ser	Ile	Asn	Pro	Leu	Ala	Gln	Gly	-	-	LEU	ARG	SER	SER	SER	GLN	THR	-	SER	ASP	LYS	PRO	VAL	ALA	HIS	VAL	VAL
COW	Glu	Gln	Val	Pro	Ser	Gly	Pro	Ser	Ile	Asn	Ser	Pro	Leu	Val	Gln	-	-	Thr	LEU	ARG	SER	SER	SER	GLN	ALA	SER	SER	ASN	LYS	PRO	VAL	ALA	HIS	VAL	VAL
RABBIT	Glu	Gln	Ser	Pro	Asn	Asn	Leu	His	Leu	Val	Asn	Pro	Val	Ala	Gln	Met	Val	Thr	LEU	ARG	SER	ALA	SER	ARG	ALA	LEU	SER	ASP	LYS	PRO	LEU	ALA	HIS	VAL	VAL
RAT	Glu	Lys	Phe	Pro	Asn	Gly	Leu	Pro	Leu	Ile	Ser	Ser	Met	Ala	Gln	Thr	Leu	Thr	LEU	ARG	SER	SER	SER	GLN	ASN	SER	SER	ASP	LYS	PRO	VAL	ALA	HIS	VAL	VAL
MOUSE	Glu	Lys	Phe	Pro	Asn	Gly	Leu	Pro	Leu	Ile	Ser	Ser	Met	Ala	Gln	Thr	Leu	Thr	LEU	ARG	SER	SER	SER	GLN	ASN	SER	SER	ASP	LYS	PRO	VAL	ALA	HIS	VAL	VAL

		20									30										40										50		
MAN	ALA	ASN	PRO	GLN	ALA	GLU	GLY	GLN	LEU	GLN	TRP	LEU	ASN	ARG	ARG	ALA	ASN	ALA	LEU	LEU	ALA	ASN	GLY	VAL	GLU	LEU	ARG	ASP	ASN	GLN	LEU	VAL	VAL	PRO	SER
PIG	ALA	ASN	VAL	LYS	ALA	GLU	GLY	GLN	LEU	GLN	TRP	GLN	SER	GLY	TYR	ALA	ASN	ALA	LEU	LEU	ALA	ASN	GLY	VAL	LYS	LEU	LYS	ASP	ASN	GLN	LEU	VAL	VAL	PRO	THR
COW	ALA	ASP	ILE	ASN	SER	PRO	GLY	GLN	LEU	ARG	TRP	TRP	ASP	SER	TYR	ALA	ASN	ALA	LEU	MET	ALA	ASN	GLY	VAL	LYS	LEU	GLU	ASP	ASN	GLN	LEU	VAL	VAL	PRO	ALA
RABBIT	ALA	ASN	PRO	GLN	VAL	GLU	GLY	GLN	LEU	GLN	TRP	LEU	SER	GLN	ARG	ALA	ASN	ALA	LEU	LEU	ALA	ASN	GLY	MET	LYS	LEU	THR	ASP	ASN	GLN	LEU	VAL	VAL	PRO	ALA
RAT	ALA	ASN	HIS	GLN	ALA	GLU	GLU	GLN	LEU	GLU	TRP	LEU	SER	GLN	ARG	ALA	ASN	ALA	LEU	LEU	ALA	ASN	GLY	MET	ASP	LEU	LYS	ASP	ASN	GLN	LEU	VAL	VAL	PRO	ALA
MOUSE	ALA	ASN	HIS	GLN	VAL	GLU	GLU	GLN	LEU	GLU	TRP	LEU	SER	GLN	ARG	ALA	ASN	ALA	LEU	LEU	ALA	ASN	GLY	MET	ASP	LEU	LYS	ASP	ASN	GLN	LEU	VAL	VAL	PRO	ALA

									60										70										80				
MAN	GLU	GLY	LEU	TYR	LEU	ILE	TYR	SER	GLN	VAL	LEU	PHE	LYS	GLY	GLN	GLY	CYS	PRO	SER	THR	HIS	VAL	LEU	LEU	THR	HIS	THR	ILE	SER	ARG	ILE	ALA	VAL	SER	TYR
PIG	ASP	GLY	LEU	TYR	LEU	ILE	TYR	SER	GLN	VAL	LEU	PHE	ARG	GLY	GLN	GLY	CYS	PRO	SER	THR	ASN	VAL	PHE	LEU	THR	HIS	THR	ILE	SER	ARG	ILE	ALA	VAL	SER	TYR
COW	GLU	GLY	LEU	TYR	LEU	ILE	TYR	SER	GLN	VAL	LEU	PHE	ARG	GLY	GLN	GLY	CYS	PRO	PRO	PRO	PRO	VAL	LEU	-	THR	HIS	THR	ILE	SER	ARG	ILE	ALA	VAL	SER	TYR
RABBIT	ASP	GLY	LEU	TYR	LEU	ILE	TYR	SER	GLN	VAL	LEU	PHE	SER	GLY	GLN	GLY	CYS	ARG	SER	TYR	-	VAL	LEU	LEU	THR	HIS	THR	VAL	SER	ARG	PHE	ALA	VAL	SER	TYR
RAT	ASP	GLY	LEU	TYR	LEU	ILE	TYR	SER	GLN	VAL	LEU	PHE	LYS	GLY	GLN	GLY	CYS	PRO	ASP	TYR	-	VAL	LEU	LEU	THR	HIS	THR	VAL	SER	ARG	PHE	ALA	ILE	SER	TYR
MOUSE	ASP	GLY	LEU	TYR	LEU	VAL	TYR	SER	GLN	VAL	LEU	PHE	LYS	GLY	GLN	GLY	CYS	PRO	ASP	TYR	-	VAL	LEU	LEU	THR	HIS	THR	VAL	SER	ARG	PHE	ALA	ILE	SER	TYR

			90										100										110										120		
MAN	GLN	THR	LYS	VAL	ASN	LEU	LEU	SER	ALA	ILE	LYS	SER	PRO	CYS	GLN	ARG	GLU	THR	PRO	GLU	GLY	ALA	GLU	ALA	LYS	PRO	TRP	TYR	GLU	PRO	ILE	TYR	LEU	GLY	GLY
PIG	GLN	THR	LYS	VAL	ASN	LEU	LEU	SER	ALA	ILE	LYS	SER	PRO	CYS	GLN	ARG	GLU	THR	PRO	GLU	GLY	ALA	GLU	ALA	LYS	PRO	TRP	TYR	GLU	PRO	ILE	TYR	LEU	GLY	GLY
COW	GLN	THR	LYS	VAL	ASN	ILE	LEU	SER	ALA	ILE	LYS	SER	PRO	CYS	HIS	ARG	GLU	THR	PRO	GLU	TRP	ALA	GLU	ALA	LYS	PRO	TRP	TYR	GLU	PRO	ILE	TYR	GLN	GLY	GLY
RABBIT	PRO	ASN	LYS	VAL	ASN	LEU	LEU	SER	ALA	ILE	LYS	SER	PRO	CYS	HIS	ARG	GLU	THR	PRO	GLU	GLU	ALA	GLU	PRO	MET	ALA	TRP	TYR	GLU	PRO	ILE	TYR	LEU	GLY	GLY
RAT	GLN	GLU	LYS	VAL	SER	LEU	LEU	SER	ALA	ILE	LYS	SER	PRO	CYS	PRO	LYS	ASP	THR	PRO	GLU	GLY	ALA	GLU	LEU	LYS	PRO	TRP	TYR	GLU	PRO	MET	TYR	LEU	GLY	GLY
MOUSE	GLN	GLU	LYS	VAL	ASN	LEU	LEU	SER	ALA	VAL	LYS	SER	PRO	CYS	PRO	LYS	ASP	THR	PRO	GLU	GLY	ALA	GLU	LEU	LYS	PRO	TRP	TYR	GLU	PRO	ILE	TYR	LEU	GLY	GLY

								130										140										150							157
MAN	VAL	PHE	GLN	LEU	GLU	LYS	GLY	ASP	ARG	LEU	SER	ALA	GLU	ILE	ASN	ARG	PRO	ASP	TYR	LEU	ASP	PHE	ALA	GLU	SER	GLY	GLN	VAL	TYR	PHE	GLY	ILE	ILE	ALA	LEU
PIG	VAL	PHE	GLN	LEU	GLU	LYS	ASP	ASP	ARG	LEU	SER	ALA	GLU	ILE	ASN	LEU	PRO	ASP	TYR	LEU	ASP	PHE	ALA	GLU	SER	GLY	GLN	VAL	TYR	PHE	GLY	ILE	ILE	ALA	LEU
COW	VAL	PHE	GLN	LEU	GLU	LYS	GLY	ASP	ARG	LEU	SER	ALA	GLU	ILE	ASN	LEU	PRO	ASP	TYR	LEU	ASP	TYR	ALA	GLU	SER	GLY	GLN	VAL	TYR	PHE	GLY	ILE	ILE	ALA	LEU
RABBIT	VAL	PHE	GLN	LEU	GLU	LYS	GLY	ASP	ARG	LEU	SER	THR	GLU	VAL	ASN	GLN	PRO	GLU	TYR	LEU	ASP	LEU	ALA	GLU	SER	GLY	GLN	VAL	TYR	PHE	GLY	ILE	ILE	ALA	LEU
RAT	VAL	PHE	GLN	LEU	GLU	LYS	GLY	ASP	LEU	LEU	SER	ALA	GLU	VAL	ASN	LEU	PRO	LYS	TYR	LEU	ASP	ILE	THR	GLU	SER	GLY	GLN	VAL	TYR	PHE	GLY	VAL	ILE	ALA	LEU
MOUSE	VAL	PHE	GLN	LEU	GLU	LYS	GLY	ASP	GLN	LEU	SER	ALA	GLU	VAL	ASN	LEU	PRO	LYS	TYR	LEU	ASP	PHE	ALA	GLU	SER	GLY	GLN	VAL	TYR	PHE	GLY	VAL	ILE	ALA	LEU

Figure 1 Comparison of TNF sequences. All polypeptide sequences were deduced from the nucleotide sequence of the cDNA genes. The heavy vertical arrow indicates where the mature sequence is cleaved off. A brace above Asn indicates a glycosylation site. Residues identical in all sequences are boxed in with full lines, those which are chemically conservative with dashed lines. References: man (Pennica et al., 1984; Marmenout et al., 1985), pig (Pauli et al., 1989), cow (Goeddel et al., 1986), rabbit (Ito et al., 1986), rat (Shirai et al., 1989), and mouse (Fransen et al., 1985; Pennica et al., 1985).

native cleavage pathway was not clear. Similar results were obtained in *Xenopus laevis* oocytes injected with TNF mRNA.

Are 26-kDa pre-TNF and possibly the intermediates biologically relevant? Kriegler et al. (1988) demonstrated that macrophages stimulated by treatment with endotoxin or phorbol ester produced, in fact, a 26-kDa integral transmembrane TNF molecule, corresponding to the unprocessed translation product of the messenger RNA. Moreover, the mature part of the TNF was exposed on the outside of the cell as it was accessible for iodination. The integral membrane 26-kDa TNF is in part a precursor form of the mature 17-kDa TNF, and a serine-type protease may

Table 1 Homology (%)

	Presequence					Mature sequence				
	Pig	Cow	Rabbit	Rat	Mouse	Pig	Cow	Rabbit	Rat	Mouse
Man	—	76.3	75.9	77.2	75.9	88.5	81.5	80.3	78.3	79.6
Pig[a]	—	—	—	—	—	—	83.4	79.0	78.3	79.0
Cow		—	72.2	70.1	70.1		—	75.2	73.9	75.2
Rabbit			—	74.7	72.2			—	78.9	80.1
Rat				—	92.4				—	94.9

[a]Note that the presequence of pig TNF was not completely determined.

actually be responsible for the cleavage reaction (Scuderi, 1989). Moreover, the membrane-bound 26-kDa TNF may also be directly responsible for cytotoxic and other functions of the producing cell. Indeed, Decker et al. (1987) demonstrated that activated macrophages exert TNF-mediated cytotoxicity by way of membrane-bound TNF. They could even fix the preparation with formaldehyde and still retained biological function (Decker et al., 1987; Espevik and Nissen-Meyer, 1987). Macrophages decorated with membrane-bound TNF may provide a local inflammatory/immune reaction without systemic release of potentially harmful TNF (Luettig et al., 1989).

Cseh and Beutler (1989) found that induced RAW 264.7 cells, a murine myeloid line, secrete, in addition to the mature TNF, larger products, the most dominant of which was an 18.5-kDa protein. This polypeptide was further analyzed and shown to be 10 amino acids longer at the N terminus, which means a cleavage between the Pro-Leu sequence (in human pre-TNF, this would correspond to cleavage between positions -9 and -8, considering that the sequence is two residues shorter in this region). It is not clear whether the 18.5-kDa form was an intermediate in the processing or a final side product. Most remarkably, this slightly elongated TNF proved to be biologically inactive. This result suggests that the small, N-terminal extension may be sufficient to block an active site on the TNF molecule. The conclusion that the material was inactive, however, was based on refolded material, and further experiments are required before this conclusion can be extended to the native form. It is quite possible that the extended TNF form described by Cseh and Beutler (1989) corresponds to the 18.5-kDa hTNF described previously by Müller et al. (1986).

III. STRUCTURE–FUNCTION OF MATURE TNF AND LYMPHOTOXIN

Earlier studies, which means in the precloning era, have mainly been carried out on "natural cytotoxins" derived either from the serum of appropriately treated animals (e.g., by treatment with BCG/endotoxin), from the supernatant of isolated white blood cells (e.g., the adherent mononuclear cell fraction), or from myeloid or lymphoblastoid cell lines (Ruff and Gifford, 1981). We now know that the serum from BCG/endotoxin-treated animals contains almost exclusively TNF, also supernatant from induced macrophages contains TNF, supernatant from antigenically or mitogenically stimulated lymphocytes contains mostly lymphotoxin, while appropriately induced cell lines may either secrete TNF (e.g., U937) or lymphotoxin (e.g., RPMI 1788) or both (e.g., HL-60). Molecular weight estimates of these natural cytotoxins were carried out almost exclusively by gel filtration. Molecular weight estimates for rabbit and human TNF were in the range 30 to 50 kDa, while that for lymphotoxin was, at least for some preparations, in the range 150 to 200 kDa (Ruff and Gifford, 1981). We now know that the exact molecular weight of human TNF is 52,068 Da, and the reason for the lower initial estimates (and the misleading assumption that TNF was a dimer, rather than a trimer) is due to retardation on the gel filtration columns because of interaction with the matrix. Too-high molecular weight estimates, especially for lymphotoxin, were due to interaction with other high-molecular-weight proteins, especially at very low concentrations of the former. Studies on the partially purified, natural material had also shown that mouse TNF is a glycoprotein (Green et al., 1976). Also, human lymphotoxin is a glycoprotein (Aggarwal et al., 1984), while there was no evidence for glycosylation in the case of rabbit or human TNF.

The characterization of these molecules became far more straightforward after the cDNA genes had been cloned and the recombinant proteins could be produced. The subunit of the mature lymphotoxin contains 171 residues (molecular weight: 18,660 Da). The mature human TNF polypeptide is 157 residues in length (Fig. 1), while that of rabbit, rat, and mouse is only 156 residues long. It may be noted that in TNF derived from natural sources the first two amino acids are often partially or completely missing (Haranaka et al., 1985; Marmenout et al., 1985; Shirai et al., 1985); the residues are very exposed (see below) and can easily be clipped off by a trypsin-type enzyme. The lymphotoxin sequence is for 30% homologous to the TNF sequence (see Chapter 3). The greater length of the lymphotoxin polypeptide relative to TNF is completely accounted for by a 17-amino-acid-long extension at the N terminus. The amino acid sequences deduced from the cloned genes also reveal that mouse and rat TNF contain a signal for N glycosylation, and the lymphotoxin genes of all species contain one N glycosylation site. It may be noted that recombinant TNF is usually produced in *Escherichia coli* cells, where it can accumulate to high concentrations; unlike many recombinant proteins, it remains soluble in the bacterial extract, from which it can readily be purified. Remarkably, although the native murine TNF is a glycoprotein, the mTNF produced in *E. coli* nevertheless also remains soluble.

Molecular weight estimates of the native protein could not really distinguish between a dimer and a trimer structure (as mentioned above, the anomalous behavior may be due to interaction with the matrix). But a number of studies have revealed that TNF is really a trimer. This can be demonstrated readily by treatment with cross-linking reagents followed by polyacrylamide gel electrophoresis under denaturing and reducing conditions. Careful physicochemical studies (e.g., by equilibrium ultracentrifugation) confirmed that native TNF is a trimer, and it remains a trimer even at very high dilution (Wingfield et al., 1987; Arakawa and Yphantis, 1987). The conclusion was that the native molecular weight of TNF was in the range 51,900 ± 900 to 52,600 ± 700 in the presence and absence of 0.1 *M* sodium chloride, respectively. These values are in excellent agreement with the exact molecular weight, 52,068 Da, deduced from the DNA sequence. No evidence for any molecular species other than the trimer was found. Also x-ray small-angle scattering spectra indicated a trimer structure with a molecular weight between 50,000 and 53,000 (Lewit-Bentley et al., 1988). Smith and Baglioni (1987) treated

TNF with a nonionic detergent (i.e., Triton X-100) and by gel filtration obtained, in addition to the trimer peak, another peak which they believed to represent monomeric TNF and which had a lower specific biological activity. However, this second peak was not further characterized (e.g., by physicochemical methods). The trimer structure was definitely confirmed by x-ray diffraction analysis of TNF crystals (Lewit-Bentley et al., 1988; Eck et al., 1988). The details of the elegant, three-dimensional structure of TNF (Jones et al., 1989; Eck and Sprang, 1989) are discussed in Chapter 5.

Mature TNF contains two cysteine residues which are in the form of a disulfide bridge (Davis et al., 1987). Treatment of TNF with sodium dodecyl sulfate in the absence of mercaptoethanol readily leads to dissociation showing that the disulfide is only intrasubunit. This conclusion is confirmed by the three-dimensional structure obtained by x-ray diffraction. A comparison between the primary structure of lymphotoxin and TNF reveals four regions of high-sequence homology; when these regions are traced in the three-dimensional structure, they turn out to form exactly the central core where the main interactions between the three subunits occur. It follows that lymphotoxin has a similar trimeric three-dimensional structure (Tavernier et al., 1989; Eck and Sprang, 1989). Although lymphotoxin interacts at high affinity with the same receptor(s) as TNF, nevertheless the exposed protein surfaces are less homologous and the residues that form the receptor interaction site are scattered among less conserved neighbors (see also below). A comparison between the different mammalian TNF sequences reported so far is given in Fig. 1, and the percentage homology is shown in Table 1. All sequences are highly homologous (73.5 to 83.5%), except for human/pig, which scores higher (88.5%) and, not unexpectedly, rat/mouse, which scores 94.9%. The intrasubunit disulfide bridge is conserved in all sequences. There are a few patches where the amino acids can apparently change freely. There seems to be a somewhat looser constraint in the region of positions 19 to 32, although even this sequence contains highly conserved residues. Other patches where the constraint is less firm are, for example, positions 6–8, 70–74, and 111–113.

Considering this high degree of sequence conservation, not only between the TNF sequences (Fig. 1), but also between TNF and lymphotoxin (see Chapter 3), it is, of course, tempting to change the primary nucleotide sequence information by site-specific mutagenesis. The first N-terminal amino acids can be deleted resulting in at most a threefold drop in activity (Mark et al., 1987; Creasey et al., 1987). This can now readily be explained on the basis of the three-dimensional structure, which reveals that indeed the N-terminal segment is a loose end dangling out, while the lysine at position 11 is essential for maintenance of the structure (Jones et al., 1989; Eck and Sprang, 1989). Remarkably, Soma et al. (1988) have reported that changing the N-terminal amino acid sequence (making it more basic) affects the cytotoxicity/systemic toxicity ratio as well as the cell specificity, rendering, for example, the normally resistant T24 bladder carcinoma cells sensitive to the mutant TNF.

The carboxyl terminal end is much more essential, as deletion of the last three residues leads to loss of biological activity (Korobko et al., 1989). Again, this is not unexpected, as the three-dimensional structure reveals that the carboxyl terminus is centrally located at the base of the triangular pyramid. Even as subtle a change as a mutation of Ile_{155} to Leu decreased cytotoxic activity. It has also been claimed that changing the C-terminal leucine residue to phenylalanine increased the differentiation-inducing activity of TNF 20-fold; this activity was quantitated by measuring the ability of treated U937 cells, for example, to reduce nitroblue tetrazolium dye (Kamijo et al., 1989).

As mentioned above, the intrasubunit disulfide bridge is highly conserved among the different TNF molecules, but it is not shared with lymphotoxin (although mouse lymphotoxin still contains the cysteine corresponding to position 69; Li et al., 1987). Conversion of either of the two cysteine residues in TNF to serine did not significantly affect the biological activity, and even the double mutant Ser_{69}–Ser_{101} still had an activity of only about 2.5-fold less than wild type. Hence the disulfide bridge helps to stabilize the structure, but is not essential (Mark et al., 1987). The two cysteine residues have also been changed to alanine or leucine, and although the overall three-dimensional structure was not much affected, the local conformation around the tryptophan residues was altered. The cytotoxic activity was decreased about fivefold in the alanine analog, and about 15-fold in the leucine mutant; macrophage activation and lipogenic activity were affected similarly (Narachi et al., 1987).

All TNF sequences contain two tryptophan residues, and these are conserved even among the lymphotoxin sequences. Each was converted by site-specific mutagenesis to a conservative phenylalanine residue; the mutants 28F and 114F had marginally reduced, biological activity (i.e., about 45% and 30% of wild type, respectively) (Van Ostade et al., 1988). Human TNF contains three histidine residues, at positions 15, 73, and 78; the residues at positions 15 and 78 are conserved not only among the TNF sequences but are also found in lymphotoxin. Histidine residues in proteins can be chemically modified by diethyl pyrocarbonate; such a treatment inactivated TNF, suggesting that at least one His residue is involved in biological activity. Changing by site-specific mutagenesis the histidines 73 and 78 into glutamine did not affect the biological activity. Changing the histidine at position 15, however, reduced the cytotoxicity to about 10 to 15% of wild type; replacing His_{15} with Asn, Lys, or Gly caused a complete loss of bioactivity (Yamamoto et al., 1989). These results strongly suggest that the histidine 15 is at or very close to the receptor-binding site of TNF, or that His_{15} is so linked to this site that changing the residue sterically alters the receptor-binding site. Especially intriguing is the observation that replacing the glutamine at position 15 by asparagine results in a drop of the biological activity by a factor of more than 10,000-fold! The authors propose that the amide N of Gen can fulfill a similar function as the $N\varepsilon 2$ of His (e.g., participate in a hydrogen bond), while the amide N of Asn would be too short relative to the peptide backbone to fulfill this function.

Another approach to the structure–function analysis is by means of antibodies with restricted specificity. Socher et al. (1987) raised antibodies against a number of synthetic TNF peptides covalently linked to a carrier. The peptides were chosen on the basis of a hydropathicity plot to have relatively higher probability of immunogenicity. Although various sera reacted not only with the immunizing peptide but also with hTNF, only one antiserum blocked binding of hTNF to its receptor, namely that obtained by the peptide 1–15. Considering that the first 10 residues are not required for biological activity, one could believe that residues 11–15 may be essential for bioactivity; however, this is not necessarily so. Antibodies provide rather broad footprints and considering the flexibility of the N-terminal segment (Jones et al., 1989; Eck and Sprang, 1989), it could be that an antibody bound to this terminus shields an active receptor-binding site somewhere in the neighborhood (see below). Peptide 1–15 antiserum not only did inhibit the TNF binding to its receptor, but also suppressed the lipoprotein lipase activity, indicating that the latter function is dependent on the same receptor interaction. Tavernier et al. (1990) studied the binding of a monoclonal antibody that neutralized human, but not murine TNF. It was shown that residue Arg_{131} was part of the epitope, as a mutation at this site to glutamine led to complete loss of binding by the monoclonal antibody, but there was no effect on the biological activity of TNF. Hence this position 131 is not part of the active center but is part of the epitope recognized by the neutralizing monoclonal antibody; the latter binds and protects an area of about 20Å, including (part of) the receptor-binding site.

To detect residues that are genuinely part of the putative receptor-binding site and also in order to find out whether there exists more than one area in the TNF molecule critical for the biological activities, a screening system was set up in order to detect mutants obtained by chemical mutagenesis of the total cDNA gene (Fiers et al., 1990; Van Ostade, Tavernier, and Fiers, in preparation). Several residues were detected, the mutation of which resulted in loss of biological activity but not in gross change of the three-dimensional structure of the molecule. For example, mutation of Ser_{86} into Phe led to a more than 10,000-fold decrease in biological activity, while the physicochemical characteristics of the mutated protein were unchanged. Hence position 86 is presumably part of the active center. An examination of the three-dimensional structure of TNF reveals that the Ser_{86} is located in one of the loops at the bottom of the triangular pyramid, close to the cleft between the individual subunits. This area, which we propose to be (part of) the receptor interaction site, is sterically sufficiently close to explain the data obtained with the monoclonal antibody (position 131) and with the N-terminal peptide antiserum (positions 1–15) as discussed above. Also, His_{15} on the neighboring subunit is in fairly close proximity. Considering that lymphotoxin and TNF bind to the same receptor, Eck and Sprang (1989) examined which residues on the surface of the molecule were conserved between TNF and lymphotoxin. This led them to suggest that the receptor-binding site was in a depression at the base of the trimer, which is lined by the sequences 11–15, 37–42, 49–57, and 155–157. This site is close to, but not identical to, the one that we propose (see above), and both may even partially overlap.

The screening for inactive mutants has provided no evidence for a TNF function other than binding to its receptor. Assuming that a TNF molecule contains three receptor-binding sites, it may be that its mechanism of action is merely to cross-link receptors. If so, one would predict that antireceptor antibody would also be able to cross-link the receptors and therefore have TNF-like activity. Indeed, this seems to be the case, as such antibodies can both exert cytotoxic activity on sensitive cells as well as mitogenic activity on FS4 cells and induction of specific genes such as IL-6 (Espevik et al., 1990).

TNF is almost not species specific. Human TNF acts readily on murine cells, and vice versa, although homologous species preference can be observed (Fransen et al., 1986; Kramer et al., 1988). When measured on the standard murine L929 cells, the specific activity of mTNF is only about threefold higher than hTNF. This conclusion is still valid, notwithstanding the recent discovery that there exist two types of human TNF receptors (Hohmann et al., 1989). Cells containing either one (e.g., Hep2 cells) or the other TNF receptor (e.g., U937) respond almost equally well to mTNF. Nevertheless, there are a number of murine systems that do respond to murine TNF and not, or much less, to hTNF. For example, the cell line PC60 can be converted to a specific cytolytic cell line by treatment with IL-2 and IL-1; the latter can be replaced by mTNF, but almost not by hTNF (Plaetinck et al., 1987). In the presence of a comitogenic stimulus, murine thymocytes proliferate in response to mTNF but not to hTNF (Ranges et al., 1988; Ehrke et al., 1988). This species specificity was also observed with a murine T-cell line, CT6, which proliferated in response to mTNF but was not affected by hTNF (Ranges et al., 1989). In the latter system, hTNF could not compete with mTNF for receptor binding. It is possible to study which segments of the highly homologous TNF sequences are responsible for this species-specific receptor interaction by the use of chimeric molecules. These can be constructed by assembling different segments of the murine and human TNF gene, and most of these chimeras retain full biological activity, at least when assayed on L929 cells (Tavernier et al., 1990).

As the human TNF receptors have recently been cloned, it is evident that the way is now open for investigating the detailed interaction between the TNF molecule and its receptor, as well as the subsequent steps in the cellular action pathway. This really will reveal at the molecular level what the structure-function relationship of TNF is.

Note Added in Proof: Yamagishi et al. (1990) have isolated and characterized about a 100 single amino-acid-substituted TNF mutants. They concluded that four regions in the primary sequence are involved in TNF receptor interaction and biological activity: regions amino acid 32 to 34, 84 to 91, 117 to 119 and 143 to 148. Similar conclusions were reached by Van Ostade et al. (1991), who reported that the mutants L29S, R32W, L36F, A84V, S86F, V91A and E146K are nearly or completely inactive, but have retained largely the native, trimeric three-dimensional structure. Some mutations may lead to inactivation because of a local distortion, but others, such as V91A and D143Y are thought to be directly involved in receptor binding. Positioning the inactive mutations on the three-dimensional structure reveals that the receptor-binding site is in the groove between two subunits with regions 29–36 and 143–148 on one side, and 84–91 on the other. Obviously, there are three receptor-binding sites per TNF molecule and this may explain functionality based on receptor clustering, as described above.

REFERENCES

Aggarwal, B. B., Moffat, B., and Harkins, R. N. (1984). Human lymphotoxin. Production by a lymphoblastoid cell line, purification, and initial characterization, *J. Biol. Chem., 259*: 686.

Aggarwal, B. B., Henzel, W. J., Moffat, B., Kohr, W. J., and Harkins, R. N. (1985). Primary structure of human lymphotoxin derived from 1788 lymphoblastoid cell line, *J. Biol. Chem., 260*: 2334.

Arakawa, T., and Yphantis, D. A. (1987). Molecular weight of recombinant human tumor necrosis factor-α, *J. Biol. Chem., 262*: 7484.

Beutler, B., Greenwald, D., Hulmes, J. D., Chang, M., Pan, Y. C., Mathison, J., Ulevitch, R., and Cerami, A. (1985). Identity of tumour necrosis factor and the macrophage-secreted factor cachectin, *Nature, 316*: 552.

Carswell, E. A., Old, L. J., Kassel, R. L., Green, S., Fiore, N., and Williamson, B. (1975). An endotoxin-induced serum factor that causes necrosis of tumors, *Proc. Natl. Acad. Sci. USA, 72*: 3666.

Creasey, A. A., Doyle, L. V., Reynolds, M. T., Jung, T., Lin, L. S., and Vitt, C. R. (1987). Biological effects of recombinant human tumor necrosis factor and its novel muteins on tumor and normal cell lines, *Cancer Res., 47*: 145.

Cseh, K., and Beutler, B. (1989). Alternative cleavage of the cachectin/tumor necrosis factor propeptide results in a larger inactive form of secreted protein, *J. Biol. Chem., 264*: 16256.

Davis, J. M., Narachi, M. A., Alton, N. K., and Arakawa, T. (1987). Structure of human tumor necrosis factor α derived from recombinant DNA, *Biochemistry, 26*: 1322.

Decker, T., Lohmann-Matthes, M. L., and Gifford, G. E. (1987). Cell-associated tumor necrosis factor (TNF) as a killing mechanism of activated cytotoxic macrophages, *J. Immunol., 138*: 957.

Eck, M. J., and Sprang, S. R. (1989). The structure of tumor necrosis factor-α at 2.6 Å resolution: implications for receptor binding, *J. Biol. Chem., 264*: 17595.

Eck, M. J., Beutler, B., Kuo, G., Merryweather, J. P., and Sprang, S. R. (1988). Crystallization of trimeric recombinant human tumor necrosis factor (cachectin), *J. Biol. Chem., 263*: 12816.

Ehrke, M. J., Ho, R. L. X., and Hori, K. (1988). Species-specific TNF induction of thymocyte proliferation, *Cancer Immunol. Immunother.*, *27*: 103.

Espevik, T., and Nissen-Meyer, J. (1987). Tumour necrosis factor-like activity on paraformaldehyde-fixed monocyte monolayers, *Immunology, 61*: 443.

Espevik, T., Brockhaus, M., Loetscher, H., Nonstad, U., and Shalaby, R. (1990). Characterization of binding and biological effects of monoclonal antibodies against a human tumor necrosis factor receptor, *J. Exp. Med., 171*: 475.

Fiers, W., Beyaert, R., Brouckaert, P., Everaerdt, B., Haegeman, G., Libert, C., Suffys, P., Takahashi, N., Tavernier, J., Van Bladel, S., Vanhaesebroeck, B., Van Ostade, X., and Van Roy, F. (1990). In vitro and in vivo action of tumor necrosis factor, *Tumor Necrosis Factor: Structure, Mechanism of Action, Role in Disease and Therapy* (B. Bonavida and G. Granger, eds.), S. Karger, Basel, p. 77.

Fransen, L., Müller, R., Marmenout, A., Tavernier, J., Van der Heyden, J., Kawashima, E., Chollet, A., Tizard, R., Van Heuverswyn, H., Van Vliet, A., Ruysschaert, M. R., and Fiers, W. (1985). Molecular cloning of mouse tumour necrosis factor cDNA and its eukaryotic expression, *Nucleic Acids Res., 13*: 4417.

Fransen, L., Ruysschaert, M. R., Van der Heyden, J., and Fiers, W. (1986). Recombinant tumor necrosis factor: species specificity for a variety of human and murine transformed cell lines, *Cell. Immunol., 100*: 260.

Goeddel, D. V., Aggarwal, B. B., Gray, P. W., Leung, D. W., Nedwin, G. E., Palladino, M. A., Patton, J. S., Pennica, D., Shepard, H. M., Sugarman, B. J., and Wong, G. H. W. (1986). Tumor necrosis factors: gene structure and biological activities, *Molecular Biology of Homo sapiens, Cold Spring Harbor Symposia Quant. Biol. 51*: 597.

Gray, P. W., Aggarwal, B. B., Benton, C. V., Bringman, T. S., Henzel, W. J., Jarrett, J. A., Leung, D. W., Moffat, B., Ng, P., Svedersky, L. P., Palladino, M. A., and Nedwin, G. E. (1984). Cloning and expression of cDNA for human lymphotoxin, a lymphokine with tumour necrosis activity, *Nature, 312*: 721.

Green, S., Dobrjansky, A., Carswell, E. A., Kassel, R. L., Old, L. J., Fiore, N., and Schwartz, M. K. (1976). Partial purification of a serum factor that causes necrosis of tumors, *Proc. Natl. Acad. Sci. USA, 73*: 381.

Haranaka, K., Satomi, N., Sakurai, A., and Nariuchi, H. (1985). Purification and partial amino acid sequence of rabbit tumor necrosis factor, *Int. J. Cancer, 36*: 395.

Hohmann, H. P., Remy, R., Brockhaus, M., and Van Loon, A. P. G. M. (1989). Two different cell types have different major receptors for human tumor necrosis factor (TNFα), *J. Biol. Chem., 264*: 14927.

Ito, H., Shirai, T., Yamamoto, S., Akira, M., Kawahara, S., Todd, C. W., and Wallace, R. B. (1986). Molecular cloning of the gene encoding rabbit tumor necrosis factor, *DNA, 5*: 157.

Jones, E. Y., Stuart, D. I., and Walker, N. P. C. (1989). Structure of tumour necrosis factor, *Nature, 338*: 225.

Kamijo, R., Takeda, K., Nagumo, M., Konno, K., Hasegawa, A., Inaka, K., and Ikehara, M. (1989). Induction of differentiation of human monoblastic and myeloblastic leukemia cell lines by TNF muteins, *Biochem. Biophys. Res. Commun., 160*: 820.

Korobko, V. G., Dobrynin, V. N., Shingarova, L. N., Filippov, S. A., Maksimova, Y. N., Chumakov, A. M., and Davydov, I. V. (1989). Protein engineering of tumour necrosis factors, *2nd International Conference on Tumor Necrosis Factor and Related Cytokines 1989*, Napa, Calif. Abstract WA 113, p. 21.

Kramer, S. M., Aggarwal, B. B., Eessalu, T. E., McCabe, S. M., Ferraiolo, B. L., Figari, I. S., and Palladino, M. A., Jr. (1988). Characterization of the in vitro and in vivo species preference of human and murine tumor necrosis factor-α, *Cancer Res., 48*: 920.

Kriegler, M., Perez, C., DeFay, K., Albert, I., and Lu, S. D. (1988). A novel form of TNF/cachectin is a cell surface cytotoxic transmembrane protein: ramifications for the complex physiology of TNF, *Cell, 53*: 45.

Kull, F. C., Jr., and Cuatrecasas, P. (1984). Necrosin: purification and properties of a cytotoxin derived from a murine macrophage-like cell line, *Proc. Natl. Acad. Sci. USA, 81*: 7932.

Lewit-Bentley, A., Fourme, R., Kahn, R., Prangé, T., Vachette, P., Tavernier, J., Hauquier, G., and Fiers, W. (1988). Structure of tumour necrosis factor by x-ray solution scattering and preliminary studies by single crystal x-ray diffraction, *J. Mol. Biol., 199*: 389.

Li, C. B., Gray, P. W., Lin, P. F., McGrath, K. M., Ruddle, F. H., and Ruddle, N. H. (1987). Cloning and expression of murine lymphotoxin cDNA, *J. Immunol., 138*: 4496.

Luettig, B., Decker, T., and Lohmann-Matthes, M. L. (1989). Evidence for the existence of two forms of membrane tumor necrosis factor: an integral protein and a molecule attached to its receptor, *J. Immunol., 143*: 4034.

Mark, D. F., Wang, A., and Levenson, C. (1987). Site-specific mutagenesis to modify the human tumor necrosis factor gene, *Methods Enzymol., 154*: 403.

Marmenout, A., Fransen, L., Tavernier, J., Van der Heyden, J., Tizard, R., Kawashima, E., Shaw, A., Johnson, M. J., Semon, D., Müller, R., Ruysschaert, M. R., Van Vliet, A., and Fiers, W. (1985). Molecular cloning and expression of human tumor necrosis factor and comparison with mouse tumor necrosis factor, *Eur. J. Biochem., 152*: 515.

Müller, R., Marmenout, A., and Fiers, W. (1986). Synthesis and maturation of recombinant human tumor necrosis factor in eukaryotic systems, *FEBS Lett., 197*: 99.

Narachi, M. A., Davis, J. M., Hsu, Y. R., and Arakawa, T. (1987). Role of single disulfide in recombinant human tumor necrosis factor-α, *J. Biol. Chem., 262*: 13107.

Pauli, U., Beutler, B., and Peterhans, E. (1989). Porcine tumor necrosis factor alpha: cloning with the polymerase chain reaction and determination of the nucleotide sequence, *Gene, 81*: 185.

Pennica, D., Nedwin, G. E., Hayflick, J. S., Seeburg, P. H., Derynck, R., Palladino, M. A., Kohr, W. J., Aggarwal, B. B., and Goeddel, D. V. (1984). Human tumour necrosis factor: precursor structure, expression and homology to lymphotoxin, *Nature, 312*: 724.

Pennica, D., Hayflick J. S., Bringman, T. S., Palladino, M. A., and Goeddel, D. V. (1985). Cloning and expression in *Escherichia coli* of the cDNA for murine tumor necrosis factor, *Proc. Natl. Acad. Sci. USA, 82*: 6060.

Plaetinck, G., Declercq, W., Tavernier, J., Nabholz, M., and Fiers, W. (1987). Recombinant tumor necrosis factor can induce interleukin 2 receptor expression and cytolytic activity in a rat x mouse T cell hybrid, *Eur. J. Immunol., 17*: 1835.

Ranges, G. E., Zlotnik, A., Espevik, T., Dinarello, C. A., Cerami, A., and Palladino, M. A., Jr. (1988). Tumor necrosis factor α/cachectin is a growth factor for thymocytes: synergistic interactions with other cytokines, *J. Exp. Med., 167*: 1472.

Ranges, G. E., Bombara, M. P., Aiyer, R. A., Rice, G. G., and Palladino, M. A., Jr. (1989). Tumor necrosis factor-α as a proliferative signal for an IL-2-dependent T cell line: strict species specificity of action, *J. Immunol., 142*: 1203.

Ruddle, N. H., and Waksman, B. H. (1967). Cytotoxic effect of lymphocyte-antigen interaction in delayed hypersensitivity, *Science, 157*: 1060.

Ruff, M. R., and Gifford, G. E. (1981). Tumor necrosis factor, *Lymphokines*, Vol. 2 (E. Pick, ed.), Academic Press, New York, p. 235.

Scuderi, P. (1989). Suppression of human leukocyte tumor necrosis factor secretion by the serine protease inhibitor p-toluenesulfonyl-L-arginine methyl ester (TAME), *J. Immunol., 143*: 168.

Shirai, T., Yamaguchi, H., Ito, H., Todd, C. W., and Wallace, R. B. (1985). Cloning and expression in *Escherichia coli* of the gene for human tumour necrosis factor, *Nature, 313*: 803.

Shirai, T., Shimizu, N., Horiguchi, S., and Ito, H. (1989). Cloning and expression in *Escherichia coli* of the gene for rat tumor necrosis factor, *Agric. Biol. Chem., 53*: 1733.

Smith, R. A., and Baglioni, C. (1987). The active form of tumor necrosis factor is a trimer, *J. Biol. Chem., 262*: 6951.

Socher, S. H., Riemen, M. W., Martinez, D., Friedman, A., Tai, J., Quintero, J. C., Garsky, V., and Oliff, A. (1987). Antibodies against amino acids 1–15 of tumor necrosis factor block its binding to cell-surface receptor, *Proc. Natl. Acad. Sci. USA, 84*: 8829.

Soma, G., Tsuji, Y., Tanabe, Y., Noguchi, K., Kitahara, N., Tanabe, Y., Gatanaga, T., Inagawa, H., Kawakami, M., and Mizuno, D. (1988). Biological activities of novel recombinant tumor necrosis factor having N-terminal amino acid sequences derived from cytotoxic factors produced by THP-1 cells, *J. Biol. Response Modif., 7*: 587.

Tavernier, J., Van Ostade, X., Hauquier, G., Prangé, T., Lasters, I., De Maeyer, M., Lewit-Bentley, A., and Fourme, R. (1989). Conserved residues of tumour necrosis factor and lymphotoxin constitute the framework of the trimeric structure, *FEBS Lett., 257*: 315.

Tavernier, J., Marmenout, A., Bauden, R., Hauquier, G., Van Ostade, X., and Fiers, W. (1990). Analysis of the structure–function relationship of tumour necrosis factor (TNF). Human/mouse chimeric TNF proteins: general properties and epitope analysis *J. Mol. Biol., 211*: 493.

Van Ostade, X., Tavernier, J., and Fiers, W. (1988). Two conserved tryptophan residues of tumor necrosis factor and lymphotoxin are not involved in the biological activity, *FEBS, Lett., 238*: 347.

Van Ostade, X., Tavernier, J., Prangé, T., and Fiers, W. (1991). Localization of the active site of human tumour necrosis factor (hTNF) by mutational analysis, *EMBO J., 10*: in press.

Wang, A. M., Creasey, A. A., Ladner, M. B., Lin, L. S., Strickler, J., Van Arsdell, J. N., Yamamoto, R., and Mark, D. F. (1985). Molecular cloning of the complementary DNA for human tumor necrosis factor, *Science, 228*: 149.

Wingfield, P., Pain, R. H., and Craig, S. (1987). Tumour necrosis factor is a compact trimer, *FEBS Lett., 211*: 179.

Yamagishi, J., Kawashima, H., Matsuo, N., Ohue, M., Yamayoshi, M., Fukui, T., Kotani, H., Furuta, R., Nakano, K., and Yamada, M. (1990). Mutational analysis of structure-activity relationships in human tumor necrosis factor-alpha, *Protein Eng., 3*: 713.

Yamamoto, R., Wang, A., Vitt, C. R., and Lin, L. S. (1989). Histidine-15: an important role in the cytotoxic activity of human tumor necrosis factor, *Protein Eng., 2*: 553.

5

Crystal Structure of TNF

E. Y. JONES and D. I. STUART
University of Oxford, Oxford, England

N. P. C. WALKER
BASF A.G., Ludwigshafen, Germany

I. INTRODUCTION

In this chapter we focus on the three-dimensional structure of human tumor necrosis factor (TNF) at close to atomic resolution as revealed by the technique of x-ray crystallography. The biological action of the cytokine TNF is dependent on its interactions with other protein molecules, such as cell surface receptors and inhibitors. These interactions are governed by the precise arrangement adopted within three dimensions by the amino acids of the linear polypeptide sequence (primary structure) on formation of the correctly folded tertiary structure. Thus to understand how the TNF molecule performs its biological function at the level of amino acid interactions, one must not only know the amino acid sequence but also the three-dimensional structure.

Structural information at a variety of levels of detail (resolution) has been reported by several authors. One very basic but crucial structural question is that of the oligomeric state of biologically active TNF. TNF has been shown to be present as a trimer in solution by analytical ultracentrifugation (Wingfield et al., 1987; Arakawa and Yphantis, 1987), small angle x-ray scattering (Lewit-Bentley et al., 1988), and gel electrophoresis (Eck et al., 1988); cross-linking studies indicate that this trimer is the active form of the protein (Smith and Baglioni, 1987). At a level up in structural detail, small-angle x-ray scattering also yielded some information on the basic shape of the molecule in solution. This indicated an elongated form for the trimer consistent with a simple bundle of three cylinders (Lewit-Bentley et al., 1988). Analysis of circular dichroism spectra placed TNF in the all-β-sheet class of proteins (Wingfield et al., 1987; Davis et al., 1987). Indeed, Davis and co-workers showed prescience by noting the similarity of the spectra to concanavalin A, which in retrospect may be seen to possess a rather similar tertiary fold. To our knowledge no analysis by ab initio structure prediction and model building based on the amino acid sequence has yielded a correct tertiary structure for TNF. Since the molecular mass of the TNF trimer is too great to allow the use of current nuclear magnetic resonance (NMR) methods, the only route to detailed structural information is x-ray crystallography.

Several different crystal forms have been reported for human recombinant TNF (Eck et al., 1988; Lewit-Bentley et al., 1988; Hakoshima and Tomita, 1988; Walker et al., 1990); in the case of Hakoshima and Tomita the protein has a two-residue N-terminal deletion. All the reported crystal forms exhibit crystallographic and/or noncrystallographic threefold symmetry indicative of the presence of TNF as trimers within the crystal. The three-dimensional structure of TNF has been solved independently from two of these different crystal forms. Jones et al. (1989) reported the structure of the TNF trimer at 2.9 Å resolution solved using trigonal crystals of space group $P3_121$ with two trimers in the asymmetric (repeating) unit. Eck and Sprang (1989) subsequently reported the structure of the TNF trimer at 2.6Å resolution from tetragonal crystals of space group $P4_12_12$ with one trimer in the asymmetric unit; the complete agreement of this structure to the original is particularly gratifying to the current authors. Eck and Sprang (1989) report a current crystallographic R-factor of 23% for their refined structure using x-ray data between 20 and 2.6Å resolution. No solvent model is included and the stereochemistry is good (rms deviation of bond lengths 0.018Å). The current R-factor for the Jones, Stuart, and Walker structure is 20% on all data from 6 to 2.9 A, with no model for the solvent structure and good stereochemistry (rms deviation of bond lengths 0.019 Å). Both these structures were built to high-quality electron density maps [an example from Jones et al. (1989) is shown in Fig. 1] and are now well refined; thus the atomic coordinates should be accurate to better than 0.4 Å. In this chapter, for reasons of familiarity, we will focus on the Jones, Stuart, and Walker data.

A well-refined crystal structure at medium resolution (3 to 2.5 Å), such as TNF, provides a wealth of information: precise atom positions, atomic interactions (H bonds, etc.), solvent accessibility, and variations in flexibility/mobility within the molecule. The environment within the crystal is still essentially that of the solvent; for the trimeric crystals used by Jones et al. (1989) TNF trimers lie in loosely packed arrays perforated by 100-Å-diameter solvent channels; the crystal solvent content is 65%. Only a small proportion of the molecular surface is involved in crystal packing contacts. Such contacts could slightly perturb a few side chains and

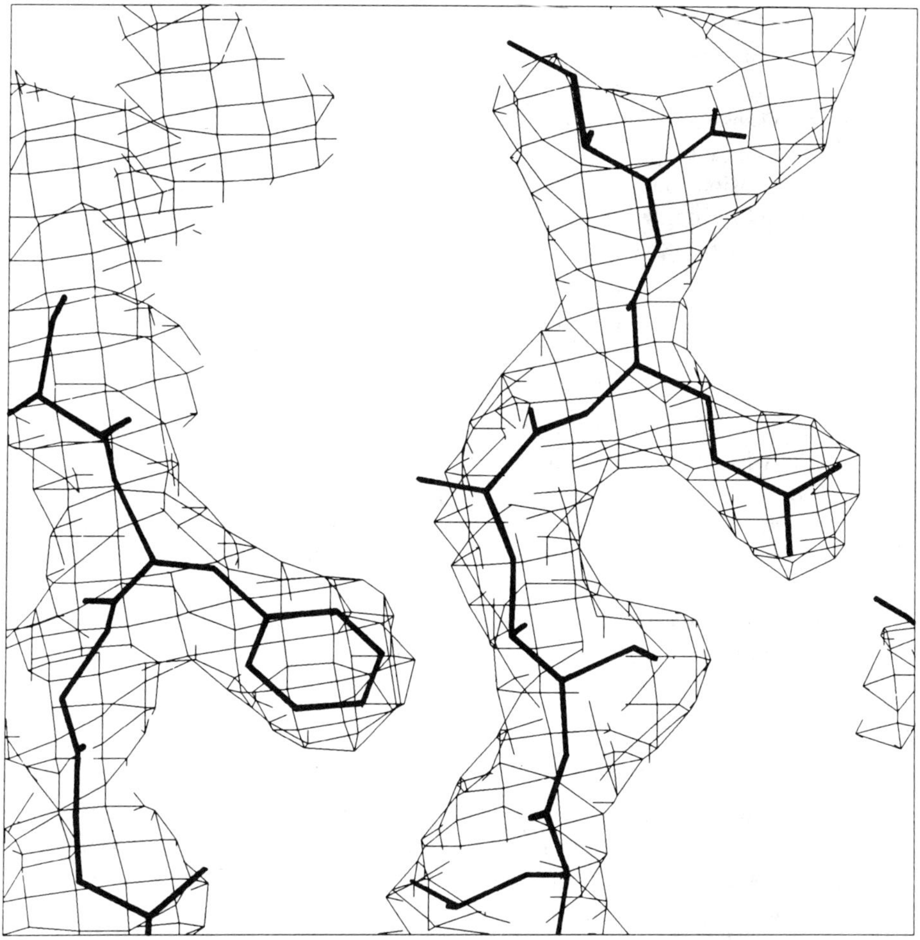

Figure 1 Portion of the electron density map (before refinement) viewed edge on to the β- sandwich. Phe 152 in β-strand I and Glu 135 in β-strand H are shown in the center of the figure. Electron density contoured at an arbitrary level is represented by chicken wire. (From Jones et al., 1989.)

perhaps even short portions of inherently flexible main chain from their preferred solution conformations, but the six independent copies of the TNF monomer in the crystals used by Jones et al. (1989) provide a very effective monitor of any such effects. The mean positional deviations between the six TNF monomers is 0.63 Å on main-chain atoms and 1.05 Å on all atoms.

In the first half of this chapter we present a review of the general topology and structural characteristics of the TNF molecule, including a discussion of its surprising structural homology to viral capsid proteins. This is followed in the later sections by a discussion, in the light of the structure, of data published by other authors on site-directed mutagenesis and antibody binding. An attempt is made to draw overall conclusions on the relationship between the detailed structure of the TNF molecule and its biological function.

II. THREE-DIMENSIONAL STRUCTURE

A. Main-Chain Fold of the TNF Monomer

The overall shape of a single 157-amino-acid subunit of the TNF trimer is wedgelike with height approximately 55Å and maximum breadth 35Å near the base. The main-chain topology is illustrated in Fig. 2; it is essentially a β-sandwich structure formed by two antiparallel β-pleated sheets. The main-chain fold conforms to that of the classic jellyroll motif (Fig. 2c) (Richardson, 1981) common in viral capsid proteins (see Section II. D). The nomenclature adopted in Fig. 2 for the labels of the secondary structural units follows the established convention for the viral structures (Rossmann et al., 1983). The standard eight β strands (B to I) are all present but with an insertion between βB and βC that adds a short β strand onto the edge of both β sheets and truncates the N-terminal half of βC. As noted in Jones et al. (1990b) a similar addition of a pair of β strands to the β barrel occurs in the comovirus, bean pod mottle virus (Chen et al., 1989).

The N terminus is highly flexible; indeed, neither Eck and Sprang (1989) nor ourselves see clear electron density for the first five residues. This region, as far as residue 10, is rather independent of the rest of the molecule, with the first few residues free to sample a variety of conformations in the solvent. In contrast, the C terminus is embedded in the base of the back β sheet and forms an integral part of this relatively flat secondary structural unit. The gradation in β-strand lengths and the insertion between β strands B and C conspire to produce a front surface formed almost entirely of loops, and it is this "masked" side of the, β sandwich, which in the trimer is presented to the solvent. The crystallographic data yield a measure of the relative flexibility of the various parts of the structure. The β strands form a fairly inflexible scaffold; in particular, the back β sheet is situated at the core of the trimer and consequently is particularly rigid. As would be expected, it is the loops that adorn the outer solvent-accessible surface of the molecule, which exhibit high levels of flexibility/mobility. Overall, there is a general decrease in rigidity as the core becomes more loosely packed in the upper half of the molecule.

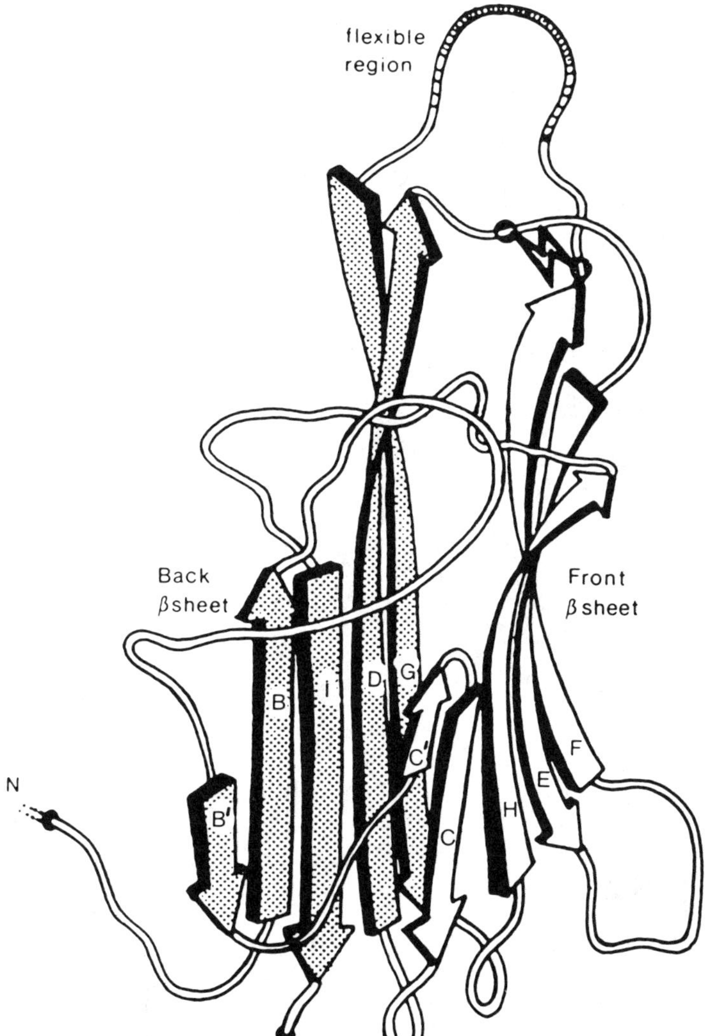

Figure 2 (a) Diagrammatic sketch of the subunit fold, β strands are shown as thick arrows in the amino-to-carboxy direction and connecting loops are depicted as thin lines. The disulfide bridge is denoted by a lightning flash and a region of high flexibility is crosshatched. The trimer threefold axis would be vertical for this orientation.

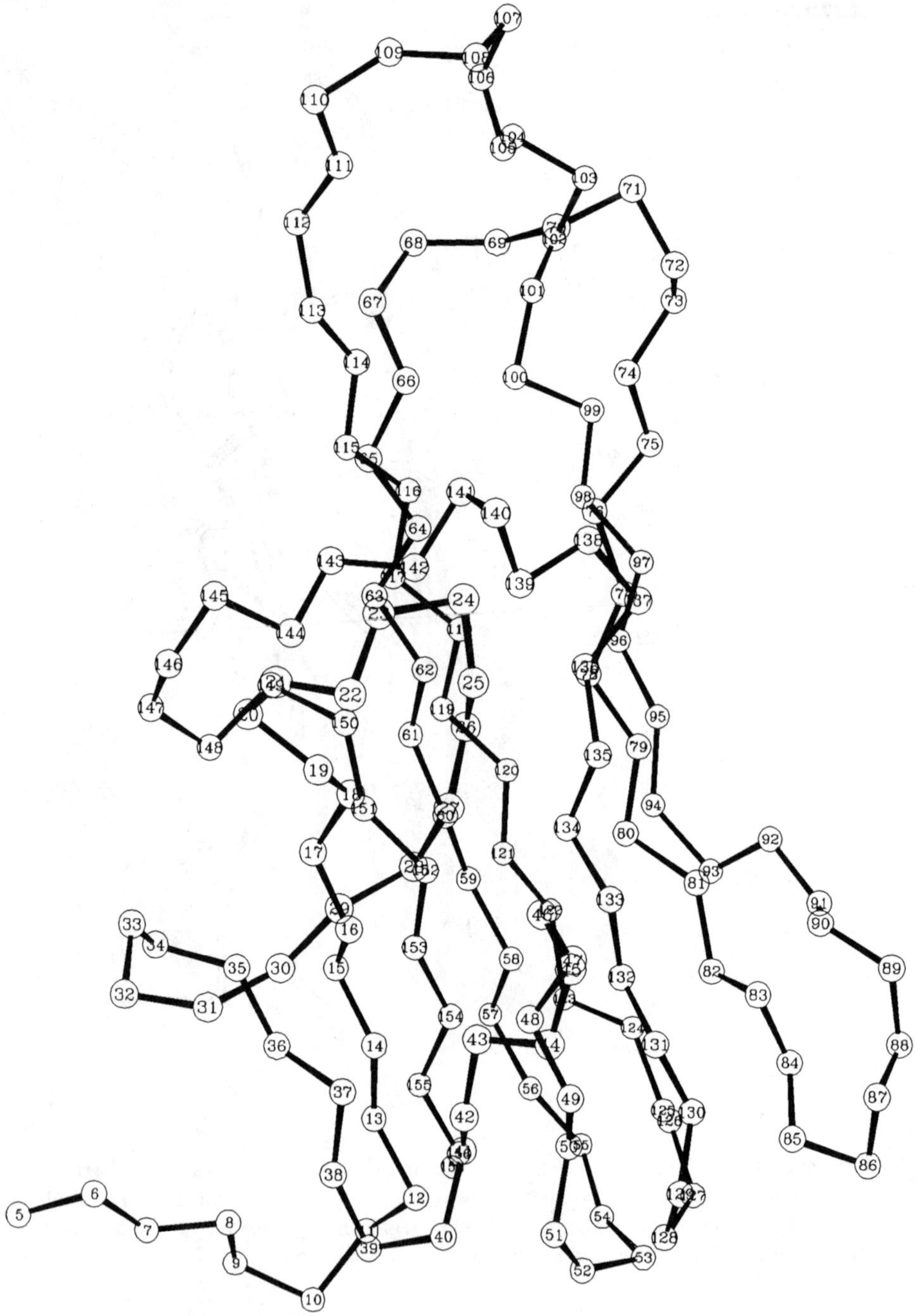

Figure 2(b) Cα chain trace. This detailed representation should be used in conjunction with part (a) to give the precise alignment of the amino acid sequence with the clearer but stylized representation of the subunit fold.

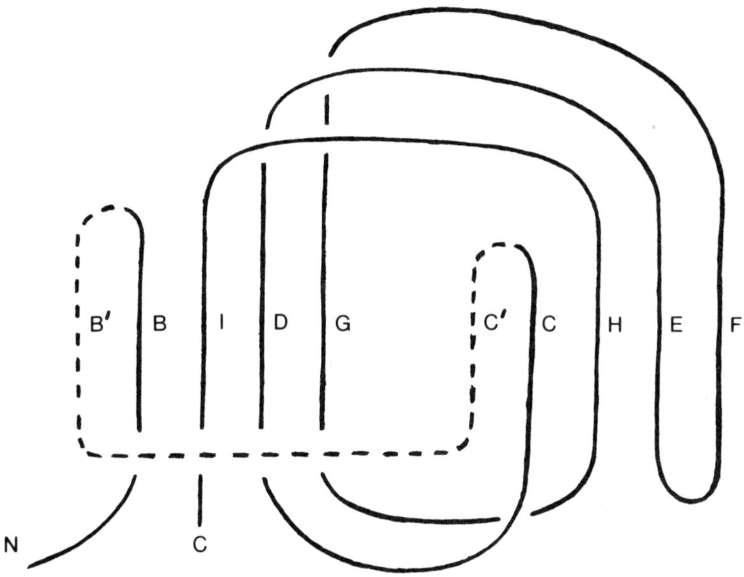

Figure 2(c) Jelly roll motif. The insertion between β strands B and C is shown in dashed lines; normally, the connection between B and C would run straight across at the top of the molecule.

B. General Topology of the TNF Trimer

Three TNF monomeric subunits associate noncovalently to form a compact, conical trimer of length about 55 Å and maximum breadth 50 Å. The β strands of the three individual β sandwiches lie approximately parallel (the tilt is about 30°) to the threefold axis of the trimer. The interaction between subunits related by the threefold axis is through a simple edge-to-face packing of the β sandwich; the edge of the β sandwich, consisting of strands F and G from one subunit, lies across the back β sheet [GDIB] of a threefold related subunit (see Fig. 3). The carboxy termini lie close to the threefold axis. The positions of the N termini, lying away from the main body of the trimer in solution, are compatible with trimer formation by TNF precursor molecules anchored to the cell membrane by a 76-amino-acid N-terminal prepeptide (Kriegler et al., 1988); an analogous situation occurs for the trimeric, membrane-bound hemagglutanin molecule of influenza (Wilson et al., 1981).

The edge-to-face mode of packing produces an extremely tight association between the subunits. Thus the core of the trimer is completely inaccessible to solvent. Loss of solvent-accessible surface area may be equated to hydrophobic free-

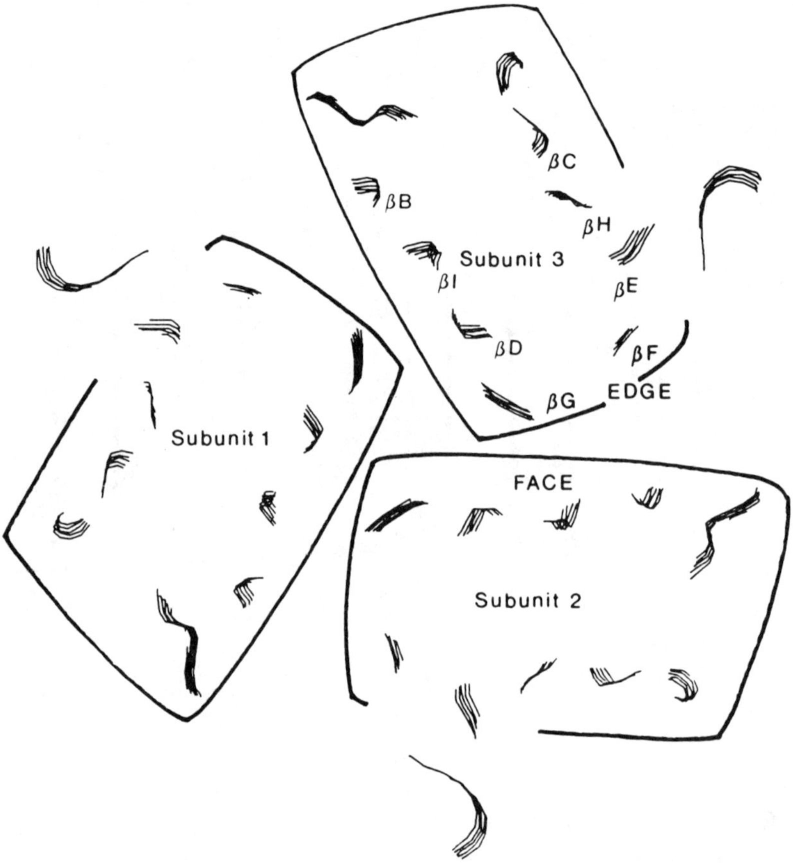

Figure 3 Edge-to-face packing of β sandwiches in the TNF trimer. The view, down the threefold axis, shows a narrow slab of the trimer with β strands represented by ribbons running into and out of the page.

energy gain. Each square angstrom of accessible surface area removed from contact with water gives a free-energy gain of approximately 25 cal · mol (Chothia, 1974). The solvent-accessible surface area buried for a single TNF subunit on formation of the trimer is over 2000 Å, the energetic equivalent of about 30 hydrogen bonds. The stability of the TNF trimer is placed in perspective if one considers that for a typical antibody-antigen complex the epitope comprises a solvent-accessible area of some 700 to 800 Å (Tulip et al., 1989).

```
            1                  20                  40                  60
                     .         .         .         .         .         .
Human       VRSSSRTPSDKPVAHVVANPQAEGQLQWLNRRANALLANGVELRDNQLVVPSEGLYLIYS
Bovine      LRSSSQASSNKPVAHVVADINSPGQLRWWDSYANALMANGVKLEDNQLVVPAEGLYLIYS
Rabbit      LRSASRALSDKPLAHVVANPQVEGQLQWLSQRANALLANGMKLTDNQLVVPADGLYLIYS
Mouse       LRSSSQNSSDKPVAHVVANHQVEEQLEWLSQRANALLANGMDLKDNQLVVPADGLYLVYS
             -- -   - -- -----      -- -    ---- ---  - -------  ---- --
                EEEeeEEbtbtbebbEEbEEEbEbEEEEEtbtebEebEeEEEebebeetbtbtbtb
                        ******                 ***   ***  ***    *******
                          B                    B'    C'   C            D

                               80                 100                 120
                     .         .         .         .         .         .
Human       QVLFKGQGCPSTHVLLTHTISRIAVSYQTKVNLLSAIKSPCQRETPEGAEAKPWYEPIYL
Bovine      QVLFRGQGCPP-PPVLTHTISRIAVSYQTKVNILSAIKSPCHRETPEWAEAKPWYEPIYQ
Rabbit      QVLFSGQGCRS-YVLLTHTVSRFAVSYPNKVNLLSAIKSPCHRETPEEAEPMAWYEPIYL
Mouse       QVLFKGQGCPD-YVLLTHTVSRFAISYQEKVNLLSAVKSPCPKDTPEGAELKPWYEPIYL
            ---- ----      ---- -- - --  --- --- ----   --- --   ------
            tbtbEbEbbEEEtbtbebebbeebEEEEEEEttttttttbbtttEEEEEEEttbtttbtb
            *******        ********       ********              ********
                              E              F                         G

                               140              157
                     .         .         .
Human       GGVFQLEKGDRLSAEINRPDYLDFAESGQVYFGIIAL
Bovine      GGVFQLEKGDRLSAEINLPDYLDYAESGQVYFGIIAL
Rabbit      GGVFQLEKGDRLSTEVNQPEYLDLAESGQVYFGIIAL
Mouse       GGVFQLEKGDQLSAEVNLPKYLDFAESGQVYFGVIAL
            ---------- -- - - - --- --------- ---
            tbtttbeEebEbbbEbEEeEebbEEEtttbtbbbtbt
            ******    ******              ******
                         H                   I
```

Figure 4 TNF sequences from various species. Absolutely conserved residues are indicated by a dash. The positions of the β strands in the human TNF molecule are shown by asterisks [the definition of residues involved in β strand follows the automatic but stringent criteria of Kabsch and Sander (1983)]. Highly solvent-accessible residues (over 50 Å of solvent-accessible area) are flagged by E and moderately accessible residues (50 to 20Å of solvent-accessible area) by e. Residues with less than 20 Å of solvent-accessible area are considered to be buried (Janin, 1979) and are classified as either t for trimer or b for β sandwich, according to whether the major loss of accessibility was on formation of the monomer or the trimer.

C. Amino Acid–Type Distribution

The overall distribution of residue types in the three-dimensional structure of TNF echoes the general rule for proteins: namely, that hydrophobic residues cluster in the core of the molecule while charged residues decorate the surface. Thus the core of the TNF β sandwich has the expected filling of tightly intercalating large apolar residues. In Fig. 4, TNF sequences from various species are aligned, the positions of the secondary structural units are indicated with respect to the human sequence, and residues are tagged as either in the core of the β sandwich or involved in the trimeric threefold interaction or exposed to solvent on the surface of the trimer. Most of the residues that are not conserved between species are situated on the surface of the molecule. Conversely, the residues that comprise the units of secondary structure are highly conserved. Such variations as occur in structurally constrained residues (categories b and t in Fig. 4) tend to be conservative (e.g., isoleucines 58 and 97 occur as valines in mouse TNF).

The detailed distribution of residue types becomes particularly noteworthy in the region near the trimeric threefold axis. Figure 5 details the residues that bury solvent-accessible area on formation of the trimer. At the top of the trimer the interaction between subunits involves charged side chains (Arg 103; Glu 104 and 116; Lys 98 and 112); toward the center it is mediated by polar side chains (Tyr 59, 115, 119, and 151; Gln 61 and 140; Ser 147; Asn 34) and at the base by a patch of large apolars (Phe 124; Ile 155; Val 13 and 123; Leu 36, 93, 94, 55, 57, and 157). The threefold interaction at the heart of the trimer is produced by the edge-to-face packing of the aromatic rings from a nest of tyrosine residues (59, 119, and 151) centered on Tyr 119. Above this point the charged interactions begin to predominate and the subunit packing is generally looser, with the possibility of solvent access down the threefold to Arg 103, testified to by the penetration into this region of the heavy atom compounds used in x-ray crystallography (Jones et al., in preparation). However, below this point the core of the trimer becomes completely inaccessible to solvent. Interspecies sequence variation is rare in the region of the most intimate interaction around and below tyrosine 119. The tightness of the threefold association in the lower half of the trimer is reflected in the general reduction of main-chain flexibility in this region. Overall, there is a gradient of increasing charge, hydrophilicity, and looseness of packing along the threefold axis.

The energetics of the system do not favor the existence of TNF in a monomeric state. For a large interface area composed of complementary residues (e.g., polar residues matched against polar residues) the loss of solvent-accessible surface area confers a considerable energetic advantage to formation of the oligomer (i.e., the trimer). The exposure to solvent of the large patch of strongly hydrophobic residues normally buried in the lower portion of the trimeric interface would also act to destabilize the TNF monomer.

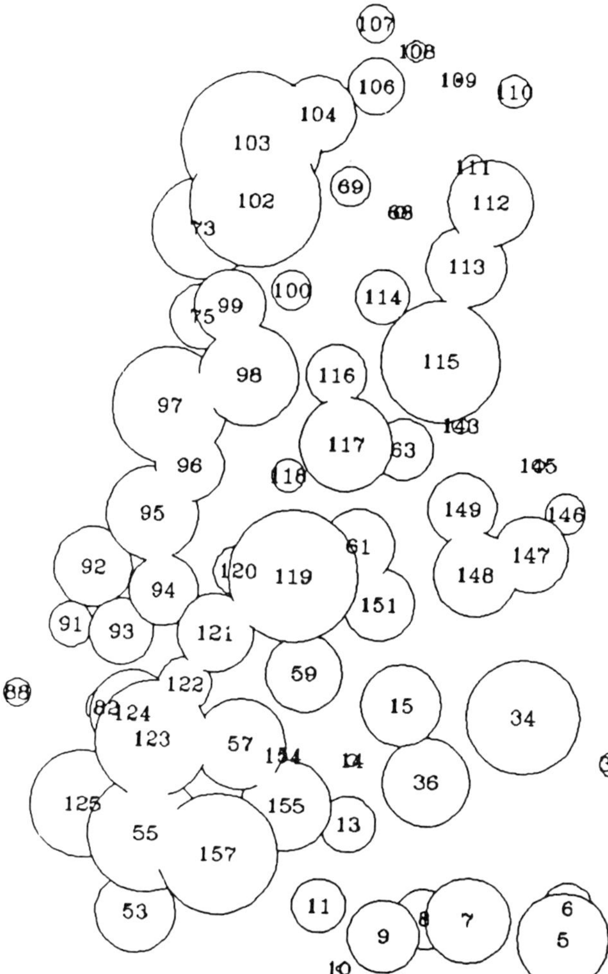

Figure 5 Residues buried at the trimeric interface. The residues for a TNF monomer are represented by spheres with area proportional to their loss of solvent-accessible area on the association of three such monomers to form a trimer. The subunit is viewed looking onto the back β sheet from the threefold axis of the trimer with the threefold axis vertical.

D. Structural Homology to Viral Capsid Proteins

TNF is the first nonviral protein shown to have a main-chain topology that conforms to the classic jellyroll motif. This type of main-chain fold is standard for the proteins that form the external shells (capsids) of small, icosahedral plant and animal RNA viruses. For animal viruses the best studied family, the picornaviridae, includes polio virus (Hogle et al., 1985), rhinovirus (the virus responsible for the common cold) (Rossmann et al., 1985), and foot-and-mouth disease virus FMDV (Acharya et al., 1989). The motif also appears in hemagglutanin, a key surface protein of influenza virus (Wilson et al., 1981), the hexon coat protein of adenovirus (Roberts et al., 1986), and the capsid protein of the SV40 virus (not yet published work by Harrison and co-workers).

The connectivity for the standard eight strands of the viral jellyroll motif and the equivalent elements of secondary structure in the TNF monomer are identical (Fig. 6). The structural similarity between TNF and the viral capsid proteins may be quantified using SHP (Stuart et al., 1979), a program that allows automatic definition of the "equivalent" residues based on a superposition of Cα positions. Typically, over 60% of TNF residues may be matched with rms deviations of less than 3.5Å (Jones et al, 1989), a level of similarity comparable to that obtained between animal and plant viruses or FMDV and hemagglutanin (Acharya et al, 1989). The closest match occurs between TNF and the simple plant virus, satellite tobacco necrosis virus (STNV) (Liljas et al., 1982); 71% of TNF residues are structurally equivalent to residues in STNV with a rms deviation of 3.3 Å.

In general, the level of sequence identity between TNF and the viral proteins is very low (less than 10% based on structural alignment), a situation that is to be expected given than there is a complete lack of measurable sequence conservation even within the viral proteins: for example, between the small RNA animal and plant viruses (Rossmann and Johnson, 1989). There are, however, many common structural features beyond that of the basic motif (Jones et al., 1990b). For the viral proteins the β strands of the [FEHC] sheet tend to be somewhat shorter than those of the [GDIB] sheet (Roberts and Burnett, 1987); this is also a feature of the TNF structure. The N-terminal region prior to βB is highly flexible in TNF, again a property often observed of its longer counterparts in the viral capsid proteins. The jellyroll motif provides a structural building block that may be used in a variety of ways (Argos et al., 1980; Roberts et al., 1986); however, the solvent-accessible outside face in the TNF trimer and in the viral capsid are equivalent sides of the jellyroll. Most strikingly, the mode of packing of jellyrolls in the capsid of adenovirus appears strongly reminiscent of the TNF trimer (R. Burnett, personal communication). The structural similarity between the capsid proteins of the small, icosahedral plant viruses, and subsequently the picornaviruses, has been taken to indicate a common evolutionary precursor (Rossmann et al., 1983, 1985). If this proposal is

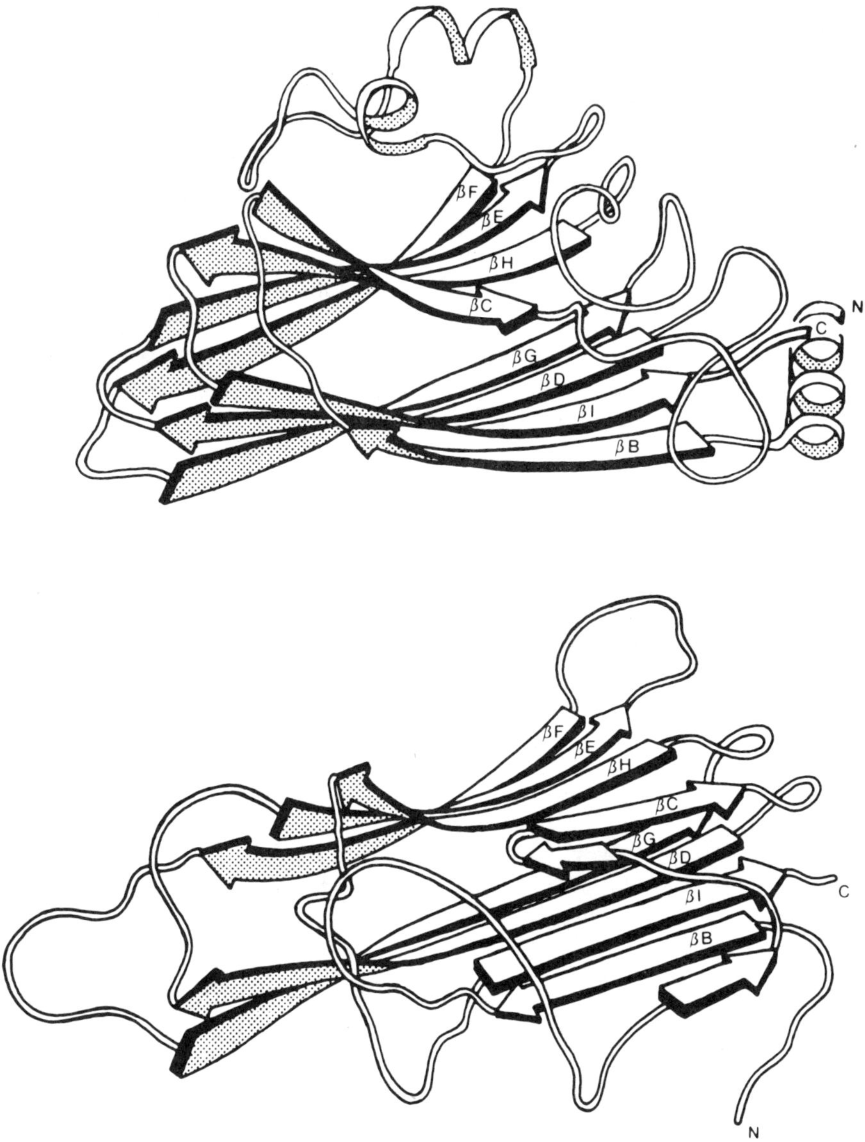

Figure 6 Diagrammatic sketch of the polypeptide fold for STNV (top) and TNF (bottom). β Strands are shown as thick arrows in the amino-to-carboxy direction and are labeled according to the viral convention. An insertion in TNF results in severe truncation of the N-terminal half of the Cβ strand and addition of short, extra β strands to the outer edges of both upper and lower sheets. The TNF trimer threefold axis would be horizontal in this orientation. (From Jones et al., 1989.)

accepted for the viral proteins, the present structural similarity points to the divergent evolution of TNF and these viral proteins from a common ancestor.

The basic antiparallel β sandwich of the jellyroll provides a very stable core arrangement of secondary structure from which connecting loops can provide a myriad of structural variations—a principle similar to that used by the topologically distinct immunoglobulin superfamily. As mentioned in Section II.A, the relative lengths of the β strands allows the solvent-accessible surface of the β sandwich to be completely covered by these loops. Such a surface will place few structural constraints on sequence variation and is thus ideal as a changeable outer surface for animal viruses that must evade the surveillance of the host immune system. TNF represents an austere version of the jelly roll, by comparison with the motif in the picornaviruses, where it is embellished by rather "baroque" loops. Possibly this is because as TNF is part of the immune system, it has nothing to evade. From this argument it is therefore not surprising that TNF most closely resembles the capsid protein of a simple plant virus (STNV) that also has no host immunological memory to evade.

The capsid proteins of the picornaviruses, and hemaglutanin in influenza, also perform the vital role of mediating the cell surface receptor recognition, which allows the virus to gain entry to the host cell. This function of the viral proteins is particularly interesting in view of the parallels with the mode of biological action of TNF, and some salient features will be drawn on in the final section of this chapter.

III. PROBES OF STRUCTURE–FUNCTION

A. TNF/Lymphotoxin Comparison

There is 28% sequence identity between sequences of TNF and lymphotoxin (Pennica et al., 1984). The primary structures of human TNF and various lymphotoxins are aligned in Fig. 7. Lymphotoxin has a longer N-terminal region than TNF (17 extra residues), but in the TNF structure this region lies out in the solvent and is essentially independent of the bulk of the molecule. A short insertion of four extra residues occurs in lymphotoxin after Cys 69 of the TNF sequence and a deletion of six residues after Cys 101 of TNF; these changes map onto the very flexible/mobile loops at the top of the TNF molecule. The majority of the residues conserved between the amino acid sequences of TNF and lymphotoxin may be classified, on the basis of the TNF structure, as internal to the β sandwich or at the trimeric interface; the conservation of the residues that form the surface buried in trimer formation is illustrated in Fig. 8. This conservation in lymphotoxin of residues that play a key structural role in TNF strongly implies the presence of the same β-sandwich motif in the lymphotoxin monomer and preservation of the edge-to-face mode of trimeric association (Jones et al., 1990a). In a simple model-building exercise (Jones and

```
                           1                  20                  40
                                    .         .         .         .
Human                      VRSSSRTPSDKPVAHVVANPQAEGQLQWLNRRANALLANG
Bovine                     LRSSSQASSNKPVAHVVADINSPGQLRWWDSYANALMANG
Rabbit                     LRSASRALSDKPLAHVVANPQVEGQLQWLSQRANALLANG
Mouse                      LRSSSQNSSDKPVAHVVANHQVEEQLEWLSQRANALLANG

Human     LPGVGLTPSAAQTARQHPKMHLAHSTLKPAAHLIGDPSKQNSLLWRANTDRAFLQDG
Bovine    LRGIGLTPSAAQPAHQQLPTPFTRGTLKPAAHLVGDPSTQDSLRWRANTDRAFLRHG
Mouse     LSGVRF--SAARTAHPLPQKHLTHGILKPAAHLVGYPSKQNSLLWRASTDRAFLRHG
                                     KP AH          L W      A    G
                               EEEeeEEbtbtbebbEEbEEEbEbEEEEEtbtebEe
                                       ******                 ***
                                         B                     B'

                             60                      80                  100
                   .         .          .            .         .         .
Human     VELRDNQLVVPSEGLYLIYSQVLFKGQGC-P---STHVLLTHTISRIAVSYQTKVNLLSAIKSP
Bovine    VKLEDNQLVVPAEGLYLIYSQVLFRGQGC-P---P-PPVLTHTISRIAVSYQTKVNILSAIKSP
Rabbit    MKLTDNQLVVPADGLYLIYSQVLFSGQGC-R---S-YVLLTHTVSRFAVSYPNKVNLLSAIKSP
Mouse     MDLKDNQLVVPADGLYLVYSQVLFKGQGC-P---D-YVLLTHTVSRFAISYQEKVNLLSAVKSP

Human     FSLSNNSLLVPTSGIYFVYSQVVFSGKAYSPKATSSPLYLAHEVQLFSSQYPFHVPLLSSQKMV
Bovine    FSLSNNSLLVPTSGLYFVYSQVVFSGRGCFPRATPTPLYLAHEVQLFSPQYPFHVPLLSAQKSV
Mouse     FSLSNNSLLIPTSGLYFVYSQVVFSGESCSPRAIPTPIYLAHEVQLFSSQYPFHVPLLSAQKSV
            L  N L  P  G Y  YSQV F G             L H        Y   V  LS  K
          bEeEEEebebeetbtbtbtbtbtbEbEbb E   EEtbtbebebbeebEEEEEEEttttttttb
           ***  ***    **************            ********       ********
            C'   C           D                      E              F

                             120                 140              157
                   .         .         .         .         .
Human     CQRETPEGAEAKPWYEPIYLGGVFQLEKGDRLSAEINRPDYLDFAESGQVYFGIIAL
Bovine    CHRETPEWAEAKPWYEPIYQGGVFQLEKGDRLSAEINLPDYLDYAESGQVYFGIIAL
Rabbit    CHRETPEEAEPMAWYEPIYLGGVFQLEKGDRLSTEVNQPEYLDLAESGQVYFGIIAL
Mouse     CPKDTPEGAELKPWYEPIYLGGVFQLEKGDQLSAEVNLPKYLDFAESGQVYFGVIAL

Human     YP--GLQE----PWLHSMYHGAAFQLTQGDQLSTHTDGIPHLVLSPS-TVFFGAFAL
Bovine    CP--GPQG----PWVRSVYQGAVFLLTRGDQLSTHTDGISHLLLSPS-SVFFGAFAL
Mouse     YP--GLQG----PWVRSMYQGAVFLLSKGDQLSTHTDGISHLHFSPS-SVFFGAFAL
                       W    Y G  F L  GD LS        L    S  V FG  AL
          btttEEEEEEEttbtttbtbtbtttbeEebEbbbEbEEeEebbEEEttbtbbbtbt
                      **************    ******              ******
                            G              H                   I
```

Figure 7 Sequence alignment for TNF and lymphotoxin. TNF sequences are given in the top four rows followed by lymphotoxin sequences in the next three. Absolutely conserved residues are indicated in a separate row. The positions of the β strands and the classifications according to solvent accessibility are given as in Fig. 4.

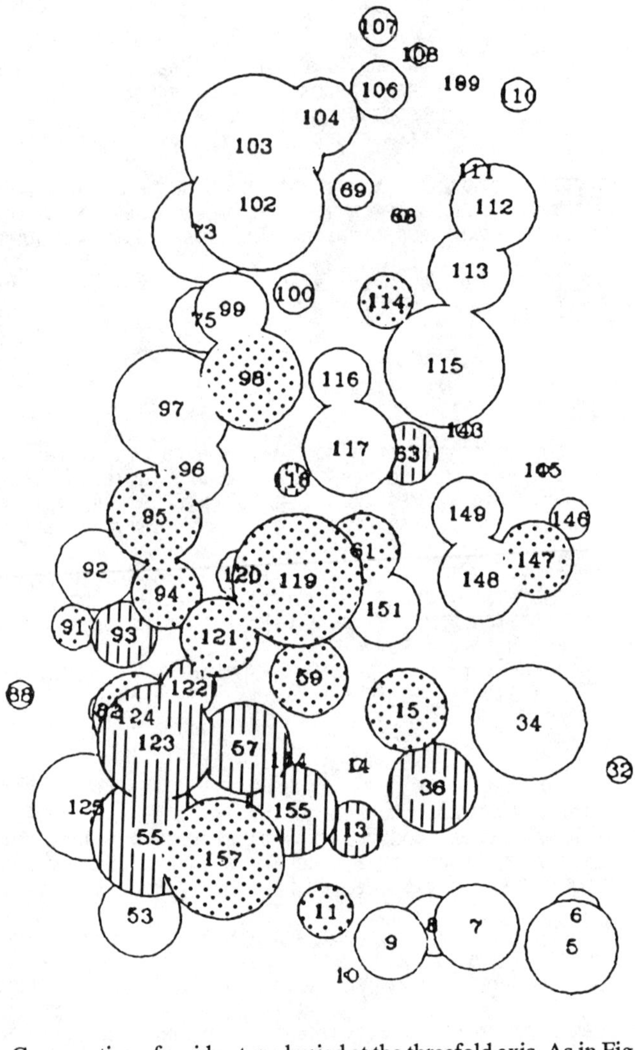

Figure 8 Conservation of residue type buried at the threefold axis. As in Fig. 5, the residues for a TNF monomer are represented by spheres with surface area proportional to their loss of solvent accessible area on trimer formation. Residues that are absolutely conserved in all TNF and lymphotoxin sequences are stippled. Residues that maintain a particular class identity (e.g., large apolars) are hatched. Variable residues remain blank.

Stuart, unpublished) the sequence alignment of lymphotoxin and TNF may be employed to position the lymphotoxin residues in accordance with the TNF main-chain fold. Lymphotoxin has a possible N-linked glycosylation site at Asn 60 (Aggarwal et al., 1985) which aligns with Asp 45 in human TNF; for the model proposed this lies at a sterically acceptable position on the surface of the lymphotoxin trimer (Fig. 9).

As pointed out by Aggarwal (1990), TNF and lymphotoxin exhibit very different properties in terms of sensitivity to proteases. A comparison of the location of trypsin cleavage sites may be made for the two molecules (Fig. 9). For TNF, analysis of the three-dimensional structure reveals several highly accessible, protease-susceptible sequences exposed on the bottom half of the molecule. In contrast, for lymphotoxin, the relevant sequences map primarily to the N-terminal region or the upper half of the molecule. The main site at which cleavage is observed for lymphotoxin (Lys 89) lies in the insertion at the flexible top of the molecule. Thus, given the contrasting distribution of potential cleavage sites, it is perhaps not surprising that the two molecules exhibit a markedly different response when exposed to trypsin. TNF is rapidly biologically inactivated and multiply cleaved by trypsin; lymphotoxin is far more robust, with biological activity unaffected by the single cleavage at the top of the molecule. Although a gross simplification, it is still noteworthy that the severity of the effects on biological activity of this structural disruption partition between the top and bottom of the molecule.

B. TNF/Antibody Interactions

The relative sizes of the TNF trimer (3 × 157 residues) and a single antibody Fab fragment (about 400 residues) are comparable (see Fig. 10); thus it is important to bear in mind that antibodies are essentially rather blunt instruments when employed to probe the properties of the TNF molecule. Nevertheless, a number of groups have reported valuable data involving the mapping of antibody binding to TNF. To relate the results of such experiments to the three-dimensional structure of TNF, it is useful to assess which parts of the molecule are available to interact with an antibody. By analogy with the solvent-accessible surface, the antibody-accessible surface of a molecule may be mapped by computer using the algorithm of Lee and Richards (1971) to test which atoms in the structure are accessible to a 10-Å-radius sphere (Novotny et al., 1986). The sphere crudely models the volume of the interactive tip of an immunoglobulin molecule (Fig. 10) and thus may be used to delineate the regions of the TNF molecular surface to which the antibody has access (Jones et al., 1990c). Thus the residues prominent in an antibodies' "eyeview" of the molecule may be highlighted.

Figure 11 provides a schematic representation of this antibody-accessible surface for TNF. The surface residues highlighted by this procedure comprise the loops connecting the β strands of the β sandwich. In particular, potential linear

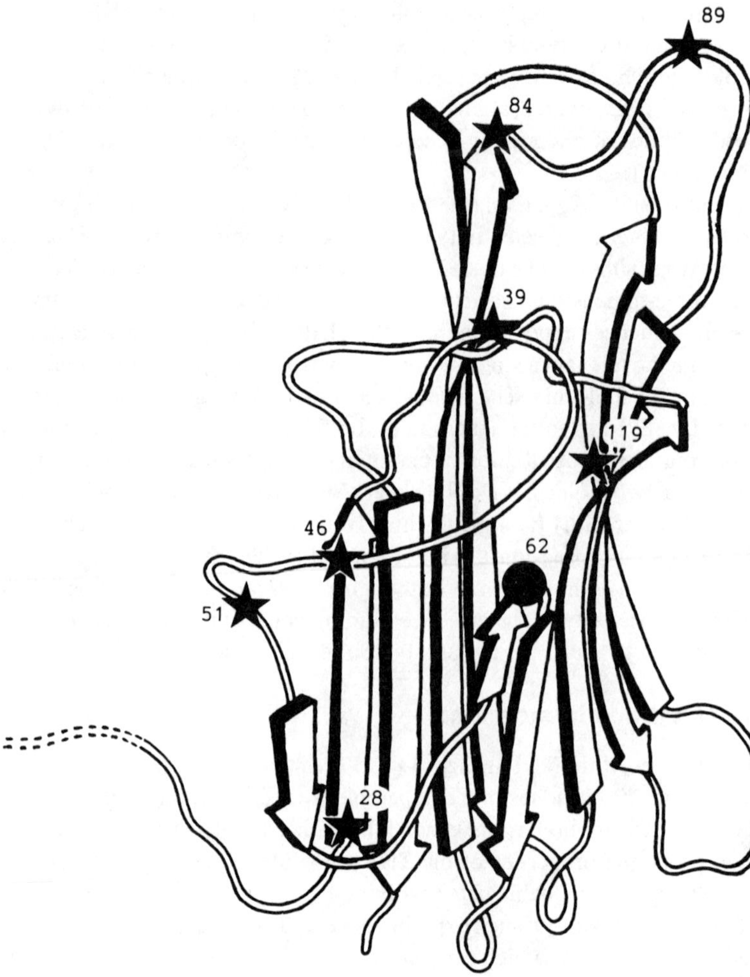

(a)

Figure 9 Proposed main-chain fold for (a) lymphotoxin compared to (b) TNF. Residues are numbered according to the lymphotoxin sequence in (a) and the TNF sequence in (b). The glycosylation site in lymphotoxin is marked by a black circle. Stars denote potential trypsin cleavage sites. Basic residues 31, 32, 44, 90, and 128 in TNF are all on very exposed parts of the polypeptide chain. None of these exposed sites are conserved on lymphotoxin. Two additional sites in the N-terminal region of TNF and lymphotoxin are not marked.

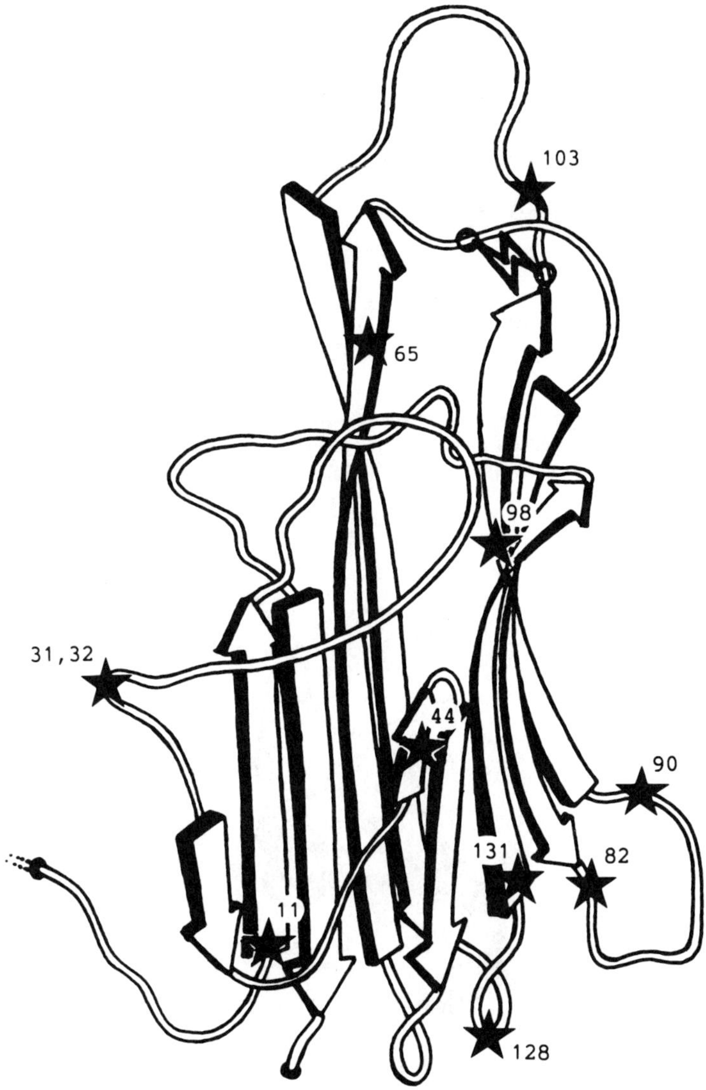

(b)

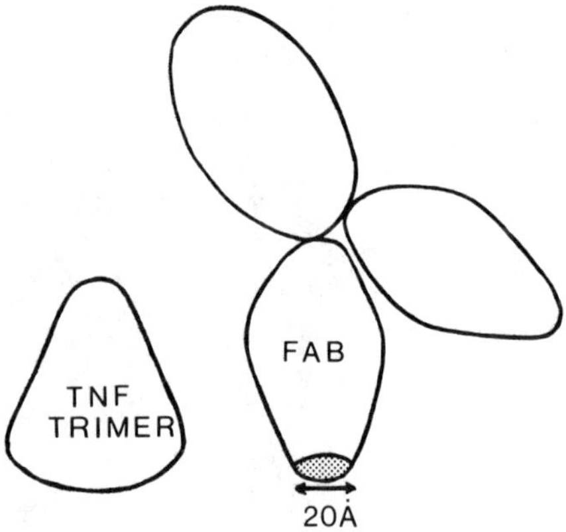

Figure 10 Relative sizes of the TNF trimer and an IgG immunoglobulin molecule. The interactive tip of one arm of the immunoglobulin molecule is stippled.

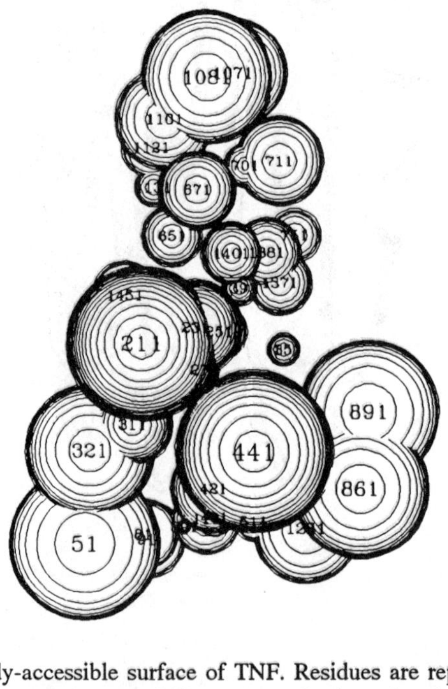

Figure 11 Antibody-accessible surface of TNF. Residues are represented by spheres with area proportional to their accessibility to an antibody molecule. Labels give residue number followed by subunit number (in this case, 1, since only one subunit of the trimer is shown).

epitopes are presented by stretches of sequence at the N terminus, residues 21 to 27, 65 to 71, 107 to 112, and 137 to 140. If the TNF structure is now assessed with respect to conformational flexibility, it is these same loop regions that display the highest structural mobility/disorder in the x-ray structure. Socher et al. (1987) raised antisera against five synthetic peptides, corresponding to residues 1 to 15, 1 to 31, 65 to 79, 98 to 111, and 124 to 141 of the human TNF sequence. All five sets of antisera responded to the native TNF molecule. On reappraisal of these data in the light of Fig. 11 it is not surprising to find that the antibodies raised against these peptides also bind to the native TNF molecule. In each case the peptide incorporates the sequence of one of the highly flexible loop regions which form potential linear epitopes prominently displayed on the surface of the native TNF structure. The combination over part of the amino acid sequence of high accessibility and flexibility allows this class of epitope to be mimicked by individual peptides (Tainer et al., 1984).

It has been observed that antibodies raised against TNF from one species (e.g., human) do not cross-react with TNF from another species (e.g., mouse) despite a sequence identity in excess of 80% and the ability of TNF to bind to the TNF receptors of other species (Fiers et al., 1987). As discussed in Section II. C, if the degree of sequence variation is mapped onto the three-dimensional structure, it is immediately obvious that the most sequence-variable regions of the molecule correspond to the antibody-accessible surface loops. The regions of highly conserved residues within the β sandwich or at the trimeric interface are effectively invisible to antibodies. Thus the epitope for an antibody against TNF will always contain some residues that will vary between species, thus abolishing antibody binding. This implies that the characteristics of the interaction between TNF and its receptor must somehow differ from those required for binding of an antibody to TNF.

The failure of the peptides of Socher et al. (1987) to compete in receptor binding points to a receptor binding site on TNF composed of residues drawn from various regions of the primary sequence (i.e., the equivalent of a discontinuous epitope for antibody binding). Neutralizing antibodies represent a small subset of the total antibody titer and have so far been mapped to two regions, amino acids 1 to 15 (Socher et al., 1987) and an epitope involving Arg 131 (Fiers et al., 1990). A possible interpretation of these results will discussed in the final section.

C. Site-Directed Mutagenesis

The role of various specific residues and regions of a molecule may be probed by replacement of those residues by different amino acids or deletion of part of the sequence using the techniques of site-directed mutagenesis. The results of a number of such experiments have recently been reported for TNF. As indicated by Goh et al. (1990), these diverse data may be brought together and interpreted in terms of the three-dimensional structure of the TNF trimer. A summary of the available data is given in Tables 1 to 4. By reference to the structure, the table is divided into sections that detail N-terminal deletions and/or mutations up to residue 10, mutations of residues internal to the β sandwich, mutations of residues involved in the interaction at the trimeric threefold axis, and mutations of residues on the surface of the trimer. The biological activity of a mutant TNF is generally assayed in terms of cytotoxicity, and this is employed in Table 1 as a measure of the impact of the structural change on function; for some of the mutants their ability to bind to the TNF receptor has been monitored directly and these data are included in the text where appropriate.

The N-terminal region is treated separately in Table 1 since it is a flexible region somewhat isolated from the major portion of the molecule. The deletion of up to eight residues from the N terminus without any deleterious effect on biological activity serves to emphasize the nonessential nature of this region for overall molecular stability. Indeed, several groups report a somewhat surprising increase in biological activity as a result of N terminal deletions, and Soma et al. (1987) report a broadening of the specificity of the cytotoxicity for TNFs with mutant N-terminal regions. Thus the N-terminal residues appear to exert an indirect, second-order effect on the biological efficacy of the TNF trimer.

From Table 2 in particular data reported by Yamagishi et al. (1989), it is clear that nonconservative mutations of the normally highly conserved residues which form the tightly packed core of the β sandwich distort the structure and hence abro-

Table 1 Site-Directed Mutagenesis on TNF: The N-Terminal Region

Nature of mutation[a]	Cytotoxicity[b]	Reference
-4	OK	Carlino et al. (1987)
-7	OK	Carlino et al. (1987)
-8	OK	Carlino et al. (1987)
-9 D10M	*	Carlino et al. (1987)
S5T D10R	WD	Soma et al. (1987)
-2	UP	Kamijo et al. (1989)
-2 S3T S4T S5T	OK	Kamijo et al. (1989)
R2K S4H T7H	OK	Kamijo et al. (1989)
-5	OK	Tsujimoto et al. (1987)
-2	OK	Masegi et al. (1989)
-7	UP	Masegi et al. (1989)
-7 P8R S9K D10R	UP	Masegi et al. (1989)

[a]-4 denotes an N-terminal deletion of four residues and D10M a mutation of Asp 10 to Met.
[b]The cytotoxicity of the mutant relative to native TNF is denoted by UP for an increase of over 200%, WD for broadened cell specificity, OK for over 50%, * for 50 to 5%, ** for less than 5%, and unfolded for incorrectly folded.

Table 2 Site-Directed Mutagenesis on TNF: Residues Internal in the Monomer

Residue	Mutation	Cytotoxicity[a]	Reference
Ala 14	Thr	Unfolded	Yamagishi et al. (1989)
Val 16	Ala	Unfolded	Yamagishi et al. (1989)
Ala 18	Val	*	Yamagishi et al. (1989)
Asn 19	Thr	Unfolded	Yamagishi et al. (1989)
Leu 26	Phe	Unfolded	Yamagishi et al. (1989)
Trp 28	Arg	Unfolded	Yamagishi et al. (1989)
Trp 28	Phe	*	Van Ostade et al. (1988)
Ala 35	His	**	Masegi et al. (1989)
Ala 38	Val	*	Yamagishi et al. (1989)
Val 50	Met	OK	Yamagishi et al. (1989)
Tyr 50	Met	OK	Yamagishi et al. (1989)
Tyr 56	Cys	Unfolded	Yamagishi et al. (1989)
Ser 60	Pro	Unfolded	Yamagishi et al. (1989)
Val 62	Asp	Unfolded	Yamagishi et al. (1989)
Phe 64	Ser	Unfolded	Yamagishi et al. (1989)
Cys 69	Ser	OK	Tsujimoto et al. (1987)
Cys 69	Ser	OK	Yamagishi et al. (1989)
Cys 69 + 101	Ala + Ala	*	Narachi et al. (1987)
Cys 69 + 101	Leu + Leu	*	Narachi et al. (1987)
His 78	Gln	*	Yamamoto et al. (1989)
Ala 84	Asp	**	Yamagishi et al. (1989)
Ala 84	His	**	Masegi et al. (1989)
Pro 100	His	OK	Yamagishi et al. (1989)
Cys 101	Ser	*	Yamagishi et al. (1989)
Trp 114	Phe	*	Van Ostade et al. (1989)
Leu 120	Gln	OK	Yamagishi et al. (1989)
Leu 126	Gln	Unfolded	Yamagishi et al. (1989)
Asp 130	Ala	Unfolded	Yamagishi et al. (1989)
Ser 133	Ile	OK	Yamagishi et al. (1989)
Ala 134	Thr	OK	Yamagishi et al. (1989)
Asp 143	Tyr	**	Yamagishi et al. (1989)
Val 150	Asp	Unfolded	Yamagishi et al. (1989)
Phe 152	Leu	Unfolded	Yamagishi et al. (1989)
Gly 153	Glu	Unfolded	Yamagishi et al. (1989)

[a]The cytotoxicity of the mutant relative to native TNF is denoted by UP for an increase of over 200%, WD for broadened cell specificity, OK for over 50%, * for 50 to 5%, ** for less than 5%, and unfolded for incorrectly folded.

Table 3 Site-directed Mutagenesis on TNF: Residues Internal in the Trimer

Residue	Mutation	Cytotoxicity[a]	Reference
His 15	Gln	*	Yamamoto et al. (1989)
His 15	Asn	**	Yamamoto et al. (1989)
His 15	Lys	**	Yamamoto et al. (1989)
His 15	Gly	**	Yamamoto et al. (1989)
His 15	Tyr	Unfolded	Yamagishi et al. (1989)
Asn 34	Tyr	**	Yamagishi et al. (1989)
Leu 36	Ile	OK	Yamagishi et al. (1989)
Gln 61	Leu	Unfolded	Yamagishi et al. (1989)
His 73	Gln	*	Yamamoto et al. (1989)
Leu 75	Pro	*	Yamagishi et al. (1989)
Ser 95	Pro	Unfolded	Yamagishi et al. (1989)
Ala 96	Thr	Unfolded	Yamagishi et al. (1989)
Ser 99	Asn	*	Yamagishi et al. (1989)
Tyr 115	Cys	*	Yamagishi et al. (1989)
Pro 117	Leu	**	Yamagishi et al. (1989)
Tyr 119	His	**	Yamagishi et al. (1989)
Val 123	Gly	Unfolded	Yamagishi et al. (1989)
Ser 147	Cys	**	Yamagishi et al. (1989)
Gly 148	Glu	**	Yamagishi et al. (1989)
Ile 155	Leu	*	Yamagishi et al. (1989)
Leu 157	Phe	UP	Kamijo et al. (1989)
Leu 157	Met	OK	Yamagishi et al. (1989)

[a]The cytotoxicity of the mutant relative to native TNF is denoted by UP for an increase of over 200%, WD for broadened cell specificity, OK for over 50%, * for 50 to 5%, ** for less than 5%, and unfolded for incorrectly folded.

gate the ability of the molecule to function. Indeed, many such muteins fail to form a stable, correctly folded molecule. The bulk of the mutations for which the molecule retains some biological activity are conservative, preserving the hydrophobic nature of the residues, if not their exact shape. Such changes in volume may be accommodated by minor rearrangement within the core, and indeed, many of the biologically viable mutations are at positions on the periphery of the core. In particular, Cys 69 and Cys 101, which form the disulfide bridge at the loosely packed top of the molecule, are relatively insensitive to changes, Ala 35 and Ala 84 have both been subjected to nonconservative changes with resultant dramatic loss of biological activity. In contrast, Leu 120, Ser 133, and Ala 134 all accommodate a change in partial charge without causing a major structural perturbation.

Table 4 Site-Directed Mutagenesis on TNF: External Residues

Residue	Mutation	Cytotoxicity[a]	Reference
Arg 31 + 32	Asn + Thr	**	Tsujimoto et al. (1987)
Arg 32	Glu	**	Masegi et al. (1989)
Ala 33	Thr	**	Yamagishi et al. (1989)
Leu 37	Pro	Unfolded	Yamagishi et al. (1989)
Asn 46	Asp	Unfolded	Yamagishi et al. (1989)
Gln 47	Pro	Unfolded	Yamagishi et al. (1989)
Ser 52	Pro	Unfolded	Yamagishi et al. (1989)
Thr 72	Tyr	OK	Yamagishi et al. (1989)
Ser 86	Phe	**	Fiers et al. (1990)
Tyr 87	His	**	Yamagishi et al. (1989)
Val 91	Ile	*	Yamagishi et al. (1989)
Thr 105	Pro	*	Yamagishi et al. (1989)
Glu 110	Lys	Unfolded	Yamagishi et al. (1989)
Gly 129	Asp	Unfolded	Yamagishi et al. (1989)
Arg 131	Gln	OK	Tavernier et al. (1990)
Glu 135	Lys	Unfolded	Yamagishi et al. (1989)
Asn 137	Asp	Unfolded	Yamagishi et al. (1989)
Arg 138	Leu	OK	Tavernier et al. (1990)
Asp 140	Tyr	Unfolded	Yamagishi et al. (1989)
Ala 145	Val	*	Yamagishi et al. (1989)
Glu 146	Lys	**	Yamagishi et al. (1989)

[a]The cytotoxicity of the mutant relative to native TNF is denoted by UP for an increase of over 200%, WD for broadened cell specificity, OK for over 50%, * for 50 to 5%, ** for less than 5%, and unfolded for incorrectly folded.

The distribution of mutated residues from Table 3 is illustrated in Fig. 12. It is apparent that any changes in the normally highly conserved residues forming the central region of the trimeric interface are disastrous in terms of biological activity. Provided that the changes are conservative (i.e., apolar to apolar), some variation is permitted within the hydrophobic patch at the bottom of the threefold axis; however, there appears to be much greater leeway in the more loosely packed region near the top of the trimer.

Ostensibly, all residues on the surface of the molecule at the aqueous interface have a considerably greater freedom to mutate without incurring disastrous structural penalties as witnessed by the proliferation of variations between species for residues in this category. Thus a drastic reduction in biological activity points to the involvement of such residues in the functional interaction of the TNF trimer with

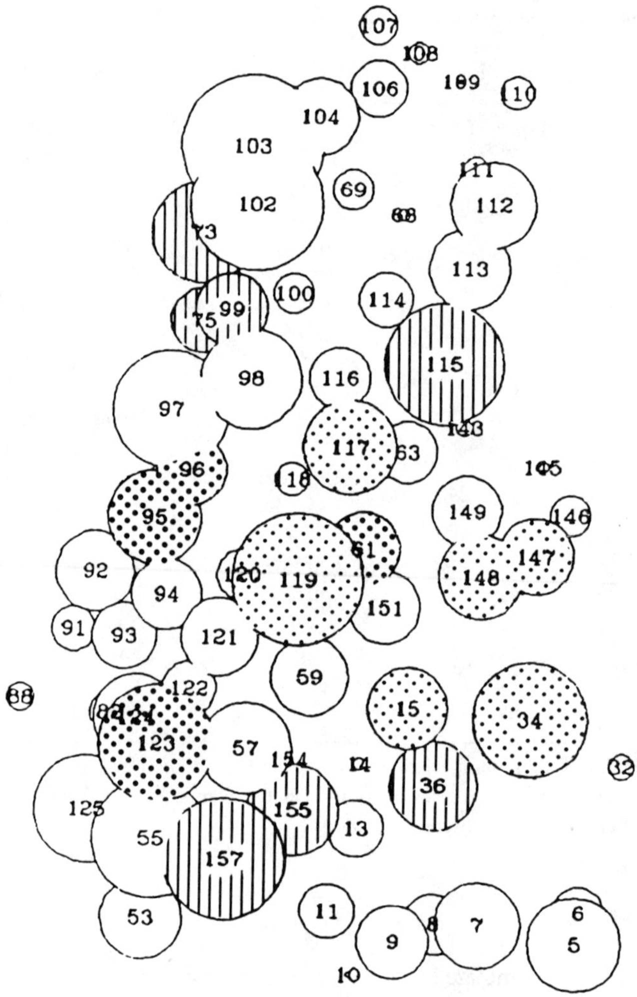

Figure 12 Distribution and biological activity of mutated residues buried at the threefold axis. As in Fig. 5, the residues for a TNF monomer are represented by spheres with area proportional to their loss of solvent-accessible area on trimer formation. Residues that when mutated obstruct correct folding are heavily stippled, those for which cytotoxicity drops to less than 5% are lightly stippled, and residues for which cytotoxicity remains greater than 5% are hatched. Residues for which there is no mutant data remain blank.

another molecule such as the receptor. For the mutations of external residues listed in Table 3, residues Arg 31, Arg 32, Ala 33, Ser 86, Tyr 87, and Glu 146 appear to comprise regions crucial for biological activity. These are illustrated in Fig. 13 and appear to fall into two distinct regions on the left-and the right-hand sides of the TNF monomer. The distribution of all deleterious mutations regardless of structural category further reinforces this picture. The existence of these "hotspots" for sensitivity of biological function to mutation has been remarked on by Yamagishi et al. (1989) and Goh et al. (1990).

IV. DISCUSSION

A rich variety of data may now be brought to bear on the specific relationship of structure to function for TNF. As reviewed in the introduction, all available evidence points to the importance of the trimer as the stable natural unit. In Fig. 14 the various pieces of evidence from the preceding sections are combined in terms of the trimer structure. It is apparent that the two hotspot regions situated on separate sides of the TNF monomer in Section III. C are brought close to each other in terms of neighboring subunits in the trimer. Thus a region of functional importance consisting of residues 31 to 35, 84–87, and 143–148 appears to be located at the interface between two subunits on the lower half of the trimer. Yamagishi et al. (1989) report loss of receptor binding ability as well as cytotoxicity for the mutation of Asp 143 to Tyr, and Tsujimoto et al. (1987) report a similar effect for Arg 31 and Arg 32 to Asn and Thr. Thus the site may be associated directly with receptor binding as well as cytotoxicity.

Secondary evidence implicating this region in receptor binding is provided by the behavior of the N terminus. It is apparent from Fig. 14 that the highly flexible N-terminal region could cause mild steric hinderance to an incoming receptor molecule and hence explain the observed benefits of a truncated N terminus. Similarly, the antibodies to the N terminus reported by Socher et al. (1987) would tend to be positioned in such a way as to block receptor binding, leading to neutralizing behavior through steric hinderance. This hypothesis can also incorporate the findings of Fiers et al. (1990), for which an antibody with an epitope involving Arg 131 neutralizes TNF. Again this antibody binds sufficiently close to the putative receptor binding site to block the receptor. It is noteworthy that this region would be unaffected by the cloaking effect of the oligosaccharide in lymphotoxin. Trypsin cleavage in TNF would be disastrous for the structural integrity of the putative receptor binding site but would not affect the corresponding region in lymphotoxin. Thus all currently available evidence fits satisfactorily with this putative binding site. However, one possible weakness in the hypothesis is the behavior of Tyr 87, which is exposed to solvent and as such would be expected to act as a site for iodination in radiolabeling experiments, yet this chemical modification within a

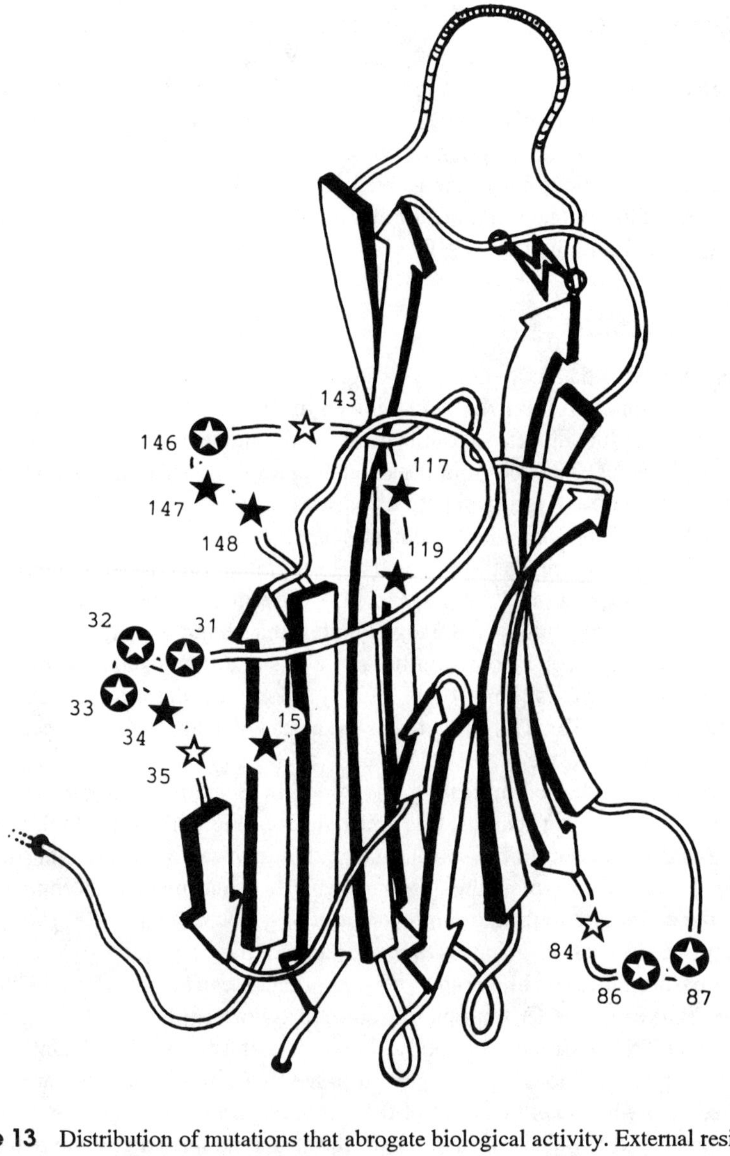

Figure 13 Distribution of mutations that abrogate biological activity. External residues are indicated by a white star on a black disk. Black stars mark residues involved in trimer stability and white stars show residues internal to the TNF monomer. Mutation of each of these residues reduces cytotoxicity to less than 5% of the native level.

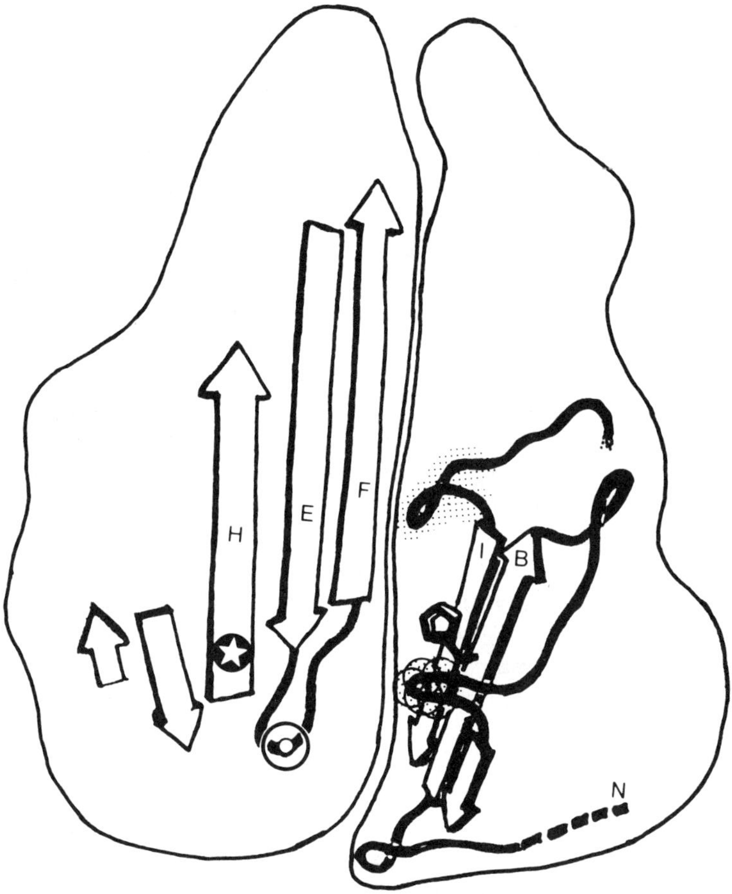

Figure 14 Putative area of receptor binding. This schematic diagram highlights the relative positions of Tyr 87 (white circle) and Arg 131 (star) on one subunit, also His 15 (pentagon), the loop comprising residues 31 to 35 (linked circles and stippling), and residues 143 to 148 (stippling) on the neighboring subunit in the trimer.

region comprising part of the putative receptor binding site does not affect biological activity.

It is interesting that the functional region of TNF appears to lie at the interface between two subunits, a situation which echoes that found in some oligomeric enzymes (e.g., phosphofructokinase) (Schirmer and Evans, 1990). Surprisingly, there is relatively low conservation of residues in this region between TNF and lymphotoxin or indeed between different TNF species; this parallels the situation in interleukine I (Priestle et al., 1989).

Eck and Sprang (1989) propose a putative receptor binding site located in a shallow depression on the base of the trimer involving residues 11 to 13, 37 to 42, 49 to 57, and 155 to 157. Their conclusions are based on their interpretation of TNF and lymphotoxin homology and the general evidence [N-terminal deletions, the neutralizing antibody of Socher et al. (1987)] cited above which points to a region of functional importance situated on the lower half of the trimer. From Table 1 to 4, mutations at residues 37, 38, 50, 52, 56, 155, and 157 fall within the Eck and Sprang site but provide no compelling evidence for biological function associated with this region. However, the hypothesis should stand, awaiting more conclusive evidence from further mutations.

The biological interactions of TNF may well prove to be particularly complex, since Hohmann et al. (1989) report more than one type of TNF receptor. Also the role of the site(s) depicted in Fig. 14 may not be restricted to receptor binding since as Tsujimoto et al. (1987) suggest, there may be at least two types of cellular responses to TNF, one of which correlates to receptor binding affinity whereas the other does not. The question of whether one or three receptor molecules bind a single TNF trimer, and if the latter, the biological role of the multiple binding, also remains open.

At this stage it is interesting to invoke a comparison with the viral capsid proteins, which also interact with receptor molecules situated on the surface of cells. The current knowledge on the location of these viral sites is transferred to the TNF main-chain fold in Fig. 15. In the common cold virus (rhinovirus) the hypothesis of a receptor binding site located in the "canyon" on VP1 (Rossmann et al., 1985), and hence inaccessible to antibody but accessible to the receptor ICAM1, is supported by the site-directed mutagenesis results of Colonno et al. (1988). In foot-and-mouth disease virus a tripeptide Arg-Gly-Asp, a recognition sequence for integrin binding, on the highly flexible FMDV loop in VP1 is implicated in receptor binding (Acharya et al., 1989). The sialic acid binding site of influenza hemagglutanin is well characterized (Weis et al., 1988). Each of these viral receptor binding sites has very individual characteristics, but comparison of Figs. 13 and 15 does show some general degree of overlap in position with the TNF hotspots. The viral proteins seek to evade antibody recognition by varying surface residues while preserving receptor binding to the same surface; this property is reminiscent of the ability of TNF from one species to bind to the receptor from another species, while the antibodies raised against TNF from one species cannot bind to TNF from a different species. Thus the principles of receptor binding for TNF may have widespread implications for a whole range of protein–receptor interactions.

In summary, the detailed three-dimensional structure for TNF serves to explain a wide range of observations on antibody binding, stability to proteases, oligomerization, and site-directed mutagenesis. When the structure is considered

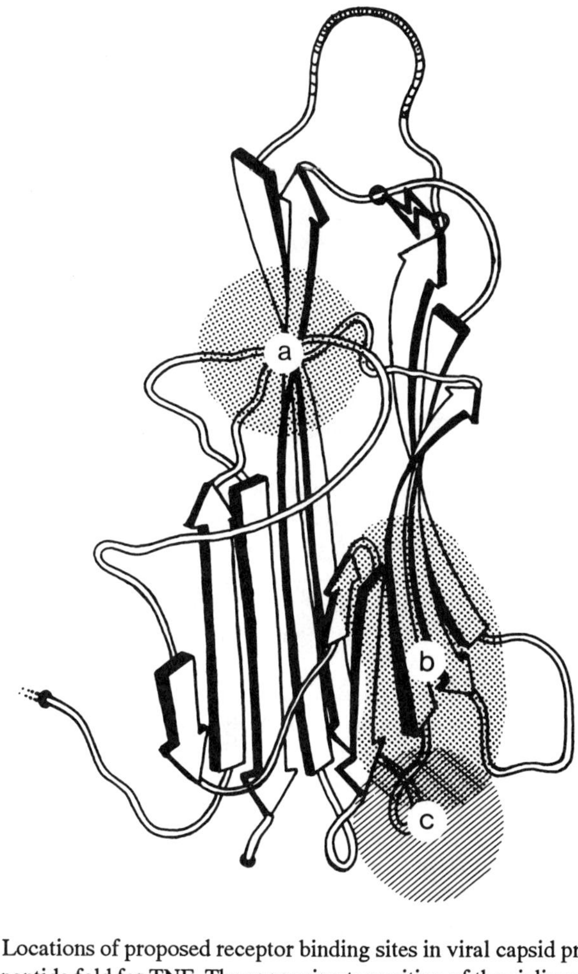

Figure 15 Locations of proposed receptor binding sites in viral capsid proteins mapped onto the polypeptide fold for TNF. The approximate position of the sialic acid binding site of influenza hemagglutanin is indicated by the stippled sphere marked a. Areas that form the canyon floor in VP1 of HRV14 (rhinovirus) are denoted by the region of dots marked b, and the region of the FMDV loop in foot-and-mouth disease virus is marked by the hatched sphere c.

in combination with recent, extensive site-directed mutants, a region of biological importance is apparent at the interface between two subunits on the lower half of the trimer.

ACKNOWLEDGMENTS

We thank Derek Logan for the use of his program Access-View in the production of Figs. 5, 8, 11, and 12, and Steven Lee for expert technical assistance in the production of all the figures.

REFERENCES

Acharya, R., Fry, E., Stuart, D. I., Fox, G., Rowlands, D., and Brown, F. (1989). The three-dimensional structure of foot-and-mouth disease virus at 2.9 Å resolution, *Nature (Lond.), 337*: 709–716.

Aggarwal, B. B. (1990). Differences in the biological responses and the structure of lymphotoxin and tumor necrosis factor, *Tumor Necrosis Factor: Structure, Mechanism of Action, Role in Disease and Therapy* (B. Bonavida and G. Grander eds.), S. Karger, Basel pp. 49–54.

Aggarwal, B. B., Eessalu, T. E., and Haas P. E. (1985a). Characterization of receptors for human tumour necrosis factor and their regulation by gamma-interferon, *Nature (Lond.), 318*: 665- 667.

Aggarwal, B. B., Henzel, W. J., Moffat, B., Kohr, W. J., and Harkins, R. N. (1985b). Primary structure of human lymphotoxin derived from 1788 lymphoblastoid cell line, *J. Biol. Chem., 260*: 2334–2344.

Arakawa, T., and Yphantis, D. A. (1987). Molecular weight of recombinant human tumor necrosis factor-β, *J. Biol. Chem., 262*: 7484–7485.

Argos, P., Tsukihara, T., and Rossmann, M. G. (1980). A structural comparison of concanavalin A and tomato bushy stunt virus protein, *J. Mol. Evol., 15*: 169–179.

Carlino, J. A., Lin, L. S., and Creasey, A. A. (1987). Use of a sensitive receptor binding assay to discriminate between full-length and truncated human recombinant tumor necrosis factor proteins, *J. Biol. Chem., 262*: 958–961.

Chen, Z., Stauffacher, C., Li, Y., Schmidt, T., Bomu, W., Kamer, G., Shanks, M., Lomonossoff, G., and Johnson, J. (1989). Protein-RNA interactions in an icosahedral virus at 3.0 Å resolution, *Science, 245*: 154–159.

Chothia, C. (1974). Hydrophobic bonding and accessible surface area in proteins, *Nature, 248*: 338–339.

Colonno, R. J., Condra, J. H., Mizutani, S., Callahan, P. L., Davies, M. -E., and Murcho, M. (1988). Evidence for the direct involvement of the rhinovirus canyon in receptor binding, *Proc. Natl. Acad. Sci. USA, 85*: 5449–5453.

Daves, J. M., Narachi, M. A., Alton, N. K., and Arakawa, T. (1987). Structure of human tumor necrosis factor β derived from recombinant DNA, *Biochemistry, 26*: 1322–1326.

Eck, M. J., and Sprang, S. R. (1989). The structure of tumor necrosis factor-β at 2.6 Å resolution : implications for receptor binding, *J. Biol. Chem., 264*: 17595–17605.

Eck, M. J., Beutler, B., Kuo, G., Merryweather, J. P., and Sprang, S. R. (1988). Crystallization of trimeric recombinant human tumor necrosis factor (cachectin), *J. Biol. Chem.*, *263*: 12816-12819.

Fiers, W., Brouchaert, P., Goldberg, A. L., Kettelhut, I., Suffys, P., Tavernier, J., Vanhaesebroeck, B., and Van Roy, F. (1987). Structure-function relationship of tumour necrosis factor and its mechanism of action, *Tumor Necrosis Factor and Related Cytotoxins*, Ciba Foundation Symposium 131 (G. Bock and J. March, eds.), Wiley, Chichester, England, pp. 109-123.

Fiers, W., Beyaert, R., Brouchaert, P., Everaerdt, B., Haegeman, G., Libert, C., Suffys, P., Takahashi, N., Tavernier, J., Van Bladel, S., Vanhaesebrock, B., Van Ostade, X., and Van Roy, F. (1990). In vitro and in vivo action of tumor necrosis factor, *Tumor Necrosis Factor: Structure, Mechanism of Action, Rose in Disease and Therapy* (B. Bonavida and G. Granger, eds.), S. Karger, Basel, pp. 77-81.

Goh, C. R., Seow, H. -F., Krishnan, L., and Porter, A. G. (1990). Structural and functional domains in human tumour necrosis factors, *New Frontiers in Biomedical Sciences*, Elsevier, Cambridge (in press).

Hakoshima, T., and Tomita, K. -I. (1988). Crystallization and preliminary x-ray investigation reveals that tumor necrosis factor is a compact trimer furnished with 3-fold symmetry, *J. Mol. Biol., 201*: 455-457.

Hogle, J. M., Chow, M., and Filman, D. J. (1985). Three-dimensional structure of polio virus at 2.9 Å resolution, *Science, 229*: 1365.

Hohmann, H. -P., Remy, R., Brockhaus, M., and Van Loon, A. P. G. M. (1989). Two different cell types have different major receptors for human tumor necrosis factor (TNF-β), *J. Biol. Chem., 264*: 14927- 14934.

Janin, J. (1979). Surface and inside volumes in globular proteins, *Nature, 277*: 491-492.

Jones, E. Y., Stuart, D. I., and Walker, N. P. C. (1989). Structure of tumour necrosis factor, *Nature, 338*: 225-228.

Jones, E. Y., Stuart, D. I., and Walker, N. P. C. (1990a). The three-dimensional structure of TNF at 2.9 Åresolution, *Tumor Necrosis Factor: Structure, Mechanism of Action, Role in Disease and Therapy* (B. Bonavida and G. Granger, eds.), S. Karger, Basel, pp. 31-37.

Jones, E. Y., Stuart, D. I., and Walker, N. P. C. (1990b). Tumor necrosis factor: a nonviral jelly roll, *Use of X-Ray Crystallography in the Design of Antiviral Agents*. (G.M.Air and W.G.Laver, eds.), Academic Press, New York, pp. 345-352.

Jones, E. Y., Stuart, D. I., and Walker, N. P. C. (1990c). The three-dimensional structure of tumour necrosis factor, *Cytokines and Lipocortins in Inflammation and Differentiation* (L. Parente and M. Melli, eds.), Alan R. Liss, New York, pp. 321-327.

Kabsch, W., and Sander, C. (1983). Dictionary of protein secondary structure: pattern recognition of hydrogen-bonded and geometric features, *Biopolymers, 22*: 2577-2637.

Kamijo, R., Takeda, K., Nagumo, M., Konno, K., Hasegawa, A., Inaka, K., and Ikehara, M. (1989). Induction of differentiation of human monoblastic and myeloblastic leukemia cell lines by TNF muteins, *Biochem, Biophys. Res. Commun., 160*:820-827.

Kriegler, M., Perez, C., DeFay, K., Albert, I., and Lu, S. D. (1988). A novel form of TNF/cachectin is a cell surface cytotoxic transmembrane protein: ramifications for the complex physiology of TNF, *Cell, 53*: 45-53.

Lee, B. K., and Richards, F. M. (1971). The interpretation of protein structures: estimation of static accessibility, *J. Mol. Biol., 33*: 319-400.

Lewit-Bentley A., Fourme R., Kahn R., Prangé, T., Vachette, P., Tavernier, J., Hauquier, G., and Fiers, W. (1988). Structure of tumour necrosis factor by x-ray solution scattering and preliminary studies by single crystal x-ray diffraction, *J. Mol. Biol., 199*: 389-392.

Liljas, L., Unge, T., Jones, T. A., Fridborg, K., Lovgren, S., Skoglund, U., and Strandberg, B. (1982). Structure of satellite tobacco necrosis virus at 3.0 Å resolution, *J. Mol. Biol., 159*: 93-108.

Masegi, T., Nakamura, S., Kitai, K., Fukuoka, M., Kato, A., and Ichikawa, Y. (1989). Fundamental studies on novel recombinant tumour necrosis factor mutants, *Abstracts, Protein Engineering '89*, Kobe, Japan, p. 252.

Narachi, M. A., Davis, J. M., Hsu, Y. -R., and Arakawa, T. (1987). Role of single disulfide in recombinant human tumor necrosis factor-β, *J. Biol. Chem., 262*: 13107-13110.

Novotny, J., Handschumacher, M., Haber, E., Bruccoleri, R. E., Carlson, W. B., Fanning, D. W., Smith, J. A., and Rose, G. D. (1986). Antigenic determinants in proteins coincide with surface regions accessible to large probes (antibody domains), *Proc. Natl. Acad. Sci. USA, 83*: 226-230.

Pennica, D., Nedwin, G. E., Hayflick, J. S., Seeburg, P. H., Derynck, R., Palladino, M. A., Kohr, W. J., Aggarwal, B. B., and Goeddel, D. V. (1984). Human tumour necrosis factor: precursor structure, expression and homology to lymphotoxin, *Nature (Lond.) 312*: 724-729.

Priestle, J. P., Schar, H. -P., and Grutter, M. G. (1989). Crystallographic refinement of interleukin 1β at 2.0 Å resolution, *Proc. Natl. Acad. Sci. USA, 86*: 9667-9671.

Richardson, J. S. (1981). Protein anatomy, *Adv. Protein Chem., 34*: 167-339.

Roberts, M. M., and Burnett, R. M. (1987). Adenovirus hexon: a novel use of the viral beta-barrel, *Biological Organization: Macromolecular Interactions at High Resolution* (R. M. Burnett and H. J. Vogel, eds.), Academic Press, Orlando, Fla., pp. 113-124.

Roberts, M. M., White, J. L., Grutter, M. G., and Burnett, R. M. (1986). Three-dimensional structure of the adenovirus major coat protein hexon, *Science, 232*: 1148-1151.

Rossmann, M. G., and Johnson, J. E. (1989). Icosahedral RNA virus structure, *Annu. Rev. Biochem., 58*: 533-573.

Rossmann, M. G., Abad-Zapatero, C., Murthy, M. R. N., Liljas, L., Jones, T. A., and Strandberg, B. (1983). Structural comparisons of some small spherical plant viruses, *J. Mol. Biol., 165*: 711-736.

Rossmann, M. G., Arnold, E., Erickson, J. W., Frankenberger, E. A., Griffith, J. P., Hecht, J. -J., Johnson, J. E., Kamer, G., Luo, M., Mosser, A. G., Rueckert, R. R., Sherry, B., and Vriend, G. (1985). Structure of a human common cold virus and functional relationship to other picornaviruses, *Nature (Lond.), 317*:145-153.

Schirmer, T., and Evans, P. R. (1990). Structural basis of the allosteric behaviour of phosphofructokinase, *Nature, 343*: 140- 145.

Smith, R. A., and Baglioni, C. (1987). The active form of tumor necrosis factor is a trimer, *J. Biol. Chem., 252*: 6951-6954.

Socher, S. H., Riemen, M. W., Martinez, D., Friedman, A., Tai, J., Quintero, J. C., Garsky, V., Oliff, A. (1987). Antibodies against amino acids 1-15 of tumor necrosis factor block its binding to cell-surface receptor, *Proc. Natl. Acad. Sci. USA, 84*: 8829-8833.

Soma, G. -I., Kitahara, N., Tsuji, Y., Kato, M., Oshima, H., Gatanaga, T., Inagawa, H., Noguchi, K., Tanabe, Y., and Mizuno, D. (1987). Improvement of cytotoxicity of tumor necrosis factor (TNF) by increase in basicity of its N-terminal region, *Biochem. Biophys. Res. Commun., 148*: 629-635.

Stuart, D. I., Levine, M., Muirhead, H., and Stammers, D. K. (1979). Crystal structure of cat muscle pyruvate kinase at a resolution of 2.6 Å, *J. Mol. Biol., 134:* 109-142.

Tainer, J. A., Getzoff, E. D., Alexander, H., Houghten, R. A., Olson, A. J., Lerner, R. A., and Hendrickson, W. A. (1984). The reactivity of anti-peptide antibodies is a function of the atomic mobility of sites in a protein, *Nature, 312*: 127-134.

Tavernier, J., Marmenout, A., Bauden, R., Hauquier, G., Van Ostade, X., and Fiers, W. (1990). Analysis of the structure-function relationship of tumor necrosis factor (TNF). 1. Human/mouse chimeric TNF proteins: general properties and epitope analysis, *J. Mol. Biol., 211*: 493-501.

Tsujimoto, M., Tanaka, S., Sakuragawa, Y., Tsuruoka, N., Funakoshi, K., Butsugan, T., Nakazoto, H., Nishihara, T., Noguchi, T., and Vilček, J. (1987). Comparative studies of the biological activities of human tumor necrosis factor and its derivatives, *J. Biochem., 101*: 919-925.

Tulip, W. R., Varghese, J. N., Webster, R. G., Air, G. M., Laver, W. G., Colman, P. M. (1989). *Cold Spring Harbor Symp. Immune Recognition*, 257-263.

Van Ostade, X., Tavernier, J, and Fiers, W. (1988). Two conserved tryptophan residues of tumor necrosis factor and lymphotoxin are not involved in the biological activity, *FEBS Lett., 238*: 347-352.

Walker, N., Marcinowski, S., Hillen, H., Machtle, W., Jones, Y., and Stuart, D. (1990). Crystallization of human tumour necrosis factor, *J. Cryst. Growth, 100*: 168-170 .

Weis, W., Brown, J. H., Cusack, S., Paulson, J. C., Skehel, J. J., and Wiley, D. C. (1988). Structure of the influenza virus hemagglutinin complexed with its receptor, sialic acid, *Nature (Lond.), 333*: 426-431.

Wilson, I. A., Skehel, J. J., and Wiley, D. C. (1981). Structure of the hemagglutinin membrane glycoprotein of influenza virus at 3 Å resolution, *Nature (Lond.), 289*: 366-373.

Wingfield, P., Pain, R. H., and Craig, S. (1987). Tumour necrosis factor is a compact trimer, *FEBS Lett., 221*: 179-184.

Yamagishi, J., Kawashima, H., Matsuo, N., Ohue, M., Furuta, R., Nakano, K., Yamayoshi, M., Fukui, T., and Yamada, M. (1989). Structure-activity analysis of human tumor necrosis factor, *Abstracts, Protein Engineering '89*, Kobe, Japan, p. 242.

Yamamoto, R, Wang, A., Vitt, C. R., and Lin, L. S. (1989). Histidine-15: an important role in the cytotoxic activity of human tumor necrosis factor, *Protein Eng., 2*: 553-558.

II

RECEPTORS AND MECHANISM OF ACTION OF TNFs

6

Characterization of TNF Receptors

RICHARD A. SMITH and CORRADO BAGLIONI
Albany Medical College and State University of New York at Albany, Albany, New York

I. INTRODUCTION

Specific high-affinity TNF receptors were reported by Rubin et al. (1985); Kull et al. (1985); Tsujimoto et al. (1985); and Baglioni et al. (1985). The same receptors bind both TNF-α and TNF-β as shown by competition binding assays with these cytokines (Aggarwal et al., 1985a). However, the response to TNF-β may differ in some cells from that to TNF-α, since only the latter induces secretion of colony-stimulating factor in macrophages (Oster et al., 1987) and of interleukin-1 from endothelial cells (Locksley et al., 1987). This different response is due to a 10-fold-lower binding affinity for TNF-β (Locksley et al., 1987).

The TNF receptors have been characterized in cells and tissues by determining their binding kinetics and subunit composition. This characterization has been carried out by affinity labeling procedures, gel filtration studies, and ligand and Western blots of TNF-receptor complexes. Finally, N- and O-glycosylation of TNF receptors has been studied using specific lectins and by enzymatic deglycosylation.

II. TISSUE DISTRIBUTION OF TNF RECEPTORS

Receptors for TNF are widely distributed throughout most cells and tissues. Injection of labeled murine TNF-α into mice results in preferential binding to certain

Table 1 Specific [^{125}I]mTNF Binding to Mouse Tissues[a]

Tissue	cpm/mg Protein
Spleen	8856
Lung	7037
Liver	3975
Testis	3481
Skeletal muscle	1250
Heart	1164
Kidney	1160

Source: Baglioni, et al. 1990.
[a]Mouse tissues were homogenized in 0.25 *M* sucrose, 0.05 *M* Tris pH 7.5 (1 g per 5 mL) with a polytron. Homogenates were centrifuged for 10 min at 1000 × *g* for 30 min to sediment membranes for the binding assay.

tissues (Beutler et al., 1985b). The highest amounts are found in liver, kidneys, and spleen, while modest amounts are found in stomach, duodenum, small bowel, pancreas, colon, and esophagus. In each of these tissues the binding of TNF-α is decreased by the injection of excess unlabeled TNF. In contrast, TNF-α bound in lungs, skin, fat, and brain is not displaced by unlabeled TNF. This finding may reflect saturable mechanisms of binding in the former tissues and unsaturatable binding in the latter.

Tissue distribution of TNF receptors is also measured by binding assays with membrane preparations (Table 1). These assays show the highest specific TNF binding in the spleen and lungs, moderate binding in liver and testis, and low binding in skeletal muscle, heart, and kidney. Since endothelial cells contain high-affinity TNF receptors (Nawroth et al., 1986), it is uncertain whether the binding of TNF-α is due to parenchymal, stromal, and vascular elements. Red blood cells do not contain TNF receptors and therefore do not contribute to TNF-α binding in whole tissues (Beutler et al., 1985; Shalaby et al., 1987; Munker et al., 1987). TNF receptors have been identified in human placenta that may be a convenient source for receptor purification (Eades et al., 1988).

III. TNF BINDING TO CELLS

Beutler et al. (1985a) initially investigated the binding of murine TNF-α to high-affinity receptors (K_d = 0.3 nM) on 3T3-L1 adipocytes and on C2 myocytes. Kull et al. (1985) also reported that murine TNF-α binds to a panel of murine, bovine, and human cells. At about the same time, Rubin et al. (1985) reported that the affinity (K_d) of TNF receptors on L(M) and HeLa cells was 0.1 nM. Baglioni et al. (1985)

reported TNF-α bound by HeLa cells is internalized and degraded, and Tsujimoto et al. (1985) reported similar findings for L929 cells and human fibroblasts.

There are contrasting reports in the literature about the molecular size of TNF. Since the concentration of ligand enters into the calculation to determine the concentration of receptor, it is important to know if monomers, dimers, or higher oligomers are active. Beutler et al. (1985a) and Rubin et al. (1985) reported for natural mTNF-α and hTNF-α M_r a vale of ~70,000 in the nondenatured state and a an M_r value of 17,000 to 19,000 under denaturing conditions of SDS-PAGE. Aggerwal et al. (1985b) described hTNF monomers of 17 kDa; these aggregate to a 45-kDa form during gel filtration chromatography. Marmenout et al. (1985) obtained for natural hTNF-α from U937 cells a 35,000 M_r by gel filtration chromatography. Shirai et al. (1985) obtained for recombinant hTNF-α an M_r value of ~45,000 by gel filtration and of 17,000 by SDS-PAGE. Recombinant mTNF was thought to be a dimer (Fransen et al., 1985). One result of the confusion about the molecular size of TNF-α is that most investigators report receptors per cell in terms of the 17-kDa TNF-α monomer. Using a higher mass for TNF-α results in fewer receptors per cell.

Equilibrium centrifugation studies by Wingfield et al. (1987) and Arakawa and Yphantis (1987) demonstrate that TNF-α exists as a stable trimer in physiological solutions, and TNF-α has also been crystalized in the trimeric form (Eck et al., 1988; Hakoshima and Tomita, 1988; Lewit-Bentley et al., 1988). Other studies have established that TNF-α trimers are active in binding to receptors (Smith and Baglioni, 1987) and that the binding site(s) near the amino termini (Socher et al., 1987) are at the base of the trimer (Eck and Sprang, 1989).

TNF-α binds to a single class of high-affinity cell surface receptors in most cells tested. Depending on the temperature and concentration of TNF-α and cells in the assay, binding reaches equilibrium after 4 to 5 h at 4°C (Fig. 1) . When binding is performed at 37°C, most of the TNF-α is internalized (Fig. 1). In competitive binding assays, varying concentrations of unlabeled TNF added with iodinated TNF give rise to competition curves. When data are analyzed by Scatchard plot, a single class of high-affinity binding is observed. Analysis by least-squares curve fitting in the LIGAND program (Munson and Rodbard, 1980) shows that the binding data fit best a mathematical model with a single high-affinity site. We and others have reported a single class of receptors for TNF-α; the K_d value is in the range of 0.3 nM and there are hundreds to thousands of receptors in different cells (Table 2).

Several investigators have reported curvilinear Scatchard plots for TNF-α binding to cells. Patton et al. (1986) described such plots for 3T3-L1 adipocytes. Creasey et al. (1987) reported that TNF-sensitive human breast carcinoma MCF-7 cells contain an additional TNF-α binding protein that is lacking in a TNF-resistant variant. The presence of this protein was correlated with a change in the affinity for TNF. Imamura et al. (1987) also observed high- and low-affinity sites in human monocytes.

Table 2 Binding Affinity and Relative Abundance of TNF Receptors

Cell	Tissue	K_D (n*M*)	Receptors per cell	Reference
3T3-L1	Adipocytes	0.33	10,000	Beutler et al. (1985a)
C2	Myotubes	0.33	10,000	Beutler et al. (1985a)
ME-180	Cervical carcinoma	0.31	2,250	Sugarman et al. (1985)
WI-38	Fetal lung	0.22	2,172	Sugarman et al. (1985)
T24	Bladder carcinoma	0.25	1,512	Sugarman et al. (1985)
U937	Histocytic leukemia	0.17	3,212	Scheurich et al. (1986)
K562	Erythroleukemia	0.16	3,623	Scheurich et al. (1986)
HL-60	Promyelocytic leukemia	0.07	1,400	Hohmann et al. (1989)
HEp-2	Epidermoid carcinoma	0.03	800	Hohmann et al. (1989)
HeLa	Cervical carcinoma	0.25	6,000	Baglioni et al. (1985)
Jurkatt	T lymphoma	0.25	1,100	Baglioni et al. (1985)
T cells	Human lymphocytes	0.06	65	Baglioni et al. (1985)
MOLT-4	Lymphoblastic leukemia	0.04	100	Baglioni et al. (1985)
CEM	Lymphoblastic leukemia	0.09	436	Baglioni et al. (1985)
THP-1	Monocytic leukemia	0.30	10,000	Yoshie et al. (1986)
FS-4	Foreskin fibroblast	0.32	7,500	Tsujimoto et al. (1986a)
L-M	Connective tissue	0.003	1,100	Kull et al. (1985)
L929	Connective tissue	0.003	770	Kull et al. (1985)
J774.1	Murine macrophage	0.003	1,100	Kull et al. (1985)
CPAE	Bovine endothelium	0.003	1,500	Kull et al. (1985)

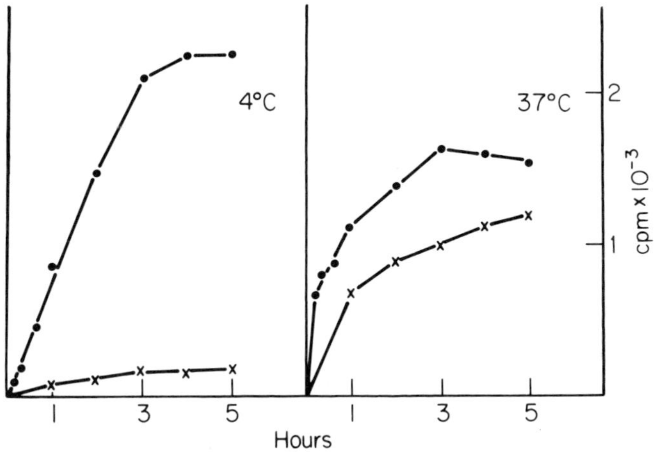

Figure 1 Time course of binding and internalization of [125I]TNF by HeLa cells at 4 and 37°C. For each experiment, 1.5 mL of cell suspension was incubated with 0.5 ng of [125I]TNF. Samples were taken at the times indicated, diluted with either saline (●) or 0.1 *M* NaCl, 50 m*M* glycine buffer, pH 3 (×), and centrifuged through phthalates oils (Baglioni et al., 1985) to measure cell-associated TNF (●) or internalized TNF (×).

Smith and Baglioni (1989) and Hohmann et al. (1989) reported that HeLa and HL-60 cells have two distinct proteins capable of binding TNF, yet Scatchard plots for TNF binding to these cells are linear. A curvilinear Scatchard plot suggests receptor heterogeneity with respect to ligand affinity. This may be explained by multiple classes of binding sites with differing affinity for TNF. Multiple classes of binding sites may arise for several reasons:

1. There may be more than one type of TNF receptor. The variety of cells exhibiting specialized responses to TNF raises the possibility that there may be cell-specific receptors with different functions. This type of heterogeneity may be expected with receptors prepared from heterogeneous cell populations, as in binding assays with membranes prepared from whole tissues, or from cells expressing different receptors.
2. TNF receptors may show heterogeneous affinity if binding is influenced by protein modifications, such as O-linked or N-linked glycosylation, proteolytic processing, or phosphorylation.
3. Receptors aggregated on the cell surface may bind with higher affinity than monomeric forms, due to cooperative binding events.

4. The affinity for TNF may be influenced by other proteins modulating receptor binding that may be present or absent in specific cell types.

IV. PHYSICAL CHARACTERIZATION OF TNF RECEPTORS

A. Affinity Labeling of TNF Receptors

Kull et al. (1985) affinity-labeled murine L-M cells and demonstrated the presence of a 95-kDa band and a faint 75-kDa band (Table 3). These results could not be easily interpreted because of the unknown contribution of TNF-α to the molecular mass of each complex. For example, either TNF monomer or dimer could be cross-linked to the 95-kDa complex. Since only a small fraction of the TNF-α added was cross-linked, these authors suggested that monomer was cross-linked. Soon thereafter, the presence of at least two affinity-labeled complexes was confirmed in L929 and HeLa cells by Smith et al. (1986), who suggested that 75- and 95-kDa components were associated in a cross-linked complex of ~350 kDa. Many investigators reported similar but slightly different results for affinity labeling of TNF receptors in different cell types, and others reported vastly different M_r values (Table 3). In particular, Creasey et al. (1987) reported the affinity labeling of a high M_r complex of 138 kDa in TNF-sensitive variant of MCF-7 breast carcinoma cells; this complex was absent from MCF-7 TNF-resistant cells. This observation suggests that a specific subunit of the receptor may be responsible for the cytotoxic activity of TNF.

Bifunctional reagents, such as disuccinimidyl suberate (DSS) and bis[2-(succinimidooxycarbonyloxy)ethyl]sulfone (BSOCOES), cross-link [^{125}I]TNF into dimers and trimers that can be resolved by SDS-PAGE (see Fig. 2). Therefore, some of the bands observed by affinity labeling may be produced by cross-linking TNF-α oligomers to receptor subunits. To examine the composition of the 75- and 95-kDa complexes, we cross-linked [^{125}I]TNF first with DSS to form dimers and small amounts of trimers; the binding to receptors of this cross-linked TNF-α is indistinguishable from that of untreated [^{125}I]TNF (Smith and Baglioni, 1989). The DSS-treated TNF-α was then cross-linked to receptors with the reversible reagent BSOCOES. Following the first-dimension SDS-PAGE, a gel strip containing the cross-linked products was excised and treated with dithiothreitol at alkaline pH to reverse the BSOCOES cross-links (Smith and Baglioni, 1989). This gel strip was mounted above a 4 to 12% gradient gel and the proteins were electrophoresed in a second dimension (Fig. 2). The 75- and 95-kDa complexes released TNF monomers, and the 95-kDa species also released TNF dimers, showing that these complexes are formed by crosslinking monomers and dimers to a 60-kDa receptor subunit. The 75- and 95-kDa complexes are in turn released from a prominent band of 150 to 175 kDa; TNF trimers are released from a band corresponding to ~116 kDa and from complexes >200 kDa.

Table 3 Affinity Labeling of TNF Receptors on Different Cells

Cell type[a]	$M_r \times 10^3$					References
L-M, L929, HEp2, MCF-7		75	95			Kull et al. (1985); Smith et al. (1986); Hohmann et al. (1989)
FS-11, KG-1, U937		74	92			Israel et al. (1986)
MCF-7	54	75	90	138		Creasey et al. (1987)
HeLa		75	90	150–175	310	Smith and Baglioni (1989)
HeLa, HT-29, U937			100			Tsujimoto et al. (1986b); Stauber et al. (1988)
HeLa, THP-1, U937			100–105			Yoshie et al. (1986)
Monocytes, U937, HL-60		75	98–100			Hohmann et al. (1989)
Monocytes			120			Bakouche et al. (1986)
K-562			93			Scheurich et al. (1986)

[a]Cells not listed in Table 2 are: FS-11, foreskin fibroblast; MCF7, breast carcinoma; and K-562, erythroleukemia.

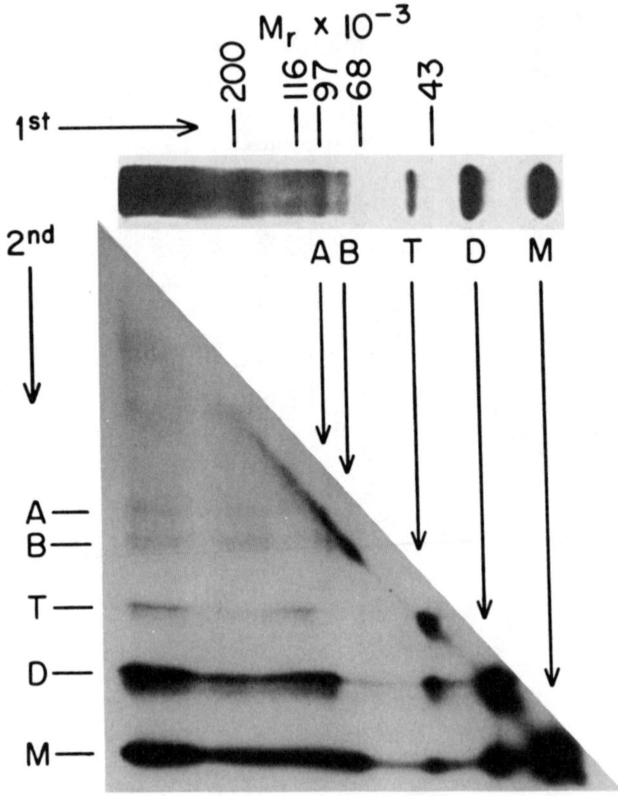

Figure 2 Cross-linking reversal in two-dimensional SDS-PAGE. TNF–receptor complexes were formed by incubating DSS-[^{125}I]TNF with HeLa cells for 4 h at 4°C. Bound TNF was cross-linked to the cells with 2 m*M* BSOCOES. Membranes were prepared and solubilized in SDS-PAGE sample buffer with 50 m*M* DTT before electrophoresis in a 4 to 12% gradient gel. The autoradiograph from this gel is mounted horizontally above the autoradiograph of the second dimension gel that was run after cross-link reversal. The positions of TNF monomers, dimers, and trimers are indicated by M, D, and T, respectively; the 95,000 and 75,000 cross-linked complexes are indicated by A and B. (From Smith and Baglioni, 1989.)

Other investigators have also reported high-M_r products of TNF cross-linking to its receptor (Creasey et al., 1987; Stauber et al., 1988). These complexes are poorly solubilized from the affinity-labeled cells due to cross-linking, but can be enriched by gel filtration chromatography from extracts of detergent-solubilized cells. Most of the cross-linked TNF–receptor complexes from affinity-labeled HeLa and L929 cells elute with 350,000 M_r (Smith et al., 1986). When these complexes are reduced and analyzed by SDS-PAGE, they dissociate into the 75- and 95-kDa components. In similar experiments with U937 cells, Stauber et al. (1988) report that some cross-linked TNF-receptor complexes elute with M_r = 480,000; SDS-PAGE of these reduced complexes shows a single band of 95 to 100 kDa. These experiments indicate that multimeric TNF–receptor complexes dissociate into 75- and 95 to 100 kDa cross-linked components and suggest that disulfide bonds may be involved in subunit association.

Multimeric TNF–receptor complexes can be also demonstrated by isolating such complexes before the cross-linking step (Smith and Baglioni, 1989). HeLa cell membranes purified over a step gradient were incubated with [^{125}I]TNF in the presence and absence of excess unlabeled TNF. After removal of unbound TNF by centrifugation, the membranes were solubilized with Triton X-100 and analyzed by gel filtration (Fig. 3). The fractions containing TNF–receptor complexes corresponded to M_r ~350,000 when compared to globular proteins. These fractions were pooled and cross-linked. SDS-PAGE and autoradiography confirmed that [^{125}I]TNF eluting in this peak was cross-linked to receptor in the predominant form of a ~310-kDa complex (Smith and Baglioni, 1989).

Disulfide bonds may stabilize high-molecular-weight TNF–receptor complexes. Smith and Baglioni (1989) solubilized cross-linked [^{125}I]TNF–receptor complexes prepared from HeLa cell membranes and analyzed fractions purified through gel filtration by SDS-PAGE before and after reduction with dithiothreitol. This analysis shows that reduction of the 310-kDa complex increases the yield of the 150- to 175-, 75-, and 95-kDa components (Fig. 4).

B. Gel Filtration, Ligand Blotting, and Immunological Studies

Solubilized TNF receptors have been also characterized by gel filtration. Stauber et al. (1988) showed that the TNF binding activity of U937 cells eluted over a broad range of molecular weights. The specific binding profile showed a shoulder at ~450 kDa and two peaks of activity centered at 230 and 60 kDa. A large fraction of the total binding activity was recovered with this 60-kDa peak. Our experiments with HeLa cells also show three peaks of binding activity. However, the predominant peak elutes at 330 kDa and significantly smaller peaks elute at 175 and 90 kDa. Scatchard plots show a K_d = 0.25 nM for TNF binding to the 330-kDa complex. We find that solubilization of membranes with high concentrations of Triton X-100

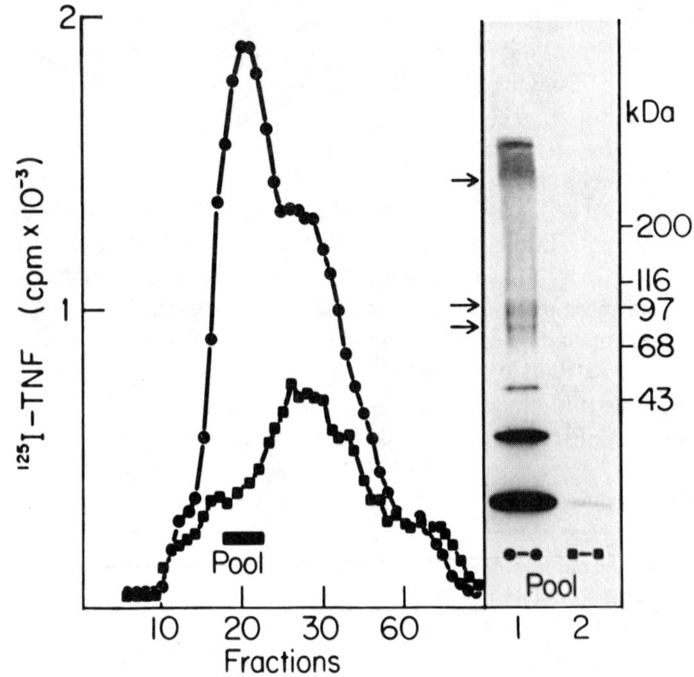

Figure 3 Affinity labeling of high-M_r TNF–receptor complexes. HeLa cell membranes were incubated for 5 h at 4°C with 15 ng of [^{125}I]TNF in the presence and absence of 100-fold excess unlabeled TNF. The membranes were centrifuged and solubilized with Triton X-100. Extracts from total binding (●) and nonspecific binding (■) assays were applied to a gel filtration column (Smith and Baglioni, 1989). Fractions 18 to 22 were pooled, cross-linked with 2 m*M* BSOCOES and compared on an equal protein basis by SDS-PAGE (inset); 1 shows the total binding pool and 2 the pool of nonspecific binding. Arrows indicate cross-linked complexes corresponding to 310, 95, and 75 kDa. (From Smith and Baglioni, 1989.)

decreases total binding and shifts the binding activity to lower molecular weights. The high-M_r receptor peak shows optimal binding, but Triton X-100 concentrations greater than 0.1% inhibits this activity.

The TNF receptors of HeLa cells have also been characterized with a ligand blotting assay (Smith and Baglioni, 1989). Cell membranes are solubilized with Triton X-100 and fractionated by SDS-PAGE in 4 to 8% gradient gels. The fractionated proteins are transferred elecrophoretically to nylon membranes and assayed: two proteins of 60 and 70 kDa bind TNF-α (Fig. 5). An additional but very

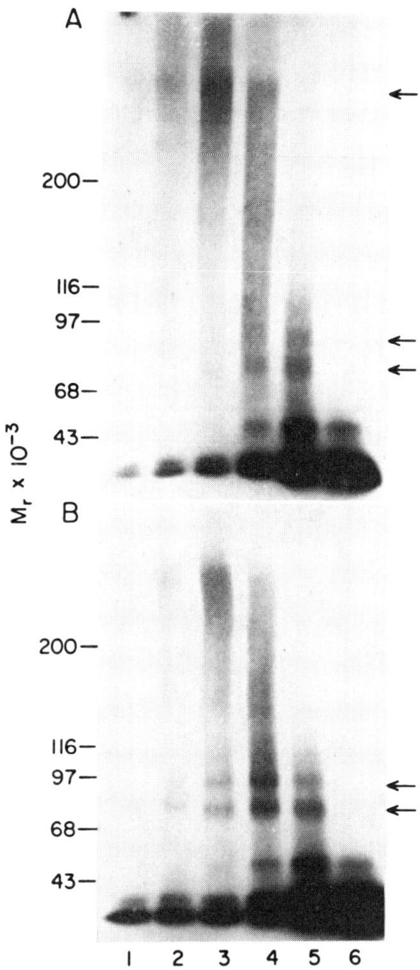

Figure 4 Dissociation of the 310,000-M_r complex by reduction. [^{125}I]TNF was incubated with HeLa cell membranes and cross-linked with 2 mM BSOCOES. The membranes were solubilized at 100°C with 2% SDS and fractionated by gel filtration. Fractions containing complexes of decreasing size (from lanes 1 to 6) were examined by SDS-PAGE unreduced (A) or after treatment with 50 mM DTT (B). The arrows indicate the 95- and 75-kDa complexes. (From Smith and Baglioni, 1989.)

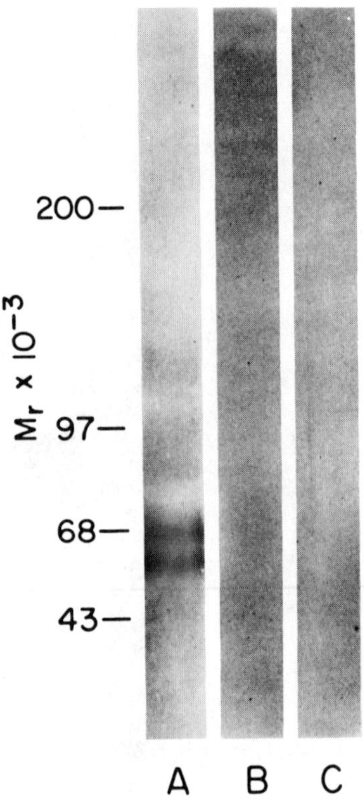

Figure 5 Ligand blot of TNF receptor from HeLa cells. HeLa membranes were solubilized with Triton X-100 in the presence of protease inhibitors, fractionated by 4 to 8% SDS-PAGE, and electrophoretically transferred to a nylon membrane. (A). Incubation with [125TNF alone. (B). Incubation with [125I]TNF and 100-fold excess unlabeled TNF. (C). Extract with 25 m*M* DTT at 4°C for 3 min before electrophoresis and incubation with [125I]TNF as in A. Positions of pre-stained M_r markers are indicated.

faint band of 135 kDa was detected in some experiments. The latter band may represent undissociated 60- and 70-kDa proteins may be related to the 150- to 175-kDa cross-linked complexes discussed above. The binding of [125I]TNF to the 60- and 70-kDa proteins is specified because it is competed by unlabeled TNF-α (Fig. 4). Inclusion of 25 m*M* dithiothreitol in SDS-PAGE sample buffer abolishes TNF-α binding, suggesting that intramolecular disulfide bridges stabilize this activity. These experiments demonstrate that there are two TNF binding proteins in HeLa membranes, each capable of specifically binding TNF. Whether they represent different forms of the same protein or two separate proteins remains to be determined.

The 60- and 70-kDa proteins are also present in the multimeric forms of TNF receptor. The 330- and 175-kDa complexes separated from gel filtration chromatography were analyzed by ligand blot assays. The same binding pattern was obtained for each complex, with both 60- and 70-kDa proteins present. This suggests that the 330-kDa complex is a dimer of the 175-kDa complex, and that the 60- and 70-kDa proteins are associated to form the TNF receptor.

Hohmann et al. (1989) have reported that a monoclonal antibody to the TNF receptor precipitates 75- and 95-kDa affinity-labeled complexes from HEp2 cells but fails to precipitate the affinity-labeled 100-kDa complex from HL-60 cells. Furthermore, this antibody fails to react with another protein that binds TNF in ligand blots. On the basis of these findings and of additional experiments demonstrating slightly different affinities for TNF, different patterns of affinity labeling and different tryptic fingerprints, Hohmann et al. (1989) suggest that the TNF receptor of epithelial cells differs from that of myeloid cells.

Several groups have purified from urine TNF binding proteins that may be soluble, proteolysis products of the TNF receptor (Engelmann et al., 1989; Seckinger et al., 1989). Engelmann et al. (1990) have purified two such proteins with different amino-terminal sequences. Polyclonal antibodies against these proteins do not cross-react, indicating that these are distinct proteins. These antibodies also inhibit TNF binding to different cell types with varying efficacy. For instance, antiserum to TNF binding protein 1 (TBP1) has no effect on U937 cells, whereas antiserum to TBP2 drastically inhibits this binding. Both antisera inhibit binding of TNF to HeLa and MCF7 cells, but antiserum to TBP1 is more effective than that to TBP2. These immunological studies have provided additional evidence for more than one receptor protein for TNF and for the expression of two types of receptors in some cells (Engelmann et al., 1990).

C. Glycosylation of TNF Receptors

Several reports have indicated that TNF receptors are glycosylated. Tsujimoto et al. (1986a) demonstrated that affinity-labeled TNF–receptor complexes are adsorbed to concanavalin A-Sepharose. Aggarwal et al. (1986) showed that both concanavalin A and wheat germ lectin increase binding of TNF-α when added to cells at 37°C; these lectins presumably bind to a glycoprotein component of the receptor and prevent receptor internalization. Hohmann et al. (1989) studied TNF receptor glycosylation using tunicamycin or glycanase; these treatments alter the mobility of affinity-labeled receptors. These studies show differences in glycosylation between cells of epidermal and myeloid origin. The 100-kDa affinity-labeled complex of HL-60 cells contain both N-linked and O-linked glycosyl groups that contribute 10 to 15 kDa to the molecular mass of the receptor. The 75- and 95- kDa affinity-labeled complexes of HEp2 cells contain N-linked glycosyl groups that contribute 15 to 20 kDa of relative mass.

V. CONCLUSIONS

High-affinity TNF receptors with K_D = 250 p*M* are found on all cell types examined, with the exception of erythrocytes. Receptors per cell range from ~50 on unstimulated T lymphocytes to ~50,000 on some U937 cell variants. Affinity-labeling studies have detected 75- and 95- to 100-kDa complexes on most cells examined. Cross-linking reversal experiments show that these complexes contain a 60-kDa subunit and TNF-α monomers or dimers, respectively. Other affinity-labeled complexes contain TNF trimers. Antibodies raised against TNF receptors or against urinary TNF binding proteins react differently with 95- or 100-kDa affinity-labeled complexes or with receptors of different cell lines, suggesting the presence of two distinct receptor proteins. These studies indicate that either one or both proteins may be expressed in different cells.

We have observed 150- to 175-kDa affinity-labeled complexes in HeLa cells. Such complexes may contain the 60-kDa and another protein subunit. Indeed, ligand blots of solubilized HeLa cell membranes show two proteins of 60 and 70 kDa that specifically bind TNF. Gel filtration studies show that solubilized receptors form multrmeric complexes. Ligand blots of the 330- and 175-kDa complexes show the presence of the 60- and 70-kDa subunits, indicating that these proteins are present in different complexes. It is not known whether the 60- and 70-kDa subunits from HeLa cells are different forms of the same protein.

Hohmann et al. (1989) have shown variation in N-linked and O-linked glycosylation of TNF receptors in different cell types and have suggested on the basis of immunological evidence that there is more than one protein that binds TNF in HL-60 cells. However, it is unclear whether all TNF receptors are composed of different subunits each capable of binding TNF-α. It seems reasonable to suggest that the TNF receptor contains at least two associated proteins in several cell types, such as in HeLa cells. In other cell types, such as in U937 cells, there may be only one TNF binding protein.

REFERENCES

Aggarwal, B. B., Eessalu, T. E., and Hass, P. E. (1985a). Characterization of receptors for human tumour necrosis factor and their regulation by gamma interferon, *Nature*, *318*: 655.

Aggarwal, B. B., Kohr, W. J., Hass, P. E., Moffat, B., Spencer, S. A., Henzel, W. J., Bringman, T. S., Nedwin, G. E., Goeddel, D. V., and Harkins, R. N. (1985b). Human tumor necrosis factor α: production, purification and characterization, *J. Biol. Chem.*, *260*: 2345.

Aggarwal, B. B., Traquina, P. R., and Eessalu, T. E. (1986). Modulation of receptors and cytotoxic response of tumor necrosis factor-α by various lectins, *J. Biol. Chem., 261*: 13652.

Arakawa, T., and Yphantis, D. A. (1987). Molecular weight of recombinant human tumor necrosis factor, *J. Biol. Chem., 262*: 7484.

Baglioni, C., McCandless, S., Tavernier, J., and Fiers, W. (1985). Binding of human tumor necrosis factor to high affinity receptors on Hela and lymphoblastoid cells sensitive to growth inhibition, *J. Biol. Chem., 260*: 13395.

Baglioni, C., Johnson, S. E., Faltynek, C. E., and Smith, R. A. (1990). Unpublished observations.

Bakouche, O., Ichinose, Y., Heicappell, R., Fidler, I. J., and Lachman, L. B. (1988). Plasma membrane-associated tumor necrosis factor: a non-integral membrane protein possibly bound to its own receptor, *J. Immunol., 140*: 1142.

Beutler, B., Mahoney, J., Le Trang, N., Pekala, P., and Cerami, A. (1985a). Purification of cachectin, a lipoprotein lipase-suppressing hormone secreted by endotoxin-induced RAW 264.7 cells, *J. Exp. Med., 161*: 984.

Beutler, B., Milsark, I. W., and Cerami, A. (1985b). Cachectin/tumor necrosis factor: production, distribution and metabolic fate in vivo, *J. Immumol., 135*: 3972.

Creasey, A. A., Yamamoto, R., and Vitt, C. R. (1987). A high molecular weight component of the human tumor necrosis factor receptor is associated with cytotoxicity, *Proc. Natl. Acad. Sci. USA, 84*: 3293.

Eck, M. J., and Sprang, S. R. (1989). The structure of tumor necrosis factor-α at 2.6 Å resolution, *J. Biol. Chem., 264*: 17595.

Eck, M. J., Beutler, B., Kuo, G., Merryweather, J. P., and Sprang, S. R. (1988). Crystallization of trimeric recombinant human tumor necrosis factor (cachectin), *J. Biol. Chem., 263*: 12816.

Engelmann, H., Aderka, D., Rubinstein, M., Rotman, D., and Wallach, D. (1989). A tumor necrosis factor-binding protein purified to homogeneity form human urine protects cells from tumor necrosis factor toxicity, *J. Biol. Chem., 264*: 11974.

Engelmann, H., Novick, D., and Wallach, D. (1990). Two tumor necrosis factor-binding proteins purified from human urine: evidence for immunological cross-reactivity with cell surface tumor necrosis factor receptors, *J. Biol. Chem., 265*: 1531.

Fransen, L., Muller, R., Marmenout, A., Tavernier, J., Van der Heyden, J., Kawashima, E., Chollet, A., Tizard, R., Van Heuverswyn, H., Van Vliet, A., Ruysschaert, M. R., and Fiers, W. (1985). Molecular cloning of mouse tumour necrosis factor and its eukaryotic expression, *Nucleic Acids Res., 13*: 4417.

Hakoshima, T., and Tomita, K. (1988). Crystallization and preliminary x-ray investigation reveals that tumor necrosis factor is a compact trimer furnished with 3-fold symmetry, *J. Mol., Biol., 201*: 455.

Hohmann, H. P., Remy, R., Brockhaus, M., and Van Loon, A. P. G. M. (1989). Two different cell types have different major receptors for human tumor necrosis factor (TNFα), *J. Biol. Chem., 264*: 14927.

Imamura, K., Spriggs, D., and Kufe, D. (1987). Expression of tumor necrosis factor receptors on human monocytes and internalization of receptor bound ligand, *J. Immunol., 139*: 2989.

Israel, S., Hahn, T., Holtmann, H., and Wallach, D. (1986). Binding of human TNF-alpha to high-affinity cell surface receptors: effect of IFN, *Immunol. Lett., 12*: 217.

Jones, E. Y., Stuart, D. I., and Walker, N. P. (1989). Structure of tumour necrosis factor, *Nature, 338*: 225.

Kull, F. C., Jr., Jacobs, S., and Cuatrecasas, P. (1985). Cellular receptor for 125-I-labeled tumor necrosis factor: specific binding, affinity labeling, and relationship to sensitivity, *Proc. Natl. Acad. Sci. USA 82*: 5756.

Lewit-Bentley, A., Fourme, R., Kahn, R., Prangé, T., Vachette, P., Tavernier, J., Hauquier, G., and Fiers, W. (1988). Structure of tumour necrosis factor by x-ray solution scattering and preliminary studies by single crystal x-ray diffraction, *J. Mol. Biol., 199*: 389.

Locksley, R. M., Heinzel, F. P., Shepard, H. M., Agosti, J., Eessalu, T. E., Aggarwal, B.B., and Harlan, J. M. (1987). Tumor necrosis α and β differ in their capacities to generate interleukin 1 release from human endothelial cells, *J. Immunol., 139*: 1891.

Marmenout, a., Fransen, L., Tavernier, J., Van Der Heyden, J., Tizard, R., Kawashima, E., Shaw, A., Johnson, M. J., Semon, D., Muller, R., Ruysschaert, M. R., Van Vliet, A., and Fiers, W. (1985). Molecular cloning and expression of human tumor necrosis factor and comparison with mouse tumor necrosis factor, *Eur. J. Biochem., 152*: 515.

Munker, R., Dipersio, J., and Koeffler, H. P. (1987). Tumor necrosis factor: receptors on hematopoietic cells, *Blood, 70*: 1730.

Munson, P. J., and Rodbard, D. (1980). LIGAND: a versatile computerized approach for characterization of ligand-binding systems, *Anal. Biochem., 107*: 220.

Nawroth, P. P., Bank, I., Handley, D., Cassimeris, J., Chess, L., and Stern, D. (1986). Tumor necrosis factor/cachectin interacts with endothelial cell receptors to induce release of interleukin 1, *J. Exp. Med., 163*: 1363.

Oster, W., Lindemann, A., Horn, S., Mertelsmann, R., and Herrmann, F. (1987). Tumor necrosis factor (TNF)-alpha but not TNF-beta induces secretion of colony stimulating factor for macrophages (CSF-1) by human monocytes, *Blood, 70*: 1700.

Patton, J. S., Shepard, H. M., Wilking, H., Lewis, G., Aggarwal, B. B., Eessalu, T. E., Gavin, L. A., and Grunfeld, C. (1986). Interferons and tumor necrosis factors have similar catabolic effects on 3T3 L1 cells, *Proc. Natl. Acad. Sci. USA, 83*: 8313.

Rubin, B. Y., Anderson, S. L., Sullivan, S. A., Williamson, B. D., Carswell, E. A., and Old, L. J. (1985). High affinity binding of 125-I-labeled human tumor necrosis factor (LuKII) to specific surface receptors, *J. Exp. Med., 162*: 1099.

Scheurich, P., Ucer, U., Kronke, M., and Pfizenmaier, K. (1986). Quantification and characterization of high-affinity membrane receptors for tumor necrosis factor on human leukemic cell lines, *Int. J. Cancer, 38*: 127.

Seckinger, P., Isaaz, S., and Dayer, J. M. (1989). Purification and biologic characterization of a specific tumor necrosis factor alpha inhibitor, *J. Biol. Chem., 264*: 11966.

Shalaby, M. R., Palladino, M. A., Hirabayashi, S. E., Eessalu, T. E., Lewis, G. D., Shepard, H. M., and Aggarwal, B. B. (1987). Receptor binding and activation of polymorphonuclear neutrophils by tumor necrosis factor-α, *J. Leukocyte Biol., 41*: 196.

Shirai, T., Yamaguchi, H., Ito, H., Todd, C. W., and Wallace, R. B. (1985). Cloning and expression in *Escherichia coli* of the gene for human tumor necrosis factor, *Nature, 313*: 803.

Smith, R. A., and Baglioni, C. (1987). The active form of tumor necrosis factor is a trimer, *J. Biol. Chem., 262*: 6951.

Smith, R. A., and Baglioni, C. (1989). Multimeric structure of the tumor necrosis factor receptor of HeLa cells, *J. Biol. Chem., 264*: 14645.

Smith, R. A., Kirstein, M., Fiers, W., and Baglioni, C. (1986). Species specificity of human and murine tumor necrosis factor: a comparative study of tumor necrosis factor receptors, *J. Biol. Chem.,*: 14871.

Socher, S. H., Riemen, M. W., Martinez, D., Friedman, A., Tai, J., Quintero, J. C., Garsky, V., and Oliff, A. (1987). Antibodies against amino acids 1–15 of tumor necrosis factor block its binging to cell-surface receptor, *Proc. Natl. Acad. Sci. USA, 84*: 8829.

Stauber, G. B., Aiyer, R. A., and Aggarwal, B. B. (1988). Human tumor necrosis factor-α receptor: pruification by immunoaffinity chromatography and initial characterization, *J. Biol. Chem., 263*: 19098.

Sugarman, B. J., Aggarwal, B. B., Hass, P. E., Figari, I. S., Palladino, M., A., and Shepard, H. M. (1985). Recombinant human tumor necrosis factor-α: effects on proliferation of normal and transformed cells, *Science, 230*: 943.

Tsujimoto, M., Yip, Y. K., and Vilček, J. (1985). Tumor necrosis factor: specific binding and internalization in sensitive and resistant cells, *Proc. Natl. Acad. Sci. USA, 82*: 7626.

Tsujimoto, M., Feinman, R., Kohase, M., and Vilček, J. (1986a). Characterization and affinity crosslinking of receptors for tumor necrosis factor on human cells, *Arch. Biochem. Biophys., 249*: 563.

Tsujimoto, M., Feinman, R., and Vilček, J., (1986b). Differential effects of type I and IFN-γ on the binding of tumor necrosis factor to receptors in two human cell lines, *J. Immunol., 137*: 2272.

Wingfield, P., Pain, R. H., and Craig, S. (1987). Tumor necrosis factor is a compact trimer, *FEBS LETT., 211*: 179.

Yoshie, O., Tada, K., and Ishida, N. (1986). Binding and crosslinking of ^{125}I-labeled recombinant human tumor necrosis factor to cell surface receptors., *J. Biochem. (Tokyo), 100*: 531.

7

Regulation of TNF Receptors

MASAFUMI TSUJIMOTO
Suntory Institute for Biomedical Research, Mishima, Osaka, Japan

NAOTO OKU
Setsunan University, Hirakata, Osaka, Japan

I. INTRODUCTION

Through recombinant DNA technology, several cytokines, including TNF, have become available during the last few years in highly purified forms and in sufficient quantities. Availability of recombinant TNF has made it possible to examine biological action of TNF, and it is now evident that TNF exerts regulatory effects on the immune system, cytotoxic action on some tumor cells, and mediation of endotoxic shock and cachexia in infections and neoplastic diseases (Beutler and Cerami, 1986).

It is well known that cytokines initiate their biological actions by binding to high-affinity receptors on the surface of target cells. Initially, it was expected that TNF receptors might serve as determinants of cellular susceptibility to cytotoxic action of TNF (Old, 1985). However, high-affinity receptors for TNF have been demonstrated in various tumor cell lines regardless of their sensitivity, and it was also shown that TNF bound to specific receptors on human FS-4 fibroblasts which were completely resistant to the cytotoxic action of TNF (Tsujimoto et al., 1985; Yoshie et al., 1986). These results suggested that the presence of specific binding sites is apparently necessary but not sufficient for cells to be sensitive to TNF cytotoxicity, and TNF receptors on cells resistant to the cytotoxic action of TNF serve to mediate the many other biological activities of TNF.

A large number of examples of receptor regulation by homologous or heterologous ligands have been reported, suggesting that the regulation of receptor number or affinity might be a prevalent mechanism of cellular regulation. Moreover, cytokines such as TNF, IL-1, and IFN-γ are often produced by the same cell population in response to the same stimuli. Therefore, the biological significance of receptor regulation might be related to synergistic or inhibitory effects observed with various combinations of cytokines.

In this chapter we describe the regulation of TNF receptor expression by various factors which might interact with TNF and modulate some inflammatory processes in vivo. We also discuss some implications of biological significance of the receptor modulation.

II. UP-REGULATION OF TNF RECEPTORS

A. IFNs

In some tumor cell lines, TNF and IFNs were shown to exert a synergistic cytotoxic action, and this effect was particularly marked with IFN-γ (Williamson et al., 1983). Moreover, it was shown that IFN-γ render some resistant cells sensitive to the cytotoxic action of TNF (Lewis et al., 1987). To elucidate the mechanism of synergistic action between TNF and IFNs, effects of IFNs on expression of TNF receptors were examined extensively.

Pretreatment of various tumor cells with IFN-γ resulted in increase of TNF binding (Aggarwal et al., 1985; Ruggiero et al., 1986; Tsujimoto et al., 1986b). Scatchard analysis showed that whereas there was no significant change in the apparent binding affinity of TNF, the number of specific binding per cell was increased by 1.3- to 2.0-fold (Fig. 1). Enhancement of TNF binding was demonstrable after 6 h of treatment with INF-γ. After removal of IFN-γ, TNF binding decreased gradually reaching to control levels by 20 h (Tsujimoto and Vilček, 1986).

Effects of IFN-α and IFN-β on TNF receptor expression were different depending on cell lines studied (Aggarwal and Eessalu, 1987a; Tsujimoto et al., 19856a). In HeLa cells, IFN-α and IFN-β increased TNF binding, whereas in HT-29 cells, these two IFNs had little effects on TNF binding. Both IFNs exerted an antagonistic effect on IFN-γ-induced stimulation of TNF receptor expression in HT-29 cells, but did not have any effects on TNF receptor induction by IFN-γ in HeLa cells.

The induction of TNF receptors by IFN-γ was observed in different cell types regardless of their sensitivity to TNF. For example, in several cell lines such as HeLa and RPMI-7272 cells, IFN-γ caused an increase in TNF binding without a concomitant increase in sensitivity to TNF cytotoxicity. Moreover, despite the inhibitory effect of IFN-β on IFN-γ-induced stimulation of TNF receptor expression, IFN-β did not inhibit synergistic enhancement of TNF cytotoxicity by IFN-γ in

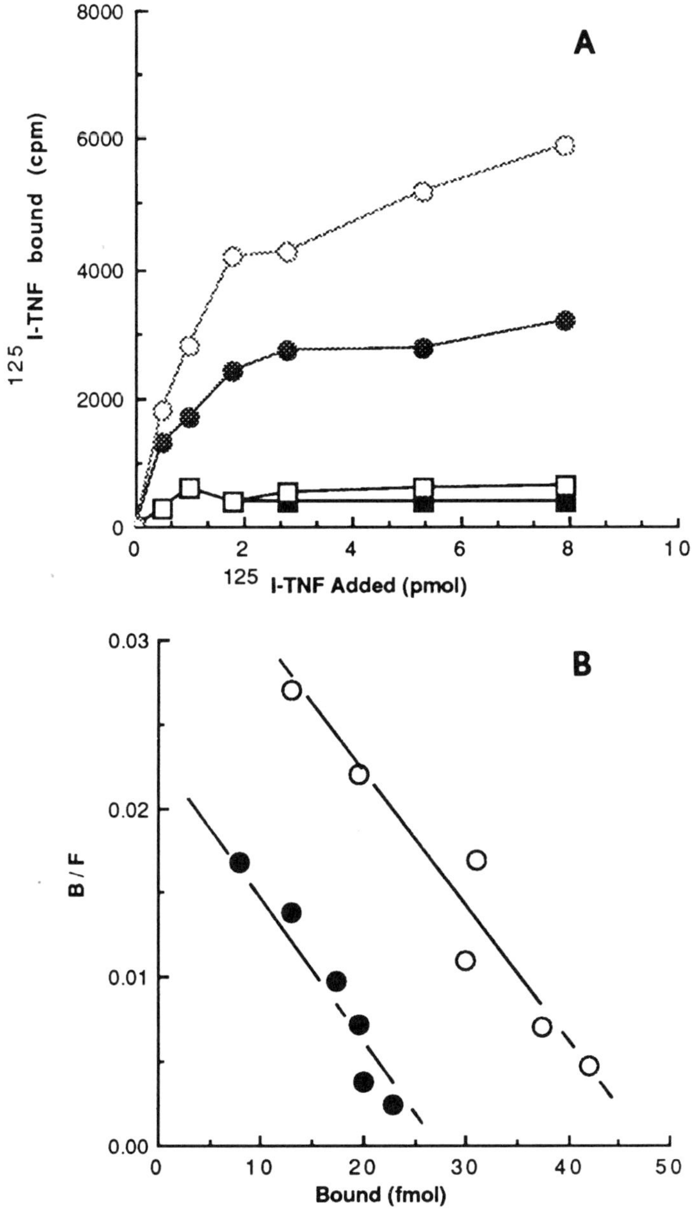

Figure 1 Effect of IFN-γ on the expression of TNF receptors on HT-29 cells. (A) HT-29 cells were incubated for 15 h with (○,□) or without (●,■) IFN-γ. Thereafter, binding of[^{125}I]TNF was determined at 4.°C. Nonspecific binding was measured in the presence of excess of unlabeled TNF(■,□). (B) Scatchard analysis of the binding data shown in (A). (From Tsujimoto et al., 1986b)

HT-29 cells. These results indicate that induction of TNF receptors by IFN-γ is not a major mechanism of synergism between TNF and IFN-γ (Aggarwal and Eessalu, 1987a; Tsujimoto et al., 1986a,b).

Mechanism of IFN-γ-induced increase of TNF receptor expression was examined employing metabolic inhibitors such as cycloheximide and actinomycin D (Ruggiero et al., 1986; Tsujimoto and Vilček, 1986). The increase of TNF receptors was completely prevented when cells were treated with IFN-γ in the presence of inhibitors. When cultures were incubated with or without IFN-γ in the presence of cycloheximide, TNF binding was increased after removal of cycloheximide in both IFN-γ-treated or untreated cultures. However, the increase was greater in the cultures incubated with IFN-γ. These results suggested that IFN-γ stimulates the synthesis of TNF receptor mRNA and that translation of this mRNA is presumably responsible for the increase of the receptors.

B. IL-2

Resting T cells do not express surface receptors for TNF. However, treatment with IL-2 resulted in specific TNF binding to lympocytes (Owen-Schaub et al., 1989). Flow cytometric analysis indicated that the receptor was induced in cytotoxic T cell, helper T cell, and NK cell populations.

Increase in TNF binding after treatment with IL-2 was rather slow, became maximal between days 5 and 9, and were maintained for 18 to 20 days in the presence of IL-2. It was also demonstrated that IL-2 concentration determined the maginitude of TNF receptor expression, influencing both the percentage of TNF-positive cells within the population and the number of receptors/cells.

After treatment with TNF, activated T cells revealed an enhanced response to IL-2 (Scheurich et al., 1987), suggesting that enhancement of TNF receptor expression was involved in the amplification of an ongoing immune response.

C. Lectins

Exposure of human cervical carcinoma cell line ME-180 to some lectins, such as concanavalin A (Con A) and wheat germ agglutinin (WGA), caused an increase in TNF receptors without significant change in their affinity constant (Aggarwal et al., 1986). In contrast with IFN-γ, this increase in receptor number did not require the synthesis of new proteins. Con A also decreased the rate of internalization and inhibited the release and degradation of TNF.

Although Con A induced the increase in the number of receptors, ME-180 cells were protected from the cytotoxic action of TNF. Because cytoskeletal-disrupting agents and inhibitors of lysosomal activities were reported to depress the sensitivity to TNF cytotoxicity (Kull and Cuatrecasas, 1981), the most likely explanation of the results was that internalization and subsequent degradation of TNF was required for cytotoxic action of TNF.

After treatment of unstimulated lymphocytes with T-cell mitogen such as phytohemaglutinin (PHA) and OKT 3 antibody, binding of TNF to surface receptor was increased (Munker et al., 1987; Scheurich et al., 1987). TNF exerted multiple stimulatory activities on TNF receptor positive T cells through mitogen-induced TNF receptors, indicating that TNF might regulate the growth and functional activities of activated T cells through mitogen-induced TNF receptors.

D. TSH

Treatment of differentiated thyroid epithelial cells (FRTL-5) with TNF blocked the TSH-stimulated uptake of iodide and thymidine on these cells, indicating that TNF affected thyroid cell function through binding to specific receptors (Pang et al., 1989b). Treatment of the cells with TSH caused an increase in TNF binding to its specific receptors (Pang et al., 1989a). Scatchard analysis indicated that the number of specific binding sites per cell for TNF were increased without significant change in apparent binding affinity.TSH-induced increase in TNF receptor expression was considered to be linked with the action of TNF on FRTL-5 cells.

III. DOWN-REGULATION OF TNF RECEPTORS

A. Phorbol Esters

Phorbol esters are known to bind and activate protein kinase C, which is involved in the signal transduction system of many growth factors. It has also been reported that PMA induces down-regulation of EGF receptors. In view of these observations, effects of PMA on expression of TNF receptors in various cells were examined by several groups.

Pretreatment of various cell lines with PMA resulted in decrease in TNF binding within 30 min. However, results of PMA effect on receptor or affinity constant was conflicting even when the same cell line was investigated. Unglaub et al. (1987) concluded that PMA reduced the affinity of cell surface receptors for TNF in U937 cells, because TNF–receptor complex in PMA-treated cells dissociated more rapidly than untreated cells. In contrast, Aggarwal and Eessalu (1987b) reported that treatment of U937 cells with PMA reduced the total receptor number without any significant change in the affinity constant of the receptors.

Using SV80 cells and HeLa cells, Holtmann and Wallach (1987) also demonstrated that PMA induced down-regulation of the receptors. The decrease in TNF binding could not be blocked by cycloheximide, suggesting that protein synthesis was not required. Scatchard analysis indicated that PMA reduced the number of receptors with no change in their affinity.

Johnson and Baglioni (1988) examined the effect of PMA on HeLa cells and found that both affinity and number of binding sites decreased with PMA treatment. Depletion or inhibition or protein kinase C antagonized PMA-induced effects on TNF binding, indicating the involvement of PMA-activated protein kinase C in down-regulation of TNF receptors.

The cytotoxic activity of TNF was greatly inhibited when sensitive cells were pretreated with PMA. Maximal inhibition of cytotoxicity occurred when cells were treated with PMA before TNF addition and the protection decreased with later addition of PMA. These results suggested that PMA interferes with one of the early step in the mechanism of TNF action. (Johnson and Baglioni, 1988).

In HeLa cells, the dose response and time course of PMA-induced decrease in TNF cytotoxicity closely paralleled the PMA-induced loss of TNF binding to cellular receptors, but in L cells and SV80 cells there was some discrepancy between the two effects of PMA (Holtmann and Wallach, 1987; Johnson and Baglioni, 1988), suggesting that receptor modulation is not the only mechanism whereby desensitization can occur. In any case, modulation of TNF sensitivity in target cells via activation of protein kinase C may play a role in some physiological or pathological processes in vivo by inducing the cells resistant to the cytotoxic action of TNF.

B. IL-1

Treatment of SV80 cells or FS-11 cells with IL-1 resulted in decrease of TNF binding to cell surface receptors (Holtmann and Wallach, 1987). Decrease in TNF binding was rapid, reaching its lowest level at about 1 h. Scatchard analysis indicated that decrease in TNF binding reflected a reduced amount of TNF receptors without a significant change in their affinity. The effect of IL-1 on TNF receptors could not be blocked by cycloheximide, suggesting that it was independent of protein synthesis.

In addition to a decrease in TNF receptors, cells treated with IL-1 exhibited a lesser vulnerability to the cytotoxic action of TNF. However, removal of IL-1 from the cultures was followed by a rapid recovery of TNF receptors but not the vulnerability to its cytotoxic effect. These results suggested that IL-1 down-regulate cellular response to TNF by inducing a decrease in the number of TNF receptors and through some additional mechanisms as well.

C. LPS

Brief preexposure of macrophages to traces of LPS rendered the cells refractory to the activation induced by TNF (Ding and Nathan, 1987). Using murine macrophage cell line RAW 264.7, the mechanism of action of LPS was examined and it was found that LPS induced a loss of surface receptors for TNF (Ding et al., 1989).

LPS-mediated down-regulation of the receptors was rapid (15 min for 50% reduction) and was temperature dependent; preexposure of the cells to LPS for 1 h at 4°C had no detectable effect on subsequent binding of TNF. Moreover, while incubation at 37°C with LPS resulted in a complete disappearance of TNF receptors on cell surface, specific binding was unchanged when measured in the presence of 0.055% digitonin. These results suggested that the cells rapidly internalize their TNF receptors in response to LPS.

The action of LPS was rather cell-type specific. Both macrophages and endothelial cells down-regulated their receptors in response to LPS, but PMN or some other tumor cells did not. These results implied that macrophages and some other host cells were resistant to the action of TNF produced during endotoxinemia, because they might internalize their TNF receptors in response to LPS before TNF was produced.

D. Glucocorticoids

Dexamethasone (DEX), a known inhibitor of phospholipase A_2, also inhibits the cytotoxic activity of TNF on some tumor cells (Kull, 1988; Tsujimoto and Adachi, 1988). Pretreatment of the cells with DEX reduced the affinity of specific cell surface receptors about three-fold while retaining the same number of binding sites (Kull, 1988). Because cytotoxic activities of TNF and TNF analogs on sensitive cells had some correlations with their receptor binding activities (Carlino et al., 1987; Tsujimoto et al., 1987), reduction in binding affinity by DEX might contribute to the inhibition of TNF cytotoxicity.

E. Oncogene (HER-2)

The HER-2 oncogene encodes a tyrosine kinase receptor-like protein ($P185^{HER\text{-}2}$) with homology to EGF receptors. It was shown that over expression of HER-2 oncogene resulted in transformation and tumorigenicity of NIH-3T3 cells and that amplification of HER-2 is often associated with aggressive human breast cancers. Therefore, it is important to elucidate the action of this oncogene.

To test the action of HER-2 gene product, HER-2 gene transfectants were prepared using NIH-3T3 cells and found that amplification of $p185^{HER\text{-}2}$ expression resulted in a parallel induction of resistance to TNF (Hudziak et al. 1988). Moreover, it was demonstrated that expression of $P185^{HER\text{-}2}$ in NIH-3T3 cells resulted in 20-fold reduction of the binding affinity of TNF receptor to the ligand. The results again indicated that resistance was accompanied by a decrease in the binding affinity between TNF and its receptors. Moreover, it also suggested that amplified expression of HER-2 oncogene not only might induce cellular transformation, but also play a role in tumor progression by suppressing some host defense mechanisms mediated by TNF.

F. TNF

TNF down-regulates its own receptors in HeLa cells (Tsujimoto and Vilček, 1987). After treatment of the cells with TNF, decrease in the number of surface receptors

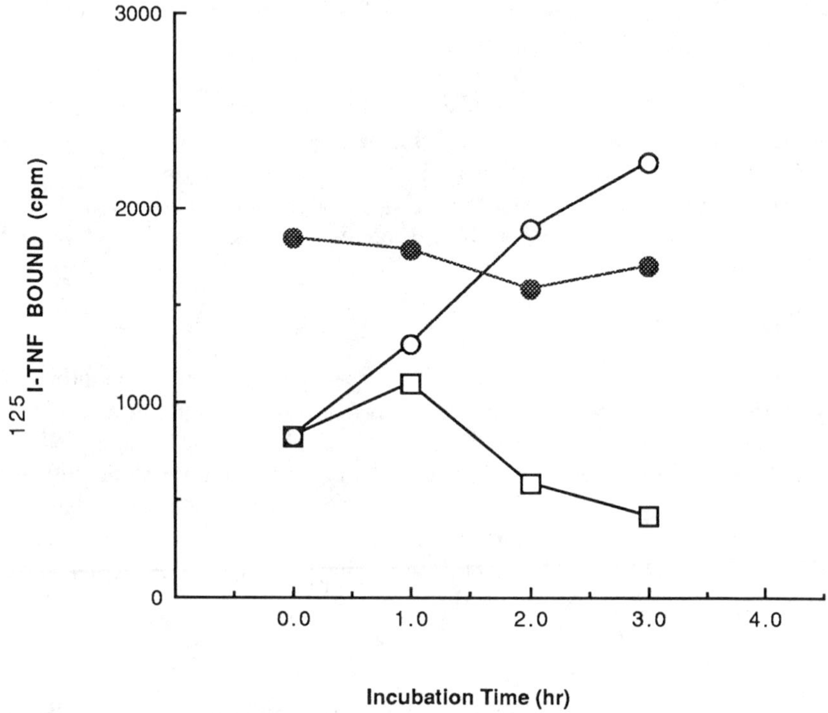

Figure 2 Recovery of ^{125}I-labeled TNF binding after prior incubation with unlabeled TNF. HeLa cells were incubated for 3 h in the presence (○,□) or absence (●) or unlabeled TNF. The cells were washed three times with culture medium and resuspended in prewarmed medium with (□) or without (●,○) cycloheximide. At the indicated times, binding of ^{125}I-labeled TNF was determined. (From Tsujimoto and Vilček, 1987.)

was rapid, reaching its lowest level at about 2 h. After removal of TNF, recovery of the amount of cell surface receptors was also rapid (Fig. 2). Full recovery required de novo synthesis of the receptors. In the presence of cycloheximide, only an initial recovery of TNF binding was observed, suggesting that some TNF receptor proteins were either replenished from an intracellular pool of receptors or recycled.

On the other hand, using breast adenocarcinoma cell line MCF-7, Vuk-Pavlovic and Kovach (1989) demonstrated that cells preincubated with TNF bound six times more TNF than did untreated cells. Preexposure of the cells to increasing concentration of TNF stimulated the binding of TNF to the cells. Analysis by compartmental models indicated that both internalization and recycling of TNF receptors were stimulated by the ligand.

In the presence of inhibitors of protein synthesis, sensitivity of tumor cells to the cytotoxic action of TNF was often increased. However, pretreatment of TNF alone with cells made the cells refractory to the cytotoxic action of TNF even in the presence of inhibitors (Wallach, 1984). Down-regulation of TNF receptors by the ligand might, at least in part, play a role in inducing the cells resistant to TNF.

IV. CONCLUDING REMARKS

In this chapter we have described various factors that regulate the cell surface number and/or affinity of TNF receptors. However, significance of the receptor modulation on the biological activities of TNF is not clear at present. In some cells, regulation of receptor number might be important for TNF actions. Because LPS completely down-regulates TNF receptors on macrophages, subsequent challenge of TNF had no effect on macrophage activation. In addition, T cells become responsible to TNF only after activated by T-cell mitogens or IL-2.

On the other hand, it was reported that induction of the receptors by IFNs was not a major mechanism for the synergistic cytotoxic action between TNF and IFNs. Indeed, occupation of a small portion of the receptor is enough for the cytotoxic action of TNF (Munker et al., 1987; Tsujimoto et al., 1985).

It is also demonstrated that TNF sensitive cells and resistant cells have similar number and affinity of receptors, indicating that postreceptor events are important for the cytotoxic action of TNF. Moreover, it was suggested that internalization and degradation of TNF is a prerequisite for the cytotoxic action of TNF. Therefore, reduction of the affinity of TNF receptors might result in the desensitization of the cells via decrease in number of TNF molecules internalized.

In an effort to elucidate the significance of TNF internalization, we and others observed that TNF caused an increase in the permeability of liposomes containing phosphatidylserine only in acidic conditions (Oku et al., 1987; Yoshimura and Sone, 1987). These results suggested the possibility that TNF bound to its cell surface receptors accumulated in lysosomes, where it was released from receptors and subsequently damaged the lysosomal membrane. Baldwin et al. (1988) also reported that the cytotoxicity of TNF and capacity of TNF to bind and penetrate phosphatidylcholine liposomes were pH dependent. They suggested that a low-pH milieu triggered conformational changes that facilitated TNF release from receptors and insertion into the membrane. In fact, we observed that increase in hydrophobicity of TNF molecules under acidic conditions. Ohsawa and Natori (1988) observed that while internalization of TNF was observed in both sensitive and resistant cells, TNF was degraded only in sensitive cells, suggesting that the degradation process is important for cytotoxic action of TNF. Moreover, they observed that the culture medium of sensitive cells contained permeability-inducing activity of liposomes composed of phosphaytidylcholine and phosphatidylserine. This activity was not detected in the culture medium of insensitive cells. They suggested that the sensitive cells contained a specific protease that degrades TNF and that degradation product released into the culture medium is responsible for the activity of liposomal damage.

From the data described above, it is tempting to speculate that internalization of TNF and its subsequent degradation and/or interaction with lysosomal membrane might be involved in the cytotoxic action of TNF. If that is the case, modulation of TNF receptors is important for the regulation of cytotoxic action of TNF by changing TNF molecules internalized. However, as discussed elsewhere, several mechanisms of the cytotoxic action of TNF have been proposed. To understand the biological significance of TNF receptor modulation, detailed analysis of mechanism of TNF actions is required.

REFERENCES

Aggarwal, B. B., and Eessalu, T. E. (1987a). Induction of receptors for tumor necrosis factor-α by interferons is not a major mechanism for their synergistic cytotoxic response, *J. Biol. Chem., 262*: 10000.

Aggarwal, B. B., and Eessalu, T. E. (1987b). Effect of phorbol esters on down-regulation and redistribution of cell surface receptors for tumor necrosis factor-α, *J. Biol. Chem., 262*: 16450.

Aggarwal, B. B., Eessalu, T. E., and Hass, P. E. (1985). Characterization of receptors for human tumor necrosis factor and their regulation by γ-interferon, *Nature, 318*: 665.

Aggarwal, B. B., Traquina, P. R., and Eessalu, T. E. (1986). Modulation of receptors and cytotoxic response of tumor necrosis factor-α by various lectins, *J. Biol. Chem., 261*: 13652.

Baldwin, R. L., Chang, M. P., Bramhall, J., Graves, S., Bonavida, B., and Wisnieski, B. J., (1988). Capacity of tumor necrosis factor to bind and penetrate membranes is pH-dependent, *J. Immunol., 141*: 2352.

Beutler, B., and Cerami, A. (2986). Cachectin and tumor necrosis factor as two sides of the same biological coin, *Nature, 320*: 584.

Carlino, J. A., Lin, L. S., and Creasey, A. A. (1987). Use of sensitive receptor binding assay to discriminate between full-length and truncated human recombinant tumor necrosis factor proteins, *J. Biol. Chem., 262*: 958.

Ding, A. H., and Nathan, C. F. (1987). Trace levels of bacterial lipopolysaccharide prevent interferon-γ or tumor necrosis factor-α from enhancing mouse peritoneal macrophage respiratory burst capacity, *J. Immunol., 139*: 1971.

Ding, A. H., Sanchez, E., Srimal, S., and Nathan, C. F. (1989). Macrophage rapidly internalize their tumor necrosis factor receptors in response to bacterial lipopolysaccharide, *J. Biol. Chem., 264*: 3924.

Holtmann, H., and Wallach, D. (1987). Down regulation of the receptors for tumor necrosis factor by interleukin 1 and 4-β-phorbol-12-myristate-13-acetate, *J. Immunol., 139*: 1161.

Hudziak, R. M. Lewis, G. D., Shalaby, R., Eessalu, T., Aggarwal, B. B., Ullrich, A., and Shepard, H. M. (1988). Amplified expression of the HER2/ERBB2 oncogene induces resistance to tumor necerosis factor-α in NIH 3T3 cells, *Proc. Natl. Acad. Sci. USA, 85*: 5102.

Johnson, S. E., and Baglioni, C. (1988). Tumor necrosis factor receptors and cytocidal activity are down-regulated by activators of protein kinase C, *J. Biol. Chem., 263*: 5686.

Kull, F. C., Jr. (1988). Reduction in tumor necrosis factor receptor affinity and cytotoxicity by glucocorticoids, *Biochem. Biophys. Res. Commun., 153*: 402.

Kull, F. C., Jr., and Cuatrecasas, P. (1981). Possible requirement of internalization in the mechanism of in vitro cytotoxicity in tumor necrosis serum, *Cancer Res., 41*: 4885.

Lewis, G. D., Aggarwal, B. B., Eessalu, T. E., Sugarman, B. J., and Shepard, H. M. (1987). Modulation of the growth of transformed cells by human tumor necrosis factor-α and interferon-γ, *Cancer Res., 47*: 5382.

Munker, R., DiPersio, J., and Koeffler, H. P. (1987). Tumor necrosis factor: receptors on hematopoietic cells, *Blood, 70*: 1730.

Ohsawa, F., and Natori, S. (1988). Selective degradation of tumor necrosis factor in sensitive cells, and production of membrane-active substance, *J. Biochem., 103*: 730.

Oku, N., Araki, R., Araki, H., Shibamoto, S., Ito, F., Nishihara, T., and Tsujimoto, M. (1987). Tumor necrosis factor-induced permeability increase of negatively charged phospholipid vesicles, *J. Biochem., 102*: 1303.

Old, L. J. (1985). Tumor necrosis factor (TNF), *Science, 230*: 630.

Owen-Schaub, L. B., Crump, W. L., III, Morin, G. I., and Grimm, E. A. (1989). Regulation of lymphocyte tumor necrosis factor receptors by IL-2, *J. Immunol, 143*: 2236.

Pang, X. -P., Hershman, J. M., Chung, M., and Pekary, A. E. (1989a). Characterization of tumor necrosis factor-α receptors in human and rat thyroid cells and regulation of the receptors by thyrotropin, *Endocrinology, 125*: 1783.

Pang, X. -P., Pekary, A. E., Mirell, C., and Hershman, J. M. (1989b). Impairment of hypothalamic-pituitary-thyroid function in rats treated with human recombinant tumor necrosis factor-α (cachectin), *Endocrinology, 125*: 76.

Ruggiero, V., Tavernier, J., Fiers, W., and Baglioni, C. (1986). Induction of the synthesis of tumor necrosis factor receptors by interferon-γ, *J. Immunol., 136*: 2445.

Scheurich, P., Thoma, B., Ücer, U., and Pfizenmaier, K. (1987). Immunoregulatory activity of recombinant human tumor necrosis factor: induction of TNF receptors on human T cells and TNF-α-mediated enhancement of T cell responses, *J. Immunol., 138*: 1786.

Tsujimoto, M., and Adachi, H. (1988). Effects of steroid hormones on the cytotoxic activity of tumor necrosis factor, *J. Biochem., 103*: 393.

Tsujimoto, M., Feinman, R., and Vilček, J. (1986a). Differential effects of type I IFN and IFN-γ on the binding of tumor necrosis factor to receptors in two human cell lines, *J. Immunol., 137*: 2272.

Tsujimoto, M., and Vilček, J. (1986). Tumor necrosis factor receptors in HeLa cells and their regulation by interferon-γ, *J. Biol. Chem., 261*: 5384.

Tsujimoto, M., and Vilček, J. (1987). Tumor necrosis factor-induced down-regulation of its receptors in HeLa cells, *J. Biochem., 102*: 1571.

Tsujimoto, M., Yip, Y. K., and Vilček, J. (1985). Tumor necrosis factor: specific binding and internalization in sensitive and resisitant cells, *Proc. Natl. Acad. Sci. USA, 82*: 7626.

Tsujimoto, M., Yip, Y. K., and Vilček, J. (1986b). Interferon-γ enhances expression of cellular receptors for tumor necrosis factor, *J. Immunol., 136*: 2441.

Tsujimoto, M., Tanaka, S., Sakuragawa, Y., Tsuruoka, N., Funakoshi, K., Butsugan, T., Nakazato, H., Nishihara, T., Noguchi, T., and Vilček, J. (1987). Comparative studies of the biological activities of human tumor necrosis factor and its derivatives, *J. Biochem., 101*: 919.

Unglaub, R., Maxeiner, B., Thoma, B., Pfizenmaier, K., and Scheurich, P. (1987). Downregulation of tumor necrosis factor (TNF) sensitivity via modulation of TNF binding capacity by protein kinase C activators, *J. Exp. Med., 166*: 1788.

Vuk-Pavlovic, S., and Kovach, J. S. (1989). Recycling of tumor necrosis-α receptor in MCF-7 cells, *FASEB. J., 3*: 2633.

Wallach, D. (1984). Preparations of lymphotoxin induce resistance to their own cytotoxic effect, *J. Immunol., 132*: 2464.

Williamson, B. D., Carswell, E. A. , Rubin, B. Y., Prendergast, J. S., and Old, L. J. (1983). Human tumor necrosis factor produced by human B-cell lines: synergistic cytotoxic interaction with human interferon. *Proc. Natl. Acad. Sci. USA, 80*: 5397.

Yoshie, O., Tada, K., and Ishida, N. (1986). Binding and crosslinking of ^{125}I-labeled recombinant human tumor necrosis factor to cell surface receptors, *J. Biochem., 100*: 531.

Yoshimura, T., and Sone, S. (1987). Different and synergistic actions of human tumor necrosis factor and interferon-γ in damage of liposome membranes, *J. Biol. Chem., 262*: 4597.

8

Purification and Structural Properties of Two Distinct TNF Receptors on Human Cells

HANSRUEDI LOETSCHER
F. Hoffmann-LaRoche Ltd., Basel, Switzerland

I. INTRODUCTION

In the last few years TNF-α and TNF-β (in this chapter jointly referred to as TNF) have been recognized as two closely related cytokines with a broad spectrum of biological activities. They share about 30% sequence homology (Aggarwal et al., 1985b; Gray et al., 1984; Pennica et al., 1984) and their genes are located in close proximity within the major histocompatibility complex in mouse and man (Mueller et al., 1987; Spies et al., 1986). Besides cytotoxic effects on certain tumor cells in vitro (Helson et al., 1975; Matthews and Neale, 1987) and in vivo (Carswell et al., 1975; Old, 1985), TNF has been found to play a role in a variety of inflammatory and immunological responses (Beutler and Cerami, 1987; 1988; Talmadge et al., 1988; Tracey et al., 1989). It appears that a complex system consisting of at least two distinct TNF receptors (Brockhaus et al., 1990; Hohmann et al., 1989) and probably additional accessory proteins (Yonehara et al., 1989) regulates cellular responses to TNF. The functional roles of TNF as mediator in intercellular communication are reviewed and discussed in more detail in other chapters of this book.

In x-ray diffraction studies TNF-α is a tightly packed trimer of 17-kDa monomers (Eck et al., 1988; Hakoshima and Tomita, 1988; Jones et al., 1989). It is assumed that the trimer is the biologically active species (Arakawa and Yphantis, 1987; Lam et al., 1988; Smith and Baglioni, 1987). In addition to the secreted

17-kDa form, a 26-kDa membrane-bound form of TNF-α has been found on monocytes (Kriegler et al., 1988). The three-dimensional structure of TNF-β has not yet been determined. Cross-linking experiments (Browning and Ribolini, 1989) as well as light-scattering and ultracentrifugation studies (H. J. Schoenfeld, and M. Zulauf, personal communication) also indicate, however, a trimeric structure for TNF-β. The potential trivalency of the ligands might have a profound functional significance. Ligand-induced microclustering of receptors on cell surfaces could activate different signal transduction pathways in different cells depending on density and lateral mobility of receptors.

The first event in the response of a cell to TNF is the interaction of the ligand with specific cell surface receptors. Several groups have identified TNF receptors on various cell types (see the references in Table 1 and Aggarwal et al., 1985a; Baglioni et al., 1985; Munker, et al., 1987; Rubin et al., 1985; Shalaby et al., 1987; Smith and Baglioni, 1989; Sugarman et al., 1985; Tsujimoto et al., 1985, 1986c). A single class of cell surface TNF binding sites with K_d values in the pM range and expressed in a few hundred to a few thousand copies per cell have been reported. TNF-α and TNF-β have been found to compete for the same cellular binding sites (Aggarwal et al., 1985a; Brockhaus et al., 1990; Stauber and Aggarwal, 1989).

In this chapter I discuss the identification and subsequent purification to homogeneity of two distinct TNF receptors of 55- and 75-kDa apparent molecular masses from different human cell lines and from human placenta in amounts sufficient for protein sequencing. Recently, the 55-kDa TNF receptor cDNA has been cloned by using oligonucleotides derived from partial amino acid sequences determined for the purified protein (Loetscher et al., 1990a). Interesting structural features of this TNF receptor are summarized at the end of this chapter.

II. IDENTIFICATION OF TNF RECEPTORS

A. Cell-Surface-Bound TNF Receptors

1. Cross-linking TNF to TNF Receptors

Various bands in SDS-PAGE analysis representing TNF-binding proteins have been found on different cells by cross-linking radiolabeled ligand to the cell surface. Table 1 summarizes molecular masses of cross-linked ligand-receptor complexes reported by different groups in the past few years using radioiodinated TNF-α and TNF-β and different human and murine cell lines. A complex structure of the TNF receptor consisting of two or even more components emerges from these data. Interestingly, the binding of TNF is not species-specific, although a certain preference of TNF-α for the homologous species in human and murine systems has been reported (Kramer et al., 1988; Smith et al., 1986). No clear correlation between TNF cytotoxicity and receptor density on the cell surfaces has been found. One study proposed, however, that the cytotoxic effects of TNF are linked to the

Table 1 Comparison of Ligand-Receptor Complexes Obtained by Cross-linking Human [^{125}I]TNF-α, Murine [^{125}I]TNF-α and Human [^{125}I]TNF-β to Different Cells

	Cross-linked with:			
Cell line	h[^{125}I]TNF-α (kDa)	m[^{125}I]TNF-α (kDa)	h[^{125}I]TNF-β (kDa)	Reference
Human				
U937	98–100,75			Hohmann et al., 1989
	100		100,120	Stauber and Aggarwal, 1989
			97,70	Hirano et al., 1989
	100			Stauber et al., 1988
	100			Yoshie, et al., 1986
	100			Tsujimoto et al., 1986a
	93			Scheurich et al., 1986
	92,75			Israel et al., 1986
HL-60	98-100,75			Hohmann et al., 1989
KG-1	92,75			Israel et al., 1986
THP-1	105			Yoshie, et al., 1986
Monocytes	98–100,75			Hohmann et al., 1989
K562	98–100,75			Hohmann et al., 1989
	93			Scheurich et al., 1986
HEp2	95,75			Hohmann et al., 1989

Table 1 (Continued)

Cell line	Cross-linked with: h[^{125}I]TNF-α (kDa)	m[^{125}I]TNF-α (kDa)	h[^{125}I]TNF-β (kDa)	Reference
MCF7	138,90,75,54			Creasy et al., 1987
	95,75			Hohmann et al., 1989
HT-29	100			Tsujimoto et al., 1986b
HeLa	95,75			Hohmann et al., 1989
	105			Yoshie et al., 1986
	100			Tsujimoto et al., 1986b
KYM	145			Niitsu et al., 1988
Murine				
L-M		95,75		Kull et al., 1985
L929			97,70	Hirano et al., 1989

presence of a particular 138-kDa TNF-binding protein (Creasy et al., 1987). Based on the biochemical characterization of proteolytic fragments of cross-linked [^{125}I]TNF-α TNF-receptor complexes from various cells, the existence of at least two distinct TNF receptors has been postulated (Hohmann et al., 1989).

2. *TNF-Receptor-Specific Monoclonal Antibodies*

To analyze TNF-biding proteins in more detail and/or assign a functionality to the individual receptors, a large effort was made to develop TNF-receptor-specific monoclonal antibodies using partially purified TNF receptors for immunization of mice (Brockhaus and Loetscher, 1990). Two sets of antibodies with different specificities were obtained, called htr and utr monoclonal antibody series, respectively (Brockhaus et al., 1990). Antibodies of the htr series completely block specific TNF-α binding to several adenocarcinoma cell lines (HEp-2, MCF-7, HeLa), whereas antibodies of the utr series have no effect on these cell lines, but partially inhibit TNF-α binding to HL-60 and U937 cells. When utr-1 and htr-9 antibodies are used in combination, however, full inhibition of TNF-α binding to HL-60 and U937 cells is observed. Specific binding of TNF-β to HEp2 and U937 cells is also inhibited by these antibodies. Flow cytometry studies show that htr-9 and utr-1 antibodies detect two distinct TNF-α binding sites on cell surfaces (Brockhaus et al., 1990). By Western blot and immunoprecipitation analyses exclusive specificity of the htr-9 and utr-1 antibodies for a 55- and a 75-Kda TNF-receptor protein, respectively, can be demonstrated. In conclusion, these results provide good evidence for the existence of two immunologically distinct TNF receptors which are expressed to different extents on various cells.

B. Solubilized TNF Receptors

To detect and quantitate the amount of solubilized TNF receptors in cell extracts and at various stages of purification, an assay for specific TNF-α binding is needed. Conditions to precipitate [^{125}I]TNF-α TNF-receptor complexes with polyethylene glycol were established and used to follow TNF-binding activity in gelfiltration studies of detergent-solubilized TNF receptors (Smith and Baglioni, 1989; Stauber et al., 1988). However, depending on buffer composition and ingredients, a considerable nonspecific coprecipitation of free ligand may occur, which makes quantitative analysis of this type of assay very difficult (Stauber et al., 1988).

A different assay type is presented in Fig. 1. In this filter-based dot blot assay samples are spotted onto nitrocellulose membranes and probed for [^{125}I]TNF-α binding. Bound radioactivity can be visualized by autoradiography or counted directly. Nonspecific [^{125}I]TNF-α binding is determined in the presence of excess unlabeled TNF-α. In the example shown in Fig. 1 crude membrane fractions prepared from placenta and two different cell lines, a cell extract and partially purified TNF receptors were analyzed for [^{125}I]TNF-α binding. Specific binding of TNF-α is evident in all samples containing TNF receptor(s). Membranes from murine EL-4 cells that are practically devoid of TNF receptors (Yoshie 1986) are included as a negative control and show mainly nonspecific binding. When specific binding of [^{125}I]TNF-α to HL-60 membranes is quantitated and analyzed according to Scatchard, a curvilinear plot is obtained suggesting a heterogeneity of binding sites with estimated K_d values in the range of about 50 and 350 pM (Loetscher et al., 1990b). In view of the fact that intact HL-60 cells display only a single class of binding sites (Hohmann et al., 1989), it is possible that the heterogeneity of sites observed with isolated membranes is caused by the disruption of the intact cell structure. Whether the two binding sites seen on isolated membranes represent in

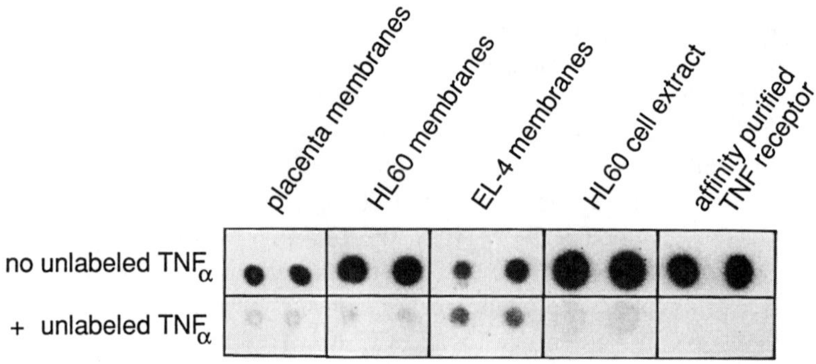

Figure 1 Filter-based dot blot assay of [^{125}I]TNF-α binding. The following samples were spotted in duplicate as 3-μL aliquots onto a prewetted sheet of a nitrocellulose filter: crude membranes prepared from human placenta, HL-60, and EL-4 cells (45 μg of membrane protein each), a total cell extract of HL-60 cells (75 μg of total protein), and a TNF-receptor preparation (113 ng of protein) partially purified from an HL-60 cell extract by TNF-α affinity chromatography. After blocking with a buffer containing 1% defatted milk powder, the filter membrane was incubated with 10 ng/mL [^{125}I]TNF-α (5×10^7 cpm/μg) in the presence or absence of 5 μg/mL unlabeled TNF-α overnight at room temperature. Bound radioactivity was visualized by autoradiography.

fact two distinct TNF receptors present on HL-60 cells (Brockhaus et al., 1990; Hohmann et al., 1989) is an intriguing question.

With the TNF receptor-specific htr and utr monoclonal antibodies a sandwich-type immunoassay has been developed to detect and quantitate solubilized TNF receptors (H. Gallati and M. Brockhaus, unpublished results). In this assay microtiter wells are first coated with a nonneutralizing anti-TNF receptor antibody and then exposed to the samples containing TNF receptors. The amount of TNF receptor captured by the first antibody is quantitated by a second antibody conjugated to horseradish peroxidase, which recognizes a different epitope. As little as 50 pg/mL TNF receptor can be detected with this method. Alternatively, ^{125}I-labeled TNF-α, biotinylated TNF-α, or biotinylated second antibody in combination with streptavidin-coupled horseradish peroxidase can be used.

III. PURIFICATION OF TNF RECEPTORS

In view of the low abundancy of TNF receptor(s) the proper choice of the source for receptor purification is important. A straightforward calculation shows that with a few thousand molecules per cell and an expected overall yield of 10 to 20%, about 10^{12} cells are required as starting material for the purification of TNF receptors to obtain amounts sufficient for protein sequencing. Such high numbers of cells can be supplied by large-scale fermentation of cell cultures. Another potential source for human TNF receptors is placenta, which in a recent report has also been used for isolation of the interferon-γ receptor in high yields (Calderon et al., 1988). In this section I discuss mainly our own approach to extract and purify TNF receptors from different sources and I refer to an alternative purification protocol reported by another group (Stauber et al., 1988). To my knowledge no other studies dealing with the isolation and purification of intact TNF receptor proteins have been published. However, several groups reported on the identification and purification of soluble TNF inhibitory proteins present in human serum and urine (Engelmann et al., 1989; 1990; Olsson et al., 1989; Peetre et al., 1988; Seckinger et al., 1988, 1989). By sequence comparison, these inhibitor proteins turn out to be soluble TNF receptor fragments (see below). I therefore refer to their purification briefly in the last part of this section.

A. Purification from Human Placenta

Preliminary experiments in our laboratory had shown that crude membrane fractions of human placenta bind [^{125}I]TNF-α specifically when analyzed in the filter-based dot blot assay (see Fig. 1). The activity has been extracted from homogenized placenta by Triton X-100 and enriched by immunoaffinity column chromatography using an htr-9 antibody column. This antibody specifically recognizes and retains the 55-kDa TNF receptor protein, whereas the 75-kDa receptor, which is present in minor amounts in the placenta extract, passes through the column. The htr-9 eluate, highly enriched for the 55-kDa TNF receptor, is further purified by TNF-α affinity chromatography and reversed-phase high-performance liquid chromatography (HPLC) in a solvent system containing 0.1% trifluoroacetic acid and 0.1% octylglucoside. An HPLC elution profile together with SDS-PAGE and ligand blot analyses of relevant fractions are presented in Fig. 2. On the silver-stained gel, two rather broad bands at about 55-kDa and 35 to 40-kDa apparent molecular mass are visible in the fractions containing most of the [^{125}I]TNF-α binding activity. In the ligand blot all these bands bind [^{125}I]TNF-α specifically. The broad band at 35 to 40 kDa seems to represent proteolytic degradation products of the 55-kDa protein, since in addition to specific TNF-α binding it also reacts with antibodies of the htr series in Western blots. The apparent heterogeneity might be due to differences in glycosylation. Starting from the extract of eight human placentas, 12 μg of pure 55-kDa TNF receptor have been recovered with a calculated enrichment factor of 1.2×10^6. Partial amino acid sequences have been determined after cyanogen bromide cleavage and HPLC fractionation (see below).

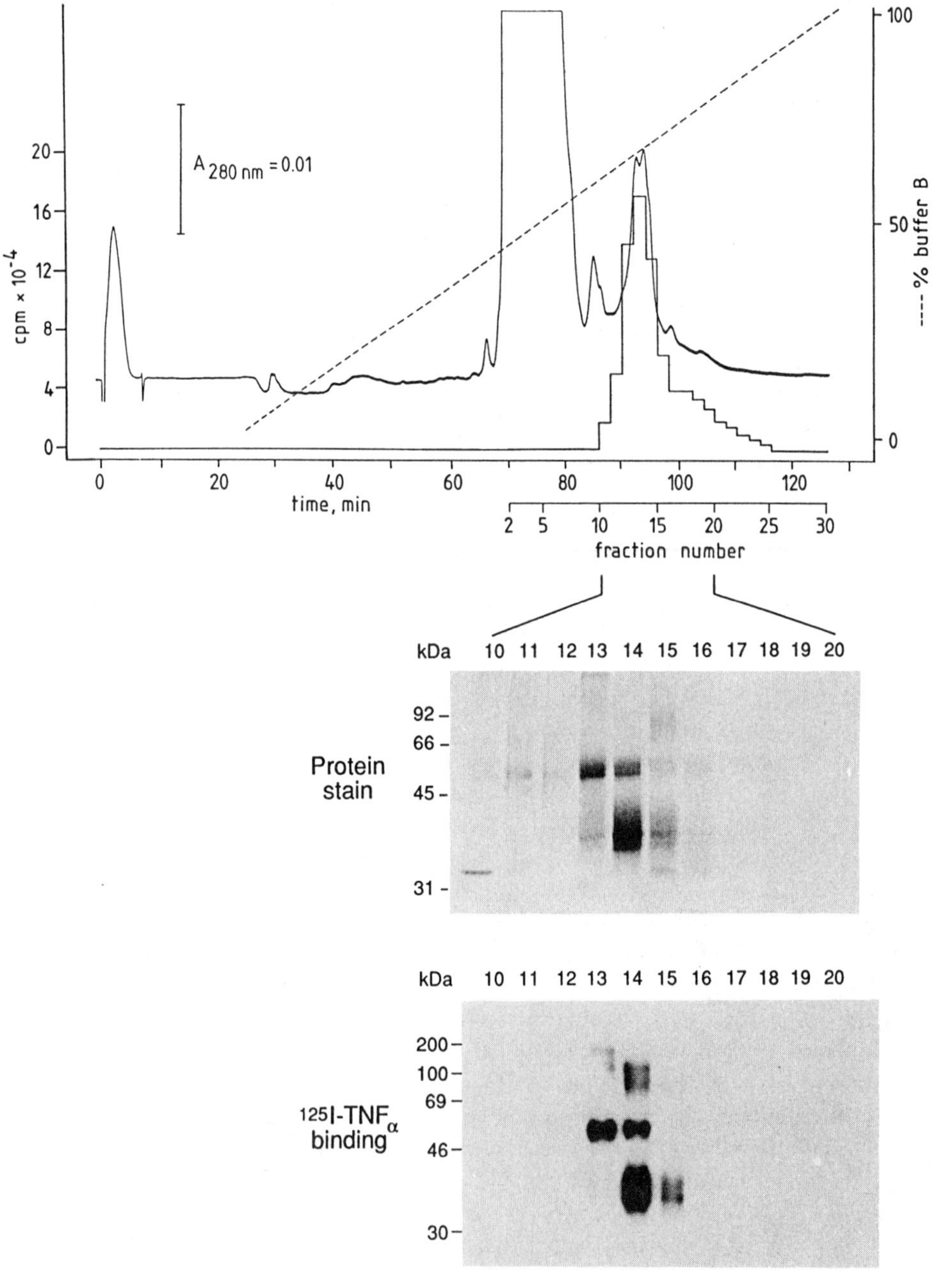
A 280 nm = 0.01
cpm × 10-4
0 4 8 12 16 20
% buffer B
0 50 100
time, min
0 20 40 60 80 100 120
fraction number
2 5 10 15 20 25 30
kDa 10 11 12 13 14 15 16 17 18 19 20
Protein stain
92 66 45 31
kDa 10 11 12 13 14 15 16 17 18 19 20
125I-TNFα binding
200 100 69 46 30

B. Purification from U937 Cells

A subclone of the human histiocytic lymphoma cell line U937 expressing up to 55,000 high-affinity TNF-α binding sites per cell has been used in a recent study as starting material for TNF-receptor purification (Stauber et al., 1988). In this purification procedure [^{125}I]TNF-α is covalently cross-linked to its receptor on the cell surface before solubilization of the cells with Triton X-100. The extract is passed over an anti-TNF-α antibody column and the TNF-α TNF-receptor-enriched fraction eluting from the antibody column is further purified by preparative SDS-PAGE. A 100-kDa cross-linked product has been obtained which after removal of the ligand by reductive cleavage migrates on SDS gels at 85-kDa apparent molecular mass. Some additional contaminating proteins are evident from gel analysis. An overall yield of about 34 ng of receptor from approximately 1.5×10^{10} U937 cells with a purity of 20% was obtained.

Another variant of U937 cells expressing about 20,000 TNF binding sites per cell (kindly provided by T. Espevik, University of Trondheim) has been used in our laboratory to isolate TNF receptors on an analytical scale. In our approach a clarified cell lysate prepared by solubilization of untreated cells with Triton X-100 is passed over a TNF-α affinity column; the bound receptor protein is eluted at low pH and rechromatographed on the same column. The TNF receptor is then subjected to reversed phase HPLC and fractions eluting from the column with an acetonitrile gradient are analyzed for specific TNF-α binding activity in the filter-based dot blot assay. Selected fractions comprising the peak of binding activity are

---

Figure 2 HPLC fractionation, SDS-PAGE, and ligand blot analysis of TNF-receptor proteins isolated from human placenta. Triton X-100 extracts prepared from eight human placentas were combined and enriched for [^{125}I]TNF-α binding activity by sequential htr-9 immunoaffinity and TNF-α ligand affinity chromatography. The low-pH eluate from the TNF-α column was subjected to HPLC fractionation on a C_1/C_8 reversed phase column (ProRPC, Pharmacia) equilibrated in 0.1% trifluoroacetic acid and 0.1% octylglucoside. The column was eluted with a linear gradient of buffer B (0.1% trifluoroacetic acid, 0.1% octylglucoside, and 80% acetonitrile) at a flow rate of 0.5 mL/min. The absorption at 280 nm was monitored and fractions of 1 mL were collected as indicated. The [^{125}I]TNF-α binding activity as determined in the filter-based dot blot assay using 2.5-μL aliquots of each fraction is represented in the histogram. As shown in the lower part, selected fractions were subjected to nonreducing SDS-PAGE and analyzed for protein and specific [^{125}I]TNF-α binding after electrophoretic transfer to a PVDF membrane. Twenty and 2 μL of the indicated fractions were applied per lane for silver staining and ligand blotting, respectively. The position of molecular weight marker proteins is indicated on the left.

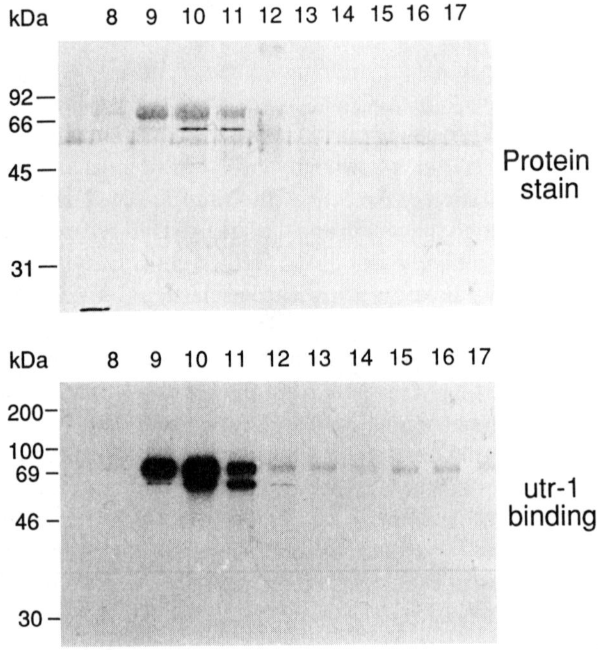

Figure 3 Analysis of TNF-receptor proteins purified from U937 cells by SDS-PAGE and Western blotting. 6×10^{10} U937 cells expressing about 20,000 TNF-receptor molecules per cell were solubilized with Triton X-100 and the extract was passed over a TNF-α affinity column. The low-pH eluate from the column was then fractionated on a C_1/C_8 reversed phase column (ProRPC, Pharmacia) using the same solvent system and elution conditions as described in the legend of Fig. 2. Fractions 8 to 17, comprising the peak of the eluted [^{125}I]TNF-α binding activity, were analyzed by SDS-PAGE and silver staining (2.5% of each fraction applied per lane) and utr-1 Western blotting (0.3% of each fraction applied per lane). Bound utr-1 antibody was detected by ^{125}I-labeled rabbit antimouse IgG and autoradiography. The position of molecular weight markers is indicated on the left.

analyzed by SDS-PAGE and silver staining. As shown in Fig. 3 the presence of a major band at 75 kDa and a minor band at 65 kDa are clearly visible in fractions 9 to 11, which both are recognized by the utr-1 monoclonal antibody in a Western blot. Since antibodies of the utr series display an exclusive specificity for the 75-kDa TNF receptor, the 75- and 65-kDa TNF-α binding proteins purified from U937 cells obviously belong to this TNF receptor type. Based on its reactivity toward TNF and the utr-1 antibody, the 65-kDa protein is most likely a proteolytic degradation product of the 75-kDa molecule.

C. Purification from HL-60 Cells

TNF-α and antibody binding studies have shown that HL-60 cells express both the 55- and 75-kDa TNF receptors with a total of about 4000 TNF binding sites per cell (Brockhaus et al., 1990; Hohmann et al., 1989). Growth conditions for HL-60 cells have been evaluated and optimized in fermentation experiments using an integrated membrane filtration system which allows continuous exchange of growth medium. With this technique cell densities of up to 4×10^7 cells/mL can be achieved, thus yielding more than 1×10^{12} HL-60 cells in 20 to 60 L of cultures. Cells from such fermentations have been used as starting material for simultaneous large-scale purification of both TNF receptors in our laboratory in order to obtain sufficient material for protein sequencing (Loetscher et al., 1990b). The important steps of the purification are summarized in the following paragraph.

The cells are lysed with 1% Triton X-100 in the presence of a protease inhibitor cocktail. Whole cells rather than isolated membranes are used because the isolation of membranes with high TNF-receptor recoveries at large scale has proven technically difficult. As a first fractionation step, the Triton X-100 extract is passed over a two-column system consisting of an htr-9 and a TNF-α column connected in tandem. According to the defined specificity of the antibody (Brockhaus et al., 1990) the htr-9 column retains the 55-kDa TNF receptor, whereas the second column with immobilized TNF-α retains the 75-kDa TNF receptor and residual 55-receptor not bound by the preceding immunoaffinity column. In some experiments a third column containing immobilized utr-1 antibody was put in between the htr-9 and TNF-α columns (Loetscher et al., 1990b). The columns are disconnected, separately washed, and eluted at low pH. Fractions with TNF-α binding activity are neutralized and pooled for each column. In a second affinity purification step the pooled relevant fractions of each of the eluates are passed repeatedly over small TNF-α affinity columns. The low pH eluates from these columns, highly enriched for TNF receptor proteins, are then subjected to fractionation by reversed phase HPLC. As already mentioned above for the receptor purification from placenta, it is essential to supplement the HPLC-solvent system with 0.1% octylglucoside in order to keep the receptors in solution and to obtain good recoveries from the column. Figure 4 shows typical HPLC-elution and TNF-α binding activity profiles obtained for protein isolates originating from the htr-9 (Fig. 4A) and TNF-α columns (Fig. 4B). In both cases the TNF-α binding activity elutes as a single, relatively broad peak at around 60% buffer B from the HPLC column. SDS-PAGE analysis and Serva blue staining of individual HPLC fractions reveals that most of the TNF-α binding activity of the sample originating from the htr-9 column elutes in fractions 11 to 13 together with two major protein bands at 55 and 51 kDa and some minor bands at 38, 36, and 34 kDa (see Fig. 5). Analysis of the sample originating from the TNF-α column shows the same protein bands in corresponding fractions and in addition a major 75-kDa and a minor 65-kDa band in fractions 8 to

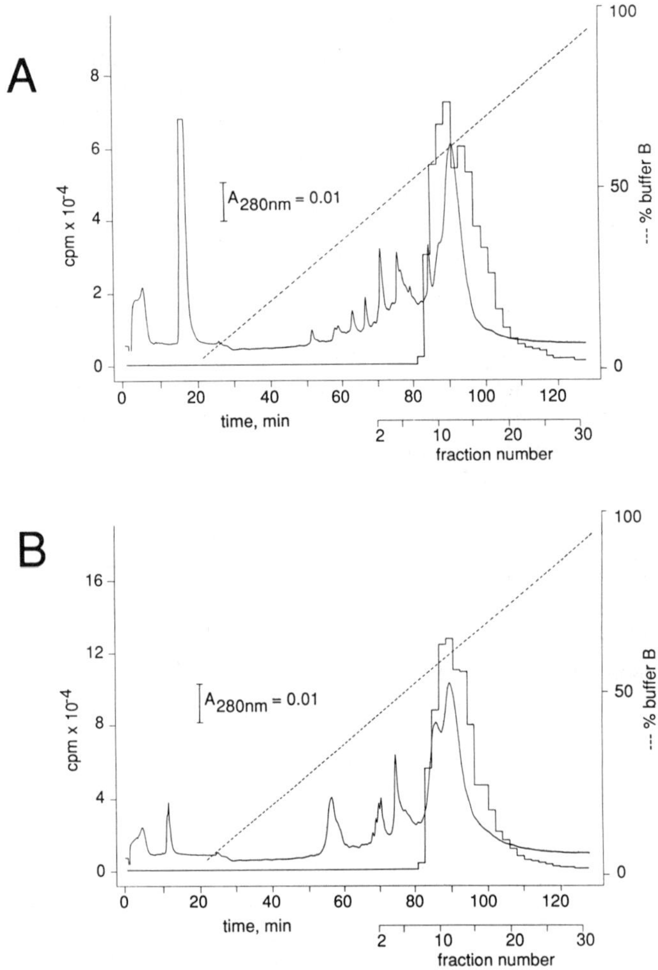

Figure 4 HPLC fractionation of TNF-receptor proteins purified from HL-60 cells. A Triton X-100 extract prepared from 1×10^{12} HL-60 cells was enriched for TNF-receptor proteins on a two-column system consisting of an htr-9 immunoaffinity and a TNF-α ligand affinity column connected in series. The columns were disconnected, washed, and eluted at low pH. In a second affinity purification step the eluates of the two columns were individually passed over small TNF-α columns, and the low-pH eluates from these columns containing highly enriched TNF-receptor proteins were then subjected to reversed phase HPLC fractionation (ProRPC column, Pharmacia). The same solvent system and elution conditions were used as described in the legend of Fig. 2. (A) HPLC elution profile monitored at 280 nm together with the [^{125}I]TNF-α binding activity (histogram) of the sample originating from the htr-9 column; (B) analogous chromatogram of the sample originating from the TNF-α column.

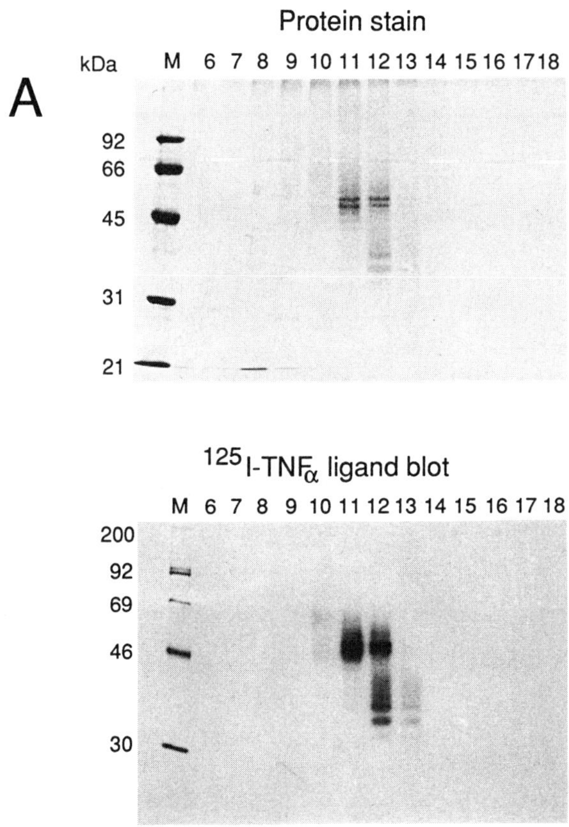

Figure 5A Analysis of HPLC fractions containing TNF-receptor proteins from HL-60 cells by SDS-PAGE and $[^{125}I]$TNF-α ligand blotting. Aliquots of fractions 6 to 18 of the HPLC separations shown in Fig. 4 were subjected to nonreducing SDS-PAGE and analyzed for protein by Serva blue staining and for specific $[^{125}I]$TNF-α binding after electrophoretic transfer to PVDF membranes. Bound ligand was visualized by autoradiography. The positions of molecular weight marker proteins (M) is indicated on left. (A) Analysis of the HPLC fractions of the TNF-receptor sample originating from htr-9 column; 25 and 0.5 μL of each fraction were applied per lane for Serva blue staining and $[^{125}I]$TNF-α ligand blotting, respectively.

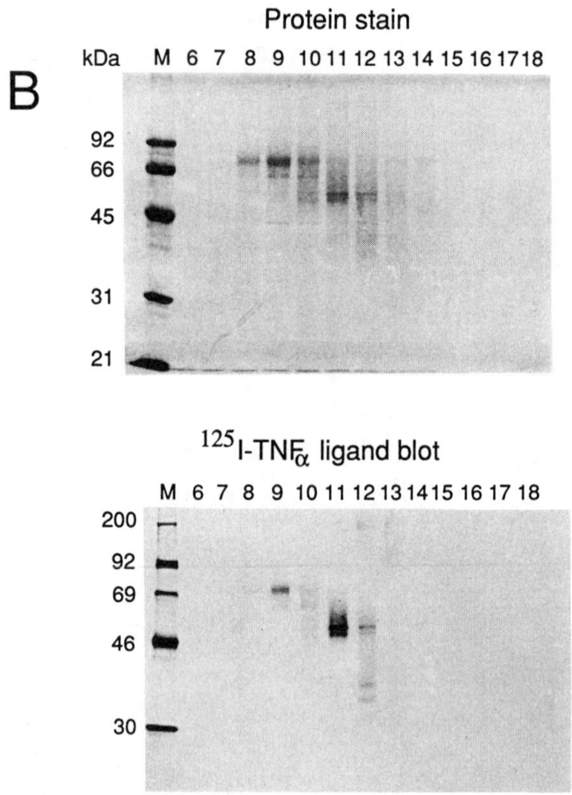

Figure 5B Analysis of the HPLC fractions of the TNF-receptor sample originating from the TNF-α column; 25 and 0.5 μL of each fraction were applied per lane for Serva blue staining and [^{125}I]TNF-α ligand blotting, respectively.

10. All these protein bands specifically bind [^{125}I]TNF-α, as demonstrated by ligand blotting experiments. Apparently, a considerable part of the 55-kDa TNF receptors passes through the htr-9 column and is only retained on the TNF-α column. This finding and the fact that the htr-9 antibody did not immunoprecipitate the 55/51-kDa TNF receptor from labeled cell lysates (Brockhaus et al., 1990) might reflect a detergent-induced affinity loss of this antibody. From the SDS-PAGE analysis of the HPLC fractions it is also evident that the two groups of proteins (i.e., the 75- and 55-kDa TNF receptor species) can be separated on the reversed phase column. As discussed earlier for the TNF-receptor proteins purified from human placenta and U937 cells, the lower-molecular-weight bands appear to be proteolytic fragments of the 55- and 75-kDa molecules, respectively. Such a re-

lation has been confirmed for the 55-, 51-, and 38-kDa protein bands by N-terminal sequence analysis (see below). Using the described purification protocol a total of 310 μg of TNF receptors (105 μg of 75-kDa protein and 205 μg of 55-kDa protein) were recovered from a cell extract of 1×10^{12} HL-60 cells with an apparent overall yield of TNF-α binding activity of 27% and a purification factor of 8.6×10^4. In a second preparation, starting from 2.6×10^{12} HL-60 cells and using a slightly modified procedure, 71 μg of the 75-kDa and 234 μg of the 55-kDa TNF-receptor protein was obtained (Loetscher et al., 1990b).

D. Purification of Soluble TNF-Receptor Fragments

Human serum and urine has been shown to contain a protein activity which protects cells from cytotoxic actions of TNF in vitro (Peetre et al., 1988; Seckinger et al., 1988). Rather than interacting with the target cell, the urinary protein inhibits the function of TNF by competing for TNF with the TNF receptor. The TNF inhibitory protein has been purified to apparent homogeneity from concentrated human urine by a combination of ion exchange, TNF-α affinity, and gel filtration chromatography and reversed phase HPLC (Engelmann et al., 1989, 1990; Olsson et al., 1989; Seckinger et al., 1989). On reducing and nonreducing SDS gels the purified protein migrates at around 30-kDa apparent molecular mass. Specific binding of TNF-α and to a lesser extent of TNF-β to the purified inhibitor has been demonstrated. Recently, a second 30-kDa TNF binding protein has been described and purified from human urine by TNF-α affinity chromatography and reversed phase HPLC (Engelmann et al., 1990). Antibodies raised against this inhibitor do not cross-react with the inhibitor protein reported in the earlier studies, and vice versa, suggesting the existence of two immunologically distinct TNF inhibitory proteins. A structural relation of the inhibitors to membrane-bond TNF receptors has been proposed (Engelmann et al., 1990). As I discuss in the following section, comparisons of partial amino acid sequence information unambiguously identify the inhibitory proteins as soluble TNF-receptor fragments.

IV. PHYSICAL AND CHEMICAL PROPERTIES OF PURIFIED 55- AND 75-kDa TNF RECEPTORS

A. Ligand and Antibody Binding to Purified Receptors

In earlier studies TNF-α and TNF-β have been found to compete for the same binding sites on the cell surface (Aggarwal et al., 1985a; Brockhaus et al., 1990; Stauber and Aggarwal, 1989). In view of the identification of two distinct TNF receptors the possibility has to be considered that the two receptors differ with regard to TNF-α and TNF-β binding. The results with purified 55- and 75-kDa receptor proteins clearly show that both receptors specifically bind TNF-α and TNF-β in ligand blots, indicating that each of the two receptors has a common binding site for

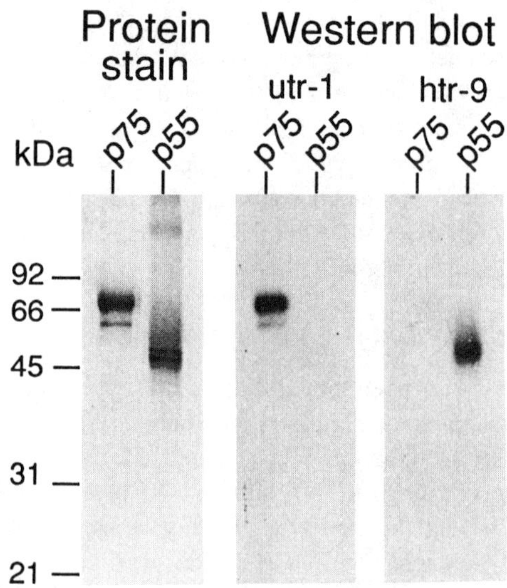

Figure 6 SDS-PAGE and Western blot analysis of 55- and 75-kDa TNF receptors purified from HL-60 cells. The purified 55- and 75-kDa TNF receptors (denoted as p55 and p75, respectively) were subjected to SDS-PAGE under nonreducing conditions. The gel was either stained with Serva blue or blotted to PVDF membranes for the antibody binding experiments. 0.75 μg of either receptor was used per lane for protein staining. Blotting was carried out with 30 ng of receptor per lane. Bound utr-1 and htr-9 antibodies were detected by radioiodinated rabbit antimouse lgG and autoradiography. Numbers on the left indicate the position of molecular weight standard proteins.

TNF-α and TNF-β. Furthermore, quantitative analysis of competitive ligand binding to either receptor in the filter-based dot blot assay has revealed identical inhibition curves for both ligands, suggesting that TNF-α and TNF-β have similar affinities (Loetscher et al., 1990b).

As documented in Fig. 6, htr-9 and utr-1 antibodies bind purified 55/51- and 75/65-kDa proteins, respectively, in Western blots, thus confirming the exclusive specificity of these antibodies previously shown by flow cytometry studies of intact cells (Brockhaus et al., 1990). In further experiments we have found that in these Western blots TNF-α abolishes binding of htr-9 antibody to the 55/51-kDa bands but has no effect on utr-1 binding to the 75/65-kDa bands. Interestingly, the binding of [^{125}I]TNF-α to the blotted 75/65-kDA bands is competed by the utr-1 antibody, whereas the htr-9 antibody does not affect the TNF-α binding to the 55/51-kDa bands (Loetscher et al., 1990b). These results are in marked contrast to studies with intact cells where mutual competition between htr-9 and TNF-α as well as between utr-1 and TNF-α has been observed (Brockhaus et al., 1990; Espevik et al., 1990). The most likely explanation is that electrophoretic separation in SDS and blotting to PVDF membranes affects the affinities of the TNF receptor proteins for ligand and antibodies.

On reducing SDS gels the 55/51- and 75/65-kDa TNF receptors migrate at slightly higher apparent molecular masses, probably due to the reduction of intramolecular disulfide bonds. All the TNF-α and the utr-1 and htr-9 antibody binding activities are completely lost upon reduction. In conclusion, the results of the ligand and Western blotting experiments suggest that ligand and antibody binding sites on either receptor are structurally closely related.

B. Receptor Glycosylation

When the 55/51- and 75/65-kDa TNF receptors purified from HL-60 cells were treated with *N*-glycanase to remove N-linked carbohydrates, reductions by about 5 to 10-kDa apparent molecular mass were observed on SDS-PAGE, demonstrating that both receptors are glycoproteins (Loetscher et al., 1990b). A similar reduction in molecular mass upon carbohydrate removal has been reported in ligand cross-linking studies with intact cells (Hohmann et al., 1989). Blotting experiments with deglycosylated 55- and 75-kDa TNF receptors partially purified from human placenta and U937 cells, respectively, indicate that N-linked sugars are not required for ligand binding (Fig. 7).

C. Peptide Mapping and Amino Acid Sequencing

1. 55- and 75-kDa TNF Receptors Are Distinct Proteins

For N-terminal amino acid sequence analysis aliquots of the 55- and 75-kDa TNF receptors, purified from HL-60 cells, were separated by SDS-PAGE and electrophoretically transferred to PVDF membranes (Loetscher et al., 1990b). As discussed earlier, the 55-kDa receptor preparation resolves into major 55- and 51-kDa and minor 38-, 36-, and 34-kDa bands. Identical N-terminal sequences are found for the 55-, 51-, and 38-kDa bands (Y.C. Pan, and H. W. Lahm, personal communication), indicating that the difference in molecular weight is probably due to truncation at the C-terminal end. When a sample of this receptor without prior electrophoretic separation was sequenced, a stretch of 28 residues could be obtained. This partial amino acid sequence has been used successfully to clone the cDNA for the 55-kDa TNF receptor (see below). The identity of the cloned cDNA has been confirmed by two additional partial amino acid sequences determined for the 55-kDa TNF receptor from human placenta after cleavage with cyanogen bromide (Y. C. Pan, and H. W. Lahm, personal communication). One stretch covers aspartic acid-12 to isoleucine-28 and the other tyrosine-205 to arginine-209 of the 55-kDa TNF-receptor cDNA sequence. An additional sequence covering serine-222 to threonine-235 has been obtained for a tryptic peptide of the 55-kDa

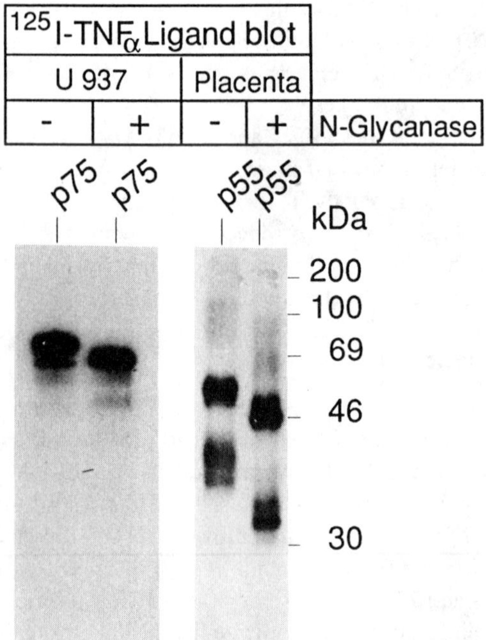

Figure 7 N-Glycanase treatment of 75- and 55-kDa TNF-receptor proteins partially purified from U937 cells and human placenta, respectively. TNF-receptor preparations partially purified by TNF-α affinity chromatography from Ug37 cells (p75) and human placenta (p55) were treated with *N*-glycanase to remove N-linked carbohydrates. After incubation overnight at 37°C, the samples were subjected to nonreducing SDS-PAGE, electrophoretically transferred to PVDF membranes, and assayed for ^{125}l]TNF-α binding in ligand blots. Bound ligand was visualized by autoradiography. Numbers on the right indicate the position of molecular weight standard proteins.

TNF receptor from HL-60 cells (Y.C. Pan, and H. W. Lahm, personal communication).

The 75-kDa TNF receptor purified from HL-60 cells was subjected to proteolytic digestion and fractionation by reversed-phase HPLC. N-terminal amino acid sequences for five tryptic peptides ranging from 5 to 18 residues were obtained by gas-phase sequencing (Loetscher et al., 1990b). None of the partial amino acid sequences for the 75/65-kDa TNF receptor is contained within the full-length amino acid sequence of the cloned 55-kDa TNF receptor (Loetscher et al., 1990a; Schall et al., 1990). This shows clearly that the 55- and 75-kDa TNF receptors are different gene products. Comparison of the complete amino acid sequences of both receptors deduced from their cDNAs confirms the distinct nature of the two proteins, albeit an extensive structural homology in the extracellular part is evident (see below).

2. *The 75/65-kDa TNF Receptor Is Modified with Ubiquitin*

Attempts to determine the N-terminal sequence of the 75-kDa TNF receptor were not successful; the N-terminal amino acid probably is modified and not accessible to Edman degradation. Sequencing of the 65-kDa band, however, reveals the presence of two different N-terminal amino acid sequences at a ratio of roughly 1:1 (Loetscher et al., 1990b). Since one of the sequences corresponds to the published N-terminal sequence of ubiquitin (Schlesinger et al., 1975), the other is assumed to be a sequence of the 75/65-kDa TNF receptor. In view of the multistep purification procedure it appears highly unlikely that ubiquitin copurifies exclusively with the 65-kDa band. It seems more likely that ubiquitin is covalently attached to the 65-kDa band, probably via an amide bond between the C-terminal carboxyl group of ubiquitin and an ε-amino group of a lysine of the receptor. Ubiquitin is known to be involved in a variety of cellular processes when it is covalently bound to cellular proteins (Hershko and Ciechanover, 1986; Rechsteiner, 1987; Wilkinson, 1987). In many cases, ubiquitination serves as a signal for intracellular degradation of the modified protein. Besides this function ubiquitin has also been postulated to play a role in chromatin condensation or cell cycle progression after reversible modification of histone molecules (Bonner et al., 1988). Modification of the lymphocyte homing receptor, originally identified as Mel 14 antigen (Gallatin et al., 1983), and the platelet-derived growth factor receptor (Yarden et al., 1986) with ubiquitin has been demonstrated. Interestingly, ubiquitin is localized in the extracellular domain of the lymphocyte homing receptor. Specific functions have been proposed for modification of cell surface proteins with ubiquitin (Siegelmann and Weissmann, 1988). The fact that the 65-kDa protein, but not the major 75-kDa protein, is ubiquitinated might indicate that this species is determined for a particular metabolic pathway.

3. *Soluble Fragments of 55- and 75-kDa TNF Receptors Are TNF Inhibitory Proteins*

Truncated soluble forms of membrane-bound receptors generated either by alternative splicing of a single transcribed gene (Gower et al., 1988; Mosley et al., 1989; Weber et al., 1984) or by proteolytic processing of the mature protein (Loughnan et al., 1988; Zupan et al., 1989) have been described. Three soluble fragments of the nerve growth factor receptor, which is structurally closely related to the 55-kDa TNF receptor (see below), have been purified from amniotic fluid and infant urine (Zupan et al., 1989). It was interesting to find that the published partial N-terminal sequence of one of the TNF inhibitor proteins (Engelmann et al., 1989) exactly matches the sequence from aspartic acid-12 to proline-16 in the 55-kDa TNF receptor sequence (Loetscher et al., 1990a; Schall et al., 1990). Moreover, the partial N-terminal sequence of the second inhibitory protein reported by Engelmann et al.,

(1990) is found in the N-terminal sequence of the 65-kDa product of the 75-kDa TNF receptor (valine-5 to proline-9) (Loetscher et al., 1990b; Dembic et al., 1990). Thus, by sequence comparison, both TNF inhibitor proteins are identified as soluble 55- and 75-kDa TNF-receptor fragments. No evidence for the existence of a distinct gene or a shorter mRNA species created by differential splicing that would code for a soluble fragment of the 55-kDa TNF receptor has been found so far (Loetscher et al., 1990a). It is more likely that the TNF inhibitory proteins are generated by proteolytic processing of the cell surface receptors. A potential physiological significance of the soluble TNF inhibitors is not yet understood. The fact that soluble fragments of several other receptors are found in serum and urine might suggest a general phenomenon for regulation/neutralization of ligand activity.

D. Primary Structure and Sequence Homology

Based on partial amino acid sequences of the purified protein a cDNA encoding the 55-kDa human TNF receptor has been cloned in our laboratory by a combination of polymerase chain reaction and conventional cloning techniques (Loetscher et al., 1990a). Simultaneously, another group also reported the cloning of the 55-kDa TNF receptor using synthetic DNA probes derived from partial sequences of a TNF inhibitory protein isolated from the serum of cancer patients (Schall et al., 1990). The open reading frame of the 55-kDa TNF receptor cDNA predicts a protein of 455 amino acids with a structure typical for a cell surface receptor: a hydrophobic leader sequence and a single transmembrane region separating extracellular and intracellular domains. Twenty-four cysteines and three potential N-glycosylation sites are located in the presumed extracellular part (Loetscher et al., 1990a; Schall et al., 1990). Recently, a cDNA clone encoding the 75-kDa TNF receptor has been isolated by direct expression screening with radiolabeled TNF-α (Smith et al., 1990). Similar to the cloning strategy of the 55-kDa TNF receptor, the cDNA coding for the 75-kDa receptor has also been identified in our group using the polymerase chain reaction in combination with conventional cloning techniques (Dembic et al., 1990). The sequence predicted from the 75-kDa TNF receptor cDNA also displays the features of a typical transmembrane protein with 21 cysteine residues and two potential N-glycosylation sites in the extracellular domain (Smith et al., 1990; Dembic et al., 1990). Analysis by a mutation data matrix (Dayhoff et al., 1979) reveals a striking sequence similarity between the two TNF receptors in the extracellular part, where four characteristic domains with regularly spaced cysteines are discovered. The first two domains are highly homologous, with an identical pattern of six cysteines in each (Dembic et al., 1990). Interestingly, alignment of the intracellular regions does not show any significant homology to each other nor to any other known mammalian sequences. However, an unusual high content of proline and serine is found in the cytoplasmic domains of both receptors. Such proline- and serine-rich structures have also been demonstrated in the cytoplasmic regions of other receptor proteins (Hatakeyama et al., 1989).

Cysteine-rich repeats have been found in the extracellular domains of receptors for epidermal growth factor (EGF), low-density lipoprotein (LDL), and insulin (Ullrich et al., 1984, 1985; Yamamoto et al., 1984) and in a number of other proteins (see Smith et al., 1990). However, these sequences show very little homology to the TNF receptor sequences. In contrast, cysteine-rich extracellular repeats of human and rat nerve growth factor (NGF) receptors (Johnson et al., 1986; Radeke et al., 1987), CDw40 (Stamenkovic et al., 1989), clone 4-1BB (Kwon and Weissman, 1989), T2 (Upton et al., 1987), and OX40 antigen (Mallett et al., 1990) show highly significant sequence similarities to the extracellular domains of both TNF receptors (Loetscher et al., 1990a; Schall et al., 1990; Smith et al., 1990; Dembic et al., 1990). It appears that the conserved domains of these molecules share common structural features presumably generated and stabilized by extensive disulfide bridging and thus define a new receptor family.

V. CONCLUDING REMARKS

The identification and subsequent purification to apparent homogeneity of two distinct TNF receptors of 55- and 75-kDa apparent molecular masses has allowed us to resolve some of the conflicting results obtained by several groups in ligand-cross-linking studies. From the data obtained with the non-cross-reactive htr and utr anti-TNF receptor monoclonal antibodies and also by Northern blot analyses it is now clear that the 55- and 75-kDa receptor proteins are expressed on various cells at different relative amounts. It is therefore not surprising that in the cross-linking experiments different cross-linked products have been identified with different cell lines. However, in most cells complexes of about 90- to 100-kDa and/or 75-kDa apparent molecular masses are found (see Table 1). Most likely, the former represents a cross-linked product between the 75-kDa TNF receptor and a TNF-α monomer and the latter between the 55-kDa TNF receptor and a TNF-α monomer. The 60-and 70-kDa monomeric TNF binding units identified in HeLa cells (Smith and Baglioni, 1989) probably represent 55-kDa TNF receptor species, because HeLa cells, as verified by antibody binding experiments, express almost exclusively this TNF receptor type (Brockhaus et al., 1990). The existence of accessory proteins associated with the TNF receptors, which may lead to additional cross-linked products under certain experimental conditions, cannot be excluded. Such a protein, the Fas antigen, has recently been characterized in several human cells with a specific monoclonal antibody (Yonehara et al., 1989). It appears that this antigen, which does not bind TNF by itself, is co-modulated with TNF receptors. In a different system, interleukin-6 has recently been shown to trigger the association of the interleukin-6 receptor with a non-ligand-binding membrane glycoprotein, gp 130 (Taga et al., 1989). Thus the association of additional membrane components with specific receptors on cell surfaces might be a common mechanism reflecting signal transduction processes that occur after ligand binding.

Despite the fact that TNF-α and TNF-β share only about 30% sequence homology, they both bind to the 55- and 75-kDa TNF receptors with comparable affinities, as demonstrated with purified receptors and intact cells. These results agree well with the observation that a variety of biological activities are shared by TNF-α and TNF-β and suggest that both ligands can stimulate both receptors in a similar way. Some biological activities, however, appear to be specific for TNF-α (Koeffler et al., 1987; Locksley et al., 1987; Oster et al., 1987) and therefore may operate through different receptor activation mechanisms. In addition, the fact that the cytoplasmic domains of the 55- and 75-kDa TNF receptors lack any significant sequence homology might indicate the existence of receptor-specific signal transduction pathways, which could be responsible, at least in part, for the diverse actions of TNF.

ACKNOWLEDGMENT

I wish to thank my colleagues M. Brockhaus, H. Gallati, H. W. Lahm, Y. C. Pan, H. J. Schoenfeld, and M. Zulauf for permission to include unpublished material in this review, and T. Espevik for providing a high expressor variant of U937 cells. I also thank W. Lesslauer and M. Steinmetz for many helpful comments on the manuscript.

REFERENCES

Aggarwal, B. B., Eessalu, T. E., and Hass, P. E. (1985a). Characterization of receptors for human tumor necrosis factor and their regulation by gamma-interferon, *Nature, 318*: 665.

Aggarwal, B. B., Kohr, W. J., Hass, P. E., Moffat, B., Spencer, S. A., Henzel, W. J., Bringman, T. S., Nedwin, G. E., Goeddel, D. V., and Harkins, R. N. (1985b). Human tumor necrosis factor: production, purification and characterization, *J. Biol. Chem., 260*: 2345.

Arakawa, T., and Yphantis, D. A. (1987). Molecular weight of recombinant human tumor necrosis factor alpha, *J. Biol. Chem., 262*: 7484.

Baglioni, C., McCandless, S., Tavernier, J., and Fiers, W. (1985). Binding of human tumor necrosis factor to high affinity receptors on HeLa and lymphoblastoid cells sensitive to growth inhibition, *J. Biol. Chem., 260*: 13395.

Beutler, B., and Cerami, A. (1987). Cachectin: more than a tumor necrosis factor, *N. Engl. J. Med., 316*: 379.

Beutler, B., and Cerami, A. (1988). Tumor necrosis, cachexia, shock, and inflammation: a common mediator, *Annu. Rev. Biochem., 57*: 505.

Bonner, W. M., Hatch, C. L., and Wu, R. S. (1988). Ubiquitinated histones and chromatin, *Ubiquitin* (M. Rechsteiner, ed)., Plenum Press, New York, p. 157.

Brockhaus, M., and Loetscher, H. (1990). Monoclonal antibodies against cytokine receptors, *Immunological Methods*, Vol. 4 (I. Lefkovits and B. Pernis, eds.), Academic Press, New York, p. 175.

Brockhaus, M., Schoenfeld, H.-J., Schlaeger, H.-J., Hunziker, W., Lesslauer, W., and Loetscher, H. (1990). Identification of two kinds of TNF receptors on human cells lines by monoclonal antibodies, *Proc. Natl. Acad. Sci. USA, 87*: 3127.

Browning, J., and Ribolini, A. (1989). Studies on the differing effects of tumor necrosis factor and lymphotoxin on the growth of several human tumor lines, *J. Immunol., 143*: 1859.

Calderon, J., Sheehan, K. C. F., Chance, C., Thomas, M. L., and Schreiber, R. D. (1988). Purification and characterization of the human interferon-gamma receptor from placenta, *Proc. Natl. Acad. Sci. USA, 85*: 4837.

Carswell, A. E., Old, L. J., Kassel, R. L., Green, S., Fiore, N., and Wiliamson, B. (1975). An endotoxin-induced serum factor that causes necrosis of tumors, *Proc. Natl. Acad. Sci. USA, 72*: 3666.

Creasy, A. A., Yamamoto, R., and Vitt, C. R. (1987). A high molecular weight component of the human tumor necrosis factor receptor is associated with cytotoxicity, *Proc. Natl. Acad. Sci. USA, 84*: 3293.

Dayhoff, M. O., Schwartz, R. M., and Orcutt, B. C. (1979). A model of evolutionary change in proteins, *Atlas of Protein Sequence and Structure* (M. O. Dayhoff, Ed.), Vol. 5, Suppl. 3, National Biomedical Research Foundation, Washington, DC, p. 345.

Dembic, Z., Loetscher, H., Gubler, U., Pan, Y. C. E., Lahm, H. W., Gentz, R., Brockhaus, M., and Lesslauer, W. (1990). Two human TNF receptors have similar extracellular, but distinct intracellular domain sequences, *Cytokine, 2*: 231.

Eck, M. J., Beutler, B., Kuo, G., Merryweather, J. P., and Sprang, S. R. (1988). Crystallisation of trimeric recombinant human tumor necrosis factor (cachectin), *J. Biol. Chem., 263*: 12816.

Engelmann, H., Aderka, D., Rubinstein, M., Rotman, D., and Wallach, D. (1989). A tumor necrosis factor-binding protein purified to homogeneity from human urine protects cells from tumor necrosis factor toxicity, *J. Biol. Chem., 264*: 11974.

Engelmann, H., Novick, D., and Wallach, D. (1990). Two tumor necrosis factor binding proteins purified from human urine, *J. Biol., Chem., 265*: 1531.

Espevik, T., Brockhaus, M., Loetscher, H., Nonstad, U., and Shalaby, R. (1990). Characterization of binding and biological effects of monoclonal antibodies against a human tumor necrosis factor receptor, *J. Exp. Med., 171*: 415.

Gallatin, W. M., Weissmann, I. L., and Butcher, E. C. (1983). A cell surface molecule involved in organ specific homing of lymphocytes, *Nature, 304*: 30.

Gower, H. J., Barton, C. H., Elsom, V. L., Thompson, J., Moore, S. E., Dickson, G., and Walsh, F. S. (1988). Alternative splicing generates a secreted form of N-CAM in muscle and brain, *Cell, 55*: 955.

Gray, P. W., Aggarwal, B. B. Benton, C. V., Bringman, T. S., Henzel, W. J., Jarrett, J. A., Leung, D. W., Moffat, B., Ng, P., Svedersky, L. P., Palladino, M. A., and Nedwin, G. E. (1984). Cloning and expression of cDNA for human lymphotoxin, a lymphokine with tumor necrosis activity, *Nature, 312*: 721.

Hakoshima, T., and Tomita, K. (1988). Crystallisation and preliminary x-ray investigation reveals that tumor necrosis factor is a compact trimer furnished with 3-fold symmetry, *J. Mol. Biol., 201*: 455.

Hatakeyama, M., Tsudo, M., Minamoto, S., Kono, T., Doi, T., Miyata, T., Miyasaka, M., and Taniguchi, T. (1989). Interleukin-2 receptor β chain gene: generation of three receptor forms by cloned human α and β chain cDNA's, *Science, 244*: 551.

Helson, L., Green, S., Carswell, E. A., and Old, L. J. (1975). Effect of tumor necrosis factor on cultured human melanoma cells, *Nature, 258*: 731.

Hershko, A., and Ciechanover, A. (1986). The ubiquitin pathway for the degradation of intracellular proteins, *Prog. Nucleic Acid Res. Mol. Biol., 33*: 19.

Hirano, K., Yamamoto, K., Kobayashi, Y., and Osawa, T. (1989). Characterization of specific high-affinity receptor for human lumphotoxin, *J. Biochem., 105*: 120.

Hohmann, H., Remy, R., Brockhaus, M., and van Loon, A. P. G. M. (1989). Two different cell types have different major receptors for human tumor necrosis factor (TNF alpha), *J. Biol. Chem., 264*: 14927.

Israel, S., Hahn, T., Holtmann, H., and Wallach, D. (1986). Binding of human TNF alpha to high affinity cell surface receptors: effect of IFN, *Immunol. Lett., 12*: 217.

Johnson, D., Lanahan, A., Buck, C. R., Sehgal, A., Morgan, C., Mercer, E., Bothwell, M., and Chao, M. (1986). Expression and structure of the human NGF receptor, *Cell, 47*: 545.

Jones, E. Y., Stuart, D. I., and Walker, N. P. C. (1989). Structure of tumor necrosis factor, *Nature, 338*: 225.

Koeffler, H. P., Gasson, J., Ranyard, J., Souza, L., Shepard, M., and Munker, A. (1987). Recombinant human TNF alpha stimulates production of granylocyte colony-stimulating factor, *Blood, 70*: 55.

Kramer, S. M., Aggarwal, B. B., Eessalu, T. E., McCabe, S. M., Ferraiolo, B. L., Figari, I. S., and Palladino, M. A. J. (1988). Characterization of the in vitro and in vivo species preference of human and murine tumor necrosis factor-alpha, *Cancer Res., 48*: 920.

Kriegler, M., Perez, C., DeFay, K., Albert, I., and Lu, S. D. (1988). A novel form of TNF/cachectin is a cell surface cytotoxic transmembrane protein: ramifications for the complex physiology of TNF, *Cell, 53*: 45.

Kull, F. C., Jacobs, S., and Cuatrecasas, P. (1985). Cellular receptor for 125l-labeled tumor necrosis factor: specific binding, affinity labeling, and relationship to sensitivity, *Proc. Natl. Acad. Sci. USA, 82*: 5756.

Kwon, B. S., and Weissmann, S. M. (1989). cDNA sequences of two inducible T-cell clones, *Proc. Natl. Acad. Sci. USA, 86*: 1963.

Lam, K., Scuderi, P., and Salmon, S. W. (1988). Analysis of the molecular organization of recombinant human tumor necrosis factor (rTNF) in solution using ethylene glycol-bis(succinimidylsuccinate) as the cross-linking reagnet, *J. Biol. Response Modif., 7*: 267.

Locksley, R. M., Heinzel, F. P., Shepard, H. M., Agosti, J., Eessalu, T. E., Aggarwal, B. B., and Harlan, J. M. (1987). Tumor necrosis factor alpha and beta differ in their capacities to generate interleukin-1 release from human endothelial cells, *J. Immunol., 139*: 1891.

Loetscher, H., Pan, Y.-C. E., Lahm, H.-W., Gentz, R., Brockhaus, M., Tabuchi, H., and Lesslauer, W. (1990a). Molecular cloning and expression of the human 55 kDa TNF receptor, *Cell, 61*: 351.

Loetscher, H., Schlaeger, E. J., Lahm, H. W., Pan, Y. C. E., Lesslauer, W., and Brockhaus, M. (1990b). Purification and partial amino acid sequence analysis of two distinct tumor necrosis factor receptors from HL60 cells, *J. Biol. Chem., 265*: 20131.

Loughnan, M. S., Sanderson, C. J., and Nossal, G. J. V. (1988). Soluble interleukin 2 receptors are released from the cell surface of normal murine B lymphoxytes stimulated with interleukin 5, *Proc. Natl. Acad. Sci. USA, 85*: 3115.

Mallett, S., Fossum, S., and Barclay, A. N. (1990). Characterization of the MRC OX40 antigen of activated CD4 positive T lumphoxytes: a molecule related to nerve growth factor receptor, *EMBO J., 9*: 1063.

Matthews, N., and Neale, M. L. (1987). Studies on the mode of action of tumor necrosis factor on tumor cells in vitro, *Lumphokines: A Forum for Immunoregulatory Cell Products* (E. Pick and M. Landy, eds.), Academic Press, London, p. 223.

Mosley, B., Beckmann, M. P., March, C. J., Idzerda, R. L., Gimpel, S. D., VandenBos, T., Friend, D., Alpert, A., Anderson, D., Jackson, J., Wignall, J. M., Smith, C., Gallis, B., Sims, J. E., Urdal, D., Widmer, M. B., Cosman, D., and Park, L. S. (1989). The murine interleukin-4 receptor: molecular cloning and characterization of secreted and membrane-bound forms, *Cells, 59*: 335.

Mueller, U., Jongeneel, C. V., Nedospasov, S. A., Fischer Lindahl, K., and Steinmetz, M. (1987). Tumor necrosis factor and lymphotoxin genes map close to H-2D in the mouse major histocompatibility complex, *Nature, 325*: 265.

Munker, R., DiPersio, J., and Koeffler, H. P. (1987). Tumor necrosis factor: receptor on hematopoietic cells, *Blood, 70*: 1730.

Niitsu, Y., Watanabe, N., Sone, H., Neda, H., Yamauchi, N., Maeda, M., and Urushizaki, I. (1988). Analysis of the TNF receptor on KYM cells by binding assay and affinity crosslinking, *J. Biol. Response Modif., 7*: 276.

Old, L. J. (1985). Tumor necrosis factor (TNF), *Science, 230*: 630.

Olsson, I., Lantz, M., Nilsson, E., Peetre, C., Thysell, H., Grubb, A., and Adolf, G. (1989). Isolation and characterization of a tumor necrossis factor binding protein from urine, *Eur. J. Haematol., 42*: 270.

Oster, W., Lindemann, A., Horn, S., Mertelsmann, R., and Herrmann, F. (1987). Tumor necrosis factor (TNF)-alpha but not TNF-beta induces secretion of colony stimulating factor for macrophages (CSF-1) by human monocytes, *Blood, 70*: 1700.

Peetre, C., Thysell, H., Grubb, A., and Olsson, I. (1988). A tumor necrosis factor binding protein is present in human biological fluids, *Eur. J. Haematol., 41*: 414.

Pennica, D., Nedwin, G. E., Hayflick, J. S., Seeburg, P. H., Derynck, R., Palladino, M. A., Kohr, W. J., Aggarwal, B. B., and Goeddel, D. V. (1984). Human tumor necrosis factor: precursor structure, expression and homology to lymphotoxin, *Nature, 312*: 724.

Radeke, M. J., Misko, T. P., Hsu, C., Herzenberg, L. A., and Shooter, E. M. (1987). Gene transfer and molecular cloning of the rat nerve growth factor receptor, *Nature, 325*: 593.

Rechsteiner, M. (1987). Ubiquitin-mediated pathways for intracellular proteolytisis, *Annu. Rev. Cell Biol., 3*: 1.

Rubin, B. Y., Anderson, S. L., Sullivan, S. A., Willamson, B. D., Carswell, E. A., and Old, L. J. (1985). High affinity binding of 125l-labeled human tumor necrosis factor (LuKll) to specific cell surface receptors, *J. Exp. Med., 162*: 1099.

Schall, T. J., Lewis, M., Koller, K. J., Lee, A., Rice, G. C., Wong, G. H. W., Gatanaga, T., Granger, G. A., Lentz, R., Raab, H., Kohr, W. J., and Goeddel, D. V. (1990). Molecular cloning and expression of a receptor for human tumor necrosis factor, *Cell, 61*: 361.

Scheurich, P., Uecer, U., Kroencke, M., and Pfizenmaier, K. (1986). Quantification and characterization of high affinity membrane receptors for tumor necrosis factor on human leukemic cell lines, *Int. J. Cancer, 38*: 127.

Schlesinger, D. H., Goldstein, G., and Niall, H. D. (1975). The complete amino acid sequence of ubiquitin, an adenylate cyclase stimulating polypeptide probably universal in living cells, *Biochemistry, 14*: 2214.

Seckinger, P., Isaaz, S., and Dayer, J. M. (1988). A human inhibitor of tumor necrossi factor alpha, *J. Exp. Med., 167*: 1511.

Seckinger, P., Isaaz, S., and Dayer, J.-M. (1989). Purification and biologic characterization of a specific tumor necrosis factor alpha inhibitor, *J. Biol. Chem., 264*: 11966.

Shalaby, M. R., Palladino, M. A., Hirabayashi, S. E., Eessalu, T., Lewis, G. D., Shepard, H. M., and Aggarwal, B. B. (1987). Receptor binding and activation of polymorphonuclear neutrophils by tumor necrosis factor alpha, *J. Leukocyte Biol., 41*: 196.

Siegelmann, M., and Weissmann, I. L. (1988). Lymphocyte homing receptors, ubiquitin, and cell surface proteins, *Ubiquitin* (M. Rechsteiner, ed.), Plenum Press, New York, p. 239.

Smith, C. A., Davis, T., Anderson, D., Solam, L., Beckmann, M. P., Jerzy, R., Dower, S. K., Cosman, D., and Goodwin, R. G. (1990). A receptor for tumor necrosis factor defines an unusual family of cellular and viral proteins, *Science, 248*: 1019.

Smith, R. A., and Baglioni, C. (1987). The active form of tumor necrosis factor is a trimer, *J. Biol. Chem., 262*: 6951.

Smith, R. A., and Baglioni, C. (1989). Multimeric structure of the tumor necrosis factor receptor of HeLa cells, *J. Biol. Chem., 264*: 14646.

Smith R. A., Kirstein, M., Fiers, W., and Baglioni, C. (1986). Species specificity of human and murine tumor necrosis factor, *J. Biol. Chem., 261*: 14871.

Spies, T., Morton, C. C., Nedospasov, S. A., Fiers, W., Pious, D., and Strominger, J. L. (1986). Genes for the tumor necrosis factors alpha and beta are linked to the human major histocompatibility complex, *Proc. Natl. Acad. Sci. USA, 83*: 8699.

Stamenkovic, I., Clark, E. A., and Seed, B. (1989). A B-lymphoxyte activation molecule related to the nerve growth factor receptor and induced by cytokines in carcinomas, *EMBO J., 8*: 1403.

Stauber, G. B., and Aggarwal, B. B. (1989). Characterization and affinity cross-linking of receptors for human recombinant lymphotoxin (tumor necrosis factor-beta) on a human histiocytic lymphoma cell line, U-937, *J. Biol. Chem., 264*: 3573.

Stauber, G. B., Aiyer, R. A., and Aggarwal, B. B. (1988). Human tumor necrosis factor-alpha receptor: purification by immunoaffinity chromatography and initial characterization, *J. Biol. Chem., 263*: 19098.

Sugarman, B. J., Aggarwal, B. B., Hass, P. E., Figari, I. S., Palladino, M. A., and Shepard, M. H. (1985). Recombinant human tumor necrosis factor-alpha: effects on proliferation of normal and transformed cells in vitro, *Science, 230*: 943.

Taga, T., Hibi, M., Hirata, Y., Yamaski, K., Uasukawa, K., Matsuda, T., Hirano, T., and Kishimoto, T. (1989). Interleukin-6 triggers the association of its receptor with a possible signal transducer, gp 130, *Cell, 58*: 573.

Talmadge, J. E., Philipps, H., Schneider, M., Rowe, T., Pennington, R., Bowersox, O., and Lenz, B. (1988). Immunomodulatory properties of recombinant murine and human tumor necrosis factor, *Cancer Res., 48*: 544.

Tracey, K. J., Vlassara, H., and Cerami, A. (1989). cachectin/tumor necrosis factor, *Lancet, 1*: 1122.

Tsujimoto, M., Yip, Y. K., and Vilček, J. (1985). Tumor necrosis factor: specific binding and internalisation in sensitive and resistant cells, *Proc. Natl. Acad. Sci. USA, 82*: 7626.

Tsujimoto, M., Feinman, R., Kohase, M., and Vilček, J. (1986a). Characterization and affinity crosslinking of receptors for tumor necrosis factor on human cells, *Arch. Biochem. Biophys., 249*: 563.

Tsujimoto, M., Feinman, R., and Vilček, J. (1986b). Differential effects of type I IFN and IFN-gamma on the binding of tumor necrosis factor to receptors in two human cell lines, *J. Immunol., 137*: 2272.

Tsujimoto, M., Yip, Y. K., and Vilček, J. (1986c). IFN-gamma enhances expression of cellular receptors for tumor necrosis factor, *J. Immunol., 135*: 2441.

Ullrich, A., Coussens, L., Hayflick, J. S., Dull, T. J., Gray, A., Tam, A. W., Lee, J., Yarden, Y., Libermann, T. A., Schlessinger, J., Downward, J., Bye, J., Whittle, N., Watefield, M. D., and Seeburg, P. H. (1984). Human epidermal growth factor receptor cDNA sequence and aberrant expression of the amplified gene in A431 epidermoid carcinoma cells, *Nature, 309*: 418.

Ullrich, A., Bell, J. R., Chen, E. Y., Herrera, R., Petruzzelli, L. M., Dull, T. J., Gray, A., Coussens, L., Liao, Y. C., Tsubokawa, M., Mason, A., Seeburg, P. H., Grunfeld, C., Rosen, O. M., and Ramachandran, J. (1985). Human insulin receptor and its relation to the tyrosine kinase family of oncogenes, *Nature, 313*: 756.

Upton, C., DeLange, A. M., and McFadden, G. (1987). Tumorigenic poxviruses: genomic organization and DNA sequence of the telomeric region of the Shope fibroma virus genome, *Virology, 160*: 20.

Weber, W., Gill, G. N., and Spiess, J. (1984). Production of an epidermal growth factor receptor-related protein, *Science, 224*: 294.

Wilkinson, K. D. (1987). Protein ubiquitinization: a regulatory post-translational modification, *Anticancer Drug Design, 2*: 211.

Yamamoto, T., Davis, C. G., Brown, M. S., Schneider, W. J., Casey, M. L., Goldstein, J. L., Russell, D. W. (1984). The human LDL receptor: a cystein-rich protein with multiple Alu sequences in its mRNA, *Cell, 39*: 27.

Yarden, Y., Escobeda, J. A., Kuang, W. J., Yang-Feng, T. L., Daniel, T. O., Tremble, P. M., Chen, E. Y., Ando, M. E., Harkins, R. N., Francke, Y., Fried, V. A., Ullrich, A., and Williams, L. T. (1986). Structure of the receptor for platelet derived growth factor helps define a family of closely related growth factor receptors, *Nature, 323*: 226.

Yonehara, S., Ishii, A., and Yonehara, M. (1989). A cell-killing monoclonal antibody (anti-Fas) to a cell-surface antigen co-downregulated with the receptor of tumor necrosis factor, *J. Exp. Med., 169*: 1747.

Yoshie, O., Tada, K., and Ishida, N. (1986). Binding and crosslinking of ^{125}I-labeled recombinant human tumor necrosis factor to cell surface receptors, *J. Biochem., 100*: 531.

Zupan, A. A., Osborne, P. A., Smith, C. E., Siegel, N. R., Leimgruber, R. M., and Johnson, E. M. J. (1989). Identification, purification, and characterization of truncated forms of the human nerve growth factor receptor, *J. Biol. Chem., 264*: 11714.

9

TNF Signal Transduction and TNF-Responsive Genes

MARTIN KRÖNKE, STEFAN SCHÜTZE, PETER SCHEURICH, and KLAUS PFIZENMAIER
Max-Planck-Society, Göttingen, Germany

I. INTRODUCTION

Tumor necrosis factor (TNF), originally defined by its antitumoral activity in vitro and in vivo, is now recognized as a polypeptide mediator of inflammation and cellular immune responses (Old, 1985; Le and Vilček, 1987; Beutler and Cerami, 1988). The cellular source of TNF are mainly macrophages and T or B lymphocytes. TNF belongs to a class of hormone-like molecules termed cytokines, a group of soluble factors that includes the interferons, interleukins, and hematopoietic growth factors (CSFs). These polypeptide mediators form a complex network of interactive signals that regulate their own production and the growth, differentiation, or function of virtually every cell type, most notably of cells of the reticuloendothelial, the hematopoietic, and the immune system. TNF has been shown to be identical to cachectin, a central mediator of the shock state in gram-negative sepsis (Beutler et al., 1985; Tracey et al., 1986). TNF also induces antiviral activity (Mestan et al., 1986; Wong and Goeddel, 1986) and may play a protective role in parasitic infections (Malik and Balkwill, 1988). On the other hand, deregulated overexpression of TNF has been implicated in the pathogenesis of cerebral malaria (Grau et al., 1989) and inflammatory tissue destruction in general (Beutler and Cerami, 1988). Clues to a subtle understanding of the biological significance of TNF may come on the one hand from studies defining the conditions of TNF gene expression in vivo, and on the other hand from investigations unraveling the multiple facets of TNF action. A salient feature of TNF action is the striking diversity of possible cellular responses; as yet, no specific biological activity of TNF could be defined that is in common to all TNF-responsive cells. Based on the apparently limited structural heterogeneity of specific TNF membrane receptors, the multitude of phenotypic and functional changes inducible by TNF, by and large, must depend on a diversification of postreceptor signaling mechanisms (Schütze et al., 1988a, b). In this chapter we discuss recent findings on cellular structures and molecules that communicate TNF signals from the cell membrane to the nucleus supporting the view of both tissue-specific and cell differentiation-dependent involvement of distinct signal transduction pathways in TNF regulation of gene expression.

II. TNF SIGNAL TRANSDUCTION ACROSS THE MEMBRANE

As for cytokines in general, the first event in triggering a cellular response is specific high-affinity interaction with membrane receptor molecules, thereby initiating a cascade of signal transfer reaction inside the cell. Today, it has become clear that different cytokines might overlap with respect to activation of certain intracellular signal pathways, while differing in others. Thus, in analogy to the extracellular cytokine network (Old, 1987), a similar picture might be drawn for intracellular signal transduction, where a limited number of pathways is differentially affected by distinct cytokine receptors upon ligand binding, resulting in apparently ligand specific cellular responses.

The most direct way of the signaling mechanism is found with receptors that themselves possess intrinsic tyrosine kinase activity in their intracellular domains (e.g., epidermal growth factor, insulin-or platelet-derived growth factor receptors) (Hunter, 1987). To date, there is no indication for tyrosine kinase activity of TNF receptors. A second mechanism includes receptor-mediated activation of phospholipases, which results in the generation of typical second messenger activities. This pathway is thought to involve guanine nucleotide binding proteins (G-proteins), similar to those controlling protein kinases A and G (Gilman, 1987; Neer and Clapham, 1988; Johnson and Dhanasekaran, 1989).

In the case of the pleiotropic cytokine TNF, several distinct, but not mutually exclusive mechanisms of signal transduction have to be considered to explain the induction of multiple biological activities: First, structural and functional heterogeneity in membrane receptors may exist, each linked to a distinct intracellular second messenger system; second, response heterogeneity may be brought about by a diversification of postreceptor signal transduction pathways; and third, membrane receptors may not only function as transmembrane signaling components, but also act as transporters of TNF, which itself, or complexed to its receptor, may exhibit intracellular signaling activity. The data summarized below show that all three aforementioned possibilities exist and eventually contribute to TNF responsiveness; however, it appears that postreceptor signal diversification plays the major role for generating response heterogeneity.

A. Role of Structural Heterogeneity of Membrane Receptors in TNF Signal Transduction

Very recently, the biochemical purification of TNF membrane receptors has revealed structural heterogeneity with two major, distinct binding proteins of 60 and 75/85 kDa (for details, see Chapter 8 of this volume). These two TNF binding proteins are coexpressed in most cell lines, although at different densities (Hohmann et al., 1989). These findings are suggestive of response heterogeneity due to distinct receptor molecules. At present, however, there are no data in support of this reasoning. In contrast, by use of an antagonistic monoclonal antibody specifically recognizing and competing for TNF binding to the p60 TNF-receptor protein, we were able to uniformly abolish in several p60/p85 TNF-receptor-positive cell lines a variety of TNF responses, including cytostasis/cytotoxicity and enhancement of HLA gene expression (Thoma et al., 1990). These data indicate that p60 is an essential component for TNF signal transduction, whereas ligand binding via p85 alone is apparently not sufficient to induce TNF responses. Although a number of distinct TNF responses were investigated of cells of epithelial, lymphoid, and myeloid origin, at present alternative signaling pathways via p85 TNF receptors cannot be ruled out. Molecular cloning and functional expression of p85 in TNF-receptor-negative cells will ultimately reveal the role of this receptor molecule in TNF signal transduction.

B. Role of Ligand Internalization for Induction of TNF Responses

Upon binding to its receptor, TNF is rapidly internalized at temperatures above 15°C and subsequently degraded with slower kinetics (Tsujimoto et al., 1985, 1986; Yoshie et al., 1986; Watanabe et al., 1989). Although it has been suggested that internalization of TNF might be important for induction of cytolysis (Kull, 1988; Watanabe et al., 1989), the question of whether or not internalization is a prerequisite for induction of TNF responses in general has been a controversial issue. Thus it is apparent that TNF can induce transmembrane signals under conditions that rule out internalization. For example, it has been shown that TNF stimulation at low temperature induces rapid phosphorylation of the cytosolic protein p26, a potential effector molecule in TNF signal transduction (see below; Schütze et al., 1989). On the other hand, experiments addressing the role of internalization by using inhibitory drugs are limited in their interpretation due to the fact that these substances usually also affect other cell functions and/or cell viability during the incubation time necessary for detection of TNF responses. However, a recent report of Smith et al. (1990) shows cytotoxic activity of microinjected TNF, suggesting, indeed, a receptor-independent intracellular function of the ligand itself. According to this view, under physiological conditions, TNF membrane receptors would serve as a ligand transporter, in addition to its function as a signal transmitter in the membrane. Whether or not this is a more general mechanism of TNF action that also applies for other than cytotoxic responses to TNF, in particular for TNF-induced gene regulation, requires further investigations and independent confirmation.

C. Guanine Nucleotide Binding Proteins

GTP binding or G-proteins provide a signal transduction coupling mechanism for many cell surface hormone receptors (Gilman, 1987; Neer and Chapham, 1988) and may also play an important role in TNF receptor signaling. G-proteins are a family of membrane-associated heterotrimeric proteins composed of alpha, beta, and gamma subunits. The two latter are structurally conserved between distinct G-proteins and provide a regulatory function, whereas alpha subunits are structurally heterogeneous and mediate distinct functional activities. Membrane receptors catalytically activate the alpha subunit by displacement of bound GDP for GTP. The GTP-bound form of the $G\alpha$ protein initiates cellular responses by altering the activity of specific intracellular effector enzymes, in particular adenylate cyclase and enzymes of phospholipid metabolism such as phospholipase A_2 and C (for a review, see Exton, 1988).

Although there exist several reports for the involvement of phospholipases in TNF signal transduction (see below), experimental evidence for the involvement of G-proteins is very limited to date. Indirect evidence for the involvement of G-proteins comes from investigations of TNF responses of endothelial cells: TNF-induced rapid permeability changes were shown to be pertussis-toxin sensitive (Brett et al., 1989). In contrast, pertussis toxin did not alter TNF-induced modulation of two endothelial cell coagulant properties (i.e., cellular responses, which take place in the order of hours). Thus provided that pertussis toxin sufficiently blocked G-proteins during these prolonged culture periods, these data suggest the existence of at least two distinct TNF signal transduction pathways effective in endothelial cells, one that is pertussis-toxin sensitive, and one that is not (Brett et al., 1989). Moreover, TNF-mediated cytolysis of L929 cells was reduced in the presence of ADP-ribosilating toxins (Hepburn et al., 1987), suggesting an involvement of G-proteins also in this TNF action. In addition, there is circumstantial evidence for the participation of G-proteins in the TNF-mediated induction of GM-CSF mRNA in mesenchymal cells (Yamato et al., 1989b).

A direct stimulation of GTPase activity by TNF as well as induction of high-affinity GTP binding was reported by Imamura et al. (1988). According to these data, a pertussis-toxin-sensitive G-protein is involved in TNF signal transduction in human myeloid HL-60 cells as well as the murine fibrosarcoma cell line L929. Based on these data, one can estimate that one ligand-activated TNF receptor molecule stimulates about 100 G-proteins (Imamura et al., 1988). At present, the nature of the G-binding proteins activated by TNF stimulation is unknown. Sensitivity to pertussis toxin suggests participation of alpha subunits of the G_i or G_o type. However, it is conceivable that TNF signaling is mediated via a novel set of PT-sensitive G-proteins distinct from those active in classical hormone signaling pathways.

D. Activation of Phospholipase A_2

Phospholipase A_2 (PL-A_2) has been demonstrated to be coupled by G-proteins to membrane receptors (Silk et al., 1989). Upon activation, PL-A_2 cleaves arachidonic acid from phospholipids. Free arachidonate may enter a number of alternative pathways: for example, the cyclooxygenase pathway, leading to formation of prostaglandins, or the lipoxygenase pathway, resulting in formation of leukotrienes (Irvine, 1982; Ford-Hutchinson, 1985). These substances are known to stimulate different genes. Arachidonate, however, may also be released from diacylglycerols by diacylglycerol lipase (Nakashima et al., 1988), which indicates that arachidonic acid release per se does not necessarily indicate PL-A_2 activation.

Data from several laboratories have demonstrated TNF-mediated activation of phospholipase A_2 in different cell types. In most systems interleukin 1 (IL-1) was also found to be effective. Due to the overlapping spectrum of bioactivities of these two cytokines, this finding was not unexpected: for example, in human synovial cells, both TNF and IL-1 induced release of radiolabeled arachidonic acid from phosphatidylserine as well as phosphatidylinositol (Godfrey et al., 1987). Release of [^{3}H]arachidonate from rat chondrocytes (Suffys et al., 1988) and of phospholipase A_2 from from rat renal mesangial cells can also be stimulated by both TNF and IL-1 (Pfeilschifter et al., 1989). Similarly, in a bovine endothelial cell line, CPAE, stimulation of [^{3}H]arachidonic acid is enhanced by TNF, presumably via activation of a pertussis-toxin-sensitive G-protein (Clark et al., 1988). Moreover, studies performed with the human myeloid cell lines U937 have shown that the phospholipase A_2 inhibitors dexamethasone and quinacrine inhibit TNF-mediated cytolysis, whereas inhibitors of the cyclo-oxygenase-, lipoxygenase-, and cytochrome P450-dependent pathways of arachidonate metabolism were ineffective in this respect (Neale et al., 1988). These data suggested that not arachidonate but rather lysophospholipids or their metabolites are effector molecules in TNF cytotoxicity.

In general, phospholipase A_2 is believed to be responsible for the increase in eicosanoid synthesis induced by TNF (Dayer et al., 1985; Bachwich et al., 1986; Clark et al., 1988). As to the induction of prostaglandin synthesis, TNF synergized in Swiss 3T3 fibroblasts with bradykinin, bombesin, thrombin, norepinephrine, and platelet-activating factor (Burch and Tiffany, 1989) and with IL-1 in resting macrophages (Bachwich et al., 1986). Prostaglandins are important mediators of inflammation and may thus enhance direct inflammatory activity of TNF. On the other hand, prostaglandins have been implicated to antagonize TNF growth stimulation of human FS-4 fibroblasts (Hori et al., 1989). However, when the role of phospholipid breakdown for either mitogenic or cytotoxic activities of TNF on BALB/c 3T3 fibroblasts was investigated in greater detail, it was noted that phospholipase activation can be associated with both growth stimulatory and inhibitory activities of TNF (Palombella and Vilček, 1989).

E. Activation of Phosphatidylcholine-Specific Phospholipase C

Initial attempts to identify classical second messengers involved in TNF signal transduction failed. Especially release of Ca^{2+} from internal stores and increase in intracellular IP_3 levels (Kobayashi et al., 1987; own unpublished observations) have not been detectable. In a recent study, however, we have obtained evidence that TNF activates a phosphatidylcholine-specific phospholipase (PC-PLC), producing diacylglycerol (DAG) from phosphatidylcholine (Schütze et al., submitted). Our data show that PC rather than PIP_2 serves as the source for TNF-induced DAG production, which is in accordance with earlier observations indicating that TNF does not induce IP_3 release. At present, the PC-specific phospholipase C thus appears to be the only TNF-induced enzyme generating 1,2-DAG.

III. TNF-SENSITIVE PROTEIN KINASES

A. Activation of Protein Kinase A

Human diploid fibroblasts (e.g., FS-4) respond to TNF with increased DNA synthesis and growth stimulation (Sugarman et al., 1985; Vilček et al., 1986). In the same cells, TNF has been noted to rapidly enhance cAMP potentially resulting in activation of PKA (Zhang et al., 1988a). Similarly, in rat mesangial cells, stimulation of cAMP levels by TNF was reported (Baud et al., 1988). TNF may either directly activate adenylate cyclase via G-proteins or, alternatively, inhibit phosphodiesterase activity. Indirect evidence for the activation of adenylate cyclase comes from studies with protein kinase C–depleted FS-4 cells, in which interleukin-6 mRNA was readily inducible by both TNF and cAMP stimulation (Zhang et al., 1988b). Moreover, TNF, similar to IL-1 and cAMP, was able to induce expression of the interleukin-2 receptor alpha chain gene (Tac antigen, p55) in the human natural killer-like cell line YT (Lee et al., 1987; Scholz and Altman, 1989). However, when applied together, TNF, IL-1, and cAMP showed synergistic effects on Tac antigen expression. These data suggest that in YT-cells distinct signal transduction pathways may be used by these agents. In fact, increase in cAMP levels by TNF per se could not be measured, although TNF enhanced forskolin-stimulated cAMP levels in the same cell line. This suggests an indirect action of TNF on cAMP levels:

for example, via activation of protein kinase C, which in turn could activate the catalytic unit of adenylatecyclase by phosphorylation (Scholz and Altman, 1989).

B. Activation of Protein Kinase C

Initial evidence for a participation of protein kinases in TNF signal transduction came from findings that protein kinase inhibitors could block TNF-mediated induction of its own gene (Hensel et al., 1987). The involvement of PKC in TNF signaling pathways was recently corroborated by monitoring the effects of TNF on the PKC activity in three human leukemic cell lines of lymphocytic (Jurkat), monocytic (U937), and erythroid (K562) lineage (Schütze et al., 1990). TNF treatment resulted in activation of PKC associated with a translocation from the cytosol to the cell membrane. Slightly different profiles of PKC translocation were observed: In U937 cells, membrane-associated PKC-activity first increased and thereafter completely vanished. In the cytosol, TNF induced a long-term down-regulation of PKC in U937 cells, thus resembling the effects of phorbol esters (PMA) on PKC activity in these cells. Interestingly, in U937 cells, TNF induced PMA-like transcriptional programs, leading to phenotypic changes such as differentiation and growth inhibition. These findings suggest that PKC may play a central role in mediating the biological effects of TNF in this cell line. With both Jurkat and K562 cells, a reversed translocation of PKC activity was observed; that is, TNF-induced translocation of PKC activity to the membranes was followed by a retranslocation to the cytosol. This TNF-induced "reversed translocation" of PKC activity is reminiscent of the effects of IL-2, IL-3, IFN-α, and IFN-γ on PKC activity in a long-term-cultured T-cell line (Farrar and Anderson, 1985) WEHI-3 cells (Farrar et al., 1985), human amniotic cells (Premecz et al., 1989), and a B-lymphoid cell line (Ostrowski et al., 1988), respectively. In addition, variable kinetics of PKC translocation were observed in primary T-lymphocytes stimulated with IL-2 at different stages of activation (Mahé et al., 1988). These different modes of activation of PKC may point to diverse functions of PKC in different cell lines; for example, TNF may activate distinct tissue-specific PKC isoenzymes (Coussens et al., 1986; Sawamura et al., 1989; Makowske et al., 1988), which may differ in activation requirements and/or substrate specificity. Alternatively, TNF may activate one single form of PKC that is coupled to different signaling pathways in different cell lines.

As to the molecular mechanism of TNF-induced PKC activation, a likely candidate would be DAG generated by PC-specific PL-C (see above and Fig. 1). It is generally accepted that DAG regulates PKC activity by reducing the Ca^{2+} requirement of this enzyme and thereby activating it. However, it has also been shown that unsaturated fatty acids, such as arachidonic acid or oleic acid, can activate PKC independently of Ca^{2+} and phospholipids (Murakami and Routtenberg, 1985). Thus TNF activation of PKC may occur through stimulation of either

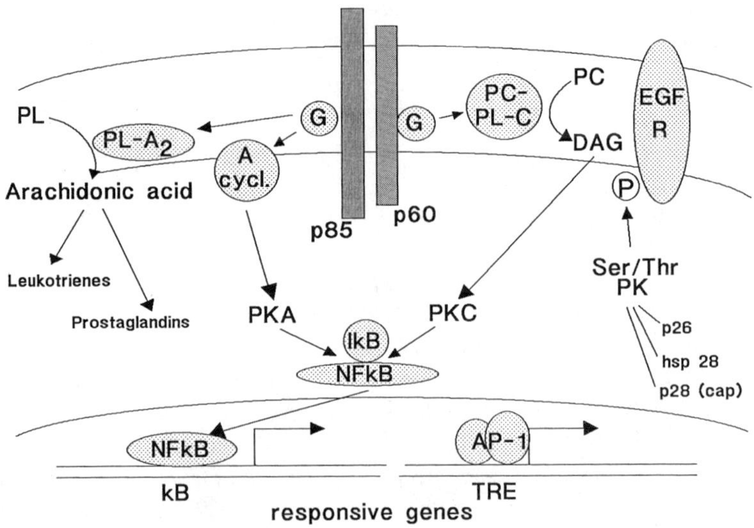

Figure 1 TNF signal transduction pathways (for details, see the text). A cycl, adenylate cyclase; DAG, diacylglycerol; EGF-R, epidermal growth factor receptor; G, GTP-binding protein; IκB, inhibitor of NF-κB protein; NFκB, nuclear factor kappa B; PC, phosphatidylcholine; PC-PL-C, PC-specific phospholipase C; PL, phospholipids; PL-A_2, phospholipase A_2; PKA, protein kinase A; PKC, protein kinase C; Ser/Thr PK, serine-threonine protein kinase; TRE, phorbol ester-responsive element.

phospholipase C, leading to increased levels of DAG, or phospholipase A_2, elevating cis-fatty acids or lysophospholipids.

IV. CELLUAR SUBSTRATES FOR TNF-INDUCED PROTEIN KINASES

The activation of protein kinases presumably will modify the phosphorylation of a discrete number of protein substrates which ultimately channel TNF signals to the transcription apparatus in the cell nucleus. Indeed, a few cytosolic proteins of low molecular weight were described to be phosphorylated within minutes after TNF treatment: with U937 cells, we have shown that TNF can induce phosphorylation of a 26-kDa cytosolic protein (p26) (Schütze et al., 1989). This process is a very rapid and transient event, as p26 phosphorylation was detectable within 20 s, peaked at 10 min, and decreased to low levels within 1 h after TNF stimulation. Dose-response studies revealed half-maximal phosphorylation of p26 at TNF concentrations of 1.8 ng/mL, which is in the range of TNF doses sufficient to induce cellular responses such as growth arrest and differentiation. p26 was phosphorylated exclusively at serine residues, indicating either the activation of a serine kinase or the inactivation of a serine phosphatase secondary to ligand–receptor interactions.

Interestingly, treatment of U937 cells with various PKC activators such as calcium inophores, mitogens, and phorbol esters (PMA) resulted in phosphorylation of a protein with the same apparent molecular weight of 26 kDa (own unpublished data). In reconciliation with the TNF-induced activation and translocation of the PKC mentioned above, it seems possible that protein kinase C may phosphorylate p26. p26 phosphorylation was also induced in some but not all other cell lines examined, indicating that p26 may be involved in a cell- or tissue-specific TNF-signal transduction pathway. As to a possible function of p26 in TNF action, the analysis of p26 phosphorylation in U937 cell subclones sharing a distinct pattern of TNF-induced responses suggested that p26 may play a role in the TNF signaling pathway linked to differentiation processes rather than to growth control (Schütze et al., 1989).

TNF-dependent protein phosphorylation has also been observed with other cell lines. For example, Hepburn et al. (1988) discovered the rapid phosphorylation of a 27-kDa protein after TNF as well as after Ca^{2+} ionophore treatment in HeLa, Me180, and bovine aortic cells, but not in murine L929 cells. Later, the same group reported the phosphorylation of a triad of 28-kDa proteins in bovine aortic endothelial cells, which again was not discernible in L929 cells (Robaye et al., 1989). In comparison to p26, the kinetics of TNF-induced phosphorylation of these proteins were slower and the isoelectric points of these three 28-kDa proteins differed, suggesting that p26 was distinct from any of the three phosphoproteins. Phosphorylation of this triad was also detected following stimulation of bovine aortic endothelial cells with bradykinin (Demolle et al., 1988) and sodium arsenite (Robaye et al., 1989) as well as under stress conditions (Kaur et al., 1989). These observations suggest that the p28 triade may belong to the family of stress proteins. Thus, in extension to the concept developed for physiological stress, the phosphorylation of the 28-kDa proteins may perhaps play a role in the cellular protective response against the cytocidal action of TNF. This hypothesis is supported by the absence of TNF-induced phosphorylation of these proteins in L929 cells that are highly sensitive to the cytotoxic action of TNF (Robaye et al., 1989).

In an independent study, Kaur and Saklatvala (1988) noted TNF-induced phosphorylation of a triade of 27-kDa cytosolic proteins with p*I* values of 5.5, 5.7, and 6.0, respectively, in human dermal fibroblasts. By use of a polyvalent antiserum specific for small heat-shock proteins, these three 27-kDa phosphoproteins of MRC-5 fibroblasts could be identified as the phosphorylated forms of the mammalian heat-shock protein hsp27 (Arrigo and Welch, 1987; Regazzi et al., 1988). These three proteins were exclusively phosphorylated at serine residues. A similar increase in phosphorylation of immunoprecipitable 27-kDa proteins was noted in U937 and HepG2 cells stimulated by TNF and by IL-1α. From these data, the authors concluded that TNF and IL-1 might act on different cell types via a similar signaling mechanism. However, the phosphorylation of hsp27 can be induced by several agents, including serum, Ca^{2+} ionophore, PMA (Welch, 1985), bradykinin (Demolle et al., 1988), and sodium arsenite (Robaye et al., 1989). Thus TNF and IL-1 may, indeed, stimulate distinct signaling pathways that share hsp27 phosphorylation.

Taken together these data suggest that two groups (Hepburn et al., 1988; Robaye et al., 1989; Kaur and Saklatvala, 1988; Kaur et al., 1989) have independently described the same triad of 27/28-kDa stress phosphoproteins. In contrast, the cytosolic 26-kDa protein phosphorylated in TNF-treated U937 cells (Schütze et al., 1989) differs from these proteins with respect to molecular weight, isoelectric point, and kinetics of phosphorylation. In addition, more recent data showed that p26 differs antigenetically from small heat-shock proteins, as it was not immunoprecipitable by a specific anti-hsp antiserum (Schütze et al., manuscript in preparation).

In addition to the cytosolic proteins described above, Marino et al. (1989) recently noted a TNF-induced rapid and transient phosphorylation of a 28-kDa protein in human cervical carcinoma cells (Me180) existing in two isoforms with p*I* values of 6.1 and 6.2. The authors could enrich this 28-kDa protein by affinity chromatography using 7-methylguanosine 5′-triphosphate-Sepharose suggesting that p28 may be an mRNA cap-binding protein. The M_r and p*I* of p28 isoforms resemble those of another cap-binding protein of the initiation factor complex eIF-4F (Duncan et al., 1987). Initiation factor complexes are necessary for the efficient translation of capped mRNA by interacting with polyribosomes (Sonenberg, 1988). Thus mRNA cap-binding proteins may be involved in the regulation of TNF action at the translational level.

A well-characterized substrate for TNF-activated protein kinases is the receptor for epidermal growth factor (EGF). TNF, like IL-1 and PMA, caused a two- to five-fold increase in EGF receptor serine and threonine phosphorylation and a rapid dose-dependent down-regulation of EGF receptor-binding capacity in human gingival fibroblasts (Bird and Saklatvala, 1989). In this work, these authors showed that in cells depleted of protein kinase C by prolonged treatment with PMA, down-regulation of EGF receptors by IL-1 and TNF was still effective. These data suggested that the phosphorylation of EGF receptors induced by either TNF or IL-1 was mediated by a kinase distinct from protein kinase C. Mapping of the EGF receptor phosphorylation site revealed that both IL-1 and TNF showed phosphate incorporation at site(s) distinct from threonine 654, whose phosphorylation was induced by PMA (Bird and Saklatvala, 1990).

In addition to EGF receptor phosphorylation, it was reported that TNF stimulates EGF receptor tyrosine kinase activity (Donato et al., 1989). The kinetics of EGF receptor tyrosine kinase activation by TNF were slower as compared to those induced by EGF itself. The precise mechanism of TNF-induced heterologous sensitization of the EGF receptor as well as the physiological significance of EGF-receptor transmodulation by TNF has yet to be elucidated.

V. TNF-INDUCIBLE TRANSCRIPTION FACTORS: THIRD MESSENGERS IN TNF SIGNALING

An especially interesting entity of cellular targets for TNF-induced protein kinases are nuclear transcription factors, which represent a crucial link in the signaling cascade from the cell membrane to the nucleus. In eukaryotic cells, the rate of transcription of many genes is altered in response to extracellular stimuli. Changes in expression of genes transcribed by RNA polymerase II in response to agents such as steroid hormones, tumor promoters, stress, growth factors, and cytokines are mediated through distinct cis-acting DNA-sequence elements. These cis-acting elements consist of so-called enhancers and promoters, which contain multiple binding sites for sequence-specific DNA-binding proteins. It is now recognized that occupation of cis-acting elements by trans-acting factors determines the transcriptional activity of both constitutively expressed and inducible genes.

Although there is increasing evidence that TNF induction of gene expression is mediated through activation of trans-acting DNA-binding nuclear proteins, little is known about the mechanism by which TNF activates nuclear transcription factors. In general, possible mechanisms include (1) the activation of DNA binding activity from an inactive precursor, (2) inducible nuclear translocation, (3) modification of an already DNA-associated factor to acquire transcription-activating competence, and (4) inactivation of repressor factors.

Recently, Lowenthal et al. (1989), Osborn et al. (1989), and Duh et al. (1989) independently reported that TNF can induce a well-known transcription factor, NF-κB. NF-κB is a pleiotropic transcription factor that controls the expression of a variety of cellular as well as viral genes (for a review, see Lenardo and Baltimore, 1989). An 11-base-pair DNA consensus sequence specifically recognized by NF-κB is present in the kappa immunoglobulin light chain gene, several other cellular genes, and in certain primate virus enhancers. NF-κB was originally described as a B-cell-specific protein, which is required for kappa enhancer function (Sen and Baltimore, 1986a; Atchinson and Perry, 1987). However, it is now recognized that NF-κB is not restricted to B cells, but is rather, inducible in a variety of cell types. Induction of NF-κB binding is independent of new protein synthesis (Sen and Baltimore, 1986b) and involves dissociation of NF-κB from a cytosolic inhibitor protein (I-κB) followed by translocation of NF-κB to the nucleus (Bäuerle and Baltimore, 1988a, b), where it binds directly to its cognate DNA sequences. Release of NF-κB can be achieved by treating cells with phorbol esters, cAMP, protein synthesis inhibitors, lipopolysaccharides, or by adding deoxycholate or formamide to cell extracts (Sen and Baltimore, 1986b; Bäuerle and Baltimore, 1988a,b; Shirakawa and Mizel, 1989). In addition, NF-κB is activated by double-stranded

RNA (Visvanathan and Goodbourn, 1989) and in cells expressing the transactivator of HTLV-I, tax1 (Lowenthal et al., 1988; Cross et al., 1987; Leung and Nabel, 1988; Ballard et al., 1988). According to a current model, the actual target of induction appears to be I-κB (Bäuerle and Baltimore, 1988a,b).

The diverse nature of NF-κB-inducing stimuli has made it difficult to define the precise molecular mechanisms of NF-κB activation and has raised the question of how physiological ligands activate NF-κB. Since TNF has been identified as one of the few naturally occurring endogenous NF-κB inducers (Osborn et al., 1989), the elucidation of the TNF-induced pathway of NF-κB activation is of particular interest. In this respect, several lines of evidence suggest the participation of protein kinases. Since NF-κB can be induced by activators of PKA and PKC, it is reasonable to hypothesize that the transcriptional activity of TNF may be channeled via one of these kinases, which in turn activates NF-κB.

In a recent study we investigated whether TNF-induced activation of PKC could be directly linked to the induction of NF-κB. We could show that TNF-induced activation of PKC and NF-κB, indeed, occurs with similar kinetics. However, unlike PMA, TNF could induce NF-κB even in the presence of inhibitors of protein kinases C. In addition, NF-κB remained TNF-inducible in Jurkat cells depleted for PKC by long-term exposure to high-dose phorbol ester, clearly indicating that NF-κB activation by TNF can occur independent of PKC (Meichle et al., 1990). Along these lines, Hohmann et al. (1990) found that in HL-60 cells, staurosporine, a potent inhibitor of protein kinases, prevented NF-κB activation by PMA or IL-1, while TNF-induced NF-κB activation was not inhibited. Together these data provide strong evidence for the existence of at least two different NF-κB activation pathways triggered by TNF.

Since NF-κB is a pleiotropic transcription factor that controls the expression of quite a number of genes in a tissue-specific manner, it is conceivable that NF-κB represents a "third messenger" of TNF signal transduction, mediating many of TNF's gene regulatory properties. For example, the pivotal role of NF-κB in TNF stimulation of mouse MHC class I gene expression has recently been elaborated by Israel et al. (1989a). The promoter of mouse MHC class I genes has already been dissected in detail and various elements responsible for basal or induced activity have been described, together with the proteins that bind to these regions. Israel et al. (1989a) were able to colocalize the TNF-responsive element with the interferon response sequence (IRS). These TNF-responsive sequence were yet distinct from IRS and included two imperfect palindromic repeats. According to the author's interpretation, the transcription factor AP-2 binds to this palindromic region in the uninduced state. Following TNF treatment, NF-κB activity is induced, which displaces AP-2 as well as another transcription factor, BF1, and binds to the two palindromes, thereby enhancing MHC gene transcription.

Besides NF-κB, TNF has been reported to induce three other transcription factors: AP-1 (Brenner et al., 1989), IRF-1 (interferon regulatory factor 1) (Fujita et al., 1989), and NF-GMa, a protein binding to the so-called CK-1 (5′GAGAT-TCCAC3′) sequence present in many hemopoietic growth factor genes (Shannon et al., 1990). Brenner et al. (1989) demonstrated that activation of the collagenase gene by TNF is mediated by an element of the gene that is responsive to the transcription factor AP-1. These authors have used chimeric plasmids containing segments of the collagenase 5′ flanking region ligated to the chloramphenicol transferase (CAT) gene. They found that TNF enhanced the activity of constructs containing one or five copies of the TPA-responsive element (TRE) of the collagenase gene constituting an AP-1 binding site. However, inhibition of protein synthesis by cycloheximide blocked induction of collagenase mRNA by TNF. Hence AP-1 activation by TNF appeared to be dependent on de novo protein synthesis.

In the same article, TNF was shown to induce both *jun* and *fos* genes, whose protein products interact by leucine zippers to form the transcription factor AP-1 (Brenner et al., 1989). According to these data, activation of AP-1 is secondary to the induction of *fos* and *jun* gene transcription and hence cannot be sensed as an immediate messenger directly conferring TNF signals to the transcription apparatus in the nucleus. It is important to emphasize that this is in contrast to NF-κB which exists as a preformed complex in the cytosol and becomes postsynthetically modified and activated by TNF.

TNF also induces the transcription factor IRF-1 (Fujita et al., 1989). IRF-1 was shown earlier to bind to cis-acting regulatory elements present in interferon (IFN)-α and IFN-β genes as well as in some IFN-inducible genes (Harada et al., 1989). As in the case of *jun* and *fos*, TNF transcriptionally activates the IRF-1 gene rather than directly activating the IRF-1 protein. Finally, like in the case of AP-1 and IRF-1, induction by TNF of the transcription factor NF-GMa appears to occur at the transcriptional level as well (Shannon et al., 1990).

In conclusion, NF-κB remains the only transcription factor so far identified that serves as a direct target in the TNF signaling pathway. In contrast, the genes encoding the transcription factors, AP-1, IRF-1, and NF-GMa, belong to the family of TNF-inducible genes at the receiving end of TNF signal transduction. Such transcription factors are newly synthesized following TNF treatment and probably stimulate the expression of a second set of genes. Further work will be necessary to identify other nuclear factors which are immediately activated by TNF and control expression of the first line of TNF-inducible genes.

VI. TNF-RESPONSIVE GENES

Cells treated with TNF respond by profound alteration of their metabolic profiles, including cessation of cellular proliferation and induction of an antiviral state. RNA transcription and protein synthesis are necessary to bring about these metabolic changes. The currently known TNF-responsive genes and the respective references are listed in Table 1. TNF has been reported to induce genes encoding soluble factors involved in hematopoiesis, inflammation, immune responses, and tissue remodeling. For example, the collagenase gene, as well as several cytokine genes, including colony-stimulating factors, interferons, IL-1, IL-6, and notable TNF itself, are induced by TNF. A variety of membrane proteins, cell surface receptors, and cellular interaction molecules are also stimulated by TNF. For example, TNF transcriptionally enhances constitutively expressed genes, directing the synthesis of cell surface HLA class I and class II antigens and costimulates IL-2 receptor expression. Further, TNF affects the expression of several genes coding for cytosolic or nuclear proteins. Genes encoding enzymes regulating fat metabolism were among the first described to be inhibitable by TNF. More recently, a TNF-mediated inhibition of other cellular genes (e.g., albumin, collagen, and thrombomodulin), as well as a direct inhibition of viral gene transcription (HSV immediate early genes), has been described (Table 1).

As to genes encoding nuclear proteins, TNF can transiently induce c-*myc*, c-*fos*, and c-*jun* gene expression in fibroblasts (Table 1). On the other hand, we as well as other have shown that TNF inhibits c-myc expression in some tumor cell lines sensitive to the growth inhibitory action of TNF (Yarden and Kimchi, 1986; Krönke et al., 1987). This inhibition was also demonstrable in the presence of cycloheximide, suggesting that this inhibition was not mediated by the induction of other proteins. It is important to note that TNF apparently can either increase or decrease expression of the same gene, depending on the target cell investigated. Furthermore, a profound plasticity of the transcriptional responses to TNF can be observed in a given cell type, particularly in cells capable to undergo differentiation. For example, the highly variable transcriptional programs induced by TNF in U937 cells can be correlated to slightly different states of U937 cell differentiation along the monocytic lineage (Schütze et al., 1988a). Similarly, in human muscle cells TNF sensitivity is within a narrow temporary window of differentiation: in myoblasts, TNF inhibits several muscle-specific genes such as actin and myosin heavy chain, whereas in differentiated myotubes, TNF has no effect on these genes (Miller et al., 1988). However, in the same cells, TNF induction of the IL-6 gene remains unaffected in the course of differentiation, allowing segregation of differentiation-dependent and differentiation-independent pathways of TNF-mediated gene activation. Accordingly, even closely related cell types can respond very differently to TNF.

Both transcriptional and translational events appear to be important in determining the level of induced gene expression. Among the best characterized TNF-inducible mRNAs and proteins are MHC class I and class II antigens. TNF does not induce MHC gene transcription from previously quiescent genes, but rather enhances either constitutive or IFN-γ-induced HLA gene expression. This is brought about by rapid modification of the preexisting transcription factor NF-κB (see

Table 1 TNF-Responsive Genes

Genes coding for:	References
Secreted proteins	
Adipsin	Min and Spiegelman, 1986
Albumin	Perlmutter et al., 1986
Alkaline phosphatase	Ng et al., 1989
Alpha-1 acidic glycoprotein	Andus et al., 1988
Collagen	Solis-Herruzo et al., 1988; Scharffetter et al., 1989
Collagenase	Nakagawa et al., 1987; Brenner et al., 1989
Complement component C3	Perlmutter et al., 1986; Katz and Strunk, 1989
Complement factor B	Perlmutter et al., 1986; Katz and Strunk, 1989
Gelatinase	Nakagawa et al., 1987
Plasminogen activator inhibitors 1 and 2	van Hinsbergh et al., 1988; Medcalf et al. 1988; Sawdey et al., 1989
Serum amyloid A protein	Woo et al., 1987
Tissue factor	Conway and Rosenberg, 1989; Scarpati and Sadler, 1989
Urokinase-type plasminogen activator (u-PA)	Georg et al., 1989
Cytokines	
G-CSF	Oster et al., 1988; Koeffler et al., 1988; Demetri et al, 1989
GM-CSF	Broudy et al., 1986; Koeffler et al., 1988; Yamato et al., 1989b
M-CSF	Oster et al., 1987
IFN-β	Jacobsen et al., 1989; Reis et al., 1989
IL-1α	Turner et al., 1989
IL-1β	Kurt-Jones et al., 1987; Turner et al., 1989; Elias et al., 1989; Yamato, 1989a
IL-6	Zilberstein et al., 1986; Kohase et al., 1986; Defilippi et al., 1987; Katz and Strunk, 1989
IL-8	Matsushima et al., 1988; Strieter et al., 1989a
MCP-1	Strieter et al., 1989b; Larsen et al., 1989
MGSA/gro	Wen et al., 1989
PDGF	Silver et al., 1989
TNF	Hensel et al., 1987; Spriggs et al., 1987; Schütze et al., 1988a
Membrane-associated proteins	
Actin	Miller et al., 1988
c-abl	Andrews et al., 1989

Table 1 (Continued)

Genes coding for:	References
C3b-receptor	Berger et al., 1988
ELAM-1	Pober, 1987, Bevilacqua et al., 1989
HLA class I	Scheurich et al., 1986; Collins et al., 1986; Pfizenmaier et al., 1987
HLA class II	Pfizenmaier et al., 1987
ICAM-1	Pober, 1987
IL-2 R alpha chain (p55)	Freimuth et al., 1989; Lowenthal et al., 1989
Lipoproteinlipase	Torti et al., 1985; Enerbaeck et al., 1988; Zechner et al., 1988
Myosin heavy chain	Miller et al., 1988
Thrombomodulin	Conway and Rosenberg, 1988; Scarpati et al., 1989
Acetyl-CoA carboxylase	Pape and Kim, 1988, 1989
Cytochrome *b*-245 heavy chain gene	Cassatella et al., 1989
Ferritin heavy chain	Torti et al., 1988
Metallothionin II	Schütze et al., 1988a
MnSOD	Wong and Goeddel, 1988; Asoh et al., 1989
MX (p78)	Goetschy et al., 1989
2′5′OASE	Mestan et al., 1988; Schütze et al., 1988a
Nuclear proteins	
c-fos	Lin and Vilček, 1987; Colotta et al., 1987; Schütze et al., 1988a
c-jun	Brenner et al., 1989; Dixit et al., 1989
c-myb	Schachner et al., 1988
c-myc	Yarden and Kimchi, 1986; Krönke, et al., 1987; Lin and Vilček, 1987; Tobler et al., 1987; Schachner et al., 1988
IRF-1	Fujita et al., 1989
NF-GMa	Shannon et al., 1990
Viral	
HIV	Duh et al., 1989; Folks et al., 1989; Griffin et al., 1989; Israel et al., 1989b; Osborn et al., 1989; Okamoto et al., 1989
HSV immediate early genes	Feduchi et al., 1989
SV40	Meichle et al., 1990; Plaetinck et al., 1989

Chapter 5) that subsequently displaces two constitutive MHC enhancer-binding proteins AP-2 and BF1 (Israel et al., 1989a). With Colo205 cells, TNF was noted to enhance HLA class I membrane expression in the absence of any changes of steady-state mRNA levels suggesting an additional regulatory action of TNF at the posttranscriptional level (Pfizenmaier et al., 1987). Very little is known about posttranscriptional enhancement of gene expression by TNF. In this respect, the observation of TNF-induced phosphorylation of a 28-kDa mRNA cap-binding protein in human cervical carcinoma cells (Marino et al., 1989) is intriguing (see above). Phosphorylation of a component of the eukaryotic initiation factor complex may represent an important control mechanism of TNF action at the translational level.

VII. CONCLUDING REMARKS

In the past few years, a number of experimental observations have been made that have provided first insight into the molecular mechanism of TNF action. A current model of TNF signal transduction pathways is illustrated in Fig. 1. Despite recent progress, several steps of TNF signal transduction are poorly understood. In particular, the mechanisms by which TNF receptors activate phosphorylcholine-dependent phospholipase C have not been elucidated. To this, important information will be available from biochemical and functional analysis of molecularly cloned TNF receptors. It is now well established that TNF initiates signal transfer reactions from the membrane to the nucleus that involve G-proteins, phosphatidylcholine-specific phospholipase C, phospholipase A_2, protein kinases A and C, and ultimately nuclear transcription factors. However, since virtually all cells contain these elements of signal transduction, an important problem in understanding the operation of these intracellular signaling systems is to explain how specificity is achieved. What differences between the action of TNF versus that of other growth factors, hormones or tumor promoters, can account for their different effects on the same cell? It is possible that while two different ligands utilize similar signal tranduction systems, differences in the magnitude and time courses of the responses triggered by these agents may be responsible for their different effects. Thus it will be especially challenging to tackle this conceptual question of how TNF signals remain specific as they cross the cell membrane. Further studies will hopefully yield a cohesive picture of the intracellular signal transduction network that links TNF cell surface receptors to nuclear transcription events.

REFERENCES

Andrews, D. F., Nemunaitis, J. J., and Singer, J. W. (1989). Recombinant tumor necrosis factor alpha and interleukin 1 alpha increase expression of c-abl protooncogene mRNA in cultured human marrow stromal cells, *Proc. Natl. Acad. Sci. USA*, *86*: 6788–6792.

Andus, T., Geiger, T., Hirano, T., Kishimoto, T., and Heinrich, P. C. (1988). Action of recombinant human interleukin 6, interleukin 1 β and tumor necrosis factor α on the mRNA induction of acute-phase proteins, *Eur. J. Immunol., 18*: 739-746.

Arrigo, A.-P., and Welch, W. J. (1987). Characterization and purification of the small 28,000-dalton mammalian heat shock protein, *J. Biol. Chem., 262*: 15359-15369.

Asoh, K., Watanabe, Y., Mizoguchi, H., Mawatari, M., Ono, M., Kohno, K., and Kuwano, M. (1989). Induction of manganese superoxide dismutase by tumor necrosis factor in human breast cancer MCF-7 cell line and its TNF-resistant variant, *Biochem. Biophys. Res. Commun., 162*: 794-801.

Atchison, M. L., and Perry, R. P. (1987). The role of the κ enhancer and its binding factor NH-κ B in the developmental regulation of κ gene transcription, *Cell, 48*: 121-128.

Bachwich, P. R., Chensue, S. W., Larrick, J. W., and Kunkel, S. L. (1986). Tumor necrosis factor stimulates interleukin-1 and prostaglandin E_2 production in resting macrophages, *Biochem. Biophys. Res. Commun., 36*: 94-101.

Ballard, D. W., Bohnlein, E., Lowenthal, J. W., Wano, Y., Franza, B. R., and Greene, W. C. (1988). HTLV-1 tax induces cellular proteins that activate the κ-B element in the Il-2 receptor α gene, *Science, 241*: 1652.

Baud, L., Perez, J., Friedlander, G., and Ardaillou, R. (1988). Tumor necrosis factor stimulates prostaglandin production and cyclic AMP levels in rat cultured mesangial cells, *FEBS Lett., 239*: 50-54.

Bäuerle, P. A., and Baltimore, D. (1988a). Activation of DNA-binding activity in an apparently cytoplasmic presursor of the NF-κ-B transcription factor, *Cell, 53*: 211-217.

Bäuerle, P. A., and Baltimore, D. (1988b). IkappaB: a specific inhibitor of the NF-κ B transcription factor, *Science, 242*: 540-546.

Berger, M., Wetzler, E. M., and Wallis, R. S. (1988). Tumor necrosis factor is the major monocyte product that increases complement receptor expression on mature human neutrophils, *Blood, 71*: 151-158.

Beutler, B., and Cerami, A. (1988). Tumor necrosis cachexia, shock and inflammation: a common mediator, *Annu. Rev. Biochem., 57*: 505.

Beutler, B. I., Milsark, I. W., and Cerami, A. C. (1985). Passive immunization against cachectin/tumor necrosis cator protects mice from lethal effect of endotoxin, *Science, 229*: 869-871.

Bevilacqua, M. P., Stengelin, S., Gimbrone, M. A., Jr., and Seed, B. (1989). Endothelial leukocyte adhesion molecule 1: an inducible receptor for neutrophils related to complement regulatory proteins and lectins, *Science, 243*: 1160-1165.

Bird, T. A., and Saklatvala, J. (1989). IL-1 and TNF transmodulate epidermal growth factor receptors by a protein kinase C-independent mechanism, *J. Immunol., 142*: 126-133.

Bird, T. A., and Saklatvala, J. (1990). Down-modulation of epidermal growth factor receptor affinity in fibroblasts treated with interleukin 1 or tumor necrosis factor is associated with phosphorylation at a site other than threonine 654, *J. Biol. Chem., 265*: 235-240.

Brenner, D. A., O'Hara, M., Angel, P., Chojkier, M., and Karin, M. (1989). Prolonged activation of jun and collagenase genes by tumor necrosis factor-α, *Nature, 337*: 661-663.

Brett, J., Gerlach, H., Nawroth, P., Steinberg, S., Godman, G., and Stern, D. (1989). Tumor necrosis factor/cachectin increases permeability of endothelial cell monolayers by a mechanism involving regulatory G proteins, *J. Exp. Med., 169*: 1977-1991.

Broudy, V. C., Kaushansky, K., Segal, G. M., Harlan, J. M., and Adamson, J. W. (1986). Tumor necrosis factor type alpha stimulates human endothelial cells to produce granulocyte/macrophage colony-stimulating factor, *Proc. Natl. Acad. Sci. USA, 83*: 7467-7471.

Burch, R. M., and Tiffany, C. W. (1989). Tumor necrosis factor causes amplification of arachidonic acid metabolism in response to interleukin 1, bradykinin, and other agonists, *J. Cell. Physiol., 141*: 85-89.

Cassatella, M. A., Hartman, L., Perussia, B., and Trinchieri, G. (1989). Tumor necrosis factor and immune interferon synergistically induce cytochrome b-245 heavy-chain gene expression and nicotinamide-adenine dinucleotide phosphate hydrogenase oxidase in human leukemic myeloid cells, *J. Clin. Invest., 83*: 1570-1579.

Clark, M. A., Chen, M.-J., Crooke, S. T., and Bomalaski, J. S. (1988). Tumor necrosis factor (cachectin) induces phospholipase A2 activity and synthesis of a phospholipase A2-activating protein in endothelial cells, *Biochem. J., 250*: 125-132.

Collins, T., Lapierre, L. A., Fiers, W., Strominger, J. L., and Pober, J. S. (1986). Recombinant human tumor necrosis factor increases mRNA levels and surface expression of HLA-A,B antigens in vascular endothelial cells and dermal fibroblasts in vitro, *Proc. Natl. Acad. Sci. USA, 83*: 446-450.

Colotta, F., Wang, J. M., Polentarutti, N., and Mantovani, A. (1987). Expression of c-fos protooncogene in normal human peripheral blood granulocytes, *J. Exp. Med., 165*: 1224-1229.

Conway, E. M., and Rosenberg, R. D. (1988). Tumor necrosis factor suppresses transcription of the thrombomodulin gene in endothelial cells, *Mol. Cell. Biol., 8*: 5588-5592.

Conway, E. M., Bach, R., Rosenberg, R. D., and Konigsberg, W. H. (1989). Tumor necrosis factor enhances expression of tissue factor mRNA in endothelial cells, *Thromb. Res., 53*: 231-241.

Coussens, L., Parker, P. J., Rhee, L., Yang-Feng, T. L., Chen, E., Waterfield, M. D., Francke, U., and Ullrich, A. (1986). Multiple, distinct forms of bovine and human protein kinase C suggest diversity in cellular signaling pathways, *Science, 233*: 859.

Cross, S. L., Feinberg, M. B., Wolf, J. B., Holbrook, N. J., Wong-Staal, F., and Leonard, W. J. (1987). Regulation of the human interleukin-2 receptor alpha chain promotor: activation of a nonfunctional promoter by the transactivator gene of HTLV-I, *Cell, 49*: 47-56.

Dayer, J. M., Beutler, B., and Cerami, A. (1985). Cachectin/tumor necrosis factor stimulates collagenase and prostaglandine$_2$ production by human synovial cells and dermal fiberoblasts, *J. Exp. Med., 162*: 2163-2168.

Defilippi, P., Poupart, P., Tavernier, J., Fiers, W., and Content, J. (1987). Induction and regulation of mRNA encoding 26-kDa protein in human cell lines treated with recombinant human tumor necrosis factor, *Proc. Natl. Acad. Sci. USA, 84*: 4557-4561.

Demetri, G. D., Zenzie, B. W., Rheinwald, J. G., and Griffin, J. D. (1989). Expression of colony-stimulating factor genes by normal human mesothelial cells and human malignant mesothelioma cell lines in vitro, *Blood, 74*: 940-946.

Demolle, D., Lecomte, M., and Boeynaems, J-M. (1988). Pattern of protein phosphorylation in aortic endothelial cells: modulation by adenine nucleotides and bradykinin, *J. Biol. Chem., 263*: 18459-18465.

Dixit, V. M., Marks, R. M., Sarma, V., and Prochownik, E. V. (1989). The antimitogenic action of tumor necrosis factor is associated with increased AP-1/c-jun proto-oncogene transcription, *J. Biol. Chem., 264*: 16905-16909.

Donato, N. J., Gallick, G. E., Steck, P. A., and Rosenblum, M. G. (1989). Tumor necrosis factor modulates epidermal growth factor receptor phosphorylation and kinase activity in human tumor cells, *J. Biol. Chem., 264*: 20474-20481.

Duh, E. J., Maury, W. J., Folks, T. M., Fauci, A. S., and Rabson, A. B. (1989). Tumor necrosis factor alpha activates human immunodeficiency virus type 1 through induction of nuclear factor binding to the NF-β B sites in the long terminal repeat, *Proc. Natl. Acad. Sci. USA, 86*: 5974-5978.

Duncan, R., Milburn, S. C., and Hershey, J. W. B. (1987). Regulated phosphorylation and low abundance of HeLa cell initiation factor eIF-4F suggest a role in translational control: heat shock effects on eIF-4F, *J. Biol. Chem., 262*: 380-388.

Elias, J. A., Reynolds, M. M., Kotloff, R. M., and Kern, J. A. (1989). Fibroblast interleukin 1 beta: synergistic stimulation by recombinant interleukin 1 and tumor necrosis factor and posttranscriptional regulation, *Proc. Natl. Acad. Sci. USA, 86*: 6171-6175.

Enerbaeck, S., Semb, H., Tavernier, J., Bjursell, G., and Olivecrona, T. (1988). Tissue-specific regulation of guinea pig lipoprotein lipase; effects of nutritional state and of tumor necrosis factor on mRNA levels in adipose tissue, heart and liver, *Gene, 64*: 97-106.

Exton, J. H. (1988). Mechanisms of action of calcium-mobilizing agonists: some variations on a young theme, *FASEBJ., 2*: 2670-2676.

Farrar, W. L., and Anderson, W. B. (1985). Interleukin-2 stimulates association of protein kinase C with plasma membrane, *Nature, 315*: 233.

Farrar, W. L., Thomas, T. P., and Anderson, W. B. (1985). Altered cytosol/membrane enzyme redistribution on interleukin-3 activation of protein kinase C, *Nature, 315*: 235.

Feduchi, E., Alonso, M. A., and Carrasco, L. (1989). Human gamma interferon and tumor necrosis factor exert a synergistic blockade on the replication of herpes simplex virus, *J. Virol., 63*: 1354-1359.

Folks, T. M., Clouse, K. A., Justement, J., Rabson, A., Duh, E., Kehrl, J. H., and Fauci, A. S. (1989). Tumor necrosis factor alpha induces expression of human immunodeficiency virus in a chronically infected T-cell clone, *Proc. Natl. Acad. Sci. USA, 86*: 2365-2368.

Ford-Hutchinson, A. W. (1985). Leukotrienes: their formation and role as inflammatory mediators, *Fed. Proc., 44*: 25-29.

Freimuth, W. W., Depper, J. M., and Nabel, G. J. (1989). Regulation of the IL-2 alpha gene: interaction of a *k* B binding protein with cell-specific transcription factors, *J. Immunol., 143*: 3064-3068.

Fujita, T., Reis, L. F. L., Watanabe, N., Kimura, Y., Taniguchi, T., and Vilček, J. (1989). Induction of the transcription factor IRF-1 and interferon-β mRNAs by cytokines and activators of second-messenger pathways, *Proc. Natl. Acad. Sci. USA, 86*: 16351-16354.

Georg, B., Helseth, E., Lund, L. R., Skandesen, T., Riccio, A., Dano, K., Unsgaard, G., and Andreasen, P. A. (1989). Tumor necrosis factor-alpha regulates mRNA for urokinase-type plasminogen activator and type-1 plasminogen activator inhibitor in human neoplasti cell lines, *Mol. Cell. Endocrinol., 61*: 87-96.

Gilman, A. G. (1987). G proteins: transducers of receptor-generated signals, *Annu. Rev. Biochem., 56*: 615-649.

Godfrey, R. W., Johnson, W. J., and Hoffstein, S. T. (1987). Recombinant tumor necrosis factor and interleukin-1 both stimulate human synovial cell arachidonic acid release and phospholipid metabolism, *Biochem. Biophys. Res. Commun., 142*: 235–241.

Goetschy, J. F., Zeller, H., Content, J., and Horisberger, M. A. (1989). Regulation of the interferon-inducible IFI-78K gene, the human equivalent of the murine Mx gene, by interferons, double-stranded RNA, certain cytokines, and viruses, *J. Virol., 63*: 2616–2622.

Grau. G. E., Piguet, P.-F., Vassalli, P., and Lambert, P.-H. (1989). Tumor-necrosis factor and other cytokines in cerebral malaria: experimental and clinical data, *Immunol. Rev., 112*: 49.

Griffin, G. E., Leung, K., Folks, T. M., Kunkel, S., and Nabel, G. J. (1989). Activation of HIV gene expression during monocyte differentiation by induction of NF-*k* B, *Nature, 339*: 70–73.

Harada, H., Fujita, T., Miyamoto, M., Kimura, Y., Maruyama, M., Furia, A., Miyata, T., and Taniguchi, T. (1989). Structurally similar but functionally distinct factors, IRF-1 and IRF-2, bind to the same regulatory elements of IFN and IFN-inducible genes, *Cell, 58*: 729–739.

Hensel, G., Männel, D. N., Pfizenmaier, K., and Krönke, M. (1987). Autocrine stimulation of TNF-alpha mRNA expression in HL-60 cells, *Lymphokine Res., 6*: 119–125.

Hepburn, A., Boeynaems, J. M., Fiers, W., and Dumont, J. E. (1987). Modulation of tumor necrosis factor-alpha cytotoxicity in L929 cells by bacterial toxins, hydrocortisone and inhibitors of arachidonic acid metabolism, *Biochem. Biophys. Res. Commun., 149*(2): 815–822.

Hepburn, A., Demolle, D., Boeynaems, J.-M., Fiers, W., and Dumont, J. E. (1988). Rapid phosphorylation of a 27 kDa protein induced by tumor necrosis factor, *FEBS Lett., 227*: 175–178.

Hohmann, H.-P., Remy, R., Brockhaus, M., and van Loon, A. P. G. M. (1989). Two different cell types have different major receptors for human tumor necrosis factor (TNFα), *J. Biol. Chem., 264*: 14927–14934.

Hohmann, H.-P., Remy, R., Kolbeck, R., and van Loon, A. P. G. M. (1990). Involvement of protein kinases A and C in NF-*k* B activation by TNF and IL-1, *J. Cell. Biochem., 14B*: 288.

Hori, T., Kashiyama, S., Hayakawa, M., Shibamoto, S., Tsujimoto, M., Oku, N., and Ito, F. (1989). Possible role of prostaglandins as negative regulators in growth stimulation by tumor necrosis factor and epidermal growth factor in human fibroblasts, *J. Cell. Physiol., 141*: 275–280.

Hunter, T. (1987). A thousand and one protein kinases, *Cell, 50*: 823–829.

Imamura, K., Sherman, M. L., Spriggs, D., and Kufe, D. (1988). Effect of tumor necrosis factor on GTP binding and GTPase activity in HL-60 and L929 cells, *J. Biol. Chem., 263*: 10247–10253.

Irvine, L. (1982). Effects of tumor promoters on arachidonic acid metabolism by cells in culture, (E. Heckner, N. E. Fusenig, W. Kunz, F. Marks, and H. W. Thielmann, eds.), vol. 7, *Carcinogenesis*, Raven Press, New York, pp. 477–494.

Israel, A., Le Bail, O., Hatat, D., Piette, J., Kieran, M., Logeat, F., Wallach, D., Fellous, M., and Kourilsky, P. (1989a). TNF stimulates expression of mouse MHC class I genes by inducing an NF *k* B-like enhancer binding activity which displaces constitutive factors, *EMBO J., 8*: 3793-3800.

Israel, N., Hazan, U., Alcami, J., Munier, A., Arenzana-Seisdedos, F., Bachelerie, F., Israel, A., and Virelizier, J. L. (1989b). Tumor necrosis factor stimulates transcription of HIV-1 in human T lymphocytes, independently and synergistically with mitogens, *J. Immunol., 143*: 3956–3960.

Jacobsen, H., Mestan, J., Mittnacht, S., and Dieffenbach, C. W. (1989). β- interferon subtype 1 induction by tumor necrosis factor, *Mol. Cell. Biol., 9*: 3037-3042.

Johnson, G. L., and Dhanasekaran, N. (1989). The G-protein family and their interaction with receptors, *Endoc. Rev., 10*: 317–331.

Katz, Y., and Strunk, R. C. (1989). IL-1 and tumor necrosis factor: similarities and differences in stimulation of expression of alternative pathway of complement and IFN-β 2/IL-6 genes in human fibroblasts, *J. Immunol., 142*: 3862–3867.

Kaur, P., and Saklatvala, J. (1988). Interleukin 1 and tumor necrosis factor increase phosphorylation of fiberoblast proteins, *FEBS Lett., 241*: 6–10.

Kaur, P., Welch, W. J., and Saklatvala, J. (1989). Interleukin 1 and tumor necrosis factor increase phosphorylation of the small heat shock protein: effects in fibroblasts, Hep G2 and U937 cells, *FEBS Lett., 258*: 269–273.

Kobayashi, Y., Utsunomiya, N., Nakanishi, M., and Osawa, T. (1987). Early transmembrane events in tumor necrosis factor and lymphotoxin-induced cytotoxicity, *Immunol. Lett., 15*: 53–57.

Koeffler, H. P., Gasson, J., and Tober, A. (1988). Transcriptional and posttranscriptional modulation of myeloid colony-stimulating factor expression by tumor necrosis factor and other agents, *Mol. Cell. Biol., 8*: 3432–3438.

Kohase, M., Henriksen-DeStefano, D., May, L. T., Vilček, J., and Sehgal, P. B. (1986). Induction of β 2-interferon by tumor necrosis factor: a homeostatic mechanism in the control of cell proliferation, *Cell, 45*: 659–666.

Krönke, M., Schlüter, C., and Pfizenmaier, K. (1987). Tumor necrosis factor inhibits MYC expression in HL-60 cells at the level of mRNA transcription, *Proc. Natl. Acad. Sci. USA, 84*: 469–473.

Kull, F. C., Jr. (1988). The TNF receptor in TNF-mediated cytotoxicity, *Nat. Immun. Cell Growth Regul., 7*: 254–265.

Kurt-Jones, E. A., Fiers, W., and Pober, J. S. (1987). Membrane interleukin 1 induction on human endothelial cells and dermal fibroblasts, *J. Immunol., 139*: 2317–2324.

Larsen, C. G., Zachariae, C. O., Oppenheim, J. J., and Matsushima, K. (1989). Production of monocyte chemotactic and activating factor (MCAF) by human dermal fibroblasts in response to interleukin 1 or tumor necrosis factor, *Biochem. Biophys. Res. Commun., 160*: 1403–1408.

Le, J., and Vilček, J. (1987). Biology of disease. Tumor necrosis factor and interleukin 1: cytokines with multiple overlapping biological activities, *Lab. Invest., 56*: 234.

Lee, J. C., Truneh, A., Smith, M. F., Jr., and Tsang, K. Y. (1987). Induction of interleukin 2 receptor (TAC) by tumor necrosis factor in YT cells, *J. Immunol., 139*: 1935–1938.

Lenardo, M. J., and Baltimore, D. (1989). NF-κ B: a pleiotropic mediator of inducible and tissue-specific gene control, *Cell, 58*: 227–229.

Leung, K., and Nabel, G. J. (1988). HTLV-1 transactivator interleukin-2 receptor expression through an NF-κ B-like factor, *Nature, 333*: 776.

Lin, J. X., and Vilček, J. (1987). Tumor necrosis factor and interleukin-1 cause a rapid and transient stimulation of c-fos and c-myc mRNA levels in human fibroblasts, *J. Biol. Chem., 262*: 11908-11911.

Lowenthal, J. W., Ballard, D. W., Boehnlein, E., and Greene, W. C. (1988). Tumor necrosis factor α induces proteins that bind specifically to κ B-like enhancer elements and regulate interleukin 2 receptor α-chain gene expression in primary human T lymphocytes, *Proc. Natl. Acad. Sci. USA, 86*: 2331-2335.

Mahè, Y., Piau, J.-P., Wakasugi, N., Tursz, T., Gacon, G., and Wakasugi, H. (1988). Comparison of interleukin 2 and 12-*O*-tetradecanoylphorbol 13-acetate as signals for protein kinase C activation in purified human T lymphocytes, *Eur. J. Immunol., 18*: 2029.

Makowski, M., Ballester, R., Cayre, Y., and Rosen, O. M. (1988). Immunochemical evidence that three protein kinase C isozymes increase in abundance during HL-60 differentiation induced by dimethylsulfoxide and retinoic acid, *J. Biol. Chem., 263*: 3402.

Malik, S., and Balkwil, F. R. (1988). Tumor necrosis factor, *Br. Med. J., 296*: 1214-1214.

Marino, M. W., Pfeffer, L. M., Guidon, P. T., Jr., and Donner, D. B. 91989). Tumor necrosis factor induces phosphorylation of a 28-kDa mRNA cap-binding protein in human cervical carcinoma cells, *Proc. Natl. Acad. Sci. USA, 86*: 8417-8421.

Matsushima, K., Morishita, K., Yoshimura, T., Lavu, S., Kobayashi, Y., Lew, W., Appella, E., Kung, H. F., Leonard, E. J., and Oppenheim, J. J. 91988). Molecular cloning of a human monocyte-derived neutrophil chemotactic factor (MDNCF) and the induction of MDNCF mRNA by interleukin 1 and tumor necrosis factor, *J. Exp. Med., 167*: 1883-1893.

Medcalf, R. L., Kruithof, E. K., and Scheuning, W. D. (1988). Plasminogen activator inhibitor 1 and 2 are tumor necrosis factor/cachectin-responsive genes, *J. Exp. Med., 168*: 751-759.

Meichle, A., Schütze, S., Hensel, G., Brunsing, D., and Krönke, M. (1990). Protein kinase C-independent activation of nuclear factor κ-B by tumor necrosis factor, *J. Biol. Chem. 265*: 8339-8343.

Mestan, J., Digel, W., Mittnacht, S., Hillen, H., Blohm, D., Möller, A., Jacobsen, H., and Kirchner, H. (1986). Antiviral effects of recombinant tumor necrosis factor in vitro, *Nature, 323*: 816-822.

Mestan, J., Brockhaus, M., Kirchner, H., and Jacobsen, H. (1988). Antiviral activity of tumor necrosis factor. Synergism with interferons and induction of oligo-2', 5'-adenylate synthetase, *J. Gen. Virol., 69*: 3113-3120.

Miller, S. C., Ito, H., Blau, H. M., and Torti, F. M. 91988). Tumor necrosis factor inhibits human myogenesis in vitro, *Mol. Cell Biol., 8*: 2295-2301.

Min, H. Y., and Spiegelman, B. M. 91986). Adipsin, the adipocyte serine protease: gene structure and control of expression by tumor necrosis factor, *Nucleic Acids Res., 14*: 8879-8892.

Murakami, K., and Routtenberg, A. (1985). Direct activation of purified protein kinase C by unsaturated fatty acids (oleate and arachidonate) in the absence of phospholipids and Ca^{2+}, *FEBS Lett., 192*: 189-193.

Nakagawa, H., Kitagawa, H., and Aikawa, Y. (1987). Tumor necrosis factor stimulates gelatinase and collagenase production by granulation tissue in culture, *Biochem. Biophys. Res. Commun., 142*: 791-797.

Nakashima, S., Nagata, K.-I., Ueeda, K., and Nozawa, Y. (1988). Stimulation of arachidonic acid release by guanine nucleotide in saponin-permeabilized neutrophils: evidence for involvement of GTP-binding protein in phospholipase A_2 activation, *Arch. Biochem. Biophys., 261*: 375-383.

Neale, M. L., Fiera, R. A., and Matthews, N. (1988). Involvement of phospholipase A2 activation in tumor cell killing by tumor necrosis factor, *Immunology, 64*: 81-85.

Neer, E. J., and Clapham, D. E. (1988). Roles of G protein subunits in transmembrane signaling, *Nature, 333*: 129-134.

Ng, K. W., Hudson, P. J., Power, B. E., Manji, S. S., Gummer, P. R., and Martin, T. J. (1989). Retinoic acid and tumor necrosis factor-alpha act in concert to control the level of alkaline phosphatase mRNA, *J. Mol. Endocrinol., 3*: 57-64.

Okamoto, T., Matsuyama, T., Mori, S., Hamamoto, Y., Kobayashi, N., Yamamoto, N., Jospehs, S. F., Wong-Staal, F., and Shimotohno, K. (1989). Augmentation of human immunodeficiency virus type 1 gene expression by tumor necrosis factor alpha, *AIDS Res. Human Retroviruses, 5*: 131-138.

Old, L. J. (1985). Tumor necrosis factor (TNF), *Science, 230*: 630-632.

Old, L. J. (1987). Tumor necrosis factor: polypeptide mediator network, *Nature, 326*: 330-331.

Osburn, L., Kunkel, S., and Nabel, G. J. (1989). Tumor necrosis factor alpha and interleukin 1 stimulate the human immunodeficiency virus enhancer by activation of the nuclear factor kappa B, *Proc. Natl. Acad. Sci. USA, 86*: 2336-2340.

Oster, W., Lindemann, A., Horn, S., Mertelsmann, R., and Herrmann, F. (1987). Tumor necrosis factor (TNF)-α but not TNF-β induces secretion of colony stimulating factor for macrophages (CSF-1) by human monocytes, *Blood, 70*: 1700-1703.

Oster, W., Lindemann, A., Riedel, D., Cicco, N. A., Mertelsmann, R., and Herrmann, F. (1988). Monokines: stimulatory and inhibitory regulator molecules of myelopoiesis in vitro, *J. Biol. Regul. Homeostatic Agents, 2*: 134-138.

Ostrowski, J., Meier, K. E., Stanton, T. H., Smith, L. L., and Bomsztyk, K. (1988). Interferon-gamma and interleukin-1α induce transient translocation of protein kinase C activity to membranes in a B lymphoid cell line, *J. Biol. Chem., 263*: 13786.

Palombella, V. J., and Vilček, J. (1989). Mitogenic and cytotoxic actions of tumor necrosis factor in BALB/c 3T3 cells: role of phospholipase activation, *J. Biol. Chem., 264*: 18128-18136.

Pape, M. E., and Kim, K. H. (1988). Effect of tumor necrosis factor on acetyl-coenzyme A carboxylase gene expression and preadipocyte differentiation, *Mol. Endocrinol., 2*: 395-403.

Pape, M. E., and Kim, K. H. (1989). Transcriptional regulation of acetyl coenzyme A carboxylase gene expression by tumor necrosis factor in 30A-5 preadipocytes, *Mol. Cell. Biol., 9*: 974-982.

Perlmutter, D. H., Dinarello, C. A., Punsal, P. I., and Colten, H. R. (1986). Cachectin/tumor necrosis factor regulates hepatic actue-phase gene expression, *J. Clin. Invest., 78*: 1349-1354.

Pfeilschifter, J., Pignat, W., Vosbeck, K., and Märki, F. (1989). Interleukin 1 and tumor necrosis factor synergistically stimulate prostaglandin synthesis and phospholipase A2 release from rat renal mesangial cells, *Biochem. Biophys. Res. Commun., 159*: 385-394.

Pfizenmaier, K., Scheurich, P., Schlüter, C., and Krönke, M. (1987). Tumor necrosis factor enhances HLA-A,B,C and HLA-DR gene expression in human tumor cells, *J. Immunol., 138*: 975-980.

Plaetinck, G., Combe, M. C., Corthesy, P., Seckinger, P., and Nabholz, M. (1989). Interleukin 1 and tumor necrosis factor enhance transcription from the SV40 early promoter in a T cell line, *Eur. J. Immunol., 19*: 897-904.

Pober, J. S. (1987). Effects of tumor necrosis factor and related cytokines on vascular endothelial cells, *Ciba Found. Symp., 131*: 170-184.

Premecz, G., Markovits, A., Bagi, G., Farkas, T., and Födes, I. (1989). Phospholipase C and phospholipase A_2 are involved in the antiviral activity of human interferon-α, *FEBS Lett., 249*: 257-260.

Regazzi, R., Eppenberger, U., and Fabbro, D. (1988). The 27,000 Daltons stress proteins are phosphorylated by protein kinase C during the tumor promoter-mediated growth inhibition of human mammary carcinoma cells, *Biochem. Biophys. Res. Commun., 152*: 62-68.

Reis, L. F., Ho Lee, T., and Vilček, J. (1989). Tumor necrosis factor acts synergistically with autocrine interferon-beta and increases interferon-beta mRNA levels in human fibroblasts, *J. Biol. Chem., 264*: 16351-16354.

Robaye, B., Hepburn, A., Lecocq, R., Fiers, W., Boeynaems, J.-M., and Dumont, J. E. (1989). Tumor necrosis factor-alpha induces the phosphorylation of 28 kDa stress proteins in endothelial cells: possible role in protection against cytotoxicity? *Biochem. Biophys. Res. Commun., 163*: 301-308.

Sawamura, S., Ase, K., Berry, N., Kikkawa, U., McCaffrey, P. G., Minowada, J., and Nishizuka, Y. (1989). Expression of protein kinase C subspecies in human leukemia-lymphoma cell lines, *FEBS Lett., 247*: 353.

Sawdey, M., Podor, T. J., and Loskutoff, D. J. (1989). Regulation of type 1 plasminogen activator inhibitor gene expression in cultured bovine aortic endothelial cells: induction by transforming growth factor-beta, *J. Biol. Chem., 264*: 10396-10401.

Scarpati, E. M., and Sadler, J. E. (1989). Regulation of endothelial cell coagulant properties: modulation of tissue factor, plasminogen activator inhibitors, and thrombomodulin by phorbol 12-myristate 13-acetate and tumor necrosis factor, *J. Biol. Chem., 264*: 20705-20713.

Schachner, J., Blick, M., Freireich, E., Gutterman, J., and Beran, M. 91988). Suppression of c-myc and c-myb expression in myeloid cell lines treated with recombinant tumor necrosis factor-alpha, *Leukemia, 2*: 749-753.

Scharffetter, K., Heckmann, M., Hatamochi, A., Mauch, C., Stein, B., Riehtmüller, G., Ziegler-Heitbrock, H. W., and Krieg, T. (1989). Synergistic effect of tumor necrosis factor-alpha and interferon-gamma collagen synthesis of human skin fibroblasts in vitro, *Exp. Cell Res., 181*: 409-419.

Scheurich, P., Krönke, M., Schlüter, C., Ûcer, U., and Pfizenmaier, K. (1986). Noncytocidal mechanisms of action of tumor necrosis factor-alpha on human tumor cells: enhancement of HLA gene expression synergistic with interferon-gamma, *Immunobiology, 172*: 291-300.

Scholz, W., and Altman, A. (1989). Synergistic induction of interleukin 2 receptor (TAC) expression on YT cells by interleukin 1 or tumor necrosis factor α in combination with cAMP inducing agents, *Cell. Signal., 1*: 367-375.

Schütze, S., Scheurich, P., Schlüter, C., Ûcer, U., Pfizenmaier, K., and Krönke, M. (1988a). Tumor necrosis factor-induced changes of gene expression in U937 cells: differentiation-dependent plasticity of the responsive state, *J. Immunol., 140*: 3000-3005.

Schütze, S., Nottrott, S., Scheurich, P., Krönke, M., and Pfizenmaier, K. (1988b). Mechanisms of TNF resistance: identification of membrane phosphoproteins associated with a dominant resistant phenotype in lymphoid-myeloid somatic cell hybrids, *Mol. Biother.*, *1*: 96–102.

Schütze, S., Scheurich, P., Pfizenmaier, K., and Krönke, M. (1989). Tumor necrosis factor signal transduction: tissue-specific serine phosphorylation of a 26-kDa cytosolic protein, *J. Biol. Chem.*, *264*: 3562–3567.

Schütze, S., Nottrott, S., Pfizenmaier, K., and Krönke, M. (1990). Tumor necrosis factor signal transduction: cell-type-specific activation and translocation of protein kinase C, *J. Immunol.*, *144* : 2604–2608.

Sen, R., and Baltimore, D. (1986a). Multiple nuclear factors interact with the immunoglobulin enhancer sequence, *Cell*, *46*: 705.

Sen, R., and Baltimore, D. (1986b). Inducibility of kappa immunoglobulin enhancer-binding protein NF kappa B by a posttranslational mechanism, *Cell*, *47*: 921–928.

Shannon, M. F., Occhiodoro, F. S., Kuczek, E. S., Pell, L. M., and Vadas, M. A. 91990). Identification of a novel transcription factor involved in TNF and IL-1 induction of G-CSF gene expression, *J. Cell. Biochem. (Suppl.)*, *14B*: 217.

Shirakawa, F., and Mizel, S. B. (1989). In vitro activation and nuclear translocation of NF kappa B catalyzed by cyclic AMP-dependent protein kinase and protein kinase C, *Mol. Cell. Biol.*, *9*: 2424–2430.

Silk, S. T., Clejan, S., and Witkom, K. (1989). Evidence of GTP-binding protein regulation of phospholipase A_2 activity in isolated human platelet membranes, *J. Biol. Chem.*, *264*: 21466–21469.

Silver, B. J., Jaffer, F. E., and Abboud, H. E. (1989). Platelet-derived growth factor synthesis in mesangial cells: induction by multiple peptide mitogens, *Proc. Natl. Acad. Sci USA*, *86*: 1056–1060.

Smith, M. R., Munger, W. E., Kung, H.-F., Takacs, L., and Durum, S. K. (1990). Direct evidence for an intracellular role for tumor necrosis factor-α: microinjection of tumor necrosis factor kills target cells, *J. Immunol.*, *144*: 162–169.

Solis-Herruzo, J. A., Brenner, D. A., and Chojkier, M. (1988). Tumor necrosis factor alpha inhibits collagen gene transcription and collagen synthesis in cultured human fibroblasts, *J. Biol. Chem.*, *263*: 5841–5845.

Sonenberg, N. (1988). Cap-binding proteins of eukaryotic messenger RNA: functions in initiation and control of translation, *Prog. Nucleic Acid Res. Mol. Biol.*, *35*: 173–207.

Spriggs, D., Imamura, K., Rodriguez, C., Horiguchi, J., and Kufe, D. W. (1987). Induction of tumor necrosis factor expression and resistance in a human breast tumor cell line, *Proc. Natl. Acad. Sci. USA*, *84*: 6563–6566.

Strieter, R. M., Phan, S. H., Showell, H. J., Remick, D. G., Lynch, J. P., Genord, M., Raiford, C., Eskandari, M., Marks, R. M., and Kunkel, S. L. (1989a). Monokine-induced neutrophil chemotactic factor gene expression in human fibroblasts, *J. Biol. Chem.*, *264*: 10621–10626.

Strieter, R. M., Wiggins, R., Phan, S. H., Wharram, B. L., Showell, H. J., Remick, D. G., Chensue, S. W., and Kunkel, S. L. (1989b). Monocyte chemotactic protein gene expression by cytokine-treated human fibroblasts and endothelial cells, *Biochem. Biophys. Res. Commun.*, *162*: 694–700.

Suffys, P., Van Roy, F., and Fiers, W. (1988). Tumor necrosis factor and interleukin 1 activate phospholipase in rat chondrocytes, *FEBS Lett., 232*: 24–28.

Sugarman, B. J., Aggarwal, B. B., Hass, P. E., Figari, I. S., Palladino, M. A., and Shepard, H. M. (1985). Recombinant human tumor necrosis factor-alpha: effects on proliferation of normal and transformed cells in vitro, *Science, 230*: 943–945.

Thoma, B., Grell. M., Pfizenmaier, U., and Scheinovich, P. (1990) Identification of a 60-KD tumor necrosis factor (TNF) receptor as the major signal transducing component in TNF responses. *J. Exp. Med., 172*: 1019–1023.

Tobler, A., Johnston, D., and Koeffler, H. P. (1987). Recombinant human tumor necrosis factor α regulates c-myc expression in HL-60 cells at the level of transcription, *Blood, 70*: 200–205.

Torti, F. M., Dieckmann, B., Beutler, B., Cerami, A., and Ringold, G. M. (1985). A macrophage factor inhibits adipocyte gene expression: an in vitro model of cachexia, *Science, 229*: 867–869.

Torti, S. V., Kwak, E. L., Miller, S. C., Miller, L. L., Ringold, G. M., Myambo, K. B., Yound, A. P., and Torti, F. M. (1988). The molecular cloning and characterization of murine ferritin heavy chain, a tumor necrosis factor-inducible gene, *J. Biol. Chem., 263*: 12638–12644.

Tracey, K. J., Beutler, B., Lowry, S. F., Merryweather, J., Wolpe, S., et al. (1986). Shock and tissue injury induced by recombinant human cachectin, *Science, 234*: 470–474.

Tsujimoto, M., Yip, K., and Vilček, J. (1985). Tumor necrosis factor: specific binding and internalization in sensitive and resistant cells, *Proc. Natl. Acad. Sci. USA, 82*: 7626–7630.

Tsujimoto, M., Feinman, R., Kohase, M., and Vilček, J. (1986). Characterization and affinity crosslinking of receptors for tumor necrosis factor on human cells, *Arch. Biochem. Biophys., 249*: 563–568.

Turner, M., Chantry, D., Buchan, G., Barrett, K., and Feldmann, M. (1989). Regulation of expression of human IL-1 alpha and IL-1 beta genes, *J. Immunol., 143*: 3556–3561.

Van Hinsbergh, V. W., Kooistra, T., van den Berg, E. A., Princen, H. M., Fiers, W., and Emeis J. J. (1988). Tumor necrosis factor increases the production of plasminogen activator inhibitor in human endothelial cells in vitro and in rats in vivo, *Blood, 72*: 1467–1473.

Vilček, J., Palombella, V. J., Henriksen-DeStefano, D., Swenson, C., Feinman, R., Hirai, M., and Tsujimoto, M. (1986). Fibroblast growth enhancing activity of tumor necrosis factor and its relationship to other polypeptide growth factors, *J. Exp. Med., 163*: 632–643.

Visvanathan, K. V., and Goodbourn, S. (1989). Double-stranded RNA activates binding of NF-κ B to an inducible element in the human β-interferon promotor, *EMBO J., 8*: 1120–1128.

Watanabe, N., Neda, H., Ohtusuka, Y., Sone, H., Yamauchi, N., Maeda, M., Kuriyama, H., and Niitsu, Y. 91989). Signalling pathway of tumor necrosis factor in normal and tumor cells, *Cancer Immunol. Immunother., 28*: 157–163.

Welch, W. J. (1985). Phorbol ester, calcium ionophore, or serum added to quiescent rat embryo fibroblast cells a1 result in the elevated phosphorylation of two 28,000 dalton mammalian stress proteins, *J. Biol. Chem., 260*: 3058–3062.

Wen, D. Z., Rowland, A., and Derynck, R. (1989). Expression and secretion of gro/MGSA by stimulated human endothelial cells, *EMBO J., 8*: 1761–1766.

Wong, G. H., and Goeddel, D. V. (1986). Tumor necrosis factor α and β inhibit virus replication and synergize with interferons, *nature, 323*: 819–822.

Wong, G. H., and Goeddel, D. V. (1988). Induction of manganous superoxide dismutase by tumor necrosis factor: possible protective mechanism, *Science, 242*: 941–944.

Woo, P., Sipe, J., Dinarello, C. A., and Colten, H. R. (1987). Structure of a human serum amyloid A gene and modulation of its expression in transfected L cells, *J. Biol. Chem., 262*: 15790–15795.

Yamato, K., el-Hajjaoui, Z., and Koeffler, H. P. (1989a). Regulation of levels of IL-1 mRNA in human fibroblasts, *J. Cell. Physiol., 139*: 610–616.

Yamato, K., El-Hajjaoui, Z., Kuo, J. F., and Koeffler, H. P. (1989b). Granulocyte-macrophage colony-stimulating factor: signals for its mRNA accumulation, *Blood, 74*: 1314–1320.

Yarden, A., and Kimchi, A. (1986). Tumor necrosis factor reduces c-myc expression and cooperates with interferon-gamma in HeLa cells, *Science, 234*: 1419–1421.

Yoshie, O., Tada, K., and Ishida, N. (1986). Binding and crosslinking of ^{125}I-labeled recombinant human tumor necrosis factor to cell surface receptors, *J. Biochem., 100*: 531–541.

Zechner, R., Newman, T. C., Sherry, B., Cerami, A., and Brewslow, J. L. (1988). Recombinant human cachectin/tumor necrosis factor but not interleukin-1 α downregulates lipoprotein lipase gene expression at the transcriptional level in mouse 3T3-L1 adipocytes, *Mol. Cell. Biol., 8*: 2394–2401.

Zhang, Y., Lin, J. X., Yip, Y. K., and Vilček, J. (1988a). Enhancement of cAMP levels and of protein kinase activity by tumor necrosis factor and interleukin 1 in human fibroblasts: role in the induction of interleukin 6, *Proc. Natl. Acad. Sci. USA, 85*: 6802–6805.

Zhang, U., Lin, J.-X., and Vilček, J. (1988b). Synthesis of interleukin 6 (interferon-β2/B cell stimulatory factor 2) in human fibroblasts is triggered by an increase in intracellular cyclic AMP, *J. Biol. Chem., 263*: 6177–6182.

Zilberstein, A., Ruggieri, R., Korn, J. H., and Revel, M. (1986). Structure and expression of cDNA and genes for human interferon-beta-2, a distinct species inducible by growth-stimulatory cytokines, *EMBO J., 5*: 2529–2537.

10

Natural Inhibitors of TNF

PHILIPPE SECKINGER and JEAN-MICHEL DAYER
University Hospital, Geneva, Switzerland

I. INTRODUCTION

Tumor necrosis factor α (TNF-α) was originally described as a monocyte product with antitumoral activity both in vitro and in vivo, but is now known to have multiple biological activities (Carswell et al., 1975; Old, 1985; Beutler and Cerami, 1986, 1988). It has cytotoxic and cytostatic effects on certain tumor cell lines, whereas normal cells are spared despite the presence of TNF-α receptors on their surface. Indeed, both sensitive and resistant cells express similar numbers of receptors with a comparable affinity for TNF-α (Sugarman et al., 1985; Kull et al., 1985; Tsujimoto et al., 1985). The mechanism of action underlying this phenomenon has still to be elucidated. Several processes seem to be involved in cytotoxicity, of which DNA fragmentation (Schmid et al., 1987; Rubin et al., 1986), alternation of arachidonic acid metabolism (Satomi et al., 1988; Matthews et al., 1987; Suffys et al., 1988), oxidative damage (Yamauchi et al., 1989), dissolution of microfilaments (Scanlon et al., 1989), and ADP ribosylation (Aggarwal et al., 1988). Moreover, it has been suggested that the cytotoxic activity of TNF-α is mediated by cell surface Fas antigen, associated with the TNF-α receptor, whereas resistance of the cells is linked to the absence of Fas antigen on the cell surface (Yonehara et al., 1989). Various experiments hint at the existence of mechanisms that confer resistance to TNF-α. Thus TNF-α-resistant cells become sensitive to the cytotoxic effect of TNF when protein synthesis inhibitor is added to the culture medium (Aderka et al., 1986; Wallach, 1986). Fusion of dominant and resistant cells results in resistant heterokaryons (Nophar et al., 1988). These observations suggest that differences in sensitivity to TNF-α cytotoxicity are due to the presence of protective proteins that are constitutively expressed in resistant cells.

TNF-α plays a key role in inflammation by stimulating prostaglandin E_2 (PGE_2) and collagenase production (Dayer et al., 1985), as well as in tissue remodeling (Vlassara et al., 1988; Brenner et al., 1989). It mediates septic shock and cachexia (Oliff et al., 1987), and nude mice inoculated with TNF-α-secreting tumor cells became progressively anaerobic and wasted. In the rat, acute toxic effects of TNF-α have been demonstrated (Tracey et al., 1986) and it was shown to cause hypotension, metabolic acidosis, transitory hyperglycemia followed by hypoglycemia, hemorrhagic infarction, pancreatic hemorrhage, acute renal tubular necrosis, and severe interstitital pneumonitis occasionally leading to respiratory arrest. These observations prove that TNF-α is sufficient to mediate endotoxic effects. Some of these phenomena, including the lethal effects of TNF-α, are tempered by the administration of cyclooxygenase inhibitors (Kettelhut et al., 1987). Thus ibuprofen blocks TNF-α-induced fever by impeding hypothalamic PGE_2 synthesis (Dinarello et al., 1986).

Nevertheless, TNF-α also has beneficial effects which might prevail over the detrimental effects. Thus it enhances HLA-A, B, C and HLA-DR gene expression in various tumor cell lines (Pfizenmaier et al., 1987). These restriction elements function as recognition structure for antigen-specific cytotoxic T lymphocytes and for the initiation of the immune response (Townsend et al., 1986; Benacerraf, 1981). In vitro, TNF-α induces neutrophils to eliminate *Candida albicans* organisms (Djeu et al., 1986); it acts synergistically with autocrine interferon-β to inhibit virus replication and increases interferon-β mRNA levels (Reis et al., 1989).

TNF-α acts as growth factor for both normal (Sugarman et al., 1985; Vilček et al., 1986) and transformed cells (Lachmann et al., 1987). As to cytotoxicity, little is known of TNF-α-mediated mitogenicity, except that it increases the number of epidermal growth factor (EGF) receptors on human fibroblasts. This observation might be correlated to the mitogenic activity of TNF-α, as EGF is a growth factor for fibroblasts (Palombella et al., 1987), and TNF-α also increases the expression of some "competence" genes, such as c-myc and c-fos, depending on target cells (Zullo et al., 1985). Since TNF-α is a growth factor, a cytotoxic and cytostatic protein associated with pathogenic disease (Grau et al., 1987; Piguet et al., 1990), it was of importance to study mechanisms whereby TNF-α could be blocked at either its level of production or that of its biological activities.

II. INHIBITION OF TNF

A. Inhibition at the Level of Induction, Synthesis, and Release

1. *Prostaglandins*

Human TNF-α is a polypeptide of 17 kDa that is secreted primarily by activated monocytes. It is first synthesized with a 76-amino-acid signal peptide into the endoplasmic reticulum, and cleavage of the signal peptide leads to elongation of a 17-kDa peptide (Pennica et al., 1984; Wang et al., 1985; Shirai et al., 1985). The protein is then secreted via normal secretory pathways. In the monocyte the signal peptide allows membrane insertion, so that TNF-α becomes also a cell surface surface cytotoxic transmembrane protein (Kriegler et al., 1988). Many processes regulate TNF-α from its induction to its release in the extracellular medium.

LPS on monocytes is a potent inducer of TNF-α, which prompts the production of PGE_2, which in turn, regulates cytokines. Thus Kunkel et al. (1988) demonstrate that exogenous PGE_2 dose-dependently suppresses LPS-induced TNF mRNA accumulation. Both Northern and in situ hybridization analyses showed a dramatic reduction in TNF-α mRNA at 100 n*M* PGE_2. Both transcriptional and posttranscriptional regulation of TNF-α mRNA by PGE_2 occurs. The capacity of PGE_2 of regulating mRNA is not restricted to TNF-α, interleukin-1 (IL-1) production also being regulated by PGE_2 (Kunkel et al., 1986), but IL-1 mRNA accumulation is not modified by high concentrations of PGE_2 (Knudsen et al., 1986) since IL-1 is regulated posttranscriptionally only at the level of production.

The hydrolysis of membrane phospholipids by phospholipase A_2 to form arachidonic acid is the rate-limiting step in prostaglandin and leukotriene synthesis (Williams and Higgs, 1988), and phospholipase is inhibited by lipocortin (Hirata et al., 1980). These arachidonic metabolites also act as second messengers in regulating TPA-induced expression of the TNF-α gene (Horiguchi et al., 1989) in the human promyelocytic leukemia cell line HL-60. Thus TPA induces TNF-α expression through the 5-lipoxygenase pathway, an effect that is inhibited by PGE_2. Inhibition of phospholipase A_2—in HL-60 or U937—by nontoxic doses of bromophenacyl bromide or quinacrine blocks the release of arachidonic acid and induction of TNF-α transcripts. These results demonstrate that arachidonic acid metabolites regulate TNF-α gene transcription by TPA. TNF-α induces the cyclooxygenase pathway, and the resulting PGE_2 down-regulates TNF-α mRNA so that the activation of the lipoxygenase pathway does not result in an overexpression of TNF-α mRNA. But PGE_2 can exert an even more sensitive regulation since at low concentrations (0.1 to 10 ng/mL) it induces TNF-α production by resident peritoneal macrophages (Renz et al., 1988). Higher concentrations of PGE_2 suppress TNF-α release, a finding that correlates with the negative-feedback inhibition reported previously (Taffet and Russell, 1980; Taffet et al., 1981; Schultz et al., 1978; Lehmann et al., 1988). The cAMP is a prime candidate in signal transduction resulting in PGE_2-induced suppression. Thus agents causing an increase in cellular cAMP, including theophyllin, isobutylmethylxanthin, dibutyryl cAMP, or cholera toxin may reduce TNF-α expression by stimulated cells. This phenomenon can be considered part of an antiregulatory pathway that controls TNF-α mRNA transcriptionally and posttranscriptionally. In contrast, induction of TNF-α mRNA by low concentrations of PGE_2 involves cGMP. The balance between cAMP and cGMP may therefore be an additional factor regulating TNF-α gene expression.

2. *Glucocorticoids*

Recent data have clearly established that the immune and neuroendocrine systems are connected, and as soon as probes for TNF-α became available, it was shown that glucocorticoids are capable of regulating TNF-α mRNA expression. Thus dexamethasone markedly suppresses the endotoxin-induced increase of TNF-α mRNA at both transcriptional and posttranscriptional levels (Beutler et al., 1986). Further studies investigating the effects of steroids on the in vitro production of TNF-α by LPS-stimulated human monocytes revealed that only the glucocorticoids, not the sex steroids or the mineral corticoids, significantly reduce TNF production (Waage and Bakke, 1988). Hydrocortisone suppresses the production of IL-1 and TNF by LPS-stimulated macrophages (Oppenheim et al., 1986; Snyder and Unanue, 1982). Of course, the present findings have in vivo implications. Having supplied evidence that TNF is the primary mediator of endotoxin-induced tumor hemorrhagic necrosis (North and Havell, 1988) the investigators demonstrated that glucocorticoids inhibit antitumoral action of endotoxin by inhibiting its ability to induce TNF production (North and Havell, 1989); this observation is also important in view of the anti-inflammatory properties of glucocorticoids.

3. *Proteases*

The primary translation product of TNF-α, synthesized by macrophages or monocytes, is a 26-kDa precursor peptide (Pennica et al., 1984; Wang et al., 1985; Shirai et al., 1985) that is converted into a low-molecular-weight form (17.5 kDa). In addition, membrane-associated TNF-α activity has been found in both monocytes (Kriegler et al., 1988) and in RAW 264.7 cells (Cseh and Beutler, 1989). The cleavage of murine propeptide occurs in RAW 264.7 cells within the propeptide fragment, 10 residues before the amino terminal leucine of the mature protein. Although secreted as a soluble product, it is biologically inactive in the L929 cell cytotoxicity assay. Inhibition of the protease that cleaves the propeptide into the fully active form could represent a potential mechanism whereby TNF-α is regulated after its synthesis.

B. Inhibition of TNF at the Level of the Target Cells

1. *Regulation of Postreceptor Events*

TNF-α mediates its cellular responses by binding to high-affinity cell surface receptors recently characterized (Aggarwal et al., 1985; Stauber et al., 1988). The second signal resulting from TNF receptor binding remains at present unclear so that no definite answer exists as to how TNF regulates gene expression after binding to its receptor. Reversible phosphorylation of intracellular proteins controlled by various protein kinases is one of the possibilities that can be linked to TNF-α transduction. Dephosphorylation of those proteins by activating specific phosphatases might be a mechanism whereby the cell resists TNF. Schütze et al. (1989) reported a TNF-α dose-dependent phosphorylation of a cytosolic protein protein with an apparent molecular mass of 26,000 Da in the promonocytic leukemia cell line U937. However, this protein seems to be associated with differentiation rather than cytotoxicity or growth control. The authors suggest that protein kinase C (PKC) or other Ca^{2+} -dependent kinases are involved in TNF-α-induced phosphorylation. Sehgal et al. (1978) and Hensel et al. (1987) reported the participation of PKC in signal transduction that can be blocked by inhibitors of PKC. The TNF transduction mechanism can also be linked by receptor coupling to GTP-binding proteins, leading to an increase or decrease of cytoplasmic cAMP through the modulation of the adenylate cyclase activity. cAMP activates the cAMP-dependent protein kinase (Aderka et al., 1989). Recently, cAMP was reported to be increased in the mesangial cell culture medium, giving credit to a TNF receptor coupled to a G-protein. Indomethacin suppresses the effect of TNF-α on prostaglandin but only reduces it on cAMP, indicating that prostaglandin production is only partially mediated by the increase in cAMP (Baud et al., 1988). A pivotal role of a pertussis-toxin-sensitive G-protein in at least some biological responses to TNF has been confirmed. Imamura et al. (Imamura et al., 1988) report that GTPγs enhances the binding of TNF to HL-60 cell membrane by increasing the affinity of the available sites. They demonstrated that TNF stimulates both high-affinity GTP binding and GTPase activity, detectable within 3 min of treatment. Moreover, ADP-ribosylation that always involves a G-protein is a necessary event in TNF-induced cytotoxicity (Aggarwal et al., 1988); this phenomenon is also pertussis-toxin sensitive. However, in contrast to the above-mentioned increase in cAMP, TNF-α had no significant effect on the basal production of cAMP on both HL-60 and L929 cell lines. These findings suggest that TNF-induced cytotoxicity is sensitive to pertussis toxin and that the TNF receptor interacts with a G-protein whose nature has to be determined. Brett et al. (1989) confirmed that a G-protein mediates TNF-α increase in the permeability of endothelial cell monolayers to macromolecules and lower-molecular-weight solutes as this biological activity is pertussis-toxin- sensitive. It appears that the TNF receptor is coupled to a G-protein that is associated with various effector proteins (e.g., adenylyl cyclase or phospholipase C). The existence of a second messenger would rather point to tissue specificity, as there is no general consensus about it. This is somewhat similar to IL-1, where different second messengers were identified, depending on the target cell. Obviously, blocking the transduction mechanism(s) would impair the mechanism of action of TNF-α but would not be specific for TNF-α itself, since it probably shares one of these mechanisms with other hormones and cytokines whose activities would consequently be affected as well.

2. *Inhibitors of Cyclooxygenase and Phospholipase A2 as Inhibitors of TNF-α-Induced Cytotoxicity*

In agreement with the previous study demonstrating the involvement of G-protein in TNF-α-induced cytotoxicity, Hepburn et al. (1987) demonstrated that the release of phospholipase A2 metabolites is also essential for cytotoxicity. Phospholipase A2 is activated through a GTP-binding protein (Burch et al., 1986). Neither blocking of cyclooxygenase nor lipoxygenase pathways had a significant effect on TNF action (Suffys et al., 1988). In contrast, inhibitors of arachidonate metabolism with a very wide range of activities, such as nordihydroguaiaretic acid and hydrocortisone, significantly inhibited TNF-α-induced cytotoxicity (Hepburn et al., 1987). Inhibitors of fatty acid metabolism in L929 caused the inhibition of TNF-induced cytotoxicity to be suppressed (Matthews et al., 1987). Taken together, these results suggest that blocking phospholipase A2 might be essential for regulating TNF cytotoxicity. The fact that various metabolite inhibitors remain rather uneffective suggests that arachidonic acid participation in cytotoxicity may rather involve a pathway other than the cyclooxygenase or lipoxygenase pathway. The lack of protective effect of dexamethasone or indomethacin observed previously (Hepburn et al., 19877) may be due to the presence of cycloheximide or actinomycin D. These agents block de novo protein synthesis, necessary for the cell to be protected from TNF-α activity. Reid et al. (1989) demonstrated the existence of two distinct mechanisms whereby TNF-α kills cells: one depending on the presence of cycloheximide, effective within 2 h, and one independent of cycloheximide, effective after 3 days. In this system, both dexamethasone and indomethacin block TNF-α-induced cytotoxicity. Taken together, these data demonstrate the key role of phospholipase A2 in cytotoxicity.

3. *Inhibitors of Proteases, Lysosomal Enzymes, and O2 Production*

Changes in the cytoskeleton are associated with cell death. The apparent dissolution of stress fibers has been studied in C3HA cells treated with TNF-α and cycloheximide and proposed as a common mechanism of TNF-mediated cytolysis (Scanlon et al., 1989). Experiments using agents that disrupt microfilaments and microtubules have shown that cell internalization and transport into lysosomes are prerequisites for the cytocidal action of TNF-α (Niitsu et al., 1985). The cytocidal action of TNF-α has been shown to involve lysomal enzymes since lysomotropic agents such as leupeptin, methylamine, ammonium chloride, and chloroquine were found to inhibit the cytotoxicity of TNF-α on L-M cells (Watanabe et al., 1988a). While decreasing sensitivity to TNF-α, chloroquine increases the number of TNF receptors on the cell surface (Watanabe et al., 1988b). Transport of [^{125}I]TNF into lysosomes after endocytosis also suggests that activation of lysosomal enzymes may play an important role in the cytocidal effect of TNF. Therefore, inhibition of lysosomal enzymes might be instrumental for the inhibition of cytotoxicity.

To elucidate the mechanism whereby TNF-α damages the cells, Watanabe et al. (1988a) demonstrated that hydroxyl-radical scavengers and inhibitors decreased cytotoxicity of TNF-α on L-M cells. Matthews et al. (1987) showed that anaerobic conditions protect the cells from cytolysis. Peroxidation of lipids is probably involved in the damage by free radicals, and TNF-α stimulates superoxide production by neutrophils (Tsujimoto et al., 1986) and hydroxyl peroxide by macrophages (Hoffman and Weinberg, 1987). It is therefore clear that hydroxyl-radical scavengers, ion chelators, and inhibitors of hydroxyl-radical production impair TNF-α cytotoxicity. It is also documented that TNF cytotoxicity can be inhibited by the addition of mitochondrial inhibitors, such as sodium azide, since the mitochondrial electron-transport chain is known to generate the hydroxyl radical. On the other hand, the arachidonic acid cascade is another pathway for the production of free radicals, demonstrating once more the pivotal role of phospholipase A_2 in TNF-α-induced cytotoxicity. Various mechanisms exist whereby cells can resist the cytotoxic action of TNF-α. Thus heat-shock proteins protect WEHI-164 cells from cytolysis (Jäätelä et al., 1989). Although the precise nature of the protective mechanism remains at present unknown, the induction of manganous superoxide dismutase definitely plays a significant role. We mentioned above that hydroxyl peroxide and oxygen-free radicals are involved in the cytotoxicity of TNF-α . Therefore, enzymes such as catalase, glutathione peroxidase, or superoxide dismutase may be essential for resistance to TNF-α. Recently, Wong and Goeddel (1988) demonstrated that TNF-α and TNF-β induce manganous superoxide dismutase mRNA by increasing transcription of the gene. Later, the authors demonstrated that this protein is involved in the protection against TNF-α (Wong et al., 1989), and overexpression of manganous superoxide dismutase confers increased resistance to TNF-α in the presence of cycloheximide on a human embryonic kidney cell line. Moreover, transfection of an antisense of the enzyme confers increased sensitivity to TNF-α, even in the absence of cycloheximide. However, this phenomenon does not account for a 100% protection to TNF-α cytotoxicity, suggesting that either other enzymes are involved or that free-radical and superoxide production is not the only mechanism by which TNF kills the cells; this would be consistent with other mechanisms of action of TNF-α described previously (Schmid et al., 1987; Rubin et al., 1986; Satomi et al., 1988; Matthews et al., 1987; Suffys et al., 1988; Scanlon et al., 1989; Aggarwal et al., 1988).

C. Viral Inhibitor of TNF-α

TNF-α exerts its antiviral activity by inducing IFN-β mRNA, which in turn synergizes with TNF-α in antiviral activity. Recently, Gooding et al. (Gooding et al., 1988) reported that adenovirus infection induces cellular susceptibility to the lytic effect of TNFα but that a product of this virus prevents lysis. A protein with a molecular weight of 14.7 kDa is involved in the resistance to TNF-α since infection with mutant viruses that do not produce it resulted in the lysis of infected cells. Whether this represents a general mechanism whereby infected cells resist TNF-α will have to be elucidated. However, virus-infected cells have been reported to produce an inhibitor of IL-1, another cytokine essential to host defense (Roberts et. al., 1986).

III. INHIBITION BY DOWN-REGULATION OF THE TNF RECEPTOR

It is a common phenomenon that various hormones or cytokines, including IFN (Branca et al., 1982), epidermal growth factor (EGF), and insulin (Schlessinger et al., 1978), down-regulate their own receptors. Holtmann et al. (Holtmann and Wallach, 1987) reported that the TNF-α receptor is down-regulated by IL-1 on SV80 cells within 2 min. PMA had a similar effect on the number of binding sites while having little effect on their affinity. Those phenomena are tissue-dependent: They were observed on human foreskin fibroblasts in response to IL-1, but U937 histiocytic lymphoma cells were unaffected. This cell line responded to PMA for the decrease in TNF-α receptor. The mechanism by which IL-2 down-regulates the TNF receptor remains unclear; PMA effects are probably mediated through enhanced phosphorylation by PKC. The importance of PKC in TNF-α expression was demonstrated in various studies, although at variance with the results of Holtmann and Wallach (1987), as PKC affects ligand affinity rather than receptor number. Thus transient TNF-α receptor on either PHA/IL-2- or IL-2-activated Tcells have been demonstrated (Scheurich et al., 1987; Owen-Schaub et al., 1989). This transient expression can be down-regulated by activators of PKC, resulting in a loss of binding of TNF-α to its receptor. This is not due to enhanced internalization of the TNF-α receptor, nor its shedding, but to the control of ligand affinity (Unglaub et al., 1987). The authors observed that while activation of PKC increases TNF-α mRNA and/or secretion, protein kinase A (PKA) acts as a negative regulator of TNF production. In contrast, TNF-α receptor is down-regulated by PKC, whereas PKA stimulation results in the enhancement of TNF-α receptor expression. Such a system allows adequate response to TNF-α.

The TNF-α receptor was more extensively investigated on the TNF-α-sensitive KYM cells derived from human myosarcoma by Watanabe et al. (1988b). The authors show that the half-life of the receptor on the surface is 2 h in the absence of TNF-α and 30 min in its presence. It can be hypothesized that this phenomenon represents a mechanism of protection against cytolysis by TNF-α. The mechanism of down-regulation involves internalization of the receptor without recycling and degradation by lysosomal enzymes. A tight regulating mechanism of cytotoxicity must exist at the level of the cells producing TNF-α to avoid "suicide." Ding et al.

(1989) reported that macrophages rapidly internalize their TNF receptors in response to LPS. The mechanism of LPS-induced internalization of the receptor modulation is unresponsiveness of the cells to the biological effects of TNF-α and TNF-β. It is therefore reasonable to speculate that induction of TNF-α internalization by LPS—a potent inducer of TNF-α—represents either a mechanism whereby macrophages protect themselves from cytotoxicity or a microbial strategy for evading host defense. Taken together, all these data demonstrate the importance and complexity of TNF-α receptor regulation, pivotal for TNF-α responsiveness.

IV. BINDING PROTEINS REGULATING TNF ACTIVITIES

Two different classes of proteins neutralizing TNF-α activities deserve our attention: antibodies and binding proteins.

A. Antibodies

Availability of recombinant molecules made it possible to raise both polyconal and monoconal antibodies against TNF-α. Thus Socher et al. (1987) raised antiserum against peptides representing the N terminal of TNF-α which blocks the association of TNF with its receptor. Both antibodies raised against the 31 and 15 N-terminal amino acid block the binding concomitantly with the biological activity. With the aid of these antibodies it was possible to identify the 9 to 15 N-terminated amino acid as being essential for receptor recognition and biological activity. Availability of blocking antibodies made it possible to investigate the role of TNF-α in various pathological situations. Thus Grau et al. (1987) demonstrated the predominant role of TNF in the pathogenesis of cerebral malaria, and almost all mice infected with *Plasmodium berghei anka* died 6 to 14 days after injection. In contrast, injection of blocking antibody to TNF-α protected mice from cerebral malaria without modifying the parasitemia. The use of anti-TNF-α antibody has allowed to define TNF-α as a major mediator of various diseases. Passive immunization of mice with polyclonal antibody to murine TNF-α 6 h before administration of lethal dose of endotoxin protected them from death (Beutler et al., 1985). Passive immunization has also been used to prevent TNF-induced development of cutaneous and intestinal lesions of the acute graft-versus-host disease (Piguet et al., 1987) as well as its role in bleomycin-induced pneumopathy and fibrosis (Piguet et al., 1989). In the development of bacterial granulomas, TNF released from macrophages in the microenvironment of developing granulomas is involved in a process of autoamplification, enhancing its own synthesis and release. Development of the disease ceased fully after the administration of anti-TNF antibodies (Kindler et al., 1989). The antibodies raised artificially differ from the autoantibodies directed against TNF-α or TNF-β. Autoantibodies are a matter of autoimmunity rather than a mechanism regulating cytokines. Jeffes et al. (1989) described the detection of naturally occurring antibodies to both TNF-α and TNF-β. Although their function is not known, they may neutralize the effect of the cytokines. Similarly, antibodies to TNF have been detected in healthy individuals and patients with inflammatory diseases and gram-negative bacterial infections (Fomsgaard et al., 1989). The relevance of the autoantibodies is not yet elucidated and we can but wonder whether they are part of a mechanism that protects from, or on the contrary, boosts circulating levels of TNF-α and TNF-β.

B. Binding Proteins: TNF Inhibitor in Urine and Plasma

1. *Inhibition of Cytotoxicity*

Contrary to the antibodies (see above) that neutralize TNF activity, TNF-inhibitory activities have been found in biological fluids such as urine and plasma. While investigating an IL-1 inhibitor in the urine of febrile patients (Balavoine et al., 1986; Seckinger et al., 1987a,b; Dayer and Seckinger, 1989) we wondered whether we might also find an activity inhibitory to TNF, both cytokines being endogenous pyrogens. Indeed, the urine of febrile patients proved to contain a TNF-α-inhibiting activity (TNF-α INH) when tested in a cytotoxic assay using the TNF-susceptible cell line L929 (Seckinger et al., 1988).

Purification to homogenity of the TNF-α inhibitory activities from urine was achieved by our group (Seckinger et al., 1989), Engelmann et al. (1989), and Olsson et al. (1989). Purification from urine and plasma yielded a protein with a novel amino acid sequence. When the protein purified to homogeneity was analyzed on SDS-PAGE and then silver-stained, a single peptide migrating with an apparent molecular weight was revealed under both reducing and nonreducing conditions (Seckinger et al., 1990a). Endoglycanase treatment reduced the molecular weight of the inhibitor by ~10 kD (Fig. 1). We demonstrated that in addition to limiting cytotoxicity, the inhibitor regulates inflammatory and immunodulatory properties of TNF-α by decreasing TNF-α-induced PGE_2 production on dermal fibroblasts, and class I HLA- and IFN-γ-induced HLA-DR class II antigen expression in the Colo 205 human cell line. The TNF inhibitor binds to the ligand itself to form a stable complex that remains stable even during gel filtration. We subsequently demonstrated that the TNF inhibitor has specificity, as it affects human TNF-α more than murine TNF-α or lymphotoxin.

Homology with TNF-α Receptor Fragments

Polyconal antibodies to the partially purified urinary TNF-α inhibitor immunoprecipitate the cross-linked TNF receptor complex, and immunofluorescence staining of activated T cells with FITC-TNF coincides with immnofluorescence staining of the same cells stained with antibodies to the TNF inhibitor, suggesting that the TNF inhibitor we purified from urine is a soluble fragment of the TNF receptor itself (Seckinger et al., 1990b).

Two different types of TNF-α receptor have been identified on the cell surface

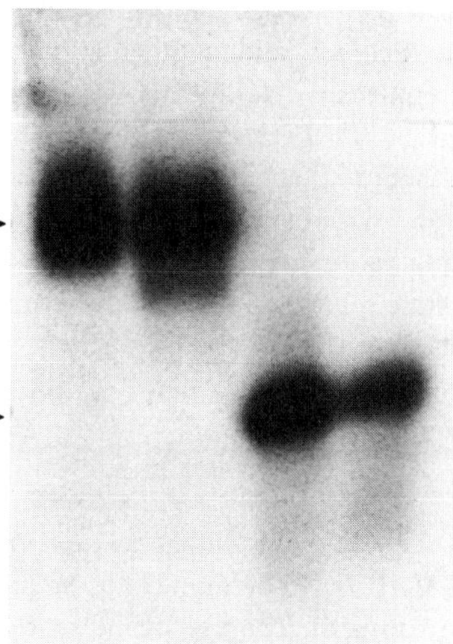

Figure 1 Purified TNF-α inhibitor (TNF-α INH) was iodinated using the chloramine-T method. [^{125}I]TNF-α INH was treated for 18 h at 37°C by either buffer alone (lane A), *O*-glycanase (lane B), *N*-glycanase (lane C), or *O*- and *N*-glycanase (lane D). The mixture was resolved on SDS-PAGE and exposed for 24 h to autoadiography.

using monoconal antibodies (Hohmann et al., 1989; Brockhaus et al., 1990). Thus it was shown that the receptor produced by myeloid cells (HL-60, U937, K562, or freshly isolated monocytes) is different from that produced by cells of epithelial origin (MCF7, HEp2, and HeLa) (Hohmann et al., 1989).

On the basis of apparent molecular mass, immunoreactivity, proteolytic fingerprints, and glycosylation, the authors suggest that TNF-α has at least two different receptors. Recently, Loetscher et al. (1990) and Schall et al. (1990) cloned and expressed the human TNF receptor of 55 kD. It is noteworthy that our TNF inhibitor was confirmed to be a soluble fragment, since the NH_2 terminal amino acid sequence of the inhibitor is similar to a sequence of the 55-kDa TNF receptor starting at aspartic acid number 12 (Seckinger et al., 1990a; Loetscher et al., 1990). This fragment can now be referred to as TNF-BPI. Englemann et al. (1990b) reported on two different proteins with different NH_2-terminal amino acid sequences that protect cells from TNF-induced cytotoxicity. Antibodies raised against the two proteins showed no immunological cross-reactivity. Hence the antibodies raised against these binding proteins have TNF-like activity, suggesting that the two proteins are soluble forms of the two receptors. The same investigators confirmed recently that antibodies to a soluble form of TNF have TNF-like activity (Engelmann et al., 1990a). These data are in agreement with the postulate that there are at least two different TNF receptors and that their soluble forms may be part of an important mechanism regulating cytokine activity. Similar data were reported recently regarding the IL-4 and IL-7 receptors (Mosley et al., 1989; Goodwin et al., 1990). The second receptor (75 kD) of TNF-α has just been cloned (Smith et al., 1990) and is probably identical with the second TNF-α binding protein, now referred to as TNF-BPII. An interesting target for the future would be the elucidation of the proteases responsible for the cleavage of the extracellular fragments of the TNF-α receptors and consequently the control of these proteases.

V. CONCLUSIONS

Numerous types of cytokine inhibitors are now known. These include (1) receptor antagonists (e.g., IL-1ra); (2) cytokine binding proteins (e.g., TNF-α-BPs), which might be soluble forms of receptor ligand; and (3) autoantibodies to cytokines, which may not necessarily be blocking antibodies. Some may even increase or mimic biological activities of the ligand. Other forms of inhibitory mechanisms include inhibitors of proteases necessary for processing and release of the ligand, specific proteases destroying the ligand, specific inhibitors of gene activation, inhibitors of cytokine release (e.g., calcium-related mechanisms, myristoylation), and down-regulation of the receptors. The concept of anticytokines or natural inhibitors of cytokines also has to be regarded as a semantic problem, since already cloned cytokines are strong antagonists of other cytokines, as in the case of IL-4 and TNF-β, which down-regulate IL-1 and TNF gene expression in human monocytes (Essner et al., 1989; Ellingsworth et al., 1988) and as such could be considered as natural inhibitors of IL-1 and TNF. Other examples exist, such as IFN-γ, which blocks the stimulation of collagen synthesis induced by TGF-β, IL-1, or TNF-α. The physiological or pathophysiological significance of the various natural inhibitors remains to be established. There is strong evidence that cytokine inhibitors are markedly elevated in diseases, including leukemia (Balavoine et al., 1986; Dayer and Seckinger, 1989), arthritis (Prieur et al., 1987; Roux-Lombard et al., 1988), and chronic lung inflammatory disease (de Rochemonteix-Galve et al., 1990; Galve-de Rochemonteix et al., 1990). In addition, the induction in vivo of IL-1 and TNF inhibitory activity in human serum after lipopolysaccharide injection has been reported (Spinas et al., 1990). Finally, since TNF-α can induce phosphorylation of the mammalian heat-shock protein hsp 28 (Arrigo, 1990), it may be hypothesized that TNF-α inhibitors interfere with this regulatory pathway.

Whatever the answer, the balance between cytokine and cytokine inhibitors is bound to be determinant for the control of manifestations and persistence of inflammatory diseases. Indeed, the lack of natural cytokine inhibitors may generate or maintain serious pathological conditions. Precise local and systematic determination of the levels of these inhibitors will be essential to understand the pathological processes.

REFERENCES

Aderka, D., Holtmann, H., Toker, L., Hahn, T., and Wallach, D. (1986). Tumor necrosis factor induction by Sendai virus, *J. Immunol., 136*: 2938.

Aderka, D., Le, J., and Vilček, J. (1989). IL-6 inhibits lipopolysaccharide-induced tumor necrosis factor production in cultured human monocytes, U937 cells, and in mice, *J. Immunol. 143*: 3517.

Aggarwal, B. B., Eessalu, T. E., and Hass, P. E. (1985). Characterization of receptors for human tumor necrosis factor and their regulation by γ-interferon, *Nature, 318*: 665.

Aggarwal, S., Drysdale, B. E., and Shin, H. S. (1988). Tumor necrosis factor-mediated cytotoxicity involves ADP-ribosylation, *J. Immunol., 140*: 4187.

Arrigo, W. -P. (1990). Tumor necrosis factor induces the rapid phosphorylation of the mammalian heat shock protein hsp28, *Mol. Cell. Biol., 10*: 1276.

Balavoine, J. F., de Rochemonteix, B., Williamson, K., Seckinger, P., Cruchaud, A., and Dayer, J. -M. (1986). Prostaglandin E_2 and collagenase production by fibroblasts and synovial cells is regulated by urine-derived interleukin-1 and inhibitor(s), *J. Clin. Invest., 78*: 1120.

Baud, L., Perez, J., Friedlander, G., and Ardaillou, R. (1988). Tumor necrosis factor stimulates prostaglandin production and cyclic AMP levels in rat cultured mesangial cells, *FEBS Lett., 239*: 50.

Benacerraf, B. (1981). Role of MHC gene products in immune regulation, *Science, 212*: 1229.

Beutler, B., and Cerami, A. (1986). Cachectin and tumor necrosis factor as two sides of the same biological coin, *Nature, 320*: 584.

Beutler, B., and Cerami, A. (1988). Tumor necrosis, cachexia, shock and inflammation: a common mediator, *Annu. Rev. Biochem., 57*: 505.

Beutler, B., Milsark, L. W., and Cerami, A. C. (1985). Passive immunization against cachectin/tumor necrosis factor protects mice from lethal effect of endotoxin, *Science, 229*: 869.

Beutler, B., Krochin, N., Milsark, I. W., Luedke, C., and Cerami, A. (1986). Control of cachectin (tumor necrosis factor) synthesis: mechanisms of endotoxin resistance, *Science, 232*: 977.

Branca, A. A., Faltynek, C. R., d'Alessandro, S. B., and Baglioni, C. (1982). Interaction of interferon with cellular receptors, *J. Biol. Chem., 257*: 13291.

Brenner, D. A., O-Hara, M., Angel, P., Chojkier, M., and Karin, M. (1989). Prolonged activation of jun and collagenase genes by tumour necrosis factor-α, *Nature, 337*: 661.

Brett, J., Gerlach, H., Nawroth, P., Steinberg, S., Godman, G., and Stern, D. (1989). Tumor necrosis factor/cachectin increases permeability of endothelial cell monolayers by a mechanism involving regulatory G proteins, *J. Exp. Med., 169*: 1977.

Brockhaus, M., Schoenfeld, H. J., Schlaeger, E. J., Hunziker, W., Lesslauer, W., and

Loetscher, H. (1990). Identification of two types of tumor necrosis factor receptors on human cell lines by monoclonal antibodies, *Proc. Natl. Acad. Sci. USA, 87*: 3127.

Burch, R. M., Luini, A., and Axelrod, J. (1986). Phospholipase A_2 and phospholipase C are activated by distinct GTP-binding proteins in response to α_1-adrenergic stimulation in FRTL5 thyroid cells, *Proc. Natl. Acad. Sci. USA, 83*: 7201.

Carswell, E. A., Old, L. J., Kassel R. L., Green, S., Fiore, N., and Williamson, B. (1975). An endotoxin-induced serum factor that causes necrosis of tumors, *Proc. Natl. Acad. Sci. USA, 72*: 3666.

Cseh, K., and Beutler, B. (1989). Alternative cleavage of the cachectin/tumor necrosis factor propeptide results in a larger, inactive form of secreted protein, *J. Biol. Chem., 264*: 16256.

Dayer, J. -M., and Seckinger, P. (1989). Natural inhibitors and antagonists of interleukin-1, *Interleukin-1, Inflammation and Disease,* Research Monographs in Cell and Tissue Physiology (R. Bomford and B. Henderson, eds.), Elsevier, Oxford, p. 283.

Dayer, J. -M., Beutler, B., and Cerami, A. (1985). Cachectin/tumor necrosis factor stimulates collagenase and prostaglandin E_2 production by human synovial cells and dermal fibroblasts, *J. Exp. Med., 162*: 2163.

de Rochemonteix-Galve, B., Dayer, J. -M., and Junod, A. F. (1990). Fibroblast-alveolar cell interactions in sarcoidosis and idiopathic pulmonary fibrosis: evidence for stimulatory and inhibitory cytokine production by alveolar cells, *Eur. Respir. J., 3*: 653.

Dinarello, C. A., Cannon, J. G., Wolff, S. M., Bernheim, H. A., Beutler, B., Cerami, A., Figari, I. S., Palladino, M. A., Jr., and O'Connor, J. V. (1986). Tumor necrosis factor (Cachectin) is an endogenous pyrogen and induces production of interleukin 1, *J. Exp. Med., 163*: 1433.

Ding, A. H., Sanchez, E., Srimal, S., and Nathan, C. F. (1989). Macrophages rapidly internalize their tumor necrosis factor receptors in response to bacterial lipopolysaccharide, *J. Biol. Chem., 264*: 3924.

Djeu, J. Y., Blanchard, D. K., Halkias, D., and Friedman, H. (1986). Growth inhibition of *Candida albicans* by human polymorphonuclear neutrophils: activation by interferon-γ and tumor necrosis factor, *J. Immunol., 137*: 2980.

Ellingsworth, L. R., Nakayama, D., Segarini, P., Dasch, J., Carillo, P., and Waegell, W. (1988). Transforming growth factor-βs are equipotent growth inhibitors of interleukin-1-induced thymocyte proliferation, *Cell. Immunol., 114*: 41.

Engelmann, H., Aderka, D., Rubinstein, M., Rotman, D., and Wallach, D. (1989). A tumor necrosis factor-binding protein purified to homogeneity from human urine protects cells from tumor necrosis factor toxicity, *J. Biol. Chem., 264*: 11974.

Engelmann, H., Holtmann, H., Brakebusch, C., Shemer Avni, Y., Sarov, I., Nophar, Y., Hadas, E., Leitner, O., and Wallach, D. (1990a). Antibodies to a soluble form of a tumor-necrosis-factor (TNF) receptor have TNF-like activity, *J. Biol. Chem., 265*: 14497 .

Engelmann, H., Novick, D., and Wallach, D. (1990b). Two tumor necrosis factor-binding proteins purified from human urine: evidence for immunological cross-reactivity with cell surface tumor necrosis factor receptors, *J. Biol. Chem., 265*: 1531.

Essner, R, Rhoades, K., McBride, W. H., Morton, D. L., and Economou, J. S. (1989). IL-4 down-regulates IL-1 and TNF gene expression in human monocytes, *J. Immunol., 142*: 3857.

Fomsgaard, A., Svenson, M., and Bendtzen, K. (1989). Auto-antibodies to tumor necrosis factor alpha in healthy humans and patients with inflammatory diseases and gram-negative bacterial infections, *Scand. J. Immunol., 30*: 219.

Galve-de Rochemonteix, B., Nicod, L. P., Junod, A. F., and Dayer, J. -M. (1990). Characterization of a specific 20- to 25-kD interleukin-1 inhibitor from cultured human lung macrophages, *Am. J. Respir. Cell Mol. Biol., 3*: 3163.

Gooding, L. R., Elmore, L. W., Tollefson, A. E., Brady, H. A., and Wold, W. S. M. (1988). A 14.700 mw protein from the E3 region of adenovirus inhibits cytolysis by tumor necrosis factor, *Cell, 53*: 341.

Goodwin, R. G., Friend, D., Ziegler, S. F., Jerzy, R., Falk, B. A., Gimpel, S., Cosman, D., Dower, S. K., March, C. J., Namen, A. E., and Park, L. S. (1990). Cloning of the human and murine interleukin-7 receptors: demonstration of a soluble form and homology to a new receptor superfamily, *Cell, 60*: 941.

Grau, G. E., Fajardo, L. F., Piguet, P. F., Allet, B., Lambert, P. H., and Vassalli, P. (1987). Tumor necrosis factor (cachectin) is an essential mediator in murine cerebral malaria, *Science, 237*: 1210.

Hensel, G., Männel, D. N., Pfizenmaier, K., and Krönke, M. (1987). Autocrine stimulation of TNF-alpha mRNA expression in HL-60 cells, *Lymphokine Res., 6*: 119.

Hepburn, A., Boeynaems, J. -M., Fiers, W., and Dumont, J. E. (1987). Modulation of tumor necrosis factor-α cytotoxicity in L929 cells by bacterial toxins, hydrocortisone and inhibitors of arachidonic acid metabolism, *Biochem. Biophys. Res. Commun., 149*: 815.

Hirata, F., Schiffmann, E., Venkatasubramanian, K., Salomon, D., and Axelrod, J. (1980). A phospholipase A_2 inhibitory protein in rabbit neutrophils induced by glucocorticoids, *Proc. Natl. Acad. Sci. USA, 77*: 2533.

Hoffman, M., and Weinberg, J. B. (1987). Tumor necrosis factor-alpha induces increased hydrogen peroxide production and Fc receptor expression, but not increased Ia antigen expression by peritoneal macrophages, *J. Leukocyte Biol., 42*: 704.

Hohmann, H., Remy, R., Brockhaus, M., and van Loon, A. P. G. M. (1989). Two different cell types have different major receptors for human tumor necrosis factor (TNF-α), *J. Biol. Chem., 264*: 14927.

Holtmann, H., and Wallach, D. (1987). Down regulation of the receptors for tumor necrosis factor by interleukin 1 and 4β-phorbol-12-myristate-13-acetate, *J. Immunol., 139*: 1161.

Horiguchi, J., Spriggs, D., Imamura, K., Stone, R., Luebbers, R., and Kufe, D. (1989). Role of arachidonic acid metabolism in transcriptional induction of tumor necrosis factor gene expression by phorbol ester, *Mol. Cell. Biol., 9*: 252.

Imamura, K., Sherman, M. L., Spriggs, D., and Kufe, D. (1988). Effect of tumor necrosis factor on GTP binding and GTPase activity in HL-60 and L929 cells, *J. Biol. Chem., 263*: 10247.

Jäätelä, M. Saksela, K., and Saksela, E. (1989). Heat shock protects WEHI-164 target cells from the cytolysis by tumor necrosis factors alpha and beta, *Eur. J. Immunol., 19*: 1413.

Jeffes, E. W. B., III, Ininns, E. K., Schmitz, K. L., Yamamoto, R. S., Dett, C. A., and Granger, G. S. (1989). The presence of antibodies to lymphotoxin and tumor necrosis factor in normal serum, *Arthritis Rheum., 32*: 1148.

Kettelhut, I. C., Fiers, W., and Goldberg, A. L. (1987). The toxic effects of tumor necrosis factor in vivo and their prevention by cyclooxygenase inhibitors, *Proc. Natl. Acad. Sci. USA, 84*: 4273.

Kindler, V., Sappino, A. P., Grau, G. E., Piguet, P. F., and Vassalli, P. (1989). The inducing role of tumor necrosis factor in the development of bactericidal granulomas during BCG infection, *Cell, 56*: 731.

Knudsen, P. J., Dinarello, C. A., and Strom, T. B. (1986). Prostaglandins posttranscriptionally inhibit monocyte expression of interleukin 1 activity by increasing intracellular cyclic adenosine monophosphate, *J. Immunol., 137*: 3189.

Kriegler, M., Perez, C., DeFay, K., Albert, I., and Lu, S. D. (1988). A novel form of TNF/cachectin is a cell surface cytotoxic transmembrane protein: ramifications for the complex physiology of TNF, *Cell, 53*: 45.

Kull, F. C., Jr., Jacobs, S., and Cuatrecasas, P. (1985). Cellular receptor for ^{125}I-labeled tumor necrosis factor: specific binding, affinity labeling, and relationship to sensitivity, *Proc. Natl. Acad. Sci. USA, 82*: 5756.

Kunkel, S. L., Chensue, S. W., and Phan, S. H. (1986). Prostaglandins as endogenous mediators of interleukin 1 production, *J. Immunol., 136*: 186.

Kunkel, S. L., Spengler, M., May, M. A., Spengler, R., Larrick, J., and Remick, D. (1988). Prostaglandin E_2 regulates macrophage-derived tumor necrosis factor gene expression, *J. Biol. Chem., 263*: 5380.

Lachmann, L. B., Brown, D. C., and Dinarello, C. A. (1987). Growth-promoting effect of recombinant interleukin 1 and tumor necrosis factor for a human astrocytoma cell line, *J. Immunol., 138*: 2913.

Lehmann, V., Benninghoff, B., and Dröge, W. (1988). Tumor necrosis factor-induced activation of peritoneal macrophages is regulated by prostaglandin E_2 and cAMP, *J. Immunol., 141*: 587.

Loetscher, H., Pan, Y. -C. E., Lahm, H. -W., Gentz, R., Brockhaus, M., Tabuchi, H., and Lesslauer, W. (1990). Molecular cloning and expression of the human 55 kd tumor necrosis factor receptor, *Cell, 61*:351.

Matthews, N., Neale, M. L., Jackson, S. K., and Stark, J. M. (1987). Tumor cell killing by tumor necrosis factor: inhibition by anaerobic conditions, free-radical scavengers and inhibitors of arachidonate metabolism, *Immunology, 62*: 153.

Mosley, B., Beckmann, M. P., March, C. J., Idzerda, R. L., Gimpel, S. D., VandenBos, T., Friend, D., Alpert, A., Anderson, D., Jackson, J., Wignall, J. M., Smith, C., Gallis, B., Sims, J. E., Urdal, D., Widmer, M. B., Cosman, D., and Park, L. S. (1989). The murine interleukin-4 receptor: molecular cloning and characterization of secreted and membrane bound forms, *Cell, 59*: 335.

Niitsu, Y., Watanabe, N., Sone, H., Neda, H., Yamauchi, N., and Urushizaki, I. (1985). Mechanism of the cytotoxic effect of tumor necrosis factor, *Jpn. J. Cancer Res., 76*: 1193.

Nophar, Y., Holtmann, H., Ber, R., and Wallach, D. (1988). Dominance of resistance to the cytocidal effect of tumor necrosis factor in heterokaryons formed by fusion of resistant and sensitive cells, *J. Immunol., 140*: 3456.

North, R. J., and Havell, E. A. (1988). The antitumor function of tumor necrosis factor (TNF). II. Analysis of the role of endogenous TNF in endotoxin-induced hemorrhagic necrosis and regression of an established sarcoma, *J. Exp. Med., 167*: 1086.

North, R. J., and Havell, E. A. (1989). Glucocorticoid-mediated inhibition of endotoxin-induced intratumor tumor necrosis factor production and tumor hemorrhagic necrosis and regression, *J. Exp. Med., 170*: 703.

Old, L. J. (1985). Tumor necrosis factor (TNF), *Science, 230*: 630.

Oliff, A., Defeo-Jones, D., Boyer, M., Martinez, D., Kiefer, D., Vuocolo, G., Wolfe, A., and Socher, S. H. (1987). Tumors secreting human TNF/cachectin induce cachexia in mice, *Cell, 50*: 555.

Olsson, I., Lantz, M., Nilsson, E. Peetre, C., Thysell, H., Grubb, A., and Adolf, G. (1989). Isolation and characterization of a tumor necrosis factor binding protein from urine, *Eur. J. Haematol., 42*: 270.

Oppenheim, J. J., Kovacs, E. J., Matsushima, K., and Durum, S. (1986). There is more than one interleukin 1, *Immunology Today, 7*: 45.

Owen-Schaub, L. B., Crump, W. L., III, Morin, G. I., and Grimm, E. A. (1989). Regulation of lymphocyte tumor necrosis factor receptors by IL-2, *J. Immunol., 143*: 2236.

Palombella, V. J., Yamashiro, D. J., Maxfield, F. R., Decker, S. J., and Vilček, J. (1987). Tumor necrosis factor increases the number of epidermal growth factor receptors on human fibroblasts, *J. Biol. Chem., 262*: 1950.

Pennica, D., Nedwin, G. E., Hayflick, J. S., Seeburg, P. H., Derynck, R., Palladino, M. A., Kohr, W. J., Aggarwal, B. B., and Goeddel, D. V. (1984). Human tumor necrosis factor: precursor structure, expression and homology to lymphotoxin, *Nature, 312*: 724.

Pfizenmaier, K., Scheurich, P., Schlüter, C., and Krönke, M. (1987). Tumor necrosis factor enhances HLA-A, B, C and HLA-DR gene expression in human tumor cells, *J. Immunol., 138*: 975.

Piguet, P. F., Grau, G. E., Allet, B., and Vassalli, P. (1987). Tumor necrosis factor/cachectin is an effector of skin and gut lesions of the acute phase of graft-vs.-host disease, *J. Exp. Med., 166*: 1280.

Piguet, P. F., Coart, M. A., Grau, G. E., Kapanci, Y., and Vassalli, P. (1989). Tumor necrosis factor/cachectin plays a key role in bleomycin-induced pneumopathy and fibrosis, *J. Exp. Med., 170*: 655.

Piguet, P. F., Collart, M. A., Grau, G. E., Sappino, A. P., and Vassalli, P. (1990). Tumor necrosis factor is required for the development of silica induced pulmonary fibrosis, *Nature, 344*: 245.

Prieur, A. M., Kaufmann, M. T., Griscelli, C., and Dayer, J. M. (1987). Specific interleukin-1 inhibitor in serum and urine of children with systemic juvenile chronic arthrities, *Lancet, ii*: 1240.

Reid, T. R., Torti, F. M., and Ringold, G. M. (1989). Evidence for two mechanisms by which tumor necrosis factor kills cells, *J. Biol. Chem., 264*: 4583.

Reis, L. F. L., Lee, T. H., and Vilček, J. (1989). Tumor necrosis factor acts synergistically with autocrine interferon-β and increases interferon-β mRNA levels in human fibroblasts, *J. Biol. Chem., 264*: 16351.

Renz, H., Gong, J. H., Schmidt, A., Nain, M., and Gemsa, D. (1988). Release of tumor necrosis factor-α from macrophages, *J. Immunol., 141*: 2388.

Roberts, N. J., Jr., Prill, A. H., and Mann, T. N. (1986). Interleukin 1 and interleukin 1 inhibitor production by human macrophages exposed to influenza virus or respiratory syncytial virus, *J. Exp. Med., 163*: 511.

Roux-Lombard, P., Modoux, C., and Dayer, J. M. (1988). Inhibitors of IL-1 and TNFα activities in synovial fluids and cultured synovial fluid cell supernatants (abstr.), *Calcif. Tissue Int., 42*: S(A47).

Rubin, B. Y., Anderson, S. L., Sullivan, S. A., Williamson, B. D., Carswell, E. A., and Old,

L. J. (1986). Nonhematopoietic cells selected for resistance to tumor necrosis factor produce tumor necrosis factor, *J. Exp. Med., 164*: 1350.

Satomi, N., Sakurai, A., Haranaka, R., and Haranaka, K. (1988). Preventive effects of several chemicals against lethality of recombinant human tumor necrosis factor, *J. Biol. Response Modif., 7*: 54.

Scanlon, M., Laster, S. M., Wood, J. G., and Gooding, L. R. (1989). Cytolysis by tumor necrosis factor is preceded by a rapid and specific dissolution of microfilaments, *Proc. Natl. Acad. Sci. USA, 86*: 182.

Schall, T. J., Lewis, M., Koller, K. J., Lee, A., Rice, G. C., Wong, G. H. W., Gatanaga, T., Granger, G. A., Lentz, R., Raab, H., Kohr, W. J., and Goeddel, D. V. (1990). Molecular cloning and expression of a receptor for human tumor necrosis factor, *Cell, 61*: 361.

Scheurich, P., Thoma, B., Ücer, U., and Pfizenmaier, K. (1987). Immunoregulatory activity of recombinant human tumor necrosis factor (TNF)-α-mediated enhancement of T cell responses, *J. Immunol., 138*: 1786.

Schlessinger, J., Shechter, Y., Willingham, M. C., and Pastan, I. (1978). Direct visualization of binding, aggregation, and internalization of insulin and epidermal growth factor on living fibroblastic cells, *Proc. Natl. Acad. Sci. USA, 75*: 2659.

Schmid, D. S., Hornung, R., McGrath, K. M., Paul, N., and Ruddle, N. H. (1987). Target cell DNA fragmentation is mediated by lymphotoxin and tumor necrosis factor, *Lymphokine Res., 6*: 195.

Schultz, R. M., Pavlidis, N. A., Stylos, W. A., and Chirigos, M. A. (1978). Regulation of macrophage tumoricidal function: a role for prostaglandins of the E series, *Science, 202*: 320.

Schütze, S., Scheurich, P., Pfizenmaier, K., and Krönke, M. (1989). Tumor necrosis factor signal transduction, *J. Biol. Chem., 264*: 3562.

Seckinger, P., Williamson, K., Balavoine, J. -F., Mach, B., Mazzei, G., Shaw, A., and Dayer, J. -M. (1987a). A urine inhibitor of interleukin 1 activity affects both interleukin 1α and 1β but not tumor necrosis factor α, *J. Immunol., 139*: 1541.

Seckinger, P., Lowenthal, J. W., Williamson, K., Dayer, J. -M., and MacDonald, H. R. (1987b). A urine inhibitor of interleukin 1 activity that blocks ligand binding, *J. Immunol., 139*: 1546.

Seckinger, P., Isaaz, S., and Dayer, J. -M. (1988). A human inhibitor of tumor necrosis factor α, *J. Exp. Med., 167*: 1511.

Seckinger, P., Isaaz, S., and Dayer, J. -M. (1989). Purification and biologic characterization of a specific tumor necrosis factor α inhibitor, *J. Biol. Chem., 264*: 11966.

Seckinger, P., Vey, E., Turcatti, G., Wingfield, P., and Dayer, J. -M. (1990a). Tumor necrosis factor inhibitor: purification, NH_2-terminal amino acid sequence and evidence for anti-inflammatory and immunomodulatory activities, *Eur. J. Immunol., 20*: 1167.

Seckinger, P., Zhang, J. H., Hauptmann, B., and Dayer, J. -M. (1990b). Characterization of tumor necrosis factor α (TNFα) inhibitor: evidence of immunological cross-reactivity with the TNF receptor, *Proc. Natl. Acad. Sci. USA, 87*: 5188.

Sehgal, P. B., Walther, Z., and Tamm, I. (1987). Rapid enhancement of β_2-interferon/B-cell differentiation factor BSF-2 gene expression in human fibroblasts by diacylglycerols and the calcium ionophore A23187, *Proc. Natl. Acad. Sci. USA, 84*: 3663.

Shirai, T., Yamaguchi, H., Ito, H., Todd, C. W., and Wallach, R. B. (1985). Cloning and expression in *Escherichia coli* of the gene for human tumor necrosis factor, *Nature, 313*: 803.

Smith, C. A., Davis, T., Anderson, D., Solam, L., Beckmann, M. P., Jerzy, R., Dower, S. K., Cosman, D., and Goodwin, R. G. (1990). A receptor for tumor necrosis factor defines an unusual family of cellular and viral proteins, *Science, 248*: 1019.

Snyder, D. S., and Unanue, E. R. (1982). Corticosteroids inhibit murine macrophage Ia expression and interleukin 1 production, *J. Immunol., 129*: 1803.

Socher, S. H., Riemen, M. W., Martinez, D., Friedman, A., Tai, J., Quintero, J. C., Garsky, V., and Oliff, A. (1987). Antibodies against amino acids 1-15 of tumor necrosis factor block its binding to cell-surface receptor, *Proc. Natl. Acad. Sci. USA, 84*: 8829.

Spinas, G. A., Bloesch, D., Kaufman, M. -T., Keller, U., and Dayer, J. -M. (1990). Induction of plasma inhibitors of interleukin-1 and tumor necrosis factor alpha activity by endotoxin administration to normal human subjects, *Am. J. Physiol., 259*: R993-R997 .

Stauber, G. B., Aiyer, R. A., and Aggarwal, B. B. (1988). Human tumor necrosis factor-α receptor, *J. Biol. Chem., 263*: 19098.

Suffys, P., Beyaert, R., van Roy, F., and Fiers, W. (1988). Reduced tumor necrosis factor-induced cytotoxicity by inhibitors of the arachidonic acid metabolism, *Biochem. Biophys. Res. Commun., 149*: 735.

Sugarman, B. J., Aggarwal, B. B., Hass, P. E., Figari, I. S., Palladino, M. A.., Jr., and Shepard, H. M. (1985). Recombinant human tumor necrosis factor-α: effects on proliferation of normal and transformed cells in vitro, *Science, 230*: 943.

Taffet, S. M., and Russell, S. W. (1980). Macrophage-mediated tumor cell killing: reduction of expression of cytolytic activity by prostaglandin E, *J. Immunol., 126*: 424.

Taffet, S. M., Pace, J. L., and Russell, S. W. (1981). Lymphokine maintains macrophage activation for tumor cell killing by interfering with the negative regulatory effect of prostaglandin E_2, *J. Immunol., 127*: 121.

Townsend, A. R. M., Rothbard, J., Gotch, F. M., Bahadur, G., Wraith, D., and McMichael, A. J. (1986). The epitopes of influenza nucleoprotein recognized by cytotoxic T lymphocytes can be defined with short synthetic peptides, *Cell, 44*: 959.

Tracey, K. J., Beutler, B., Lowry, S. F., Merryweather, J., Wolpe, S., Milsark, I. W., Hariri, R. J., Fahey, T. J., III, Zentella, A., Albert, J. D., Shires, G. T., and Cerami, A. (1986). Shock and tissue injury induced by recombinant human cachectin. *Science, 234*: 470.

Tsujimoto, M., Yip, Y. K., and Vilček, J. (1985). Tumor necrosis factor: specific binding and internalization in sensitive and resistant cells, *Proc. Natl. Acad. Sci. USA, 82*: 7626.

Tsujimoto, M., Yokota, S., Vilček, J., and Weissman, G. (1986). Tumor necrosis factor provokes superoxide anion generation from neutrophils, *Biochem. Biophys. Res. Commun., 137*: 1094.

Unglaub, R., Maxeiner, B., Thoma, B., Pfizenmaier, K., and Scheurich, P. (1987). Downregulation of tumor necrosis factor (TNF) sensivity via modulation of TNF binding capacity by protein kinase C activators, *J.Exp. Med., 166*: 1788.

Vilček, J., Palombella, V. J., Henriksen-DeStefano, D., Swenson, C., Feinman, R., Hirai, M., and Tsujimoto, M. (1986). Fibroblast growth enhancing activity of tumor necrosis factor and its relationship to other polypeptide growth factors, *J. Exp. Med., 163*: 632.

Vlassara, H., Brownlee, M., Manogue, K. R., Dinarello, C. A., and Pasagian, A. (1988). Cachectin/TNF and IL-1 induced by glucose-modified proteins: role in normal tissue remodeling, *Science, 240*: 1546.

Waage, A., and Bakke, O. (1988). Glucocorticoids suppress the production of tumor necrosis factor by lipopolysaccharide-stimulated human monocytes, *Immunology, 63*: 299.

Wallach, D. (1986). Cytotoxins (tumor necrosis factor, lymphotoxin and others): molecular and functional characteristics and interactions with interferons, *Interferon*, *7*: 89.

Wang, A. M., Creasey, A. A., Ladner, M. B., Lin, L. S., Strickler, J., van Arsdell, J. N., Yamamoto, R., and Mark, D. F. (1985). Molecular cloning of the complementary DNA for human tumor necrosis factor, *Science*, *228*: 149.

Watanabe, N., Niitsu, Y., Neda, H., Sone, H., Yamauchi, N., Maeda, M., and Urushizaki, I. (1988a). Cytocidal mechanism of TNF: effects of lysosomal enzyme and hydroxyl radical inhibitors on cytotoxicity, *Immunopharmacol. Immunotoxicol., 10*: 109.

Watanabe, N., Kuriyama, H., Sone, H., Neda, H., Yamauchi, N., Maeda, M., and Niitsu, Y. (1988b). Continuous internalization of tumor necrosis factor receptors in a human myosarcoma cell line, *J. Biol. Chem., 263*: 10262.

Williams, K. I., and Higgs, G. A. (1988). Eicosanoids and inflammation: review, *J. Pathol., 156*: 101.

Wong, G. H. W., and Goeddel, D. V. (1988). Induction of manganous superoxide dismutase by tumor necrosis factor: possible protective mechanism, *Science, 242*: 941.

Wong, G. H. W., Elwell, J. H., Oberley, L. W., and Goeddel, D. V. (1989). Manganous superoxide dismutase is essential for cellular resistance to cytotoxicity of tumor necrosis factor, *Cell, 58*: 923.

Yamauchi, N., Kuriyama, H., Watanabe, N., Neda, H., Maeda, M., and Niitsu, Y. (1989). Intercellular hydroxyl radical production induced by recombinant human tumor necrosis factor and its implication in the killing of tumor cells in vitro, *Cancer Res., 49*: 1671.

Yonehara, S., Ishii, A., and Yonehara, M. (1989). A cell-killing monoclonal antibody (anti-Fas) to a cell surface antigen co-downregulated with the receptor of tumor necrosis factor, *J. Exp. Med., 169*: 1747.

Zullo, J. N., Cochran, B. H., Huang, A. S., and Stiles, C. D. (1985). Platelet-derived growth factor and double-stranded ribonucleic acids stimulate expression of the same genes in 3T3 cells, *Cell, 43*: 793.

III

BIOLOGICAL ACTIONS OF TNFs

11

Antiproliferative and Antitumor Activity of TNF In Vitro and In Vivo

SALEEM T. A. MALIK and FRANCES R. BALKWILL
Biological Therapies Laboratory, Imperial Cancer Research Fund, London, England

I. INTRODUCTION

The term *tumor necrosis factor* was originally coined to describe a putative macrophage-derived protein that was induced by endotoxin administration in mice primed with BCG or other agents known to cause reticuloendolethial hyperplasia (Carswell et al., 1975). Injection of serum from BCG primed and endotoxin challenged animals into mice bearing the Meth A sarcoma led to a hemorrhagic necrosis of the tumor. These experiments demonstrated that the phenomenon of hemorrhagic necrosis, hitherto ascribed to a direct action of endotoxin on tumor cells (Shear et al., 1943) or the hemodynamic perturbations caused by endotoxin (Algire et al., 1952), was due to a host-derived protein released as a consequence of immunological priming and endotoxin challenge. The tumor necrosis factor was active against a range of murine tumors in vivo and had cytostatic or cytotoxic activity for tumor cell lines and transformed cells in vitro, but no growth-inhibitory effects on murine embryo fibroblasts. Nearly 10 years later, Pennica et al. (1984) reported the cloning of the cDNA for the protein that is now known as tumor necrosis factor (TNF or TNF-α) and the production of recombinant TNF. Subsequent experiments have confirmed that recombinant TNF had identical activities in the Meth A sarcoma model to the factor described by Carswell et al. (Palladino et al., 1987). A second cytokine, lymphotoxin LT or TNF-β), originally characterized as a soluble mediator in delayed-type hypersensitivity reactions (Ruddle and Waksman, 1968), was also cloned (Gray et al., 1984) and shown to have antitumor and cell regulatory effects essentially similar to those of TNF. Although many of the antiproliferative actions of LT and TNF overlap, more data are available from laboratory and clinical studies on TNF (TNF-α), in this review we concentrate on these data.

It is now evident that the actions of TNF are not restricted to cytotoxic/cytostatic effects on tumor cells, but include other effects, such as modulation of MHC antigen expression (Pfizenmaier et al., 1987), induction of cell surface adhesion molecules such as ICAM-1 (Rothstein et al., 1988), induction of enzyme inhibitors (Georg et al., 1989), and induction of differentiation (Trinchieri et al., 1986). In addition, TNF has wide-ranging effects on normal cell populations of hemopoietic and non-hemopoietic origin and has been implicated not only as a mediator in the pathophysiology of infectious diseases, autoimmune disease, and inflammatory conditions (reviewed in Balkwill, 1989), but also as a potential mediator in physiological processes such as cell differentiation (Fillipak et al., 1988; Pillai et al., 1989), bone resorption (Bertolini et al., 1987), angiogenisis (Fráter-Schröder et al., 1987). and tissue remodeling (Vlassara et al., 1988). The range of cells know known to be capable of TNF production include macrophages, T lymphocytes, B lymphocytes, and mast cells, and also diverse nonhemopoietic cells such as smooth muscle cells, astroglial cells, and Paneth cells in the gut (Warner and Libby, 1989; Sawada et al., 1989; Keshave et al., 1990). Constitutive and induced TNF production by nonhemopoietic tumor cell lines has been demonstrated in vitro (Rubin et al., 1986, Spriggs et al., 1987, Krönke et al., 1988; Niitsu et al., 1988), and TNF mRNA and protein has been detected in fresh human tumor tissue taken from patients (Balkwill et al., 1987a; Beissert et al., 1989; Hsu and Hsu, 1989; Naylor et al., 1990). Therefore, increasing attention is being focused on the role of TNF produced by tumor cells or tumor associated stromal cells in the pathophysiology of cancer. Studies with TNF tranfected cell lines have suggested a potential role of this cytokine in cancer cachexia, anemia, hypercalcemia, and tumor metastasis (Oliff et al., 1987; Johnson et al., 1989; Malik et al., 1989). Thus the potentially harmful effects of tumor necrosis factor cachetin emphasized by the work Beutler and Cerami and others (reviewed in Beutler and Cerami, 1989) seem to be gaining in importance. On the other hand, studies of the synergistic antitumor activity of TNF in combination with other cytokines, cytotoxic drugs, and hyperthermia in animal models offer new therapeutic options for the cancer patient. In this chapter we review some of the data that have been gathered on a variety of aspects of TNF and cancer, mainly on the mechanisms of cytotoxicity and resistance to TNF in vitro and in vivo, but also in the role of endogenously produced TNF in tumor pathophysiology.

II. ACTIONS OF TNF IN VITRO

A. Is TNF Selectively Cytoxic/Cytostatic for Tumor Cells?

The landmark paper by Carswell et al.(1975) demonstrated that TNF had selective toxicity for tumor cells and transformed cell lines (e.g. the murine L929 fibroblasts). Sugarman et al.(1985) showed an antiproliferative response of TNF in 16 out of 34 tumor cell lines, while the growth of normal human cell lines from the colon, fetal skin, and lung was not inhibited. Selective antiproliferative effects of TNF on tumor cells were also reported by others (Fransen et al., 1986a). Subsequent studies with recombinant material demonstrated that TNF can have either growth stimulatory or antiproliferative actions on normal cells and tumor cells (Lewis et al., 1987), depending on the in vitro conditions. TNF has antiproliferative effects on normal cell populations such endothelial cells and smooth muscle cells (Sato et al., 1986, Schuger et al., 1989), adipocyes (Kawakami et al., 1989), fibroblasts (Palombela and Vilček, 1989), keratinocytes (Pillai et al., 1989), and hemopoietic progenitor cells (Broxmeyer et al., 1986). Some of these studies have revealed parameters that are of relevance to the effects of TNF on tumor cell lines. For example, it was shown that TNF stimulated the growth of human fibroblasts or mouse 3T3 fibroblasts in vitro, and that this effect was enhanced by epidermal growth factor and platelet-derived growth factor (Vilček et al., 1986, Palombella and Vilćek, 1989). Similarly, Sugarman et al., (1987) noted that other growth factors (EGF, TGF-α, and TGF-β) modulated the antiproliferative effects of TNF on tumor cell lines in vitro. In a subsequent study recombinant murine TNF was shown to be cytotoxic for 3T3 fibroblasts in subconfluent cultures, but in confluent cultures a dose-dependent increase of DNA synthesis was observed (Palombella and Vilćek, 1989). Subconfluent cultures of endolethial cells were more sensitive than confluent cells to the inhibitory effects of TNF, assessed by inhibition of thrombomodulin and tissue factor synthesis, and the disruption of cytoskelatal structures (Gerlach et al., 1989). Similarly, TNF was more growth inhibitory for confluent keratinocyte cultures (Pillai et al., 1989), and the cytotoxic effect of TNF in adipocyte cell lines was related to the state of differentiation (Kawakami et al., 1989).

Overall, therefore, studies with nontumorigenic cells do not support the absolute dictum that TNF is selectively toxic for tumor cells, but emphasize that the cytotoxicity of TNF in vitro depends on variables such as the state of confluence of cultures and the composition of the media used for such experiments. Indeed, the toxicity of TNF for normal cells, particularly endolethial cells, may be an essential component of the antitumor effects seen in vivo. However, there is unquestionably some degree of selectivity when tumor cells and normal cells from the same tissue are examined. Dollbaum et al. (1988) showed that in short-term culture TNF did not inhibit the growth of normal mammary epithelial cells but inhibited clonal growth of 13 out of 18 samples of malignant breast epithelium. Dealtry et al.

(1987a) also showed that normal mammary epithelial cells were resistant to TNF, whereas SV40 transformed mammary epilethial cells became increasingly sensitive to the antiproliferative effect of TNF with progression of the malignant phenotype. Motoo et al. (1986) showed that while TNF was cytostatic for a human hepatoma cell line, it had no antiproliferative activity on nontumorigenic liver cells.

B. Mechanisms Involved in TNF Cytotoxicity and Resistance

It has been estimated that approximately 40% of tumor cell lines are growth inhibited or lysed by TNF in vitro (Goeddel et al., 1986). The sensitivity of different cell lines to TNF shows considerable variation; for example, murine L929 and WEHI 164 cell lines are lysed by concentrations of TNF in the fentimolar range, whereas the sensitive human MCF-7 breast carcinoma cell line requires exposure to 10 times as much TNF to achieve a similar degree of lysis. The heterogentiy of cellular response to TNF also applies to the gross manifestations of its cytocidal effect (e.g., TNF can induce either apoptotic or necrotic forms of cell death in different tumor cell lines) (Laster et al., 1989). This indicates that TNF has different modes of action or that the effect of TNF is related to the biological characteristics of different cell populations. Although much of the evidence that will be presented indicates that the response to TNF is dictated by the constitutive properties of cells, Reid et al.,(1989) have shown that two distinct or overlapping mechanisms may be involved in TNF-mediated cytotoxicity in adipocyte cell lines. The parent adipocyte cell line was not sensitive to TNF but was lysed by a combination of TNF and cyclohexamide, while a cloned cell line was resistant to TNF and cycloheximide but lysed by TNF alone.

A variety of cellular targets and metabolic/molecular changes have been linked to the cytotoxic effect of TNF. The issue is complicated by the finding that TNF can simultaneously activate cellular mechanisms that can abrogate its own cytocidal effects (Wallach, 1984), explaining the potentiation of TNF cytotoxicity by inhibitors of protein and DNA synthesis. Studies on fused heterokaryons of TNF sensitive and TNF resistant cells have shown that TNF resistance is inherited as a dominant trait, and underline the importance of protective mechanisms in determining the cellular response to TNF (Nophar et al., 1988). In the following sections we consider some of the parameters and cellular characteristics that have been linked to the mechanisms of cytotoxicity and resistance to TNF in vitro.

1. *Phenotypic Characteristics of Cells*

Fletcher et al. (1987) reported the correlation of TNF resistance with the presence of gap junctions between cells. Gap junction competent cells such as Chinese hamster ovary cells were sensitized to TNF cytolysis by rendering them gap-junction deficient by treatment with a phorbol ester (12-*o*-tetredecanoylphorbyl-13-acetate). In addition, TNF-sensitive murine cell lines became resistant to the cytolytic effects of TNF following induction of gap junctions between the cells by treatment with 8-bromo-cyclic adenosine monophosphate. Comparison of TNF-sensitive and TNF-resistant L929 and U937 cells revealed that resistant cells differed by forming tighter colonies and showing increased plastic adherence (Matthews and Neale, 1989), although the resistant cells remained gap-junction deficient. Thus cell–cell communication may diminish the susceptibility of tumor cell lines to the cytocidal effects of TNF. Subsequently, it has been shown that resistant U937 cells have a different glycoform of an integral cell surface glycoprotein from TNF-sensitive cells, and are less metastatic than the parent cell line (Matthews et al. 1990). The importance of intercellular contact in determining the in vitro sensitivity to TNF lysis is also evident from the increased susceptibility of subconfluent cell cultures of normal and transformed cell lines, compared to confluent cultures (see Gerlach et al., 1989; Pillai et al., 1989; Patek et al., 1989).

2. *Membrane–Receptor Interactions*

TNF interacts with specific cell surface receptors and the binding of TNF to those receptors is generally thought to be essential to its cell regulatory effects (e. g., down regulation of the receptor by phorbol esters protects the cell against TNF cytotoxicity) (Johnson and Bagliono, 1988). The TNF receptor complex is internalized via classical receptor-mediated endocytosis pathway, followed by lysosomal degradation of the receptor complex and extrusion of degraded protein into the extracellular space (Kull et al., 1985; Tsujimoto et al., 1985; Mosselmans et al., 1988). There is conflicting evidence on the nonspecific membrane effects of TNF from studies with liposomal membranes. Yoshimura and Sone (1987) noted that TNF increased the permeability of liposomes at low pH, whereas another study found that TNF did not induce damage of liposomes (Roozemond et al., 1998). Indeed, it has been shown that although TNF binding to cell membranes was enhanced by low pH, stabilization of cell membranes occurred (Baldwin et al., 1988). Other lines of evidence also indicate that the cytocidal effects of TNF differ from those of pore-forming agents (e.g., the perforins) (Hasegawa and Bonavida, 1989).

Circumvention of cell surface interaction by microinjection of TNF into cells has been shown to have cytotoxic effects, suggesting that intracelluar delivery of TNF is important (Smith et al., 1990). Intriguingly, this study also showed that intracellular delivery of TNF was cytocidal for normal macrophages. It is possible, therefore, that some effects of TNF can be dissociated at the membrane level; for example, intracellular TNF may be cytocidal for macrophages because membrane interaction activates protective mechanisms. Major differences in receptor number or affinity, or subsequent degradation of the TNF-receptor complex, have not been found to account for the differential sensitivity of tumor cell lines to the cytocidal effects of TNF (Kull et al., 1985; Tsujimoto et al., 1985; Sugarman et al., 1985).

However a few reports have noted differences in these parameters between TNF sensitive and resistant cell lines (Ohsawa and Natori, 1988; Remels et al., 1989).

A receptor for TNF has been cloned recently (Loetscher et al., 1990, Schall et al., 1990), and it is likely that at least one other form of TNF receptor exists. The relationship between binding of TNF to different receptors and its antiproliferative effects are as yet undefined. Cross-linking studies in endothelial cells in various stages of confluence (Gerlach et al, 1989) and in tumor cell lines of hemopoietic epithelial origin (Hohmann et al., 1989) have suggested the existence of different classes of receptors or a single class of receptor associated with different membrane proteins. Creasey et al. (1987) reported the detection of a 138-kDa protein in a MCF-7 cells that were sensitive to the antiprolierative effects of TNF. This protein was not detected in resistant MCF-7cells or other cell lines that were not growth inhibited by TNF but nevertheless responded to the mitogenic effects of TNF. They suggested that the TNF receptor may be noncovalently associated with different membrane proteins that could determine the end response of TNF–receptor interaction. A high-molecular-weight (220=kDa) cell membrane protein (Fas) distinct from the TNF receptor was shown to be down-regulated in tandem with the TNF receptor in TNF-susceptible but not TNF-resistant cell lines. Binding of specific monoclonal antibodies to this protein mimicked the cytocidal effects of TNF (Yonehara et al., 1989). The authors suggested that interaction of TNF with its receptor and the Fas protein may be a crucial step in TNF cytotoxicity. However, more data are needed on the role of this protein in other cell regulatory effects of TNF.

An important finding has been the description of membrane-bound 26-kDa TNF as a precursor of the released 17-kDa free TNF molecule (Kriegler et al., 1988). There appears to be some conflict as to whether it is the integral membrane-bound TNF moeity, released 17-kDa TNF, that has subsequently bound to surface TNF receptors, or both that mediate cytotoxic effects (Bakouche et al., 1988). However, membrane-bound TNF can be cytocidal (Decker et al., 1987) and may act differently from free TNF. For example, it has been suggested that membrane-bound TNF abrogates the need for internalization of TNF in order to have a cytotoxic effect (Hofsli and Niessen-Meyer, 1989) and that cells resistant to free TNF are lysed by membrane-bound TNF (Peck et al, 1989). These findings may have considerable implications for TNF as an anticancer agent.

3. *Phospholipase A_2 (PLA_2) and Arachadonic Acid*

An essential step in the cytotoxic effect of TNF may be the involvement of arachadonic acid (AA) metabolism (Suffys et al., 1987; Neale et al., 1988). TNF activates PLA_2 with release of AA and prostaglandins from cells that are lysed by TNF, but not from their resistant sublines. Inhibition of PLA_2 activity by dexamethasone and quinacrine abrogates not only TNF cytotoxicity, but also the mitogenic effects of TNF (Palombell and Vilček, 1989). Therefore, the essential difference between sensitive and resistant cell lines must lie elsewhere, possibly related to the subsequent metabolism of AA by the lipoxygenase, cyclogenase, or the cytochrome P450 pathways. Inhibition of the lipoxygenase and cyclooxygenase pathways does not abrogate TNF cytotoxicity. Inhibitors of cytochrome P450 such as SKF525A and benzphetamine do inhibit TNF cytotoxicity, but by-products of the activation of this pathway have been difficult to detect and the specificity of the inhibitors is debatable, (Matthews et al., 1987). Further evidence for the involvement of AA in the cytotoxic effect of TNF was provided by the demonstration that exogenous AA rendered a TNF resistant cell line sensitive to TNF lysis, (Hori et al., 1989). TNF susceptibility was not, however, related to the amount of AA generated by the exposure of cells to TNF, as resistant and sensitive cell lines released comparable amounts of AA, nor was a high concentration of AA toxic per se. More likely was the possibility that the provision of sufficient quantities of AA allowed the participation of AA in metabolic pathways that led to the overwhelming of the protective mechanisms of the cell, and generation of metabolic intermediates that led to cell death. The other by-products of PLA_2 activation (i.e., the lysophospholipids) were not cytotoxic for TNF susceptible cell lines, and there is little evidence that continued PLA_2 activation leads to membrane damage (N. Mathews, personal communication). Free radicals generated at the membrane or the mitochondria during AA metabolism may cause cellular damage. Matthews et al. (1987) compared the time course of release of malonyldealdehyde (MDA), and end product of lipid peroxidation, and cell death in TNF-susceptible cells. They concluded that the increased production of MDA in the cells was a late secondary event rather than an early step in the cytolytic process. Overall, it is still possible that PLA_2 activation is not directly related to the cytolytic processes evoked by TNF, and that other mechanisms are being activated simultaneously.

4. *Free-Radical Generation*

Earlier investigations with rabbit tumor necrosis serum suggested a role for free-radical generation in the cytotoxic effect of TNF with the mitrochondrion as a selected intracellular target (Matthews, 1983). This issue has yet to be settled satisfactorily—scavengers of reactive oxygen species added to in vitro cultures have had variable inhibitory effects on TNF cytotoxicity (Matthews et al., 1987; Suffys et al., 1987), but other lines of evidence continue to keep the free-radical hypothesis alive. Zimmerman et al. (1989) looked at intracellular glutathione and oxidized glutathione levels in TNF-resistant and TNF-sensitive cell lines, Susceptibility to TNF lysis and oxidative damage to cellular DNA correlated with the relative levels of oxidized and reduced glutathione, (i.e., the buffering capacity of the cell). However, Meth A sarcoma cells were not lysed by TNF, despite having a low radical-scavenging capacity. The generation of the hydroxyl radical, an extremely potent oxidant, has been implicated in studies showing inhibition of TNF cytotoxicity by hydroxyl radical scavengers of varying specificity, such as desferroxamine, promethazine, and 2,2′-bipyridine (Matthews et al., 1987; Suffys et al., 1987; Yamamauchi et al., 1989). Direct measurement of hydroxyl radical generation correlated with the time course of TNF cytotoxicity in TNF-susceptible cell lines and increase in hydroxyl radical production was not detected in TNF-resistant cells (Yamauchi et al., 1989). Perhaps the most compelling evidence for the involvement of free radicals in TNF cytotoxicity is the demonstration that the protection induced to the cytolytic effects of TNF by prior exposure to TNF or IL-1 (Wallach, 1984) can be correlated to TNF and IL-1 induced synthesis of manganese superoxide dimutase (MnSOD) (Wong and Goeddel, 1988), a mitochondrial antioxidant enzyme that protects cells from reactive oxygen species. Elegant experiments showed that transfection of a human embryonic kidney cell line with the MnSOD gene with or without antisense MnSOD cDNA decreased or increased susceptibility in proportion to the expression of MnSOD by the cells (Wong et al., 1989). Modulation of MnSOD levels in clones of the ME180 cervical carcinoma cell line gave similar results. However, the induction of MnSOD did not fully abrogate TNF cytotoxicity or totally parallel the protective effect of prior exposure to TNF in these cell lines. This suggested that other TNF-induced proteins, such as ferritin (Torti et al., 1988), may contribute to neutralization of reactive oxygen species. However, these results do indicate that the mitochondrion is an important cellular target for TNF in some cell lines supporting earlier data (Matthews, 1983) and more recent findings showing the inhibition of electron transfer in TNF-susceptible cell lines (Lancaster et al., 1989).

5. *Lysosomes, Proteases, and DNA Damage*

Other biochemical events that have been linked to the cytotoxic effect of TNF include the activation of lysomal enzymes, endonucleases, proteases, and ADP ribosylation. The cytotoxic effect of TNF can be inhibited by a variety of protease inhibitors (Baglioni et al., 1987). More recent data indicate that activation of a serine protease is involved in TNF-susceptible cells as a late rather than an early event in the cytotoxic cascade initiated by the TNF (Suffys et al., 1988). The source of the protease is not known, but apparently it was not of lysomal origin, as lysosomotropic amines (ammonium chloride or chloroquine) did not inhibit the lysis of ME-180 cells by TNF and cyclohexamide (Baglioni et al., 1987). Other investigators have suggested an important role of lysosomal activation in TNF induced cytolysis (Watanabe et al., 1988a). The early uptake of the lysosomotropic probeacridine orange into lysosomes was shown to correlate with TNF sensitivity in a panel of cell lines (Haranaka et al., 1987a). Liddil et al.(1989) showed that TNF cytolysis of L929 cells was inhibited by a variety of lysosomotropic agents, including ammonium chloride and more specifically, by a β-glucuronidase inhibitor (D-saccharic acid lactone). In addition, they demonstrated that the basal levels of β-glucuronidase were greater in TNF-sensitive compared to TNF-resistant 19229 cells and could not confirm that TNF sensitivity was related to intracellular thiol levels, ATP depletion, or DNA strand damage. DNA strand damage has, however, been noted in L929 cells (cf. Zimmerman et al., 1989) and other cell lines (Dealtry et al., 1987b), and these differing results may indicate technical variation in different studies. Two mechanisms of DNA strand damage have been proposed—free-radical-induced damage and the activation of endonucleases. The evidence for the latter is based on the inhibition of TNF cytotoxicity by Zn^{2+} (but not other divalent cations), a known inhibitor of endonucleases (Dealtry et al., 1987b; Flieger et al., 1989). There is also as yet unpublished data showing direct activation of endonucleases in cell cytosol by TNF (see Smith et al., 1990). ADP ribosylation has been linked to the cytotoxic action of TNF in L929 cells, although it is not known whether this was observed as a consequence of DNA fragmentation or whether this process is involved in the generation of other protein intermediates in the cytotoxic process (Aggarwal et al., 1988).

6. *Miscellaneous Mechanisms*

Other mechanisms may be involved in the cytotoxic effects of TNF, as suggested by the increased susceptibility of cells to TNF lysis by transfection of NIH-3T3 fibroblasts with adenovirus E1A oncogene (but not *ras* or c-*myc* oncogenes) (Chen et al., 1987), but this effect may not be specific to TNF cytotxicity only (Cook et al., 1989). The expression of the viral gene product pp60$^{v\text{-}src}$ correlated with the loss of gap junctions in a normal rat kidney cell line and increased susceptibility to TNF cytotoxicity. Conversely, transfection of NIH-3T3 cells with the HER/ERBB2 oncogene was shown to confer resistance to TNF, but the underlying mechanism is not known (Hudziak et al., 1988). Reports of the synergistic effects of other cytokines (γ-interferon and IL-1) (Sugarman et al., 1985, Fransen et al., 1986b; Ruggiero and Baglioni, 1987) and inhibitors of DNA topoisomerase II (Coffman et al., 1989) may yet uncover other mechanisms of TNF toxicity. Induction of heat-shock proteins in tumor cells may also lead to TNF resistance (Jäättelä et al., 1989), although the potentiation of TNF cytotoxicity by increased temperatures has been reported more commonly (Gromkowski et al., 1989; Dubois et al., 1989).

The overall impression from in vitro studies of the mechanisms of TNF cytotoxicity is one of heterogeneity between different cell lines and the dependence on the experimental conditions. For example, microfilament lattice dissolution has been shown to be an early event in the cytotoxicity of TNF in a mouse fibroblast cell line (Scanlon et al., 1989). The potentiation of TNF cytotoxicity by microfilament disrupting agents such as cytochalasin B in this cell line is not, however, seen in other cell lines, where these agents have been found to inhibit TNF cytotoxicity (Watanabe et al., 1988a). The presence of growth factors also affects the antiproliferative effects of TNF (Sugarman et al., 1987). Cytokines induced by TNF (e.g. IL-6) (Kohase et al., 1988) may also modulate its cell regulatory effects. Indeed, the induction of TNF in cell lines exposed to TNF has been linked to the development of TNF resistance (Rubin et al., 1986, Spriggs et al., 1987) but is not a necessary prerequisite for TNF resistance in all cell lines (Pfreundshuh et al., 1989).

III. ANTITUMOR ACTIVITY OF TNF IN VIVO

A large body of data has been collected on the antitumor activities of TNF in experimental murine tumor models and human tumor xenograft models in nude mice. In addition to direct antiproliferative effects on tumor cells, TNF can activate other antitumor mechanisms such as tumoricidal macrophages (Talmadge et al., 1987; Watanabe et al., 1988b), cytotoxic T cells (Nakano et al., 1989) natural killer cells (Ostensen et al., 1987), and neutrophils (Shalaby et al., 1985; Shau, 1988). Furthermore, TNF can affect the interaction of the host and tumor by effects on host stromal cell populations and induce the release of other cytokines (e.g., IL-1 and IL-6) that may have antitumor effects. Some of the major findings from studies in both murine cancer models and in human tumor xenograft models are discussed in the following sections.

The classical tumor used for the study of the antitumor effects of TNF is the Meth A sarcoma mouse model (Carswell et al., 1975; Haranaka et al., 1984; Sohmura et al., 1986; Creasey et al., 1986; Palladino et al., 1987; Manda et al., 1987). Intravenous or intratumoral injection of tumor necrosis serum or recombinant TNF leads to hemorrhagic necrosis of subcutaneous Meth A tumors within 24 h. The antitumor effect was dose dependent and the cure rates of tumor-bearing mice increased with higher doses and increased frequency of administration of TNF (Creasey et al., 1986; Tamura et al., 1989). As the growth of Meth A sarcoma cells is not inhibited by TNF in vitro, the antitumor effect of TNF in vivo is mediated indirectly, and the induction of hemorrhagic necrosis suggests a profound effect on tumor vasculature. Early damage to tumor vasculature was detected by following the metabolic changes in Meth A tumors by nuclear magnetic resonance studies. The changes seen were very similar to those seen in ischaemic necrosis (Shine et al., 1989). In addition, only well-established Meth A subcutaneous tumors underwent necrosis after TNF administration, while intraperitoneal and early Meth A tumors were resistant to the effects of TNF (Palladino et al., 1987; Manda et al., 1987). These observations indicate that the development of tumor vasculature or a host immune response to the tumor is essential to the phenomenon of hemorrhagic necrosis in this model. Thus the picture that has emerged in the Meth A sarcoma model is one of TNF-induced vasculature damage, due to a direct effect of TNF on tumor vasculature and/or indirectly by activation of host cells, with concomitant induction of intravascular thrombosis and fibrin deposition (Naworth et al., 1988). This process is facilitated by the procoagulant activities of TNF on vascular endolethium (reviewed in Pober, 1987). The end result is ischemic necrosis of the central portions of the tumor. Large tumors may subsequently regrow at the periphery unless TNF administration is replaced or initiated with higher doses (Tamura et al., 1989). Palladino et al.(1987) have also shown that mice cured of Meth A tumors by TNF are subsequently resistant to challenge by the tumors and that this effect is mediated by T cells. This confirmed the observations of Haranaka et al.(1984) that hemorrhagic necrosis of Meth A tumors was more difficult to elicit in nude mice. Additional mechanisms that may be operative in this model are the suppression of tumor cell TGF-β production (Figari et al., 1989), and TNF-induced release of IL-1 and IL-6 (Nakamura et al., 1986; Mule et al., 1990).

The marked effects of TNF on tumor vasculature have been noted in other murine tumor models. Using the murine SA1 sarcoma, Havell et al. (1988) showed that the extravasation of red cells into tumor following intravenous TNF injection was an early event and was partially T-cell dependent. Intravenous TNF was also shown to lead to a rapid decrease of tumor blood flow in murine colon 26 tumors, and endogenous TNF produced following administration of flavone acetic acid acted similarly (Madhevan et al., 1990). Vascular effects of TNF administration have been described in a rat carcinosarcoma model (Kalllinowski et al., 1989) and in Friend leukemia cell tumors in mice (Proetti et al., 1988). Therefore, it would appear that the antitumor effect in vivo is based on the ability of TNF to damage tumor vasculature selectively. The observation that TNF was cytotoxic for early endothelial cultures in vitro suggests that newly developing vasculature is especially vulnerable to TNF (Gerlach et al., 1989). Kawai et al. (1987) showed that TNF-induced hemorrhagic necrosis in normal granulation tissue. In another study TNF did not cause damage of the nascent vasculature of autologuous or semiallogenic skin grafts (McIntosh et al.,1990). Thus there may be inherent differences between newly formed tumor and normal endothelium to explain the selective effect of TNF on tumor vasculature. An alternative mechanism proposed by Naworth et al.(1988) is the production of tumor-derived soluble proteins that enhance the procoagulant action of TNF on tumor endothelium.

The relevance of murine tumors to the assessment of the therapeutic potential of TNF in the treatment of human cancer has been questioned because of the immunogenicity of chemically induced tumors such as the Meth A sarcoma. Immunogenicity of tumors is undoubtedly a major factor in determining the antitumor activity of TNF in vivo. A comparative study of the effect of TNF in chemically induced tumors of varying immunogenicity showed that the antiproliferative effects of TNF and hemorrhagic necrosis were significantly greater in mice with immunogenic tumors than those with tumors of low immunogenicity (Asher et al., 1987).

The limitations of murine tumor models has led to investigations of the antitumor activity of TNF in human tumor xenograft models in nude mice. These are clearly limited by the absence of a T-cell repertoire. However, as TNF is essentially nonspecies specific, the interaction of the tumor and the host can be observed at other levels. Most studies have investigated the effect of TNF on subcutaneous hu-

Table 1 Studies of TNF in Human Tumor Xenograft Models

Study	Tumors	Reference
1	Melanoma Colon cancer Testicular cancer	Helson et al., 1979
2	Gastric cancer Melanoma Nasopharangeal cancer	Haranaka et al., 1984
3	Breast Colorectal cancer Ovarian cancer	Balkwill et al., 1986
4	Ovarian cancer	Creasey et al., 1986
5	Melanoma Lung cancer Neuroblastoma	Sohmura et al., 1986
6	Intraperitoneal ovarian cancer	Balkwill et al., 1987 (b)
7	Gastric carcinoma	Haranaka et al., 1984
8	Ovarian carcinoma Uterine carcinoma	Suzumori et al., 1987
9	Gastric cancer Breast cancer Gallbladder cancer Esophageal cancer Liposarcoma	Nosoh et al., 1988

man tumor xenografts of varying origin (see Table 1). Early studies showed that mouse tumor necrosis serum had growth inhibitory effects on subcutaneous human tumor xenografts established from tumor cell lines of diverse origin, including malignant melanomas, gastrointestinal cancer, nasopharyngeal cancer, lymphoma, and cancer of the cervix (Helson et al., 1979; Haranaka et al., 1984). The results indicated that after early necrosis of tumors, tumor regrowth occurred and repeated administration of tumor necrosis serum was necessary for continued suppression of tumor growth. This finding has been confirmed using recombinant TNF in several studies, and in some studies where the treatment duration has been extended, complete tumor regression has been noted (Nosoh et al., 1987). All the studies that have looked at dose-response relationships and routes of administration have noted that high doses and intratumoral injection are most effective (Sohmura et al., 1986;

Suzumori et al., 1987; Nosoh et al., 1987; Balkwill et al., 1987a) Hemorrhagic necrosis of human tumor xenografts following TNF administration has been reported (Nosoh et al., 1987).

The antitumor efficacy of local/locoregional administration of TNF against subcutaneous human tumor xenografts has led to the study of the antitumor effects of intracavity TNF administration, particularly intraperitoneal human ovarian cancer xenograft models (Balkwill et al., 1987b; Creasey et al., 1986; Manetta et al., 1989; Rubin et al., 1989). In a study of the intraperitoneal therapy of three intraperitioneal human ovarian cancer xenografts, survival of nude mice was prolonged significantly in mice bearing two of the the three tumors (Balkwill et al., 1987b). TNF has been shown to be effective in curing intraperitoneal ovarian cancer established in nude mice following intraperitoneal injection of the NIH OVCAR-3 cell line if given intraperitioneally (Manetta et al., 1989) but not intravenously (Creasey et al., 1986), confirming that high local concentrations are needed to achieve an antitumor effect. In summary, the antitumor actions of TNF in human tumor xenograft models indicate that TNF does have dose-dependent growth inhibitory effects, particularly if given intratumorally. The precise mechanisms of these effects have not been fully elucidated and are likely to involve indirect actions of TNF on the host-tumor interactions. The effect on tumor vasculature in the nude mouse-human tumor xenograft models has not been studied as extensively as in murine tumor models, but the overall impression is that the phenomenon of hemorrhagic necrosis is less pronounced. This may reflect the absence of T-cell mediated mechanisms in these models rather than a real difference between murine and human tumors.

IV. TNF IN COMBINATIONS WITH OTHER TREATMENT MODALITIES

A. Cytokines

The direct antiproliferative effects ofTNF on tumor cells in vitro can be enhanced by cytokines such as γ-interferon (INF-γ) (Sugarman et al., 1985: Fransen et al., 1986b), and IL-1 (Ruggiero and Baglioni, 1987). TNF can also potentiate the tumoricidal mechanisms activated by other cytokines; for example, the generation of lymphokine-activated (LAK) killer cells by interleukin-2 (IL-2) (Owen-Schaub et al., 1988), and the activation of tumoricidal macrophages and polymorphonuclear leuocyctes by IFN-γ (Hori et al., 1987; Shalaby et al., 1985). Several investigators have looked at the antitumor effects of combinations of TNF and other cytokines in vivo. Brouckaert et al.(1986) reported additive effects of murine recombinant IFN-γ and human recombinant TNF in the treatment of subcutaneous B16BL6 murine melanoma tumors, and Marquet et al. (1987) showed similar effects in a rat colon cancer model using recombinant murine TNF and recombinant rat IFN-γ. Both groups commented on the toxicity of the combination, which could be reduced by simultaneous administration. Balkwill et al. (1987b) reported on the synergistic effects of human recombinant IFN-γ and recombinant human TNF given intraperitoneally in the therapy of intraperitoneal human ovarian cancer xenografts. In further studies (unpublished data), it has been shown that the synergistic effect can also be seen with murine recombinant IFN-γ, showing that the synergy can occur because of direct effects on tumor cells, or by potentiation of host antitumor mechanisms. Other studies have reported additive/synergistic effects of IFN-γ and TNF in human ovarian cancer xenograft models (Rubin et al., 1989; Manetta et al., 1989).

The additive antitumor effects of TNF in combination with IL-2 in murine tumor models have been reported in studies in murine tumor models. Winkelhake et al. (1987) showed that TNF in combination with IL-2 completely inhibited subcutaneous tumor takes of five different murine tumors, although either cytokine administered alone had little activity. The maximal antitumor effects were seen when the maximal tolerated dose of TNF was given, whereas the IL-2 dose could be reduced by 90% of the maximal tolerated dose. The combination was less effective against intraperitoneal tumors, but did inhibit the development of melanoma pulmonary metastases if administered early after tumor injection. The antitumor effects of TNF in combination with IL-2 were reported against established MCA-induced sarcoma pulmonary metastases (Agah et al., 1988). The effects were diminished in immunosuppressed mice and were maximal when IL-2 was administered before TNF. McIntosh et al. (1988) also reported on the synergistic antitumor effects of TNF and IL-2 against subcutaneous murine sarcomas and noted that the antitumor activities were minimal against nonimmunogenic sarcomas. In contrast to the study of Agah et al. (1987), they showed that IL-2 could be administered after TNF and still show significant additive antitumor effects. In a subsequent study they confirmed the importance of tumor immunogenicity to the antitumor effect of TNF and IL-2 and showed that further cures and prolongation of survival were achieved by the addition of IFN-α (McIntosh et al., 1989). Nishimura et al., (1987) showed TNF/IL-2 synergy in the treatment of intradermal mouse MBL-2 lymphoma when the cytokines were administered intratumorally. Mice cured of tumor were developed immunity to rechallenge with the tumor, and splenocytes from cured mice demonstrated cytotoxic activity against MBL-2 tumor cells. Most of the investigations of TNF/IL-2 synergy in vivo showed that this was dependent on the presence of T cells and immunogenic tumors. Although the induction of LAK activity has been reported in athymic mice, TNF did not potentiate the antitumor effect of IL-2 in nude mice bearing murine tumors (Winkelhake et al., 1987).

A recent report of the synergistic actions of high-dose recombinant IL-6 in combination with TNF against several murine tumors (Mule et al., 1990) is of considerable interest, as this cytokine is induced by TNF in vivo. IL-6 was less toxic than

IL-2 in these experiments, and the antitumor effect was abolished by prior sublethal irradiation of the mice. Other cytokines could theoretically enhance the antitumor effects of TNF (e. g., IL-1 and the colony-stimulating factors), but there are no reported studies of their use in vivo.

B. Cytoxic Drugs and Other Agents

The additive antiproliferative effects of cytotoxic drugs that inhabit DNA topoisomerase II was reported in vitro and in a murine bladder cancer model in vivo (Alexander et al., 1987 a, b). Subsequent studies have shown additive antitumor effects of other classes of cytotoxic drugs and TNF in murine tumor models (Nakata et al., 1986; Regenass et al., 1987; Haranaka et al., 1987b: Krosnick et al., 1989). These studies have suggested that the interactions between cytotoxic drugs and TNF can also diminish it by suppressing immune effector mechanisms, increasing toxicity, and inhibiting the development of TNF sensitive targets, (e.g. tumor vasculature). TNF has also been noted to have increased antitumor effects in vivo when combined with hyperthermia (Haranaka et al., 1984b; Watanabe et al., 1988c) and antibody-drug conjugates (Smyth et al., 1988) in murine tumor models.

V. TNF AND TUMOR METASTASIS

A small number of studies of TNF in experimental metastasis models have been reported (Talmadge et al., 1987: Tomazic et al., 1988; Scheringa et al., 1989; Nishiyama et al., 1989). In the B16-BL6 mouse melanoma model moderate but significant dose-dependent inhibition of spontaneous and experimental metastasis was observed with intravenous administration of recombinant human TNF (Talmadge et al., 1987), while in a rat liver metastasis model high-dose TNF administered by continuous infusion was only minimally effective (Scheringa et al., 1989). Nishiyama et al.(1989) noted that continuous 10-day administration of TNF following the injection of mouse colon-26 tumor cells into the superior mesentric vein of CDF1 mice led to an increase in the number of liver metastases. Only pretreatment of mice with TNF prior to tumor injection was shown to decrease the number of liver metasteses. Interestingly, the antimetastatic effects of TNF were noted only after early intravenous injection in a study of the number of lung metastases following the intravenous injection of a chemically induced murine fibrosarcoma (Tomazic et al., 1988). These studies suggest that TNF is not a very effective agent in preventing tumor metastasis and indeed can occasionally enhance metastasis.

We have conducted a detailed analysis of the effects of intraperitoneal TNF in ovarian cancer xenografts and noted that while TNF led to necrosis of ascitic tumor, it also promoted the adhesion and establishment of solid tumor implants on the peritoneal surface and the intraabdominal viscera (Malik et al., 1989) (Fig. 1). Furthermore, the promotion of peritoneal metastases was shown to be independent of antitumor activity. In subsequent studies we have shown that the antitumor effect and the enhancement of peritoneal metastasis of TNF in these models are not related to the pronounced neutrophil infiltration of the peritoneal cavity following TNF injection. Two factors that we have identified as potential contributors to the TNF-induced enhanced peritoneal implantation are the increased adherence of tumor cells to the peritoneal surface and the stromal proliferation caused by intraperitoneal injection of recombinant TNF. Increased adhesiveness of tumor cells to endothelium after exposure to TNF has also been described (Rice et al., 1988).

The findings in our ovarian cancer xenograft models have led us to study the metastatic behavior of cell lines that constitutively secrete TNF. Chinese hamster ovary (CHO) cells that had been transfected with the human TNF gene (CHO/TNF cells) or the transfection vector alone (CHO/NEO cells)(Oliff et al., 1987) were injected intraperitoneally into nude mice and histological examination of mouse tissues conducted at 4 to 14 days after injection. There was a distinct difference in behavior of the TNF transfectant compared to the CHO/NEO cells. Mice injected with the former died earlier of ascitic disease and mice in the latter group died of solid abdominal tumors. Microscopic examination of the nude mouse tissues revealed marked invasion of the peritoneal and hepatic surfaces with CHO/TNF cells, while tissues taken at the same time points from mice injected with CHO/NEO cells were normal. The enhanced invasiveness of the TNF producing cells was confirmed by localizing radiolabeled cells after intraperitoneal injection (Fig. 2). These studies have also shown that CHO/TNF cells were able to metastasize to the lungs (data not shown). Metastasis to the lungs and the invasion of the peritoneal and liver surfaces was specifically inhibited by anti-TNF antibodies (Malik et al., 1990).

VI. CONCLUSIONS

The last few years have yielded a considerable amount of information on the antiproliferative effects of TNF in vitro and in vivo. TNF has been used in several clinical trials (Blick et al., 1987; Creaven et al., 1987; Kimura et al., 1987; Selby et

Figure 1 Peritoneal biopsies from nude mice with intraperitoneal ovarian cancer xenograph (OS) treated for 3 weeks with daily intraperitoneal injections of (a) diluent and (b) recombinant human TNF (1 μg/day). Tumor cells stained for tumor-associated antigen (HMFG 2) by indirect immunoperoxidase method. Note free-floating tumor cells in (a) and peritoneal implanation of tumor cells (arrows) in (b). P, peritoneal surface.

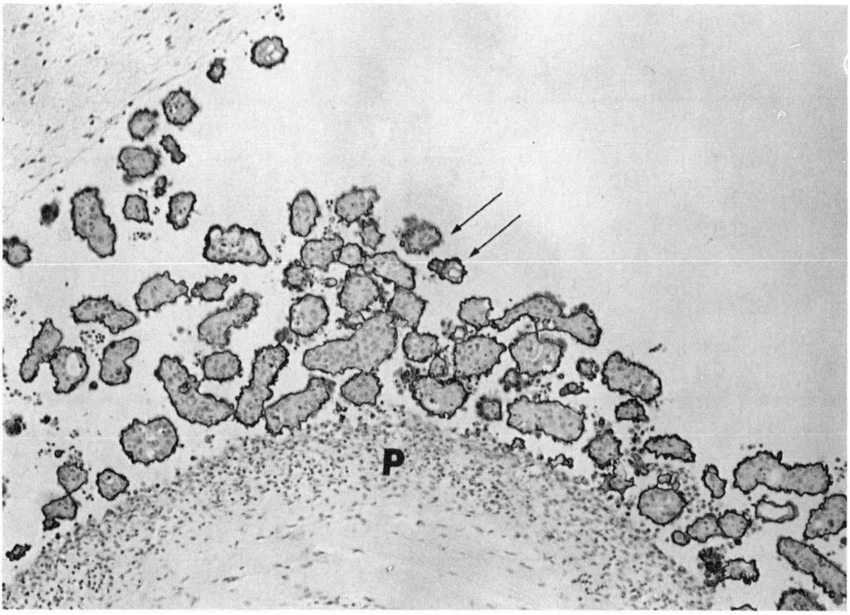

(a)

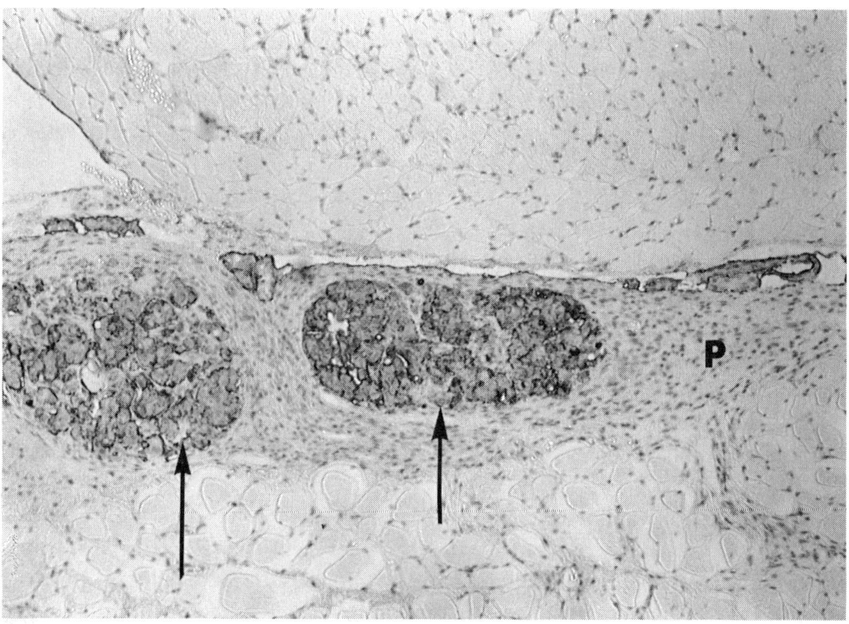

(b)

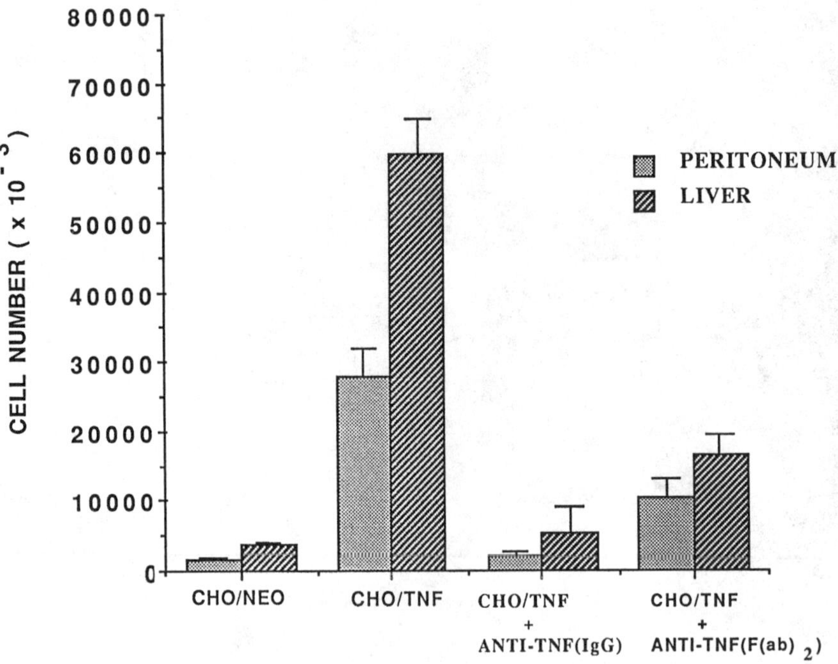

Figure 2 Localization of ^{125}I-radiolabelled CHO/NEO cells and CHO/TNF cells in the peritoneum and liver 1 week after intraperitoneal injection of 5×10^6 cells. The localization of CHO/TNF cells is reduced by concomitant injection of anti-TNF monoclonal antibody [whole IgG or $F(ab)_2$ fragment].

al., 1987; Feinburg et al., 1988; Spriggs et al., 1988). Although most reported trials are phase I studies, the overall response rate of approximately 1% is not promising. The few small phase II trials that have been reported are also disappointing (Lenk et al., 1989). It has been pointed out that based on experimental animal data, the optimal doses of TNF needed for antitumor activity have not been given (Frei and Spriggs, 1989). The response rates of 40 to 50% noted in some clinical trials of intratumoral TNF tend to confirm the dose dependency of the antitumor effect of TNF in vivo (Taguchi et al., 1987; Diehl et al., 1987). However, intratumoral TNF is of limited clinical use, and its efficacy has not been confirmed by others (Retsas et al., 1989).

Other issues relevant to the clinical use of TNF have been raised by experimental studies. A recent study showed that the TNF-sensitive WEHI 164 murine fibrosarcoma cell line, exquisitely sensitive to TNF in vitro, became rapidly resistant after transplantation into mice. (Lattime and Stutman, 1989). Wong and Goeddel (1988) have shown that MnSOD can be induced by TNF in vivo. A significant proportion of patients entered into TNF trials are likely to have been exposed to endogenous TNF released as a result of the infectious complications of standard therapy. Therefore, the poor response rates seen thus far may be due to the induction of TNF resistance by the prior therapy of such patients. Increasing interest is therefore likely to be directed at trials of recombinant TNF or its muteins (Gatanga et al., 1989), in combination with other cytokines (such as the interferons, interleukins-2, IL-1, and IL-6) or cytotoxic drugs. Such cytokine cocktails may yet achieve impressive response rates seen with Coley's toxins (Coley-Nauts et al., 1953). However, it is equally evident that the roles of TNF in cancer pathophysiology, for example, as a possible autocrine growth factor and a promoter of metastatic (Cordingley et al., 1988; Malik et al, 1990), or as a mediator of metabolic and hematological disturbances in cancer (Oliff et al., 1987; Johnson et al., 1989; Lindemann et al., 1989), will need to be studied further. The seemingly perverse possibility that some future cancer therapies may be based in neutralization of TNF activity cannot be discounted.

REFERENCES

Agah, R., Malloy, B., Sherrod, A., Bean, P., Girgis, E., and mazumder, A., (1989). Therapy of dissemated NK-resistant tumor by the synergistic effects of recombinant interleukin-2 and tumor necrosis factor, *J. Biol. Response Mod.* *7*:140–151.

Aggarwal, S., Drysdale, B. E., and Shin, H. S. (1988).Tumor necrosis factor-mediated cytotoxicity involves ADP-ribosylation, *J. Immunol., 140*: 4187–4192.

Algire, G. H., Legallais, F. Y., Anderson, B. F. (1952). Vascular reactions of normal and malignant cells in vivo. V. Role of hypotension in action of bacterial polysaccharide on tumors, *J. Natl. Cancer Inst., 12*:1279–1295.

Alexander, R. B., Nelson, W. G., and Coffey, D. S. (1987a). Synergistic enhancement by tumor necrosis factor of in vitro cytotoxicity from chemotherapuetic agents targeted at DNA toopisomerase II, *Bancer Res., 47*:2403-2406.

Alexander R. B., Isaacs, J. D., and Coffey, D. S. (1987b). Tumor necrosis factor enhances the in vitro and the in vivo efficacy of cytotoxic drugs targeted at DNA topoisomerse II in the treatment of murine bladder caner, *J. Urol., 138*:427–429.

Asher, A., Mule, J. J., Reichert, C. M., Shiloni, E., and Rosenberg, S. A. (1987). Studies on the antitumor efficacy of systemically administered recombinant tumor necrosis factor against several murine tumors in vivo, *J. Immunol. 138*: 963-974.

Bakouche, O., Ichinise, Y., Heicappell, R., Fidler. I. J., and Lachman, L. B. (1988). Plasma membrane-associated tumor necrosis factor: a non-intregral membrane protein possibly bound to its own receptor, *J. Immunol. 140*:1142–1147.

Baglioni, C., Ruggero, V., Latham, K., and Johnson, S. E. (1987). Cytocidal activity of tumor necrosis factor: protection by protease inhibitors, *Ciba Found. Symp. 131*:52–61.

Baldwin, R. L., Chang, M. P., Bramhall, J., Graves, S., Bonavida, B., and Wisieski, B. J., (1988). Capacity of tumor necrosis factor to bind and penetrate membranes is pH dependent. *J. Immunol., 141*:2352–2357.

Balkwill, F. R. (1989). *Cytokines in Cancer Therapy*, Chap 8, Oxford University Press, Oxford.

Balkwill, F. R., Lee, A., Aldam, G., Moodie, E., Thomas, A.., Tavernier, J., and Fiers, W. (1986). Human tumor xenografts treated with recombinant human tumor necrosis factor alone or in combination with interferons. *Cancer Res., 46*: 3990–3993.

Balkwill F., Osborne, R.., Burke, F., Naylor, S., Talbot, D., Durbin, H., Tavernier, J., and Fiers, W. (1987a). Evidence for tumor necrosis factor/cachetin production in cancer, *Lancet,* 2: 1229–1232.

Balkwill, F. R., Ward, B. G., Moodie, E., and Fiers, W., (1987b). Therapeutic potential of tumor necrosis factor alpha and gamma interferon in experimental human ovarian cancer, *Cancer Res., 47*:4755–4758.

Beissert, S., Bergholz, M., Waase, I., Lepsien, G., Schauer, A., Pfizenmaier, K., and Kronke, M., (1989). Regulation of tumor necrosis factor gene expression in colorectal adenocarcinoma in vivo analysis by in situ hybridization. *Proc. Natl. Acad. Sci. USA, 86*: 5064–5068.

Bertolini, D. R., Nedwin, G. E., Bringman, T. S., Smith, D. D., and Mundy, G. R. (1986). Stimulation of bone resorption and inhibition of bone formation in vitro by human tumor necrosis factors. *Nature, 319*:516–518.

Beutler, B., and Cerami, A., (1989). The biology of cachectin/TNF—a primary mediator of the host response, *Ann. Rev Immunol. 7*:625–655.

Blick, M., Sherwin, S. A.., Rosenblum, M., and Gutterman, J. (1987). Phase I study of recombinant tumor necrosis factor in cancer patients, *Cancer Res. 47*: 2986–2989.

Brouckaert, P. G. G., Leroux-Roels, G. G., Guisez, Y., Tavernier, J., and Fiers, W. (1986).In vivo antitumor activity of recombinant human and murine TNF, alone and in combination with murine IFN-g on a synergenic murine melanoma, *Int. J. Cancer, 38*:763–769.

Carswell, E. A., Old, L. J., Kassel, R. J., Green, S., Fiore, N. and Williamson, B. (1975). An endotoxin-induced serum factor that causes necrosis of tumors, *Proc. Natl. Acad. Sci. USA, 72*:3666–3670.

Chen, M. J., Holskin, B., Strickler, J., Gorniak, J., Clark, M. A. , Johnson, P. J., Mitcho, M., and Shalloway, D. (1987). Induction by E1A oncogene expression of cellular susceptibility to lysis by TNF, *Nature, 330*: 581–583.

Coffman, F. D., Green, L. M., Godwin, A., Ware, C. F. (1989).Cytotoxicity mediated by tumor necrosis factor in variant subclones of the ME-180 cervical carcinoma line: modulation by specific inhibitors of DNA topoisomerase II, *J. Cell. Biochem., 39*:95–105.

Cook, J. L., May, D. L., Wilson, B. A., Holskin, B., Chen, M. J., Shalloway, D., and Walker, T. A. (1989). Role of tumor necrosis factor alpha in E1A oncogene induced susceptibility of neoplastic cells to lysis by natural killer cells and activated mcarophages, *J. Immunol., 142*:4527–34.

Coley-Nauts, H., Fowler, G. A., and Bogatko, F. H. (1953). A review of the influence of bacterial and of bacterial products (Coley's toxims) on maliganant tumors in man, *Acta Med. Scand. (suppl.)*, (7): 729–97.

Cordingley, F. T., Bianchi, A., Hoffbrand, A. V., Reittie, J. E., Heslop, H. E., Vyakarnam, A., Turner, M., Meager, A., Brenner, M. K., (1988). Tumor necrosis factor as an autocrine tumor growth factor for chronic B-cell malignancies. *Lancet, 1*:969–971.

Creasey, A. A., Reynolds, M. T., and Laird, W. (1986). Cures and partial regression of murine and human tumors by recombinant human tumor necrosis factor. *Cancer Res. 465*: 687-5690.

Creasey, A. A., Yamamoto, R., and Vitt, C. R. (1987). A high molecular weigh component of the human tumor necrosis factor receptor is associated with cytotoxicity, *Proc. Natl. Acad. Sci. USA, 84*: 3293-3297.

Creaven, P. J., Plager, J. E., Dupere, S., Huben, R. P., Takita, H., Mittelman, A., and Proefrock, A. (1987). Phase I clinical trial of recombinant human tumor necrosis factor, *Cancer Chemother. Pharamacol, 20*:223-229.

Dealtry, G. B., Naylor, M. S., Fiers, W., Balkwill, F. R. (1987a). The effect of recombinant tumor necrosis factor on the growth and macromolecular synthesis of human epithelial cells, *Exp. Cell. Res., 170*: 428-438.

Dealtry, G. B., Naylor, M. S., Fiers, W. and Balkwill, F. R. (1987b). DNA fragmentation and cytotoxicity caused by tumor necrosis factor is enhanced by interferon-γ, *Eur. J. Immunol. 17*: 689-693.

Decker, T., Lohmann-Mattes, M. and Gifford, G. E. (1987). Cell-associated tumor necrosis factor (TNF) as a killing mechanism of activated cytotoxic macrophages, *J. Immunol., 138*: 957-962.

Diehl, V., Pfreundschuh, M., Steinmetz, M. T., and Schaadt, M. (1987). Phase I studies of recombinant human tumor necrosis factor in patients with advanced cancer, *Tumor Necrosis Factor and Related Cytokines* B. Bonavida, G. Clifford, H. Kirchner, and L. J. Old, (eds.) S. Karger, Basel; pp. 183-188.

Dollbaum, C., Creasey, A. A., Dairkee, S. H., Hiller, A. J., Rudolph, A. R., Lin, L., Vitt, C., and Smith, H. S. (1988). Specificity of tumor necrosis factor toxicity for human mammary carcinomas relative to normal mammary epithelium and correlation with response to doxorubicin, *Proc. Natl. Acad. Sci. USA 85*: 4740-4744.

Dubois, M. F., Ferrieux, C., and Lebon, P. (1989). Synergistic cytotoxic effects of recombinant human necrosis factor, interferons, and heat stress, *Cancer Res., 49*:5618-5622.

Feinberg, B., Kurzrock, R.., Talpaz, M., Blick, M., Saks, S., and Gutterman J. U. (1988). A phase I trial of intravenously-administered recombinant tumor necrosis factro-alpha in cancer patients, *J. Clin. Oncol., 6*:1328-1334.

Figari, I. S., Rice, G. C., Palladino, M. A. (1989). Possible mechanisms mediating recombinant tumor necrosis factor-alpha induced rejection of Meth A sarcoma: role of transforming factor beta and class I expression, *Proc. Am. Assoc. Cancer Res., 30*:406 (Abstract 1611).

Fillipak, M., Sparks, R. L., Tzen, C., and Scott, R. E. (1988). Tumor necrosis factor inhibits the terminal event in mesenchymal stem cell differentation, *J. Cell. Physiol., 137*: 367-373.

Fletcher, W. H., Shiu, W. W., Ishida, T. A.., Haviland, D. L., and Ware, C. F. (1987). Resistance to the cytolytic action of lymphotoxin and tumor necrosis factor coincides with the presence of gap junctions uniting target cells, *J. Immunol, 139*:956-962.

Fliegar, D., Reithmuller, G., Ziegler, B., and Heitbrock, H. W. (1989). Zn^{++} inhibits both tumor necrosis factor mediated DNA fragmentation and cytolysis, *Int. J. Cancer, 44*: 315-3199.

Fransen, L., Ruysschaert, M. R.., Van der Heyden, J., and Fiers, W. (1986a). Recombinant tumor necrosis factor: species specificity for a variety of human and murine transformed cell lines.

Fransen, L., Van der Heyden, J., Ruysschaert, R., and Fiers, W., (1986b). Recombinant tumor necrosis factor: its effect and its synergism with interferon-gamma on a variety of normal and transformed human cell lines, *Eur. J. Cancer. Clin. Oncol. 4*: 419–424.

Fráter-Schröder, M., Risau, W., Hallmann, R., Gautschi, P., and Bohlen, P. (1987). Tumor necrosis factor type alpha, a potent inhibitor of endolethial cell growth in vitro is angiogenic in vivo, *Proc. Natl. Acad. Sci. USA 84*: 5277–5281.

Frei, E. III, Spriggs, D., (1989). Tumor necrosis factor: still a promising agent, *J. Clin. Oncol., 7*: 291–294.

Gatanaga, T., Noguchi, K., Tanabe, Y., Inagawa, H., Soma, G., and Mizuno, D. (1989). Antitumor effect of systemic administration of novel recombinant tumor necrosis factor (rTNF-S) with less toxicity than conventional rTNF-alpha in vivo, *J. Biol. Response Mod., 8* : 278–286.

Georg, B., Helseth, E., Lund, L. R., Riccio, A., Dano, K., Unsgaard, G. and Andreasen, P. A. (1989). Tumor necrosis factor-alpha regulates mRNA for urokinase type plasminogen activator and type-1 plasminogen activator inhibitor in human neoplastic cell lines, *Mol. Cell. Endocrinol., 61*:87–96.

Gerlach, H., Lieberman, H., Bach, R., Godman, G., Brett, J., and Stern, D., (1989). Enhanced responsiveness of endolethium in the growing/motile state to tumor necrosis factor/cathectin, *J. Exp. Med., 170*: 913-931.

Goeddel. D. V., Aggarwal, B. B., Gray, P. W., Leung, D. W., Nedwin, G. E., Palladino, M.A., Patton, J. S., Pennica, D., Shepard, H. M., Sugarman, B. J., and Wong, G. H. W. (1986). Tumor necrosis factors: gene structure and biological activities, *Cold Spring Harbor Symp. Quant. Biol. 51*:597–609.

Gray, P. W., Aggarwal, B. B., Benton, C. V., Bringman, T. S., Henzel, W. J., Jarett, J. A., Leung, D. W., Moffat, B. N. P., Suedersky, L. P., Palladino, M. A.., and Nedwin, G. E. (1984). Cloning and expression of cDNA for human lymphotoxin, a lymphokine with tumor necrosis activity, *Nature, 312*: 721–724.

Gray, P. W., Aggarwal, B. B., Benton, C. V., Bringman, T. S., Henzel, W. J., Jarett, J. A., Leung, D. W., Moffat, B., NP., Suedersky, L. P., Palladino, M. A., and Nedwin, G.E. (1984). Cloning and expression of cDNA for human lymphotoxin, a lymphokine with tumor necrosis activity, *Nature, 312*: 721–724.

Gromkowski, S. H., Yagi, J., and Janeway, C. A.. Jr. (1989). Elevated temperature regulates tumor necrosis factor-mediated immune killing, *Eur. J. Immunol., 19*: 1709–1714.

Haranaka, K., Satomi, N., and Sakurai, A. (1984). Antitumor activity of murine tumor necrosis factor (TNF) against transplanted murine tumors and heterotransplanted human tumors in nude mice, *Int. J. Cancer, 34*: 263–267.

Haranaka, K., Satomi, N., Sakurai, A., and Haranaka, R., (1987a). Antitumor effects of tumor necrosis factor: cytotoxic or necrotizing activity and its mechanism, *Ciba Found. Symp., 131*:140–153.

Haranaka, K., Satomi, N., and Sakurai, A. (1987b). Antitumor activity of tumor necrosis factor in combination with hyperthermia, chemotherapy or immunotherapy, *J. Biol. Resp. Modif. 6*: 379–391.

Hasegawa, Y., and Bonavida, B., (1989), Calcium-independent pathway of tumor necrosis factor-mediates lysis of target cells, *J. Immunol., 142*: 2670–2676.

Havell, E. A., Fiers, W., and North, R. J. (1988). The antitumor function of tumor necrosis factor (TNF). 1. Therapeutic action of TNF against an established murine sarcoma is indirect, immunologically dependent, and limited by severe toxicity, *J. Exp. Med., 167*:1067–1085.

Helson, L., Helson, C., and Green, S. (1979). Effects of murine tumor necrosis factor in heterotransplanted tumors, *Exp. Cell. Biol., 47*: 53–56.

Hofsli, E., and Nissen-Meyer, J. (1989). Recombinant tumor necrosis factor (TNF) fixed to cell monolayers retains its cytotoxic and growth-stimulatory activity: evidence that internalization of TNF is not necessary for induction of biological effects, *Scand. J. Immunol., 29*: 57–63.

Hohmann, H., Remy, R., Brockhaus, M., and van Loon, A. P. G. M. (1989). Two different cell types have different major receptors for human tumor necrosis factor (TNF-α), *J. Biol. Chem., 264*: 14927–14934.

Hori, K., Ehrke, M. J., Mace, K., Mihich, E. (1987). Effect of recombinant tumor necrosis factor in tumoricidal activation of murine macrophages: synergism between tumor necrosis factor and γ-interferon, *Cancer Res., 47*: 5868–5874.

Hori, T., Kashiyama, S., Hayakaw, M., Shibamoto, S., Tsujimoto, M., Oku, N., and Ito, F., (1989). Possible role of prostaglandins as negative regulators in growth stimulation by tumor necrosis factor and epidermal growth factor in human fibroblasts, *J. Cell. Physiol., 141*: 275–280.

Hsu, P. L. and Hsu, S. M., (1989). Production of tumor necrosis factor-alpha and lymphotoxin by cells of Hodgkins's neoplastic cell lines HDLM-1 and KM-H2, *Am. J. Pathol., 135*: 735–745.

Hudziak, R. M., Lewis, G. D., Shalaby, M. R., Eessalu, T. E., Aggarwal, B. B., Ullrich, A., and Shepard, H. M. (1988). Amplified expression of the HER2/ERBB2 oncogene induces resistance to tumor necrosis factor in NIH 3T3 cells, *Proc. Natl. Acad. Sci. USA, 85*: 5102–5106.

Jäättälä, M., Saksela, K., and Saksela, E., (1989). Heat shock protects WEHI 164 target cells from the cytolysis by tumor necrosis factors alpha and beta, *Eur. J. Immunol. 19*: 1413–1417.

Johnson, R. A., Boyce, B. F., Mundy, G. R., and Roodman, G. D., (1989). Tumors producing human tumor necrosis factor induced by hypercalcemia and osteoclastic bone resorption in nude mice. *Endocrinology, 124*: 1424–1427.

Johnson, S. E., and Baglioni, C., (1988). Tumor necrosis factor receptors and cytocidal activity are down-regulated by activators of protein kinase C, *J. Biol. Chem. 263*: 5686–5692.

Kallinowskim F., Schaefer, C., Tyler, G., and Vaupel, P. (1989). In vivo targets of recombinant human tumor necrosis factor-α: blood flow, oxygen, consumption ang growth of isotransplanted rat tumors, *Br. J. Cancer, 60*: 555–560.

Kawai, T., Satomi, N., Sato, N., and Haranaka, K., (1987). Necrotising activity of tumor necrosis factor: histopathological investigations using Meth A and granulation tissue, *Virchows Arch. B. Cell Pathol. Incl. Mol. Pathol. 52*:489–500.

Kawakami, M., Watanabe, N., Ogawa, H., Kato, A., Sandom H., Yamada, N., Murase, T., Takaku, F., Shibata, S., and Oda, T. (1989). Cachetin/TNF kills or inhibits the differentiaton of 3T3-Li cells according to developmental stage. *J. Cell. Physiol., 138*: 1–7.

Keshav, S., Lawson, L., Ping Chung, L., Stein, M., Perry, V. H., and Gordon, S. (1990). Tumor necrosis factor mRNA localised to Paneth cells of normal murine intestinal epithelium by in situ hybridisation. *J. Exp. Med., 171*: 327–332.

Kimura, K., Taguchi, T., Urushizaki, I., Ohno, R., Abe, O., Furue, H., Hattori, T., Ichihashi, H., Inoguchi, K., Majima, H., Niitani, H., Ota, K., Saito, T., and Suga, S. (1987). Phase I study of recombinant human tumor necrosis factor, *Cancer Chemother. Pharmacol., 20*: 223–229.

Kohase, M., Henriksen-Destefano, D., May, L. T., Vilček, J., and Shegal, P. B. (1988). Induction of b2-interferon by tumor necrosis factor: a homeostatic mechanism in the control of cell proliferation, *Cell, 45*: 659–666.

Kriegler, M., Perez, C., Defay, K., Albert, I., and Lu, S. D. (1988). A novel form of TNF/cachectin is a cell surface cytotoxic transmembrane protein: ramifications for the complex physiology of TNF, *Cell, 53*:45–53.

Krönke, M., Hensel, G., Schuluter, C., Scheurich, P., Schutze, S., and Pfizenmaier, K. (1988). Tumor necrosis factor and lymphotoxin gene expression in human tumor cell lines, *Cancer Res. 48*: 5417–5421.

Krosnick, J. A.,, Mule, J. J., McIntosh, J. K., and Rosenberg, S. A. (1989). Augmentation of antitumor efficacy by the combination of tumor necrosis factor and chemotherapeutic agents in vivo. *Cancer Res. 49*: 3729–3733.

Kull, F. C., Jacobs, S., and Cuatrecasas, P. (1985). Cellular receptor for ^{125}I-labeled tumor necrosis factor: specific binding, affinity labelling, and relationship to sensitivity, *Proc. Natl. Acad. Sci. USA, 82*: 5756–5760.

Lancaster, J. R. Jr., Laster, S. M. and Gooding, L. R.. (1989). Inhibition of target cell mitochondrial electron transfer by tumor necrosis factor, *FEBS Lett., 248*: 169–174.

Laster, S. N., Wood, J. G., and Gooding, L. R. (1988). Tumor necrosis factor can induce both apoptic and necrotic forms of cell lysis, *J. Immunol. 141*: 2629–2634.

Lattime, E. C., and Stutman, O. (1989). Tumor growth in vivo secrets for resistance to tumor necrosis factor, *J. Immunol. 143*:4317–4323.

Lenk, H., Tanneberger, S., Muller, U., Ebertm J., and Shiga, T. (1989). Phase II clinical trial of high-dose recombinant human tumor necrosis factor, *Cancer Chemother. Pharmacol., 24*: 391–392.

Lewis, G. D., Aggarwal, B. B., Eessalu, T. E., Sugarman, B. J., and Shepard, H. M. (1987). Modulation of the growth of transformed cells by human tumor necrosis factor-alpha and interferon-gamma, *Cancer Res., 47*: 5382–5385.

Liddil, J. D., Dorr, R. T., and Scuderi, P. (1989). Association of lysosomal activity with sensitivity and resistance to tumor necrosis factor in murine L929 cells, *Cancer Res., 49*: 2722–2728.

Lindemann, A., Ludwig, W., Oster, W., Mertelsman, R., and Hermann, F. (1989). High level secretion of tumor necrosis factor-alpha contributes to haematopoietic failure in hairy cell leukaemia, *Blood, 73*:880–884.

Loetscher, H., Pan, Y. C. E., Lahm, H. W., Gentz, R., Brockhaus, M., Tabuchi, H., and Lesslaer, W., (1990). Molecular cloning and expression of the 55kd tumor necrosis factor receptor, *Cell, 61*: 352–359.

Madhevan, V., Malik, S. T. A., Maeger, T., Fiers, W., and Hart, I. (1990). Role of tumour necrosis factor in flavone-aceticacid-induced tumour vasculative shutdown, *Cancer Res., 50*: 5537–5542.

Malik, S. T. A., Griffin, D. B., Fiers, W., and Balkwill, F. R.. (1989). Paradoxical effects of tumor necrosis factor in experimental ovarian cancer, *Int. J. Cancer, 44*: 918–925.

Malik, S. T. A., Naylor, M. S., Oliff, A., and Balkwill, F. R.. (1990). Cells secreting tumor necrosis factor show enhanced metastasis in nude mice, *Eur. J. Cancer, 26*: 1031-1034.

Manda, T., Shimomura, K., Mukumoto, S., Kobayashi, K., Mizota, T., Hirai, O., Matsumoto, S., Oku, T., Nishigakim F., Mori, J., and Kikuchi, H., (1987). Recombinant tumor necrosis factor-α: evidence of an indirect mode of activity, *Cancer Res., 47*: 3707-3711.

Manda, T., Nishigaki, F., and Shimomura, K. (1988).Important role of serotonin in the antitumor effects of recombinant human tumor necrosis-α in mice, *Cancer Res., 48*: 4250-4255.

Manetta, A., Podczaski, E., Zaino, R. J., and Satyaswaroop. P. G. (1989). Therapeutic effect of recombinant human tumor necrosis factor in ovarian carcinoma xenograft in nude mice, *Gynecol. Oncol., 34*: 360-364.

Marquet, R. L., Ijzermans, J. N., DeBruin, R. W., Fiers. W., and Jeekel, J. (1987). Antitumor activity of mouse tumor necrosis factor in colon cancer in rates is promoted by recombinant rat interferon gamma: toxicity is reduced by indomethacin, *Int. J. Cancer, 40*: 550-553.

Matthews, N. (1983). Antitumor cytoxin produced by human monocytes: studies on its mode of action, *Brit. J. Cancer 48*: 405-410.

Matthews, N., and Neale, M. L. (1989). Relationship between tumor cell morphology, gap junctions and susceptibility to cytolysis by tumor necrosis factor, *Br. J. Cancer, 59*: 189-193.

Matthews, N., Fiera, R. A., and Neale, M. L., (1990). Tumor cells which develop resistance ot cytolysis by tumor necrosis factor have a different glycoform of a 105-kDa glycoprotein and lose the capacity to invade and metastasise, *Int. J. Cancer, 45*: 203-208.

Matthews, N., Neale, M. L., Jackson, S. K., and Stark, J. M. (1987). Tumor cell killing by tumor necrosis factor: inhibition by anaerobic conditions, free-radical scavengers and inhibitors of arachidonate metabolism, *Immunology, 62*: 153-155.

McIntosh, J., Mule, J. J., Krosnick, J. A., and Rosenberg, S. A., (1989). Combination cytokine therapy with tumor necrosis factor α, interleukin-2, and α-interferon and its synergistic antitumor effects in mice, *Cancer Res., 49*: 1408-1414.

McIntosh, J., Mule, J. J., Travis, W. D., and Rosenberg, S. A. (1990). Studies of effects of recombinant tumor necrosis factor on autochonous tumor and transplanted normal tissue in mice, *Cancer Res., 50*: 2463-2469.

Mosselmans, R., Hepburn, A., Dumint, J. E., Fiers, W., and Galandm P. (1988). Endocytic pathway of recombinant murine tumor necrosis factor in L-929 cells, *J. Immunol., 141*: 3096-3100.

Motoo, Y., Hill, N. O., Mahmoudi, M.m and Osther, K. (1986). Antitumor effect of human tumor necrosis factor in human hepatoma cells PLC.PRF/5, *Jpn. J. Exp. Med., 56*: 151-154.

Mule, J. J., McIntosh, J. K., Hablons, D. M., and Rosenbergm S. A.. (1990). Antitumor effect of recombinant interleukin 6 in mice, *J. Exp. Med., 171*: 629-636.

Nakamura, S., Nakata, K., and Kashnoto, S. (1986). Antitumor effect of recombinant interleukin alpah against murine synergeneic tumors, *J. Cancer Res., 77*: 767-773.

Nakano, K., Okugawa, K., Furuichi, H., Matsui, Y., and Sohmura, Y., (1989). Augmentation of the generation of cytotoxic T lymphocytes against synergenic tumor cells by recombinant human tumor necrosis factor, *Cell Immunol., 120*: 154-164.

Nakata, K., Yoshida, H., Kashimotom S., Sohmura, Y., Nakamura, S., and Taguchim T., (1986). Combined effect of recombinant human tumor necrosis factor and antitumor drugs on syngenic murine tumors, *Gan. To. Kagaku Ryoho, 13*: 3186–3193.

Naworth, P. D., Hanafley, G., Matsueda, R., DeWaal, H., Gerlach, H., Blohm, D., and Stern, D. (1988). Tumor necrosis factor/cachectin induced intravascular fibrin formation in meth A sarcoma, *J. Exp. Med., 168*: 637–643.

Naylor, M. S., Malik, S. T. A., Jobling, T., Stamp, G., and Balkwill, F. (1990). Demonstration of tumor necrosis factor in human ovarian cancer in situ hybridisation, *Eur. J. Cancer, 26*: 1027–1030.

Neale, M. L., Fiera, R. A., and Matthews, N. (1988). Involvement of phospholipase A2 activation in tumor cell killing by tumor necrosis factor, *Immunology, 64*: 81–85.

Niitsu, Y., Watanabe, N., Neda, H., Yamaauchi, N., Maeda, M., Sone, H., and Kuriyama, H. (1988). Induction of synthesis of tumor necrosis factor in human and murine cell lines by exogenous recombinant human tumor necrosis factor, *Cancer Res., 48*:5407–5410.

Nishimura, T., Ohta, S., Sato, N., Togashi, Y., Goto, M., and Hashimoto, Y. (1987). Combination tumor immunotherapy with recombinant tumor necrosis factor and recombinant interleukin 2 in mice, *Int. J. Cancer, 40*: 255–261.

Nishiyama, Y., Fuchimoto, S., Orita, K.. (1989). Preventative and antiproliferative effects of tumor necrosis factor against experimental hepatic metastases of mouse colon-26 tumor, *Jpn. J. Cancer Res., 80*: 366–372.

Nophar, Y., Holtmann, H., Ber, R., and Wallach, D. (1988). Dominance of resistance to the cytocodal effect of tumor necrosis factor in heterokaryons formed by the fusion of resistant and sensitive cells, *J. Immunol. 140*: 3456–3460.

Nosoh, Y., Toge, T., Nishiyama, M., Yamaguchi, M., Hirabayashi, N., Niimoto, M., and Hattori, T. (1987). Antitumor activity of recombinant human tumor necrosis factor against human tumor xenografts transplanted into nude mice. *Jpn. J. Surg., 17*: 51–54.

Ohsawa, F., and Natori, S. (1988). Selective degradation of tumor necrosis factor in sensitive cells, and production of membrane-active substance. *J. Biochem. Tokoyo, 103*: 730–734.

Oliff, A., Defeo-Jones, D., Boyer, M., Martinez, D., Kiefer, D., Voucolo, G., Wolfe, A., and Socher, S. H. (1987). Tumors secreting human TNF/cachetin induce cachexia in mice, *Cell, 50*: 555–563.

Ostensen, M. E., Thiele, D. L., and Lipsky, P. E. (1987). Tumor necrosis factor-α enhances activity of human natural killer cells, *J. Immunol., 138*: 4185–4191.

Owen-Schaub, L B., Gutterman, J., and Grimm, E. A. (1988). Synergy of tumor necrosis factor and interleukin-2 in activation of human cytotoxic lymphocytes: effects of tumor necrosis factor a and interleukin 2 in generation of human lymphokine activateds killer activity, *Cancer Res., 48*: 788–792.

Palladino, M. A. Jr., Refaat Shalaby, M.m Kramer, S. M., Ferraiolo, B. L., Baughman, R. A., Deleo, A. B., Crase, D., Marafino, B., Aggarwal, B. B., and Figari, I. S. (1987). Characterization of the antitumor activities of human tumor necrosis factor alpha and the comparison with other cytokines: induction of tumor-specific immunity, *J. Immunol., 138*: 4023–4032.

Palombella, V. J., and Vilček, J. (1989). Mitogenic and cytotoxic actions of tumor necrosis factor in BALB/c 3T3 cells: role of phospholipase activation, *J. Biol. Chem., 264*: 18128–18136.

Patek, P. Q., Lin, Y., and Case, P. G. (1989). Cell lines cultured at high density are reistant to lysis by tumor necrosis factor and natural cytotoxic cells, *Proc. Soc. Exp. Biol. Med., 190*(3): 234–239.

Peck, R., Brockhaus, M., and Frey, J. R. (1989). Cell surface tumor necrosis factor (TNF) accounts for monocyte- and lymphocyte-mediated killing of TNF-resistant target cells, *Cell Immunol., 122*: 1–10.

Pennica, D., Nedwin, G. E., Hayflick, J. S., Seeburg, P. H., Derynck, R., Palladino, M. A. and Kohur, W. J., Aggarwal, B. B., and Goeddel, D. V. (1984). Human tumor necrosis factor: precursor structure, expression and homology to lymphotoxin, *Nature 312*: 724–729.

Pfizenmaier, K., Scheurich, P., Schulter, C., and Kronke, M. (1987). Tumor necrosis factor enhances HLA A, B, C, and HLDA DR gene expression in human tumor cells, *J. Immunol. 138*: 975–980.

Pfreundshuh, M., Genth, B., Kirchner, H., Scheurich, P., Lindemann, A., Steinmetz, H. T., and Schaadt, M. (1989). Mechanism of resistance to tumor necrosis factor, *Onkologie, 12*: 128–130.

Pillai, S., Bilke, D. D., Eessalu, T. E., Aggarwal., B. B., and Elias, P. M. (1989). Binding and biological effects of tumor necrosis factor alpha on cultured human neonatal foreskin keratinocytes, *J. Clin. Invest., 83*: 816–821.

Pober, J. S. (1987). Effects of tumor necrosis factor and related cytokines on vascular endolethial cells, *Ciba. Found. Symp., 131*: 170–184.

Proetti, E., Belerdelli, F., Carpinelli, G., Di Vito, M., Woodrow, D., Moss, J., Sestili, P., Fiers, W., Gresser, I., and Podo, F. (1988). Tumor necrosis factor-α induces early morphologic and metabolic alterations in Friend leukaemia cell tumors and fibrosarcomas in mice, *Int. J. Cancer, 42*: 582–591.

Regenass, U., Muller, M., Curschellas, E., and Matter, A. (1987). Antitumor effects of tumor necrosis factor in combination with chemotherapeutic agents, *Int. J. Cancer, 39*: 266–273.

Reid, T. R., Torti, F. M., and Ringold, G. M. (1989). Evidence for two mechanisms by which tumor necrosis factor kills cells, *J. Biol. Chem., 264*: 4583–4589.

Remels, L., Neirynck, A., Brys, L., Vercauteren, E., and De-Baetselier, P. (1989). TNF-α mediated selection of macrophage-resistant gene-regulatory tumor variants, *Clin. Exp. Metastasis, 7*: 493–506.

Retsas, S., Leslie, M., and Bottomley, D. (1989). Intralesional tumor necrosis factor combined with interferon gamma in metastatic melanoma, *Br. Med. J., 298*: 1290–1291.

Rice, G. E., Gimborne, M. A., and Bevilacqua, M. P. (1988). Tumor cell endolethial interactions: increased adhesion of human melanoma cells to activated vascular endothelium, *Am. J. Pathol., 133*: 204–210.

Roozemond, R. C., Urli, D. C., Jansen, J., and Bonavida, B. (1989). Liposomes can function as targets for natural killer cytotoxic factor but not for tumor necrosis factor, *J. Immunol., 142*: 1209–1216.

Rothstein, R., Czajkowski, M., O'Neill, M. M., Marlin, S. D., Mainoff, E., and Merluzzi, V. J., (1988). Induction of intercellular adhesion molecule 1 on primary and continuous cell lines by pro-inflammatory cytokines: regulation by pharmacologic agents and neutralizing antibodies, *J. Immunol., 141*: 1665–1669.

Rubin, B. Y., Anderson, S. L., Sullivan, S. A., Williamson, B. D., Carswell, E. A., and Old,

L. J. (1986). Nonhaemopoietic cells selected for resistance to tumor necrosis factor produce tumor necrosis factor, *J. Exp. Med., 164*: 1350–1356.

Rubin, S. C., Hoskins, W. J., Markman, M., Federici, M., Lloyd, K. O., and Lewis, J. L. (1989). Synergistic activity of tumor necrosis factor and interferon in a nude mouse model of human ovarian cancer, *Gynecol. Oncol., 34*(3): 353–356.

Ruddle, N. H., and Waksman, B. H. (1968). Cytotoxicity mediated by soluble antigen and lymphocytes in delayed sypersensitivity. III. Analysis of mechanism, *J. Exp. Med., 128*: 1267–1279.

Ruggerio, V., and Baglioni, C. (1987). Synergistic anti-proliferative activity of interleukin 1 and tumor necrosis factor, *J. Immunol., 138*: 661–663.

Sato, N., Goto, T., Haranaka, K., Satomi, N., Nariuchi, H., Mano-Hirano, Y., and Sawasaki, Y. (1986). Actions of tumor necrosis factor on cultured vascular endolethial cells: morphologic modulation, growth inhibition, and cytotoxicity, *J. Nat. Cancer Inst., 76*: 1113–1119.

Sawada, M., Kondo, N., Suzamura, A., and Narunouchi, T. (1989). Production of tumor necrosis factor alpha by microglia and astrocytes in culture, *Brain Res., 491*: 394–397.

Scanlon, M., Laster, S. M., Wood, J. G., and Gooding, L. R. (1989). Cytolysis by tumor necrosis factor is preceded by a rapid and specific dissolution of microfilaments, *Proc. Natl. Acad. Sci. USA, 86*: 182–186.

Schall, T. J., Lewis, M., Koller, K. J., Lee, A., Rice, G. C., Wong, G. H. W., Gatanaga, T., Granger, G. A., Lentz, R., Raab, H., Kohr, W. J., and Goeddel, D. V. (1990). Molecular cloning and expression of a receptor for human tumor necrosis factor, *Cell, 61*: 361–370.

Scheringa, M., Keizer, A., Jeekel, J., and Marquet, R. L. (1989). Antitumor effect of recombinant murine TNF-alpha (rMuTNFa) given by continuous i. v. infusion as compared to repeated i. v. injections in a rat liver metastasis model, *Int. J. Cancer. 43*: 905–909.

Schuger, L., Varani, J., Marks, R. M., Kunkel, S. L., Johnson, K. J., and Ward, P. A. (1989). Cytotoxicity of tumor necrosis factor alpha for human umbilical vein endothelial cells, *Lab Invest., 61*: 62–68.

Selby, P., Hobbs, S., Viner, C., Jackson, E., Jones, A., Newell, D., Calvert, A. H., Mclwain, T., Fearon, K., Humphreys, J., and Shinga, T. (1987). Tumor necrosis factor in man: clinical and biological observations, *Br. J. Cancer, 56*: 803–808.

Shalaby, M. R., Aggarwal, B. B., Rinderknecht, L., Svedersky, B., Finkle, S., and Palladino, M. A. (1985). Activation of human polymorphonuclear neutrophils by gamma interferon and tumor necrosis factors, *J. Immunol., 135*: 2069–2074.

Shau, H. (1988). Cytostatic and tumoricidal activities of tumor necrosis factor-treated neutrophils, *Immunol. Lett., 17*: 47–51.

Shear, M. J., Turner, F. C., Perrault, A., and Shovelton, T. (1943). Chemical treatment of tumors. V. Isolation of the haemmorrhage producing fraction from *Serratia marcescens* (*Bacillus prodiogosus*) culture filtrates, *J. Natl. Cancer Inst., 4*: 81–97.

Shine, N., Palladino, M. A. Jr., Patton, J. S., Deisserworth, A., Karczmar, G. S., Matson, G. B., and Weiner, M. W. (1989). Early metabolic response to tumor necrosis factor in mouse sarcoma: a phosphorus-31 nuclear magnetic resonance study, *Cancer Res., 49*: 2123–2127.

Smith, M. R., Munger, W. E., Kung, H., Takacs, L., and Durum, S. K. (1990). Direct evidence for an intracellular role for tumor necrosis factor, *J. Immunol., 144*: 162–169.

Smyth, M. J., Pieteresz, A., McKenzie, I. F. C. (1988). Increased antitumour effect of immunoconjugates and tumour necrosis factor in vivo. *Cancer res., 48*: 3607–3712.

Sohmura, Y., Nakata, K., Yoshida, H., Kashimoto, S., Matsui, Y., and Furuichi, H. (1986). Recombinant human tumor necrosis factor. II. Antitumor effect on murine and human tumors transplanted in mice, *Int. J. Immunopharmacol., 8*(3): 357–368.

Spriggs, D., Imamura, K., Rodriguez, C., Horiguchi, J., and Kufe, D. W. (1987). Induction of tumor necrosis factor expression and resistance in a human breast tumor cell line, *Proc. Natl. Acad. Sci. USA, 84*: 6563-6566.

Spriggs, D. R.., Sherman, M. L., Michie, H., Arthur, K. A. A., Imamura, K., Wilmore, D., Frei, E., and Kufe, D. W. (1988). Recombinant human tumor necrosis factor administered as a 24-hour intravenous infusion: a phase I and pharmacologic study, *J. Nat. Cancer Inst., 80*: 1039-1044.

Suffys, P., Beyaert, R., Van-Roy, F., and Fiers, W. (1987). Reduced tumor necrosis factor-induced cytotoxicity by inhibitors of the arachidonic acid metabolism, *Biochem. Biophys. Res. Commun., 149*: 735–743.

Suffys, P., Beyaert, R., Van-Roy, F., and Fiers, W. (1988). Involvement of a serine protease in tumor-necrosis-factor-mediated cytotoxicity, *Eur. J. Biochem., 178*: 257–265.

Sugarman, B. J., Aggarwal, B. B., and Hass, P. E. (1985). Recombinant human tumor necrosis factor alpha: effects of proliferation on normal and transformed cells in vitro, *Science, 230*: 943–945.

Sugarman, B. J., Lewis, G. D., Eessalu, T. E., Aggarwal, B. B., and Shepard, H. M. (1987). Effects of growth factors on the antiproliferative activity of tumor necrosis factors, *Cancer Res., 47*: 780–786.

Suzumori, K., Yasui, Y., Yagami, Y., and Kimura, K. (1987). Antitumor activity of tumor necrosis factor against human gynaecological carcinoma transplanted into nude mice, *Gan To Kagaku Ryoho, 14*: 2341–2346.

Taguchi, T., Kimoto, Y., and Tanji, Y. (1987). Clinical studies of recombinant human tumor necrosis factor, *Tumor Necrosis/Cachectin and Related Cytokines* B. Bonavida, G. Clifford, H. Kirchner, and L. J. Old (eds.) Karger, Basel, pp.196–204.

Talmadge, J. E., Phillips, H., Schneider, M., Rowe, T., Pennington, R., Bowersox, O., and Lenz, B. (1987). Immunomodulatory properties of recombinant murine and human necrosis factor, *Cancer Res., 48*: 544–550.

Tamm, I., Cardinale, I., Krueger, J., Murphy, J. S., May, L., and Seghal, P. B., (19??). Interleukin 6 decreases cell-cell association and increases motility of ductal breast carcinoma cells, *J. Exp. Med. 170*: 1649-1669.

Tamura, K., Aso, H., Nakamura, T., Hemmi, H., and Ishida, N. (1989). Evaluation of recombinant human tumor necrosis factor by scheduled intratumoral administration in mice bearing transplantable tumors, *Tohuku J. Exp. Med., 157*: 107–118.

Tomazic, V. J., Farha, M., Loftus, A., and Elias, E. G. (1988). Antitumor activity of recombinant tumour necrosis factor on mouse fibrosarcoma in vivo and in vitro, *J. Immunol., 140*: 4056–4061.

Torti, S. V., Kwak, E. L., Miller, S. C., Miller, L. L., Ringold, G. M., Myambo, K. B., Young, A. P. and Torti, F. (1988). The molecular cloning and characterisation of murine ferritin heavy chain, a tumor necrosis factor inducible gene, *J. Biol. Chem. 263*: 12638–12644.

Trinchieri, G. M., Koyabashi, M., Rosen, M., London, R., Murphy, M., and Perussia, B.

(1986). Tumor necrosis factor and lymphotoxin indice differentiation of human myeloid cell lines in synergy with immune interferon, *J. Exp. Med. 164*: 1206–1212.

Tsujimoto, M., Yip, Y. K., and Vilček, J. (1985). Tumor necrosis factor: specific binding and internalisation in sensitive and resistant cells, *Proc. Natl. Acad. Sci. USA, 82*: 7626–7630.

Vilček, J., Palombella, V. J., Henriksen-DeStefano, D., Swenson, C., Feinman, R., Hirai, M., Tsujimoto, M. (1986). Fibroblast growth enhancing activity of tumor necrosis factor and its relationship to other polypepetide growth factors, *J. Exp. Med., 163*: 632–643.

Vlassara, H., Brownlee, M., Manogue, K. R., Dinarello, C. A., and Pasagian, A. (1988). Cachectin/TNF and IL-1 induced by glucose-modified proteins: role in tissue remodelling, *Science, 240*: 1546–1548.

Wallach, D. (1984). Preparations of lymphotoxins induce resistance to their own cytocidal effect, *J. Immunol., 132*: 2464–2469.

Warner, S. J., and Libby, P. (1989). Human vascular smooth muscle cells: target for and source of tumor necrosis factor, *J. Immunol., 142*: 100–109.

Watanbe, N., Niitsu, Y., Neda, H., Sone, H., Yamauchi, N., Maeda, M., and Urushizaki, I., (1988a). Cytocidal mechanism of TNF: effects of lysosomal enzyme and hydroxyl radical inhibitors on cytotoxicity, *Immunopharmacol. Immunotoxicol., 10*: 109–116.

Watanabe, N., Umetsu, T., Sone, H., Neda, H., Yamauchi, N., Umeno, H., Maeda, M., and Niitsu, Y. (1988b). Stimulation of antitumorigenic cytotoxicity in macrophages by tumor necrosis factor, *Cancer J. 2*: 165–168.

Watanbe, N., Niitsu, Y., Umeno, H., Sone, H., Neda, H., Yamauchi, N., Maeda, M., and Urushizaki, I., (1988c). Synergistic cytotoxic and antitumor effects of recombinant human tumor necrosis factor and hyperthermia effects. *Cancer Res. 48*: 650–653.

Winkelhake, J. L., Stampfl, S., and Zimmerman, R. J. (1987). Synergistic effects of combination therapy with human recombinant interleukin-2 and tumor necrosis factor in murine tumor models, *Cancer Res., 47*: 3948–3953.

Wong, G. H. W. and Goeddel, D. V. (1988). Induction of manganous superoxide dismutase by tumor necrosis factor: possible protective mechanism, *Science, 242*: 941–943.

Wong, G. H. W., Elwell, J. H., Oberley, L. W., and Goeddel, D. V. (1989). Manganese superoxide dismutase is essential for cellular resistance to cytotoxicity of tumor necrosis factor, *Cell, 58*: 923–931.

Yamauchi, N., Kuriyama, H., Watanabe, N., Neda, H., Maeda, M., and Niitsu, Y. (1989). Intracellular hydroxyl radical production induced by recombinant human tumor necrosis factor and its implication in the killing of tumor cells in vitro, *Cancer Res., 49*: 1671–1675.

Yonehara, S., Ishii, A., and Yonehara, M. (1989). A cell-killing monoclonal antibody (anti-Fas) to a cell surface antigen co-downregulated with the receptor of tumor necrosis factor, *J. Exp. Med., 169*; 1747–1756.

Yoshimura, T., and Stone, S., (1987). Different and synergistic actions of human tumor necrosis factor and interferon-gamma in the damage of liposome membranes, *J. Biol. Chem., 262*:4597–4561.

Zimmerman, R. J., Marafino, B. J., Jr., Chan, A., Landre, P., and Winkelhake, J. L. (1989). The role of oxidant injury in tumor cell sensitivity to recombinant human tumor necrosis factor in vivo: implications for mechanisms of action, *J. Immunol., 142*: 1405–1409.

12

TNF as a Growth Factor

JAN VILČEK
New York University Medical Center, New York, New York

VITO J. PALOMBELLA
Harvard University, Cambridge, Massachusetts

I. INTRODUCTION

TNF*was first described as the mediator of LPS-induced hemorrhagic necrosis of tumors in intact animals (Carswell et al., 1975). This action of TNF can be ascribed to an indirect effect on the tumor vasculature. Early studies also suggested that TNF exerts a direct growth-inhibitory effect on transformed cell lines but fails to affect the growth of normal cells in culture (Ruff and Gifford, 1981). For many years the direct and indirect antitumor actions of TNF were its only recognized functions. As a result of the successful cloning of the TNF gene, pure recombinant TNF became widely available around 1985. Availability of pure TNF enticed several groups to analyze more thoroughly the actions of TNF on cell growth. Very soon it became clear that the results did not support the original concept of TNF as a highly selective antitumor agent in the intact organism and a selective inhibitor of the growth of transformed cells in vitro (see also Chapter II in the present volume). Many unexpected important biological actions of TNF were discovered, as reviewed in other chapters in this volume.

*In this chapter the term *TNF* generally means TNF-α. The term *TNF-β* or *lymphotoxin* is used when specific reference is made to this form of TNF.

Among the newly recognized actions of TNF was a stimulatory action on the growth of some cells, especially normal human fibroblasts (Sugarman et al., 1985; Vilček et al., 1986). Even earlier, in studies with highly purified natural human lymphotoxin, Lee et al. (1984) made the unexpected observation that rather than inhibiting cell growth, lymphotoxin actually increased the density of cultured human fibroblasts and murine B16 melanoma cells. Gradually, it became apparent that the growth factor–like actions of TNF are at least as important as its ability to inhibit cell growth.

In this chapter we review information on the growth-promoting actions of TNF. We concentrate on what is known about the mechanisms involved and the possible significance of TNF's mitogenic actions in pathophysiology.

II. GROWTH-STIMULATORY ACTIONS OF TNF IN DIFFERENT CELL TYPES

The effect of recombinant human TNF on the viability and growth of a large variety of transformed cell lines was examined by Sugarman et al. (1985). Of 22 tumor cell lines examined, 7 showed a significant reduction (≥ 25%) in cell number after exposure to TNF for 72 h. No significant effect was seen in the remaining tumor cell lines. However, in several lines of normal human fibroblasts (including the well-characterized WI-38 line of fetal lung cells) TNF increased the cell number. A marked growth-stimulatory action of TNF was also seen in the FS-4 line of normal human foreskin fibroblasts (Vilček et al., 1986). In addition, many other types of cells originating from various tissues were found to be responsive to the growth-stimulatory action of TNF (Table 1).

The stimulatory action of TNF on cell growth is not limited to normal cells, as TNF was reported to be mitogenic for several cell lines derived from various tumor tissues (Table 1). It appears, however, that the growth-stimulatory action of TNF is less readily demonstratable in tumor cell lines than in normal cells. Thus human fibroblasts lost their responsiveness to the mitogenic action of TNF after their transformation by SV40 (Sugarman et al., 1985; J. Wolchok and J. Vilček, unpublished data). In some tumor cell lines TNF was stimulatory only at low concentrations and became inhibitory at higher doses (Lewis et al., 1987; Feinman et al., 1987). In contrast, in normal human fibroblasts the growth-stimulatory action of TNF increased in a dose-dependent manner and a plateau level was reached when the optimal TNF dose was exceeded (Sugarman et al., 1985; Vilček et al., 1986; Palombella et al., 1988). In another instance, growth of the osteosarcoma line HOS-1 was increased by TNF only when the concentration of serum in the medium was reduced from 10% to 0.5% (Kirstein and Baglioni, 1988). This observation contrasts with the increased responsiveness of normal human FS-4 fibroblasts or rat chondrocytes to the mitogenic action of TNF with increasing concentrations of fetal bovine serum (Vilček et al., 1986; Ikebe et al., 1988). It is possible that tumor

Table 1 Growth-Stimulatory Actions Observed with Recombinant TNF in Different Types of Cells

Cell type or cell line	Reference
Normal human colon (CCD-18C0), fetal skin (Detroit 551), lung (LL24 and WI-003), and fetal lung (WI-38) fibroblasts	Sugarman et al., 1985
Normal human foreskin fibroblasts (FS-4, FS-7, FS-49)	Vilček et al., 1986
Human synovial fibroblasts	Butler et al., 1988
Human smooth muscle cells	Kahaleh et al., 1988
Human mesangial cells	Silver et al., 1989
Normal human B cells	Jelinek and Lipsky, 1987
Normal human T cells	Yokata et al., 1988
Murine thymocytes	Ranges et al., 1988
Murine T-cell line	Ranges et al., 1989
Murine bone marrow macrophages	Branch et al., 1989
Rat costal chondrocytes	Ikebe et al., 1988
Normal and leukemic human granulocyte-macrophage progenitors	Piacibello et al., 1990
Human cervical carcinoma (ME-180neo line)	Lewis et al., 1987
Human astrocytoma (U373)	Lachman et al., 1987
Human osteosarcoma (HOS-1)	Kirstein and Baglioni, 1987
Murine fibroblasts (BALB/c 3T3)	Palombella and Vilček,1989
Murine fibroblasts (3T3-L1)	Cornelius et al., 1990
Murine fibroblasts (Swiss 3T3)	Kohno et al., 1990
Rat fibroblasts (NRK)	Palombella, 1989

cells (but not normal cells) grown in the presence of high serum concentrations already are maximally stimulated and the addition of TNF (and perhaps any other growth factor) cannot further increase the rate of cell growth. In addition, in normal cells TNF appears to partially overcome the constraints of contact inhibition (Fig. 1), whereas tumor cells are not contact inhibited.

Some normal cells too are stimulated to grow by TNF only under certain conditions. Piacibello et al. (1990) found that granulocyte-macrophage progenitors were stimulated to grow by TNF in the presence of GM-CSF, but the same doses of TNF inhibited the growth of granulocyte-macrophage progenitors grown in the pres-

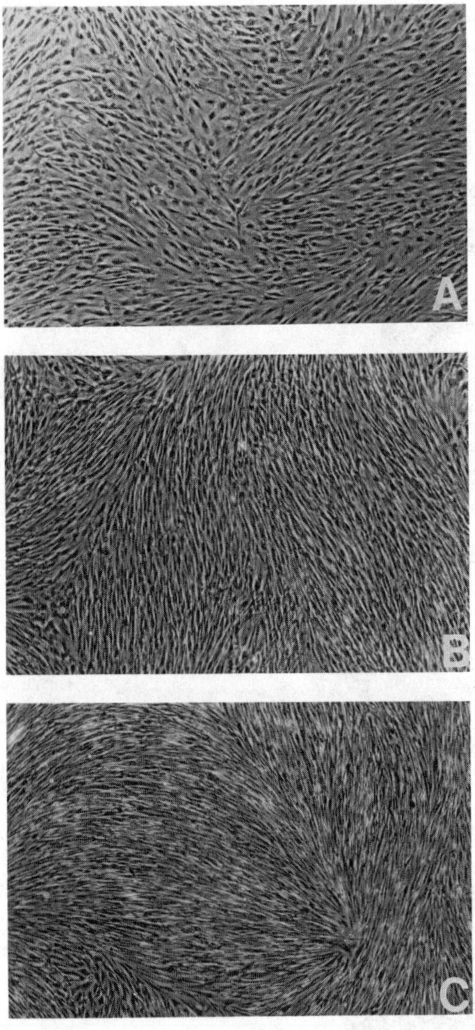

Figure 1 Effect of TNF on the growth and morphology of human FS-4 fibroblasts. FS-4 cells were seeded into six-well plates (3.5×10^5 cells per well) in minimal essential medium with 5% FBS. One day later the cells were treated with medium alone (A), 10 ng/mL TNF (B), or 100 ng/ml TNF (C). Photomicrographs of the cultures were taken with the aid of a phase-contrast microscope 7 days after the addition of TNF. Magnification ×60. (From Palombella, 1989.)

ence G-CSF. In murine BALB/c 3T3 fibroblast the action of TNF depended on the culture conditions; when added to confluent growth-arrested cultures, TNF was mitogenic, whereas in subconfluent actively growing cells it was cytostatic or (at higher concentrations) cytotoxic (Palombella and Vilček, 1989). These few examples will suffice to support the general conclusion that the outcome of TNF's action on cell growth is very much dependent on the specific conditions (e.g., the density of the cells, the stage of the cell cycle, the presence of other growth factors or cytokines, etc.). These examples also illustrate how difficult it is to decide which of TNF's opposing actions on cell growth (i.e., the growth-stimulatory or cytostatic/ cytotoxic action) is more important and more relevant to the role of TNF in the intact organism.

III. MECHANISMS OF TNF'S MITOGENIC ACTION

A. General Considerations

The regulation of cell division is a complex process involving a network of various nutrients and growth factors. The ability of serum to supply many of the necessary factors has long been recognized and many serum components responsible for growth have been isolated and characterized (Olashaw and Pledger, 1985). However, the intracellular mechanisms triggered by these factors and responsible for cell growth are only beginning to be understood.

In studying the regulation of cell division and the progression of nontransformed cells through the cell cycle, many groups have made use of a murine cell line, BALB/c 3T3, which is very sensitive to *contact inhibition* of cell division (Todaro and Green, 1963; Todaro et al., 1965). The addition of serum to quiescent, density-inhibited BALB/c 3T3 cells stimulates these cells to initiate DNA synthesis (Todaro et al., 1965). Pledger et al. (1977, 1978) showed that the induction of DNA synthesis in confluent quiescent BALB/c 3T3 cells follows an ordered sequence of events that can be separated into two discrete phases, each controlled by different serum components. The first phase is the acquisition of *competence*, induced by platelet-derived growth factor (PDGF), and the second phase is the *progression* of competent cells into the cell cycle promoted by factors in platelet-poor plasma (PPP). Since then, insulin-like growth factor-1 (IGF-1), or hyperphysiological concentrations of insulin, together with epidermal growth factor (EGF) have been shown to replace the progression activity of PPP (Stiles et al., 1979; Leof et al., 1983). In addition, other competence factors have been identified, e.g., fibroblast growth factor, FGF, and $Ca_3(PO_4)$ (Stiles et al., 1979). The sequential or simultaneous addition of a competence and of progression factors to quiescent BALB/c 3T3 cells stimulates the cells to traverse G_0/G_1 and enter S phase, after a lag of approximately 12 h (reviewed by Olashaw and Pledger, 1985).

In contrast to these findings in BALB/c 3T3 cells, Westermark and Heldin (1985) have reported that in human diploid fibroblasts the addition of PDGF or EGF alone is sufficient to stimulate DNA synthesis. In addition, they reported that EGF and PDGF are very similar in their actions in the prereplicative phase of human fibroblasts. It has also been reported that PDGF or FGF can stimulate DNA synthesis and cell division in quiescent Swiss 3T3 cells in the absence of any other mitogenic agents, while other growth factors must be present in specific combinations in order to produce an efficient stimulation of DNA synthesis (reviewed by Rozengurt, 1986). It is apparent from these data that the control of cell division depends not only on the interaction of different growth factors with the cell, but also on the nature of the target cell itself.

In addition to PDGF, IGF-1, EGF, and insulin, many other polypeptide growth factors/modulators have been identified, purified, and characterized. These include, among others, acidic and basic FGF, transforming growth factor (TGF) α (an EGF-like molecule), TGF-β, interferon (IFN)-β, bombesin, and vasopressin (reviewed by Sporn and Roberts, 1988). Furthermore, many factors elaborated from monocytes/macrophages and lymphoid cells can stimulate or inhibit the growth of fibroblasts (Wahl and Wahl, 1981; Gillespie et al., 1985). These factors include some of the "classical" growth factors mentioned above in addition to other distinct cytokines/lymphokines. Interleukin (IL)-1, elaborated by activated macrophages and similar to TNF in many of its actions (Le and Vilček, 1987), can stimulate the growth of normal human fibroblasts (Schmidt et al., 1982) and BALB/c 3T3 cells (Estes et al., 1984; Singh et al., 1988). In contrast, IFN-α and IFN-β, also produced by macrophages, and IFN-γ, from activated T lymphocytes, can inhibit the proliferation of most mesenchymal cell types (reviewed by Vilček, 1990).

Polypeptide growth factors/modulators interact with their target cell through specific high-affinity receptors. The binding of these factors to their receptors stimulates the generation of many intracellular signals, the type and magnitude of which depends on the target cell and the factor/receptor initiating the response (reviewed by Rozengurt, 1986). Reversible phosphorylation of proteins is known to be one of the major mechanisms by which cells respond to external stimuli (i.e., growth factors, hormones, cytokines). There are several phosphorylating systems involved in the control of cell growth (reviewed in Czech et al., 1990). The principal actions of many growth factors involve the modulation of gene transcription; these actions are mediated by the activation or inactivation of a variety of nuclear transcription factors. These diverse signaling pathways eventually lead to a common event (i.e., DNA synthesis and cell division).

B. Interactions of TNF with Other Growth Factors

As is evident from the foregoing discussion, the action of all growth factors and cytokines is *contextual*, that is it is influenced by the presence of other effector molecules and receptors (Sporn and Roberts, 1988). An evaluation of the mitogenic action of TNF in the human diploid FS-4 foreskin fibroblast line has elucidated the interrelationships of TNF with several other growth factors (Vilček et al., 1986; Palombella et al., 1988; Palombella, 1989).

The growth-promoting action of TNF on FS-4 cells is readily seen when TNF is added to the complete serum-containing medium. Cells cultured in the presence of TNF appear manifestly denser and more spindle shaped (Fig. 1). The increase in cell density suggests a partial loss of contact inhibition. To quantitate the growth stimulation, cells were stained and the amount of dye taken up by the cells (as a measure of cell density) was determined by spectrophotometer (Vilček et al., 1986). Alternatively, the rate of DNA synthesis was measured by pulse labelling with [^{3}H] thymidine. A dose-dependent increase in both of these parameters was seen after the exposure of FS-4 cells to TNF (Vilček et al., 1986; Palombella et al., 1988).

As mentioned earlier, the growth-stimulatory action of TNF was more pronounced and more sustained in the presence of optimal concentrations of fetal bovine serum (FBS) than with suboptimal serum concentrations (Vilček et al., 1986). This difference was especially marked upon the addition of TNF to growth-arrested FS-4 cells in which the addition of TNF with 5% FBS exerted a strong synergistic effect on cell growth. TNF alone was a weak mitogen in G_0-arrested cells, and serum as well as EGF or PDGF stimulated DNA synthesis much more efficiently than did TNF (Palombella et al., 1988). However, TNF was synergistic not only with serum but also with EGF or PDGF in stimulating DNA synthesis in quiescent cells. Thus even though TNF was an inefficient mitogen in growth-arrested cells, it appeared to act as a powerful modulator of the actions of both EGF and PDGF. A more detailed analysis of the synergistic action of TNF and EGF suggested that TNF acts earlier than EGF in the prereplicative phase of FS-4 cells.

The interaction of TNF with several other growth factors/cytokines was studied in FS-4 cells, and the salient results are summarized in Table 2. In addition to EGF or PDGF, TNF was synergistic in its mitogenic action with TGF-β and basic FGF and, under some conditions, with insulin (Palombella et al., 1988; Palombella, 1989). A synergistic growth-stimulatory effect was also seen in FS-4 cells with dexamethasone (Kohase et al., 1987). In other studies the cyclooxygenase inhibitor indomethacin was found to increase the mitogenic effect of TNF in FS-4 cells or human synovial cells, whereas the addition of prostaglandins suppressed the stimulatory action of TNF in these cells (Hori et al., 1989; Butler et al., 1988).

The outcome of many of these interactions depends on the cell type and conditions employed. In growth-arrested murine BALB/c 3T3 cells, as in FS-4 cells, the

Table 2 Interactions of TNF with Other Growth Factors/Cytokines in Human FS-4 Fibroblasts[a]

Growth factor added together with TNF	Mitogenic effect with TNF in FS-4 cells: In medium with serum	In serum-free medium	In growth-arrested cultures
Insulin	ND[b]	Synergy/additive	ND
IL-1 α	Additive	ND	ND
Dexamethasone	Synergy	ND	ND
TGF-β	Additive	ND	Synergy
EGF	Additive	Synergy	Synergy
PDGF	ND	ND	Synergy
Basic FGF	ND	ND	Synergy
IL-6	No effect	ND	No effect
IFN-β	Inhibitory	ND	Inhibitory
IFN-γ	Inhibitory	ND	Inhibitory

Source: Data from Palombella et al. (1988), Palombella (1989), and Kohase et al. (1987). Adapted from Palombella (1989).

[a]Mitogenic action of TNF was evaluated in the presence or absence of various other growth factors in FS-4 cells grown in serum containing or serum-free defined medium, or in growth-arrested cells, The table presents a qualitative summary of the mitogenic action seen with TNF plus growth factor, relative to the mitogenic action seen with TNF or respective growth factor alone.

[b]ND, not determined.

mitogenic action of TNF was synergistic with either EGF or PDGF (Palombella and Vilček, 1989). However, in the same BALB/c 3T3 cultures that showed a stimulation of DNA synthesis in response to TNF, high doses of murine TNF were also cytotoxic as demonstrated by a decrease in the number of viable cells. It appeared that a portion of the cells in culture was killed in response to a high TNF dose, whereas another portion of the cells was stimulated to undergo DNA synthesis and to divide. This difference in the cell response could be due to a heterogeneity in the BALB/c 3T3 cell population with respect to the expression of TNF receptors or some other important parameter. There also appear to be cell-type-specific differences in the response to TNF and TGF-β. Whereas in FS-4 cells the mitogenic actions of TNF and TGF-β were additive to synergistic (Palombella, 1989), TGF-β inhibited the growth-stimulatory action of TNF in WI-38 human fetal lung fibroblast (Kamijo et al., 1989).

Interesting interactions between TNF and hematopoietic colony-stimulating factors have been reported. In primary murine bone marrow macrophages, TNF alone allowed only a weak mitogenic action, but it significantly boosted the stimulation of DNA synthesis by CSF-1 (Branch et al., 1989). In either normal or chronic myeloid leukemia granulocyte-macrophage progenitors, TNF greatly enhanced GM-CSF-dependent cell growth; this stimulatory effect was also seen in the absence of accessory cells, suggesting that TNF acted directly on the progenitors (Piacibella et al., 1990). Interestingly, the growth of the same cells was inhibited by TNF when G-CSF was present instead of GM-CSF.

C. Effects of TNF on Growth Factor Receptors

Several studies were devoted to the transmodulation of EGF receptors by TNF. To examine the possible role of EGF in the mitogenic action of TNF in human FS-4 fibroblasts, Palombella et al. (1987) examined the effect of TNF on the expression of EGF receptors. Treatment with TNF resulted in a dose-dependent increase in the number of EGF binding sites, with no change in binding affinity. The increase in EGF binding was seen after a 12-h incubation of FS-4 cells with TNF and became maximal (about 50 to 100% increase over control) by 24 h. Immunoprecipitation with anti-EGF receptor antibody showed a concomitant increase in the synthesis of EGF receptor protein; in fact, the increase in newly synthesized receptor protein was much greater than the increase in cell surface binding sites. Dose-response and kinetic data suggested that the increased expression of EGF receptors could contribute to the mitogenic action of TNF in the presence of EGF. However, increased EGF receptor expression is clearly not the sole pathway of TNF's mitogenic action because in the absence of added EGF, the mitogenic action of TNF was not reduced by the addition of potent blocking anti-EGF receptor monoclonal antibody (Palombella et al., 1988).

Effects of TNF on the EGF receptor were also examined by Bird and Saklatvala (1989) in a line of normal human gingival fibroblast (HuGi). The authors found that treatment with TNF caused a rapid and very transient decrease in EGF binding (maximal after 15 min of TNF treatment), apparently due to a decrease in binding affinity. These results are not contradictory to our own data reported earlier (Palombella et al., 1987), in which an increase in EGF binding was seen in FS-4 cells after 12 to 24 h of treatment with TNF. In fact, we too noticed an initial decrease in EGF binding at 2 to 4 h after TNF treatment in FS-4 cells, but this drop did not appear to be statistically significant. Bird and Saklatvala (1989) also examined EGF receptor phosphorylation in HuGi cells after TNF treatment. There was a two to five fold increase in the phosphorylation of the immunoprecipitated EGF receptor after 15 min of TNF treatment. This increase was accounted for by phosphorylation of serine and threonine residues; incorporation into phosphotyrosine was actually decreased by TNF treatment. A transient decrease in the basal level of phosphotyrosine in the EGF receptor was also seen in A431 cells after TNF treatment (Palombella, 1989).

In contrast to the data in HuGi (Bird and Saklatvala, 1989), FS-4, and A431 (Palombella, 1989) cells, in which no increase tyrosine phosphorylation could be detected after TNF treatments, Donato et al. (1989a,b) reported that in the ME-180 cervical carcinoma line, TNF enhanced the EGF receptor tyrosine phosphorylation. In the latter cells TNF also increased tyrosine protein kinase activity of the EGF receptor itself in a manner similar to that reported for EGF. Curiously, TNF was cytotoxic rather than growth stimulatory in the ME-180 cell line. No increase in tyrosine protein kinase activity was seen in the T24 bladder carcinoma line, resistant to TNF cytotoxicity. An interesting conclusion offered by the authors is that some early events in the action of TNF are similar to the early events in the growth-stimulatory action of EGF.

Kohno et al. (1990) reported that in human FS-4 and murine Swiss 3T3 cells TNF induced, within 5 min, tyrosine phosphorylation of two cytosolic 41- and 43-kDa proteins. Increased tyrosine phosphorylation of these two proteins is commonly seen in fibroblast stimulated with growth factors, including EGF, PDGF, and FGF. The reports of increased phosphorylation on tyrosine after TNF treatment by Kohno et al. (1990) and by Donato et al. (1989a,b) are intriguing in view of the absence of discernible tyrosine kinase domains on the recently established sequences of the p55 and p75 TNF receptors (Dembic et al., 1990). It seems that kinase activity would have to reside in a protein separate from the two known TNF receptors.

Not much is known about the action of TNF on receptors for other growth factors or cytokines. Hori et al. (1988) reported that in FS-4 cells TNF induced a modest stimulation of transferrin binding, peaking at 2 min after TNF treatment; EGF caused a similar increase in the expression of transferrin receptors. TNF was also found to up-regulate the expression of interferon (IFN)-γ receptors in a human carcinoma cell line (Raitano and Korc, 1990). The latter finding is interesting because many earlier studies found that IFN-γ causes up-regulation of TNF receptors in a variety of cell lines (see Chapter 7 in the present volume). In addition, IFN-γ is known to stimulate TNF production in monocytes/macrophages (Beutler et al., 1986; Collart et al., 1986). This mutually stimulatory relationship involving both the receptors and cytokines themselves could be functionally significant in some pathophysiological situations. Since IFN-γ tends to act as an antagonist of TNF's mitogenic action, the ability of TNF to increase the expression IFN-γ receptors (if confirmed in a wider variety of cell types) could act to reduce the growth-stimulatory action of TNF.

D. Direct and Indirect Modes of Action

Three general mechanisms might account for TNF's mitogenic activity. First, TNF could be inducing responsiveness to other growth factors (either autocrine or exogenous). Examples of such actions have been reported for other growth factors (reviewed in Baserga, 1985). Second, TNF could be inducing intracellular events in the target cell that lead to the activation of genes mediating G_0/G_1 transition and/or progression through the cell cycle. Finally, TNF might produce a growth stimulation through the induction of other autocrine growth factors. It appears that all three of the above-mentioned mechanisms can contribute to TNF's mitogenic action and that the relative importance of the individual mechanisms depends on the nature of the target cell and specific conditions.

We have already explained that in promoting fibroblast growth, TNF acts synergistically with serum, insulin, EGF, PDGF, and TGF-β (Table 2). [Synergy with TGF-β possibly may be mediated by an autocrine EGF-like molecule (Palombella, 1989).] In the FS-4 cell line increased responsiveness of cells to the mitogenic action of EGF correlated with an increased expression of EGF receptors in TNF-treated cells. Therefore, it is apparent that TNF can modulate the growth-stimulatory actions of other growth factors.

There is also evidence that TNF can trigger intracellular events leading to DNA synthesis and cell division. In FS-4 cells TNF induces a rapid increase in steady-state levels of c-*fos* and c-*myc* mRNA (Lin and Vilček, 1987). These proto-oncogenes are often activated in response to growth-promoting agents. However, the kinetics of c-*myc* mRNA induction were different from those seen with other growth factors in that TNF produced a much more transient elevation (peaking at 30 min after TNF addition) than EGF or serum. A similar transient c-*myc* mRNA induction was seen in a line of human osteosarcoma cells whose growth was enhanced by TNF (Kirstein and Baglioni, 1988). The very transient nature of c-*myc* activation may be related to the fact that by itself TNF is only a weak mitogen in growth-arrested cells (Palombella et al., 1988). It is significant that c-*myc* mRNA expression was inhibited in cells in which TNF was cytostatic (e.g., in HeLa cells) (Yarden and Kimchi, 1986). Proto-oncogenes c-*jun* and *jun*-B were also induced in some cell lines, due mainly to transcriptional activation (Brenner et al., 1989; Cornelius et al., 1990). Some other early events associated with growth factor actions shown to be activated by TNF include a stimulation in glucose transport activity in 3T3-L1 fibroblasts (Cornelius et al., 1990), the phosphorylation of cytosolic proteins in Swiss 3T3 and FS-4 cells (Kohno et al., 1990), increase in phospholipase activity in BALB/c 3T3 cells (Palombella and Vilček, 1989), a rapid and transient increase in the cAMP level and protein kinase activity in FS-4 cells (Zhang et al., 1988), and activation of protein kinase C in some cell lines (Brenner et al., 1989). These results suggest that at least in some situations, TNF actions are similar to classical growth factors.

The third general mechanism by which TNF might stimulate cell growth is via the induction of autocrine growth factors. This mechanism was shown to be responsible for the mitogenic response to some other agents. For instance, Leof et al. (1986) showed that TGF-β stimulates DNA synthesis in AKR-2B cells through the induction of PDGF. Similarly, IL-1 stimulates the growth of fibroblasts and smooth muscle cells via the synthesis of PGGF-AA (Raines et al., 1989). TNF too has been reported to induce PDGF in endothelial cells and monocytic cell lines (Hajjar et al., 1987; Alitalo et al., 1987).

Our results suggest that in the extensively studied FS-4 cell line, TNF does not stimulate cell growth through the induction of some other secreted factor. We have virtually ruled out the role of autocrine PDGF and EGF or TGF-α with the aid of specific antisera, and we have also ruled out the possible involvement of TGF-β (Palombella et al., 1987; Palombella, 1989). Le et al. (1987) have shown that TNF can induce membrane-associated IL-1 in FS-4 cells, and IL-1 is mitogenic for FS-4 cells (Le and Vilček, 1987; Kohase et al., 1987; Palombella and Vilček, unpublished observations). However, the mitogenic effect of TNF apparently does not depend on the generation of IL-1 because dexamethasone blocks TNF-induced IL-1 synthesis in FS-4 cells (Le et al., 1987) but does not block the mitogenic effect of TNF (Kohase et al., 1987). An additional argument against the rule of an autocrine factor is that in growth-arrested FS-4 cells the induction of DNA synthesis by TNF does not show delayed kinetics as would be expected if the stimulation were indirect (Palombella et al., 1988). In addition, we also could not detect any secreted mitogenic factor in the culture medium from TNF-treated FS-4 cells (Palombella, unpublished data).

Even though available evidence does not support the view that TNF acts by inducing an autocrine growth factor in human FS-4 fibroblasts, our data suggest that TNF may be producing a mitogenic response indirectly in rat NRK fibroblasts (Palombella, unpublished data). TNF stimulates DNA synthesis in quiescent NRK cells, with a peak of DNA synthesis occurring 40 h after the addition of TNF. In contrast, the peak of EGF-induced DNA synthesis occurs 20 h after EGF addition. This suggests that TNF may be stimulating NRK cells to produce some other autocrine mitogenic factor. The mitogenic action of TNF in human mesangial cells was recently shown to be mediated by the generation of PDGF (Silver et al., 1989).

IV. SIGNIFICANCE

At first it appeared that the mitogenic action of TNF is an interesting laboratory phenomenon with little or no relevance to the functions of TNF in the intact organism. In fact, since TNF was long thought to be a specific antitumor agent and selective growth inhibitor or cytotoxic agent, the initial findings of TNF's growth-stimulatory actions were somewhat disturbing. We proposed the idea —unorthodox at the time—that "TNF is primarily a growth factor, and that its direct cytostatic or cytotoxic effects on transformed cells are in fact the results of an anomalous growth signal transduction in cells lacking the constraints of normal growth control mechanisms" (Vilček et al., 1986).

While the primary function of TNF remains uncertain, it is now clear that the growth-stimulatory effects of TNF are relevant to the actions of TNF in the intact organism. As is the case with many other manifestations of TNF actions, the mitogenic effect could be beneficial in some circumstances and detrimental in others. First of all, TNF is almost certainly involved in connective tissue repair and wound healing. Many studies have shown that monocytes/macrophages produce substances with growth-stimulatory activity for mesenchymal cells, including fibroblasts (Wahl and Wahl, 1981; Gillespie et al., 1985). These monocyte-derived substances include IL-1, TGF-α, TGF-β, PDGF, EGF, and IGF-1 (Schmidt et al., 1982; Lynch et al., 1987; Assoian et al., 1987; Rappolee et al., 1988). Austgulen et al. (1987) identified TNF as a major contributor to the monocyte-derived fibroblast growth-stimulatory activity. Addition of a monoclonal antibody to TNF drastically reduced the mitogenic activity of monocyte supernatants on human fibroblasts. Related to its fibrogenic activity is the recently demonstrated ability of TNF to stimulate fibroblast chemotaxis (Postlehwaite and Seyer, 1990). The latter action too is likely to be beneficial in tissue repair.

Since TNF is a major product of activated monocytes, and monocytes represent a major component in mononuclear infiltrates accompanying inflammation, TNF is also likely to be involved in the generation of fibrotic and granulomatous lesions in a variety of pathophysiological processes. Indeed, Piguet al. (1989) have demonstrated that TNF plays a key role in the alveolitis and fibrosis induced by bleomycin in mice, because passive immunization with anti-TNF IgG blocked these effects of bleomycin. It is interesting that IFN-γ was earlier shown to ameliorate the effects of bleomycin-induced lung fibrosis in mice (Giri et al., 1986), and it is known that the growth-stimulatory effect of TNF can be blocked by IFN-γ (Vilček et al., 1986; Sugarman et al., 1985). TNF was also shown to play a key role in silica-induced pulmonary fibrosis (Piguet et al., 1990). An elegant recent study has demonstrated that TNF is an essential mediator of granuloma formation in the liver of mice injected with Bacillus Calmette-Guérin (Kindler et al., 1989). In addition, TNF may play a role in rheumatoid arthritis, because TNF stimulates the growth of synovial cells (Butler et al., 1988) and increases glycosaminoglycan synthesis and hyaluronate synthetase production in fibroblasts (Elias et al., 1988). Moreover, TNF could play a role in sarcoidosis (reviewed by Elias et al., 1988). In fact, mononuclear cells from patients with sarcoidosis appear to secrete TNF spontaneously (Bachwich et al., 1986).

TNF may also play a role in other inflammatory disorders where fibrosis is a major pathological feature. For example, viruses can induce TNF (Aderka et al., 1986; Wong and Goeddel, 1986; Berent et al., 1986) and the local production of TNF could be involved in the fibrosis associated with chronic viral disease (i.e., hepatitis B virus-induced cirrhosis of the liver). Aderka and Levo (1988) have suggested that TNF also may play a role in hepatocyte regeneration. The actions of TNF in these disorders are likely to be contextual; that is, they may depend on the interaction of TNF with other growth factors/cytokines (Lynch et al., 1987; Sporn and Roberts, 1988).

In addition, TNF has angiogenic activity in vivo (Leibovich et al., 1987; Fráter-Schröder et al., 1987). The ability of TNF to promote neovascularization may be due to a direct effect of TNF on endothelial cells or may occur indirectly through the activation of mononuclear cells to synthesize and secrete angiogenic growth factors (i.e., FGF, TGF-α). An indirect mechanism is more likely in view of the fact that TNF was actually shown to inhibit the proliferation of isolated capillary endothelial cells cultured in vitro (Fráter-Schröder et al., 1987; Schweigerer et al., 1987).

The demonstration that TNF can exert a simultaneous cytotoxic and mitogenic effect in BALB/c 3T3 cells (Palombella and Vilček, 1989) may also be relevant to the actions of TNF in the intact organism. Piguet et al. (1987) have implicated TNF in the pathophysiology of graft-versus-host disease (GVHD) in mice. The characteristic alterations seen in the skin and gut of mice with GVHD consist of both isolated epithelial cell necrosis and acceleration of epithelial cell renewal (increased number of mitoses). Both necrosis and increased proliferation were completely prevented by passive immunization with anti-TNF immunoglobulin.

ACKNOWLEDGEMENTS

We thank Ilene Toder for help with the preparation of the manuscript. Work from the authors' laboratory was supported by NIH Grants CA-47304 and AI-12948 and by a predoctoral fellowship to V.J.P. from the National Cancer Center, Plainview, NY.

REFERENCES

Aderka, D., and Levo, Y. (1988). Does tumor necrosis factor play a role in the pathogenesis of fulminant hepatitis? *Med. Hypotheses, 27*: 193.

Aderka, D., Holtmann, H., Toker, L., Hahn, T., and Wallach, D. (1986). Tumor necrosis factor induced by Sendai virus, *J. Immunol., 136:* 2938.

Alitalo, R., Andersson, L. C., Betsholtz, C., Nilsson, K., Westermark, B., Heldin, C. -H., and Alitalo, K. (1987). Induction of platelet-derived growth factor gene expression during megakaryoblastic and monocytic differentiation of human leukemia cell lines, *EMBO J., 6*: 1213.

Assoian, R. K., Fleurdelys, B. E., Stevenson, H. C., Miller, P. J., Madtes, D. K., Raines, E. W., Ross, R., and Sporn, M. B. (1987). Expression and secretion of type beta transforming growth factor by activated human macrophages, *Proc. Natl. Acad. Sci. USA, 84*: 6020.

Austgulen, R., Espevik, T., and Nissen-Meyer, J. (1987). Fibroblast growth-stimulatory activity released from human monocytes: the contribution of tumour necrosis factor, *Scand. J. Immunol., 26*: 621.

Bachwich, P. R., Lynch, J. P., III, Wiggins, R., and Kunkel, S. L. (1986). Tumor necrosis factor-like activity in normal and sarcoid alveolar macrophages, *Am. Rev. Respir. Dis., 133*: A244.

Baserga, R. (1985). *The Biology of Cell Reproduction*, Harvard University Press, Cambridge, Mass.

Berent, S. L., Torczynski, R. M., and Bollon, A. P. (1986). Sendai virus induces high levels of tumor necrosis factor mRNA in human peripheral blood leukocytes, *Nucleic Acids Res., 14*: 8997.

Beutler, B., Tkacenko, V., Milsark, I., Krochin, N., and Cerami, A. (1986). Effect of gamma interferon on cachectin expression by mononuclear phagocytes: reversal of the *Ips*^{d} (endotoxin resistance) phenotype, *J. Exp. Med., 164*: 1791.

Bird, T. A., and Saklatvala, J. (1989). IL-1 and TNF transmodulate epidermal growth factor receptors by a protein kinase C-independent mechanism, *J. Immunol., 142*: 0126.

Branch, D. R., Turner, A. R, and Guilbert, L. J. (1989). Synergistic stimulation of macrophage proliferation by the monokines tumor necrosis factor-alpha and colony-stimulating factor 1, *Blood, 73*: 307.

Brenner, D. A., O'Hara, M., Angel, P., Chojkier, M., and Karin, M. (1989). Prolonged activation of *jun* and collagenase genes by tumor necrosis factor-alpha, *Nature, 337*: 661.

Butler, D. M., Piccoli, D. S., Hart, P. H., and Hamilton, J. A. (1988). Stimulation of human synovial fibroblast DNA synthesis by recombinant human cytokines, *J. Rheumatol., 15*: 1463.

Carswell, E. A., Old, L. J., Kassel, R. L., Green, S., Fiore, N., and Williamson, B. (1975). An endotoxin-induced serum factor that causes necrosis of tumors, *Proc. Natl. Acad. Sci. USA, 72*: 3666.

Collart, M. A., Belin, D., Vassali, J. -D., De Kossodo, S., and Vassali, P. (1986). Gamma interferon enhances macrophage transcription of the tumor necrosis factor/cachectin, interleukin 1, and urokinase genes, which are controlled by short-lived repressors, *J. Exp. Med., 164*: 2113.

Cornelius, P., Marlowe, M., Lee, M. D., and Pekala, P. H. (1990). The growth factor-like effects of tumor necrosis factor-alpha: stimulation of glucose transport activity and induction of glucose transporter and immediate early gene expression in 3T3-L1 preadipocytes, *J. Biol. Chem., 265*: 20506.

Czech, M. P., Clairmont, K. B., Yagaloff, K. A., and Corvera, S. (1990). Properties and regulation of receptors for growth factors, *Peptide Growth Factors and Their Receptors, Handbook of Experimental Pharmacology*, Vol. 95/I (M.A. Sporn and A. B. Roberts, eds.), Springer-Verlag, Berlin, p. 37.

Dembic, Z., Loetscher, H., Gubler, U., Pan, Y. -C. E., Lahn, H. -W., Gentz, R., Brockhaus, M., and Lesslauer, W. (1990). Two human TNF receptors have similar extracellular, but distinct intracellular, domain sequences, *Cytokine, 2*: 231.

Donato, N. J., Gallick, G. E., Steck, P. A., and Rosenblum, M. G. (1989a). Tumor necrosis factor modulates epidermal growth factor receptor phosphorylation and kinase activity in human tumor cells, *J. Biol. Chem., 264*: 20474.

Donato, N. J., Ince, C., Rosenblum, M. G., and Gallick, G. E. (1989b). Early events in the antiproliferative action of tumor necrosis factor are similar to the early events in epidermal growth factor growth stimulation, *J. Cell. Biochem., 41*: 139.

Elias, J. A., Krol, R. C., Freundlich, B., and Sampson, P. M. (1988). Regulation of human lung fibroblast glycosaminoglycan production by recombinant interferons, tumor necrosis factor, and lymphotoxin, *J. Clin. Invest., 81*: 325.

Estes, J. E., Pledger, W. J., and Gillespie, G. Y. (1984). Macrophage-derived growth factor for fibroblast and interleukin-1 are distinct entities, *J. Leukocyte Biol., 35*: 115.

Feinman, R., Henriksen-DeStefano, D., Tsujimoto, M., and Vilček, J. (1987). Tumor necrosis factor is an important mediator of tumor cell killing by human monocytes, *J. Immunol., 138*: 635.

Fráter-Schröder, M., Risau, W., Hallmann, R., Gautschi, P., and Bohlen, P. (1987). Tumor necrosis factor type alpha, a potent inhibitor of endothelial cell growth in vitro, is angiogenic in vivo, *Proc. Natl. Acad. Sci. USA, 84*: 5277.

Gillespie, G. Y., Estes, J. E., and Pledger, W. J. (1985). Macrophage-derived growth factors for mesenchymal cells, *Lymphokines*, Vol. 11, (E. Pick, ed.), Academic Press, New York, p. 213.

Giri, S. N., Hyde, D. M., and Marafino, B. J., Jr. (1986). Ameliorating effect of murine interferon-gama on bleomycin-induced lung collagen fibrosis in mice, *Biochem. Med. Metab. Biol., 36*: 194.

Hajjar, K. A., Hajjar, D. P., Silverstein, R. L., and Nachman, R. L. (1987). Tumor necrosis factor-mediated release of platelet-derived growth factor from cultured endothelial cells, *J. Exp. Med., 166*: 235.

Hori, T., Kashiyama, S., Oku, N., Hayakawa, M., Shibamoto, S., Tsujimoto, M., Nishihara, T., and Ito, F. (1988). Effects of tumor necrosis factor on cell growth and expression of transferrin receptors in human fibroblast, *Cell Struct. Funct., 13*: 425.

Hori, T., Kashiyama, S., Hayakawa, M., Shibamoto, S., Tsujimoto, M., Oku, N., and Ito, F. (1989). Possible role of prostaglandins as negative regulators in growth stimulation by tumor necrosis factor and epidermal growth factor in human fibroblasts, *J. Cell. Physiol., 141*: 275.

Ikebe, T., Hirata, M., and Koga, T. (1988). Effects of human recombinant tumor necrosis factor-alpha and interleukin 1 on the synthesis of glycosaminoglycan and DNA in cultured rat costal chondrocytes, *J. Immunol., 140*: 827.

Jelinek, D. F., and Lipsky, P. E. (1987). Enhancement of human B cell proliferation and differentiation by tumor necrosis factor-alpha and interleukin 1, *J. Immunol., 139*: 2970.

Kahaleh, M. B., Smith, E. A., Soma, Y., and LeRoy, E. C. (1988). Effect of lymphotoxin and tumor necrosis factor on endothelial and connective tissue cell growth and function, *Clin. Immunol. Immunopathol., 49*: 261.

Kamijo, R., Takeda, K., Nagumo, M., and Konno, K. (1989). Suppression of TNF-stimulated proliferation of diploid fibroblasts and TNF-induced cytotoxicity against transformed fibroblasts by TGF-beta, *Biochem. Biophys. Res. Commun., 158*: 155.

Kindler, V., Sappino, A. -P., Grau, G. E., Piguet, P. -F., and Vassalli, P. (1989). The inducing role of tumor necrosis factor in the development of bactericidal granulomas during BCG infection, *Cell, 56*: 731.

Kirstein, M., and Baglioni, C. (1988). Tumor necrosis factor stimulates proliferation of human osteosarcoma cells and accumulation of c-*myc* messenger RNA, *J. Cell. Physiol., 134*: 479.

Kohase, M., Henriksen-DeStefano, D., Sehgal., P. B., and Vilček, J. (1987). Dexamethasone inhibits feedback regulation of the mitogenic activity of tumor necrosis factor, interleukin-1 and epidermal growth factor in human fibroblasts, *J. Cell. Physiol., 132*: 271.

Kohno, M., Nishizawa, N., Tsujimoto, M., and Nomoto, H. (1990). Mitogenic signalling pathway of tumour necrosis factor involves the rapid tyrosine phosphorylation of 41 000-M_r and 43 000-M_r cytosol proteins, *Biochem. J., 267*: 91.

Lachman, L. B., Brown, D. C., and Dinarello, C. A. (1987). Growth-promoting effect of recombinant interleukin 1 and tumor necrosis factor for a human astrocytoma cell line, *J. Immunol., 138*: 2913.

Le, J., and Vilček, J. (1987). Tumor necrosis factor and interleukin 1: cytokines with multiple overlapping biological activities, *Lab. Invest., 56*: 234.

Le, J., Weinstein, D., Gubler, U., and Vilček, J. (1987). Induction of membrane-associated interleukin 1 by tumor necrosis factor in human fibroblast, *J. Immunol., 138*: 2137.

Lee, S. H., Aggarwal, B. B., Rinderknecht, E., Assisi, F., and Chiu, H. (1984). The synergistic anti-proliferative effect of gamma-interferon and human lymphotoxin, *J. Immunol., 133*: 1083.

Leibovich, S. J., Polverini, P. J., Shepard, H. M., Wiseman, D. M., Shively, V., and Nuseir, N. (1987). Macrophage-induced angiogenesis is mediated by tumor necrosis factor-alpha, *Nature, 329*: 630.

Leof, E. B., Van Wyk, J. J., O'Keefe, E. J., and Pledger, W. J. (1983). Epidermal growth factor (EGF) is required only during the traverse of early G_1 in PDGF stimulated density-arrested BALB/c-3T3 cells, *Exp. Cell Res., 147*: 202.

Leof, E. B., Proper, J. A., Goustin, A. S., Shipley, G. D., DiCorleto, P. E., and Moses, H. L. (1986). Induction of c-*sis* mRNA and activity similar to platelet-derived growth factor by transforming growth factor-beta: a proposed model for indirect mitogenesis involving autocrine activity, *Proc. Natl. Acad. Sci. USA, 83*: 2453.

Lewis, G. D., Aggarwal, B. B., Eessalu, T. E., Sugarman, B. J., and Shepard, H. M. (1987). Modulation of the growth of transformed cells by human tumor necrosis factor-alpha and interferon-gamma, *Cancer Res., 47*: 5382.

Lin, J. -X., and Vilček, J. (1987). Tumor necrosis factor and interleukin-1 cause a rapid and transient stimulation of c-fos and c-myc mRNA in human fibroblast, *J. Biol. Chem., 262*: 11908.

Lynch, S. E., Nixon, J. C., Colvin, R. B., and Antoniades, H. N. (1987). Role of platelet-derived growth factor in wound healing: synergistic effects with other growth factors, *Proc. Natl. Acad. Sci. USA, 84*: 7696.

Olashaw, N. E., and Pledger, W. J. (1985). Mechanisms initiating cellular proliferation, *Mediators of Cell Growth and Differentiation* (R. J. Ford and A. L. Maizel, eds), Raven Press, New York, p. 31.

Palombella, V. (1989). Mitogenic action of tumor necrosis factor in fibroblasts, Ph.D. thesis, New York University.

Palombella, V. J., and Vilček, J. 91989). Mitogenic and cytotoxic actions of tumor necrosis factor in BALB/c 3T3 cells: role of phospholipase activation, *J. Biol. Chem., 264*: 18128.

Palombella, V. J., Yamashiro, D. J., Maxfield, F. R., Decker, S. J., and Vilček, J. (1987). Tumor necrosis factor increases the number of epidermal growth factor receptors on human fibroblasts, *J. Biol. Chem., 262*: 1950.

Palombella, V. J., Mendelsohn, J., and Vilček, J. (1988). Mitogenic action of tumor necrosis factor in human fibroblasts: interaction with epidermal growth factor and platelet-derived growth factor, *J. Cell. Physiol., 135*: 23.

Piacibello, W., Sanavio, F., Severino, A., Morelli, S., Vaira, A. M., Stacchini, A., and Aglietta, M. (1990). Opposite effect of tumor necrosis factor alpha on granulocyte colony-stimulating factor and granulocyte-macrophage colony-stimulating factor-dependent growth of normal and leukemic hemopoietic progenitors, *Cancer Res., 50*: 5065.

Piguet, P. -F., Grau, G. E., Allet, B., and Vassalli, P. (1987). Tumor necrosis factor/cachectin is an effector of skin and gut lesions of the acute phage of graft-vs. -host disease, *J. Exp. Med., 166*: 1280.

Piguet, P. -F., Collart, M. A., Grau, G. E., Kapanci, Y., and Vassalli, P. (1989). Tumor necrosis factor/cachectin plays a key role in bleomycin-induced pneumopathy and fibrosis, *J. Exp. Med., 170*: 655.

Piguet, P. -F., Collart, M. A., Grau, G. E., Sappino, A. -P., and Vassalli, P. (1990). Requirement of tumor necrosis factor for development of silica-induced pulmonary fibrosis, *Nature, 344*: 245.

Pledger, W. J., Stiles, C. D., Antoniades, H. N., and Scher, C. D. (1977). Induction of DNA synthesis in BALB/c 3T3 cells by serum components: re-evaluation of the commitment process, *Proc. Natl. Acad. Sci. USA, 74*: 4481.

Pledger, W. J., Stiles, C. D., Antoniades, H. N., and Scher, C. D. (1978). An ordered sequence of events is required before BALB/c-3T3 cells become committed to DNA synthesis, *Proc. Natl. Acad. Sci. USA, 75*: 2839.

Postlethwaite, A. E., and Seyer, J. M. (1990). Stimulation of fibroblast chemotaxis by human recombinant tumor necrosis factor alpha (TNF-alpha) and a synthetic TNF-alpha 31-68 peptide, *J. Exp. Med., 172*: 1749.

Raines, E. W., Dower, S. K., and Ross, R. (1989). Interleukin-1 mitogenic activity for fibroblasts and smooth muscle cells is due to PDGF-AA, *Science, 243*: 393.

Raitano, A. B., and Korc, M. (1990). Tumor necrosis factor up-regulates gamma-interferon binding in a human carcinoma cell line, *J. Biol. Chem., 265*: 10466.

Ranges, G. E., Zlotnik, A., Espevik, T., Dinarello, C. A., Cerami, A., and Palladino, M. A., Jr. (1988). Tumor necrosis factor alpha/cachectin is a growth factor for thymocytes: synergistic interactions with other cytokines, *J. Exp. Med., 167*: 1472.

Ranges, G. E., Bombara, M. P., Aiyer, R. A., Rice, G. G., and Palladino, M. A., Jr. (1989). Tumor necrosis factor-alpha as a proliferative signal for an IL-2-dependent T cell line: strict species specificity of action, *J. Immunol., 142*: 1203.

Rappolee, D. A., Mark, D., Banda, M. J., and Werb, Z. (1988). Wound macrophages express TGF-alpha and other growth factors in vivo: analysis by mRNA phenotyping, *Science, 241*: 708.

Rozengurt, E. (1986). Early signals in the mitogenic response, *Science, 234*: 161.

Ruff, M. R., and Gifford, G. E. (1981). Tumor necrosis factor, *Lymphokines*, (Vol. 2, (E. Pick, ed.), Academic Press, New York, p. 235.

Schmidt, J. A., Mizel, S. B., Cohen, D., and Green, I. (1982). Interleukin 1, a potential regulatory of fibroblast proliferation, *J. Immunol., 128*: 2177.

Schweigerer, L., Malerstein, B., and Gospodarowicz, D. (1987). Tumor necrosis factor inhibits the proliferation of cultured capillary endothelial cells, *Biochem. Biophys. Res. Commun., 143*: 997.

Silver, B., Jaffer, F. E., and Abboud, H. E. (1989). Platelet-derived growth factor synthesis in mesangial cells: induction by multiple peptide mitogens, *Proc. Natl. Acad. Sci. USA, 86*: 1056.

Singh, J. P., Adams, L. D., and Bonin, P. D. (1988). Mode of fibroblast growth enhancement by human interleukin-1, *J. Cell. Biol., 106*: 813.

Sporn, M. B., and Roberts, A. B. (1988). Peptide growth factors are multifunctional, *Nature, 332*: 217.

Stiles, C. D., Capone, G. T., Scher, C. D., Antoniades, H. N., Van Wyk, J. J., and Pledger, W. J. (1979). Dual control of cell growth by somatomedins and platelet-derived growth factor, *Proc. Natl. Acad. Sci. USA, 76*: 1279.

Sugarman, B. J., Aggarwal, B. B., Hass, P. E., Figari, I. S., Palladino, M. A., Jr., and Shepard, H. M. (1985). Recombinant human tumor necrosis factor-alpha: effects on proliferation of normal and transformed cells in vitro, *Science, 230*: 943.

Todaro, G. J., and Green, H. (1963). Quantitative studies of the growth of mouse embryo cells in culture and their development into established lines, *J. Cell. Biol., 17*: 299.

Todaro, G. J., Lazar, G. K., and Green, H. (1965). The initiation of cell division in a contact-inhibited mammalian cell line, *J. Cell Comp. Physiol., 66*: 325.

Vilček, J. (1990). Interferons, *Peptide Growth Factors and Their Receptors; Handbook of Experimental Pharmacology*, Vol. 95/II (M. A. Sporn and A. B. Roberts, eds.), Springer-Verlag, Berlin, p. 3.

Vilček, J., Palombella, V. J., Henriksen-DeStefano, D., Swenson, C., Feinman, R., Hirai, M., and Tsujimoto, M. (1986). Fibroblast growth-enhancing activity of tumor nerosis factor and its relationship to other polypeptide growth factors, *J. Exp. Med., 163*: 632.

Wahl, S. M., and Wahl, L. M. (1981). Modulation of fibroblast growth and function by monokines and lymphokines, *Lymphokines*, Vol. 2, (E. Pick, ed.), Academic Press, New York, p. 179.

Westermark, B., and Heldin, C. -H. (1985). Similar action of platelet-derived growth factor and epidermal growth factor in the prereplicative phase of human fibroblasts suggests a common intracellular pathway, *J. Cell. Physiol., 124*: 43.

Wong, G. H. W., and Goeddel, D. V. (1986). Tumor necrosis factors alpha and beta inhibit virus replication and synergize with interferons, *Nature, 323*: 819.

Yarden, A., and Kimchi, A. (1986). Tumor necrosis factor reduces c-*myc* expression and cooperates with interferon-gamma in HeLa cells, *Science, 234*: 1419.

Yokota, S., Geppert, T. D., and Lipsky, P. E. 91988). Enhancement of antigen- and mitogen-induced human T lymphocyte proliferation by tumor necrosis factor-alpha, *J. Immunol., 140*: 531.

Zhang, Y., Lin, J. -X., Yip, Y. K., and Vilček, J. (1988). Enhancement of cyclic AMP levels and of protein kinase activity by TNF and IL-1 in human fibroblasts: role in the induction of IL-6, *Proc. Natl. Acad. Sci. USA, 85*: 6802.

13

Effects of TNF and Lymphotoxin on the Hematopoietic System

GIORGIO TRINCHIERI

The Wistar Institute, Philadelphia, Pennsylvania

I. INTRODUCTION

The homeostasis of the hematopoietic system is maintained by a series of complex cellular interactions and feedback mechanisms. These cellular interactions are often mediated by release of soluble factors which directly affect hematopoietic cell proliferation and differentiation, regulate the emargination and migration ability of hematopoietic cells and their adherence to stromal cells, and modulate the production by accessory cells of other factors affecting hematopoiesis (Metcalf, 1989; Trinchieri et al., 1987a). Alteration in the balance of the regulatory cell types, in the production of the various factors, or in the ability of hematopoietic and stromal cells to respond to them results in pathologic alteration of homeostasis. Soluble products (cytokines) of cells involved in regulation of hematopoiesis include, among others, pluripotent and lineage-specific colony-stimulating factors (CSF), interferons (IFN), differentiation-inducing factors (DIF), growth and transforming factors, and cytotoxins. Many of these cytokines were originally identified and named on the basis of specific biologic activities, often linked to their role in the host defense against pathogens (e.g., antiviral or antitumor activity). Subsequent studies have shown that these cytokines can exert additional effects and that they represent hormone-like physiologic regulators.

The cytotoxins tumor necrosis factor (TNF) and lymphotoxin (LT) were originally defined and measured on the basis of their antitumor toxic effect. However, the cytotoxic activity of cytotoxins represents only one facet of their pleomorphic activity and the cytotoxins, in both physiologic and pathologic conditions, might be important regulators of hematopoiesis of cellular energy metabolism and of host defenses, acting primarily on the hematopoietic effector cells of nonadaptive resistance against pathogens (Old, 1985; Sherry and Cerami, 1988). TNF and LT interact with hematopoietic cells at every stage of differentiation, inhibiting or enhancing proliferation of hematopoietic precursor cells, inducing differentiation of immature myelomonocytic cells, and activating terminally differentiated granulocytes and monocyte/macrophages. In many of these nontoxic effects on hematopoietic cells, TNF and LT synergize with IFN-γ. TNF and LT also affect hematopoietic cells by inducing, alone or together with other stimuli, secretion of various factors, including CSF, from stromal cells(fibroblasts, keratinocytes, endothelial cells) and from lymphocytes and macrophages and by affecting emargination, migration, and adhesion of hematopoietic cells to tissue cells.

Because of the many different mechanisms by which TNF and LT can affect hematopoiesis, it is very difficult to extrapolate from in vitro results on isolated cell preparations to possible in vivo effects of TNF/LT. However, the in vitro dissection of the various mechanisms of action of TNF/LT on hematopoietic cells is a necessary step for the interpretation of the often paradoxical in vivo observations.

The final effect of TNF/LT on in vivo hematopoietic homeostasis depends on many different parameters, such as dose and length of in vivo endogenous production or exogenous treatment, localization of TNF/LT-producing cells, gradient of concentration in various tissues, and antagonistic or synergistic interaction with other cytokines. TNF and LT are themselves products of hematopoietic cells and represent important molecules involved in certain effector functions of lymphocytes and macrophages. Although TNF and LT genes are present in tandem organization within the MHC complex on human chromosome 6 (Spies et al., 1986), they are activated in different cell types and independently regulated. LT is produced only by T and B lymphocytes and the LT gene promoter is inactive in mouse macrophages (Jongeneel et al., 1989). Natural killer (NK) cells were the first lymphocyte type recognized to produce TNF, a cytokine previously considered a product of monocyte/macrophage only (Degliantoni et al., 1985a). Peripheral blood lymphocytes (PBL) were then demonstrated to produce both TNF and LT and the regulation of these two closely linked genes shown to be independent, because (1) different inducers preferentially induce production of either cytotoxin, and (2) with most inducers, accumulation of TNF mRNA and TNF production was observed at earlier times than accumulation of LT mRNA and LT production (Cuturi et al., 1987).

The original observations of the role of TNF/LT in regulation of hematopoiesis came from studies directed to identify the soluble mediators by which activated NK or T cells suppress proliferation of hematopoietic precursor cells (Degliantoni et al., 1985a) and by which the supernatant fluids from mitogen-activated T cells induce differentiation of myeloid cells (Trinchieri et al., 1986).

II. EFFECT OF TNF AND LT ON PROLIFERATION/DIFFERENTIATION OF HEMATOPOIETIC PRECURSOR CELLS IN VITRO

Evidence that TNF and LT were able to inhibit formation of hematopoietic colonies in vitro was initially obtained during studies investigating the role of soluble factors in the inhibition mediated by activated T cells and NK cells. Purified NK cells from human peripheral blood inhibit colony formation by hematopoietic precursor cells when preincubated with bone marrow cells before plating in semisolid medium (Hansson et al., 1982; Degliantoni et al., 1985b). Although cell-mediated cytotoxicity requiring cell contact may play a role in this inhibitory effect, Degliantoni et al. (1985b) demonstrated that NK cells, during contact with bone marrow cells or with NK-sensitive target cell lines, such as the erythromyeloid leukemia cell line K562, release a soluble inhibitor of colony formation (NK-derived colony-inhibiting activity, NK-CIA). Degliantoni et al. (1985a) subsequently identified NK-CIA as TNF, thus demonstrating that TNF can be produced by lymphocytes and is a potent suppressor of hematopoiesis in vitro. Recombinant TNF (and NK-CIA) were shown to induce 50% inhibition of early precursors of granulocyte-macrophage colony-forming units (early CFU-GM, forming colonies in semisolid medium around day 14) at concentrations of 1 U/mL (0.1 ng/mL), whereas late CFU-GM (forming colonies around day 7) were inhibited only at concentrations higher than 10 U/mL. IFN-γ strongly synergized with rTNF in inhibiting late CFU-GM (Degliantoni et al., 1985a).

Murphy et al. (1986) showed that the colony-inhibiting activity present in the supernatant of mitogen-activated tumor T cells, previously attributed to IFN-γ alone, was due to the synergistic effect of LT and IFN-γ, whereas the two factors separately at the concentrations produced by T cells had no or minimal inhibiting activity. LT was shown to have an inhibitory effect on CFU comparable to that of TNF (Broxmeyer et al., 1986; Murphy et al., 1986). Although TNF and LT show an almost identical effect on late CFU-GM (50% inhibition at >10 U/mL), unlike TNF, LT did not inhibit early CFU-GM at doses as high as 100 U/mL, but synergized with IFN-γ in this effect (Murphy et al., 1986, 1988). In the presence of 10 U/mL of IFN-γ, equivalent concentrations of TNF and LT induced similar inhibition of early CFU-GM. This (Murphy et al., 1986) was the first reported example of one of the rare cases of different biologic activity between TNF and LT, two highly homologous cytokines acting through identical cellular receptors.

T cells, depending on the stimulus and on the length of the culture period, produce both LT and TNF (Cuturi et al., 1987) and are therefore able to inhibit colony formation by production of either cytokines. T and NK cells, by producing both IFN-γ and cytotoxins, factors synergizing in inhibition of CFU, are potent suppressors of hematopoiesis in vitro and possibly in vivo; however, T and NK cells, due to their ability to produce also several hematopoietic stimulator factors (Cuturi et al., 1989) and due to the complex effects of all these lymphokines directly on precursor cells or indirectly on accessory and stromal cells, probably play a much more complex role in vivo in the regulation of hematopoiesis than suggested by the experiments of inhibition of colony formation.

Monocytes, unlike T and NK cells, do not produce IFN-γ, but enhance IFN-γ-induced inhibition of myeloid precursor cell growth by a cell-contact-independent mechanism involving secretion of TNF (Cannistra et al., 1988). IFN-γ induces or enhances TNF production by monocyte-macrophages (Cannistra et al., 1988; Herrmann et al., 1989; Celada et al., 1989). Production of TNF by marrow adherent cells was also shown to be responsible for the synergistic inhibition of CFU-GM by different types of IFN and prostaglandin E (PGE) (Pelus et al., 1988). Interestingly, TNF itself, alone or in combination with IL-1, induces production of PGE by fibroblasts or other stromal cells (Dayer et al., 1985; Elias et al., 1987), suggesting a new complex series of interaction involving PGE and TNF between various cellular types and humoral factors affecting hematopoiesis.

TNF and LT, with equivalent efficiency, also inhibit erythroid colonies (burst forming unit-erythroid, BFU-E, and CFU-erythroid, CFU-E) and colonies formed by pluripotent precursor cells (CFU-granulocyte, erythrocyte, monocyte, megakaryocyte, CFU-GEMM) (Broxmeyer et al., 1986; Murphy et al., 1988). In the various studies 50% inhibition was observed with TNF/LT concentrations in the range 10 to 50 U/mL. IFN-γ had always a more than additive effect on the inhibition mediated by TNF and LT.

The mechanism of suppression of colony growth by TNF and LT is unknown but unlikely to be dependent on a direct cytotoxic effect on precursor cells. Although Broxmeyer et al.(1986) reported that 60 min treatment was sufficient to induce inhibition, other studies (Akahane et al., 1987; Murase et al., 1987) showed that the presence of TNF in culture for more than 24 h is required in order to obtain efficient inhibition, suggesting a nontoxic effect. One possible mechanism that may play a role in inhibition of proliferation is the ability of TNF to induce differentiation along the macrophage lineage of myeloid cells, with suppression of the proliferative potential of the cells (Trinchieri et al., 1986; Takeda et al., 1986). Consistent with this mechanism is the observation by Murphy et al. (1988) and Beran et al. (1988a) that while TNF induces inhibition of granulocyte colonies, at low doses it induces a modest increase in macrophage colonies. The mechanism of synergism between TNF/LT and IFN-γ is also not known. Although on certain cell lines IFN-γ was shown to increase slightly the number of TNF receptors (Aggarwal et al., 1985; Tsujimoto et al., 1986a), this effect does not seem to account completely for the synergistic effects between the two cytokines (Ruggiero et al.,

1986), also taking into consideration that TNF receptors are expressed on all hematopoietic cells and that their density does not correlate with sensitivity of the cells to the toxic or growth regulatory effect of TNF (Munker et al., 1987). In other systems, the synergism between TNF and IFN-γ was observed not only for toxicity on cell lines, but also for the differentiation-inducing activity of TNF on myeloid cells (Trinchieri et al., 1986) as well as for the induction of specific gene expression (Cassatella et al., 1989).

The exact determination of the effect of TNF and LT on proliferation and differentiation of hematopoietic precursor cells was initially hampered by the use of non-purified preparation of precursor cells and of crude preparations of CSF. Some of the studies illustrated above, indicating various mechanisms by which lymphocytes and monocytes can affect the inhibition mediated by TNF on the hematopoietic cells, clearly indicate the necessity of using purified cellular preparations. Crude preparations of CSF can contain other factors that are active on precursor cells or act indirectly by stimulating accessory cells: The best example is provided by the conditioned medium of mitogen-activated lymphocytes, a commonly used source of CSF, which also contain IFN-γ and often LT and/or TNF (Murphy et al., 1986; Cuturi et al., 1987). Broxmeyer et al. (1986) used human bone marrow cells depleted of monocyte/macrophage and T cells, whereas Murphy et al. (1988) used human bone marrow cells depleted of monocyte/macrophages, T and NK cells, erythroid cells, and myeloid cells: The ability of TNF in these two studies to inhibit various types of CFU at similar concentrations suggests that TNF is directly acting on precursor cells. The use of highly purified (cloning efficiency 0.84) murine bone marrow precursor cells has allowed Williams et al. (1988) to confirm the direct effect of TNF on precursor cells, although in that study inhibition of CFU-GM was observed at doses of human TNF (100 to 1000 U/mL) much higher than those required for inhibition of human progenitor cells. Similarly, Akahane et al. (1987) have observed almost no inhibition of murine CFU-GM by human TNF, although inhibition of erythroid colonies burst forming units-erythroid (BFU-E) and CFU-erythroid (CFU-E) was observed. The possibility that these results can be explained by a partial species specificity in the effect of TNF against bone marrow cells is suggested by the study of Eliason and Vassalli (1988) that showed inhibition of murine CFU by recombinant murine TNF at doses similar to those required for human TNF to inhibit human bone marrow hematopoietic cells. Eliason and Vassalli (1988) also showed that in long-term bone marrow culture, TNF induces a prolonged inhibition of cell production by acting on stromal cells and inducing a detachment of the precursor cells. TNF inhibition of hematopoiesis occurs therefore at the level of both progenitor cells and stromal cells.

In the original studies on the effect of TNF and LT on CFU in vitro crude preparations of CSF were used, often containing more than one type of CSF. However, it became soon apparent that the ability of TNF and LT to inhibit CFU depends not only on the type of CFU analyzed but also on the type of CSF which induces colony formation. For example, late CFU-GM induced by giant cell condition medium (GTC) or by rGM-CSF were relatively resistant to the effect of TNF on LT in the absence of IFN-γ (Degliantoni et al., 1985a; Murphy et al., 1988), but they were very sensitive to the inhibition by TNF when colony formation was induced by supernatant fluid of the bladder carcinoma cell line 5637, mostly containing granulocyte CSF (G-CSF) (Broxmeyer et al., 1986; Murphy et al., 1988). Barber et al. (1987) using a limiting dilution assay showed that both TNF and LT almost completely inhibited the response of bone marrow cells to G-CSF, whereas the frequency of cells able to form colonies in culture stimulated with GM-CSF was unaltered. GM-CSF in some cases was also shown to protect progenitor cells from the inhibitory effect of TNF (Munker et al., 1987; Peetre et al., 1986). On murine bone marrow, CSF-1-induced CFU were shown to be inhibited by TNF in a study by Eliason and Vassalli (1988), whereas Williams et al. (1988) showed that TNF enhances macrophage colony formation induced by CSF-1. Recent studies by Caux et al. (1990) showed that TNF and LT in liquid cultures strongly potentiate the growth of highly purified CD34$^+$ human hematopoietic progenitor cells in response to interleukin-3 (IL-3) or GM-CSF, whereas they inhibit the growth-promoting effect of G-CSF, which acts on a more committed subpopulation of CD34$^+$ cells different from that recruited by IL-3. In analogy to the effects described on other normal or malignant cells (Sugarman et al., 1985; Vilček et al., 1986), TNF has therefore both stimulating and inhibitory effects on the growth of hematopoietic precursor cells and appears to enhance the early stages of hematopoiesis, in which proliferation is joined to little or no differentiation, whereas it has a suppressor effect on the proliferation of more mature hematopoietic precursor cells. Hematopoietic cells at different stages of differentiation might have constitutively a different sensitivity to the effect of TNF, or alternatively, TNF might specifically affect the proliferative signal induced by certain CSF (e.g., G-CSF). It should be pointed out that the somewhat contrasting results obtained in the experiments of limiting dilution or of liquid cultures versus those obtained in the experiments of colony formation are not necessarily contradictory. The end point of colony formation measures the appearance of detectable colonies of differentiated cells during a period of up to 14 days and the inhibition mediated by TNF could take place at different stages during the formation of the colony and not necessarily at the level of the single precursor cell. Consistent with this hypothesis are the observations that large colony formation is much more sensitive to the inhibition by TNF than the formation of small clusters (Broxmeyer et al., 1986; Beran et al., 1988b) and the several studies (Akahane et al., 1987; Murase et al., 1987) showing that to inhibit colony formation TNF needs to be present in the culture for periods longer than 24h. Unlike colony formation, liquid culture experiments measure proliferation of the precursor cells in the first few days of culture, often before terminal differentiation takes place, evaluating more accurately the effect of TNF at the level of early precursor cells.

Early studies on the effect of TNF on leukemic precursor cells from patients with chronic or acute myelogenous leukemia (CML, AML) indicated that colonies or clusters formed by leukemic cells from most patients were more sensitive to the inhibitory effect of TNF than those formed by early normal precursor cells or even than those formed by more differentiated precursor cells (Broxmeyer et al., 1986; Beran et al., 1988b; Munker and Koeffler, 1987; Murase et al., 1987). Significant inhibition of leukemic colonies were observed at doses of 0.1 to 1 U/mL of TNF. TNF was also shown (Nagata et al., 1989) to inhibit the self-renewal capacity of leukemic blast progenitors in AML. Although these data generated some interest for the possible therapeutic utilization of TNF in patients with leukemia, the interpretation of the data was hampered by the utilization in most studies of crude preparations of CSF, often in the form of conditioned media containing more than one type of CSF together with other cytokines. Hoang et al. (1989) using pure recombinant CSF showed that TNF antagonizes the mitogenic effect of G-CSF and IL-3 on AML blasts, but enhances the proliferation induced by GM-CSF and the cell density-dependent proliferation of AML blasts. Therefore, TNF acts on the same AML cells with unique capacity to either support or inhibit cell proliferation, depending on the growth signaling context. Whereas on the AML cells TNF only augments the proliferation induced by other factors, it was shown to be directly mitogenic in vitro for neoplastic B cells from chronic lymphocytic leukemia patients (Digel et al., 1989). The density-dependent growth of AML blasts indicates the ability of these cells to produce autocrine growth factors (Oster et al., 1989; Hoang et al., 1989). TNF itself is one of the factors produced by the leukemic cells with a possible role in the autocrine control of their growth (Oster et al., 1989). Hairy cell leukemia cells were shown by Lindemann et al. (1989) to secrete a high level of TNF that is responsible for the decreased ability of patients' bone marrow cells to form colonies in vitro and possibly for the hematopoietic failure in vivo observed in these patients.

III. EFFECT OF TNF AND LT ON DIFFERENTIATION OF MYELOID CELLS AND ACTIVATION OF TERMINALLY DIFFERENTIATED MYELOMONOCYTIC CELLS

Supernatant fluids from activated lymphocytes induce differentiation of human leukemic myeloid cell lines, fresh myeloid leukemia cells, and bone marrow myeloid cells, to cells with phenotypic characteristics of mature monocyte/macrophages (Elias et al., 1980; Dayton et al., 1983). IFN-γ was found to be necessary for the differentiation-inducing activity of the leukocyte-conditioned medium, acting in synergism with other differentiation-inducing factors (Dayton et al., 1985; Perussia et al., 1983). TNF and LT were identified by Trinchieri et al., (1986) and Takeda et al. (1986) as the differentiation-inducing factors present in the leukocyte-conditioned medium and acting in synergism with IFN-γ. Recombinant TNF and LT at concentrations of 10^{-11} *M* induce monocytic differentiation of the human myeloid cell lines HL-60, ML-1, ML-3, U937, and THP-1 (Trinchieri et al., 1986; Takeda et al., 1986; Takuma et al., 1987; Hemmi et al., 1987). After 5-d culture in the presence of TNF or LT, a significant proportion of the cells expresses monocyte differentiation antigens (e.g., CD14, CD11b) and nonspecific esterase activity, mediates antibody-dependent cytotoxicity, and responds to various stimuli with respiratory burst. The expression of these markers and functions of differentiated cells are maximally induced when IFN-γ is present together with the cytotoxins, and the combined effect of IFN-γ and TNF or LT is highly synergistic (Trinchieri et al., 1986). A decrease in cell proliferation accompanies induced differentiation and is not due to the cytotoxic properties of TNF or LT, because arrest of proliferation and accumulation in G1 is observed late in the culture period only in those cells expressing markers of terminal differentiation (Trinchieri et al., 1986). TNF actually induces an increase of [^{3}H] thymidine uptake in HL-60 cells at 20 to 24 h of culture due in part to a modest increase of cells in S phase (Trinchieri et al., 1986) and in part to stimulation of thymidine kinase (Elias, 1988).

The differentiation effect of TNF on myeloid cells is potentiated by several other cytokines or substances with or without differentiation-inducing ability of their own. TNF and LT synergize with retinoic acid in inducing differentiation and growth inhibition of the human myeloid cell lines HL-60 and THP-1 (Hemmi et al., 1987; Trinchieri et al., 1987b; Tobler et al., 1987a). Retinoic acid alone induces a partial differentiation of HL-60 cells to granulocytes (Breitman et al., 1980), whereas TNF induces differentiation along the monocytic/macrophagic pathway: The combination of the two substances potentiate both effects, inducing cells with morphology of polymorphonucleated cells and with differentiation markers of both granulocytes and monocytes (Trinchieri et al., 1987b). Retinoic acid synergizes with TNF in inhibiting clonal growth in vitro of myeloid leukemic cells from about half of patients, whereas it reverses the inhibitory effect of TNF on the growth of normal CFU-GM and of leukemic cells from the other half of patients, suggesting that TNF and retinoic acid interact in a complex manner with normal and leukemic hematopoietic cells (Tobler et al., 1987a). TNF also cooperates with 1α, 25-dihydroxyvitamin D_3. (Trinchieri et al., 1987c; Katakami et al., 1988), transforming growth factor-β (DeBenedetti et al., 1990), and with PGE_2 (Hosoi et al., 1989). Interestingly, 1α, 25-dihydroxyvitamin D_3 transcriptionally up-regulate TNF mRNA in HL-60 cells, but in the absence of other stimuli does not regulate translation or secretion of active TNF (Steffen et al., 1988). TNF has also been shown to induce differentiation of the mouse myeloid leukemic cell line M1 in synergism with IL-1 with a mechanism of action that might involve IFN-β as an autocrine differentiation factor (Onozaki et al., 1988). Interleukin-6 (IL-6) is a potent inducer of differentiation of the murine M1 cell lines (Chen et al., 1988); IL-6 has only minimal effect on human myeloid cell lines, but it was reported to synergize with TNF (Chen et al., 1988; Takeda et al., 1988).

TNF was shown to induce monocyte/macrophage differentiation in blast cells from patients with AML or myeloid blast crisis of CML (Geissler et al., 1989). Myeloid cells from peripheral blood of patients with CML are induced to differentiate to monocyte/macrophages by IFN-γ (Perussia et al., 1983), but TNF has only a minimal effect. The inefficacy of TNF in inducing differentiation of CML cells is possible due to the constitutive and TNF-γ-inducible expression of the TNF gene in CML patients, with an autocrine effect on cell differentiation and proliferation (Cassatella et al., 1989; Duncombe et al., 1989).

The mechanism of action by which TNF induces differentiation alone and in synergism with IFN-γ remains largely unknown. TNF in human myeloid cell lines was shown to induce phosphorylation rapidly at serine residues of a 26-kDa protein (Schütze et al., 1989) and at both serine and tyrosine residues of a 75-kDa protein (Evans et al., 1990). Whereas phosphorylation of the 26-kDa protein appears relatively specific for myeloid cells stimulated by TNF only, phosphorylation of the 75-kDa protein is also induced by other cytokines, such as GM-CSF or IFN-γ. Phospholipase A_2 activation is commonly observed within a few minutes of interaction of TNF with cells (Clark et al., 1988) and phospholipase A_2 inhibitors block the TNF-mediated induction of TNF gene expression in human myeloid cell lines (Kubin and Trinchieri, unpublished observation). TNF also rapidly induces increased activity in myeloid cell line nuclei of proteins binding to the DNA elements kB and AP-1 (Griffin et al., 1989; Flynn and Trinchieri, unpublished observation); because kB-type enhancers are involved in transcriptional activation of the TNF gene (Shakhov et al., 1990), induction of nuclear factors binding to κB (NF-κB) could be the mechanism of the autocrine induction of the TNF gene by TNF. In myeloid cells TNF rapidly induces transcription of both c-fos and c-jun (Squinto et al., 1989; Bertani et al., 1984). TNF could therefore regulate the AP-1-binding complex c-fos/c-jun at the transcriptional level, although the appearance of AP-1-binding activity (and of NF-κB) within minutes of TNF treatment suggests that the induction of the DNA-binding activities could be at least initially due to posttranslational or posttranscriptional modification of existing nuclear factors. Inhibition of cellular proliferation by TNF in myeloid cells follows inhibition of c-myc expression at the transcriptional level (Krönke et al., 1987; Tobler et al., 1987b), although in transformed fibroblasts TNF was shown to inhibit c-myc and v-mos expression by decreasing message stability (Selinger et al., 1988), suggesting that TNF is affecting oncogene expression acting at both the transcriptional and posttranscriptional levels. No information is yet available on the effect of the synergism of TNF and IFN-γ on these early events.

To analyze the mechanism of action of the cytokines in inducing differentiation of myeloid cell lines, studies of regulation of expression of genes encoding myelomonocytic differentiation markers were initiated. Because induction of the ability to respond to external stimuli with a respiratory burst was one of the hallmarks of differentiation in the cell lines, expression of the genes encoding cytochrome *b*-245, a component of the NADPH oxidase of phagocytic cells, was analyzed (Cassatella et al., 1989). TNF and IFN-γ induce, within 6 h, accumulation of transcripts of the X-CGD gene, encoding the 91-kDa heavy chain of cytochrome *b*-245 and increased accumulation is observed with IFN-γ up to 5 days. The combined effect of the two cytokines is more than additive. TNF and IFN-γ induces X-CGD gene expression in the myeloid cell lines acting, at least in part, at the transcriptional level, as shown in nuclear run-on experiments. The gene encoding the 22-kDa light chain of cytochrome *b*-245 is constitutively expressed in the human myeloid cell lines and the accumulation of its transcripts is affected by neither TNF nor IFN-γ. TNF and IFN-γ act synergistically in inducing the cell lines to express the cytochrome *b*-245 heterodimer (as evaluated by its visible absorbance spectrum) and to produce NADPH oxidase activity and H_2O_2 upon stimulation with phorbol diesters (Cassatella et al., 1989). TNF also rapidly induces accumulation in human myeloid cell lines or transcripts of the gene coding for p47, one of the cytoplasmatic components participating in the NADPH oxidase system; IFN-γ also induces accumulation of p47 mRNA, although not as efficiently as TNF, and synergizes with TNF in this effect (Cassatella, Gupta, and Trinchieri, unpublished observations).

Accumulation of transcripts of the X-CGD and p47 genes is induced by TNF and IFN-γ at early times of culture before phenotypic differentiation is demonstrable, and at those early times TNF is a more efficient inducer than IFN-γ. Expression of the gene encoding the high-affinity receptor for Fc of IgG (CD64 or FcR-I) is also induced at very early times, but in this case IFN-γ is much more efficient than TNF (Cassatella et al., 1990). High-level expression of other genes, such as IL-1 and the low-affinity receptor for Fc of IgG (CD32 or FcR-II), is observed only when the lines are cultured in the presence of both TNF and IFN-γ and at a time (3 to 5 days) when phenotypic evidence of cell differentiation is demonstrable (Cassatella et al., 1990). Kinetic analysis of expression of various genes during monocytic differentiation of HL-60 cell line induced by TNF and IFN-γ combined distinguishes three groups of myelomonocytic differentiation markers: those induced in few hours, before terminal differentiation of the cells (e.g., X-CGD and FcR-I); those induced maximally at 4 days of culture, when monocytic differentiation is observed (IL-1, FcR-II, receptor for C3b or CR-1); and those the expression of which is down-regulated during monocytic differentiation (β-glucuronidase and elastase) (Cassatella et al., 1990). Induction of TNF mRNA accumulation is biphasic: An early (1 to 2 h) accumulation induced by TNF is transient and minimally affected by IFN-γ; TNF and IFN-γ synergistically induce a later persistent accumulation of TNF mRNA, starting at 4 to 6 h of incubation (Hartman and Trinchieri, unpublished observations). Therefore, the expression of genes encoding certain markers of myelomonocytic cells appears to be modulated by TNF and/or IFN-γ directly at a time preceding differentiation of the cells and possibly independently of differentiation, whereas the expression of genes encoding other markers is concomitant with cell differentiation and possibly dependent on an ordered and regulated pathway of gene expression, leading to terminal differentiation.

TNF and LT are also potent activators of terminally differentiated myelomonocytic cells with molecular mechanisms of action that in some cases are identical or overlapping with those responsible for their differentiating effects on immature myelomonocytic cells. The activating effects of TNF on neutrophils and macrophage have a central role in the control by TNF of inflammatory responses (Sherry and Cerami, 1988). TNF enhances phagocytosis, cytotoxicity, aggregation, and adherence of neutrophils following binding to its receptor (Shalaby et al., 1985; Perussia et al., 1987; Klebanoff et al., 1986; Larrick et al., 1987; Gamble et al., 1985). TNF also induces neutrophil degranulation; directly stimulates release of reactive oxygen intermediates, including superoxide anion and hydrogen peroxidase; and primes neutrophils for oxidative burst response to other stimuli such as chemotactic peptides (Klebanoff et al., 1986; Tsujimoto et al., 1986b; Perussia et al., 1987; Nathan, 1989). LT has similar effects on neutrophils as TNF, although it is active at higher concentrations and induces somewhat lower maximal levels of activation (Kapp et al., 1989). TNF also activates macrophages, possibly acting in an autocrine fashion, enhancing their cytotoxic potential and increasing production of IL-1 and PGE_2 (DeTitto et al., 1986; Philip and Epstein, 1986; Bachwich et al., 1986). TNF alone, and additively together with IFN-γ, also increases severalfold, within a few hours, the level of acid phosphatase and β-glucuronidase activity in murine peripheral macrophages (Pierangeli and Sonnenfeld, 1989); interestingly, this effect of TNF contrasts strongly with that observed in human myeloid cell lines, on which TNF significantly down-regulate the accumulation of β-glucuronidase mRNA (Cassatella et al., 1990). Another important aspect of TNF in inflammation is its ability to be chemotactic for both monocytes and neutrophils (Ming et al., 1987; Ferrante et al., 1988), and its local production at the site of inflammation may play a major role in both attracting and activating these cell types. Other authors (Mrowietz et al., 1988, 1989; Yonemazu et al., 1989), however, failed to demonstrate a chemotactic effect of TNF alone. Yonemazu et al. (1989) showed that in the presence of zymosan-activated serum, TNF at low concentrations increases neutrophil chemotaxis, whereas at high concentrations it causes a decrease that might contribute to retaining neutrophils at the sites of inflammation.

IV. TNF AND LT TREATMENT OF VARIOUS CELL TYPES INDUCES OR ENHANCES PRODUCTION OF CYTOKINES AFFECTING HEMATOPOIESIS

As discussed in the previous sections, the effect of TNF and LT in vitro or in vivo on hematopoietic cells could be direct or mediated by other soluble factors produced by the hematopoietic cells themselves or by stromal cells. TNF was shown by Kohase et al. (1986) to induce production by fibroblasts of IL-6, a factor with profound effects on hematopoiesis in addition to those on B and T cells. TNF was approximately threefold more effective than LT in inducing IL-6 production (Akashi et al., 1990). Induction of IL-6 by TNF or LT does not depend on activation of protein kinase C (Zhang et al., 1988; Akashi et al., 1990), but may be dependent on activation of cAMP-dependent protein kinase (Zhang et al., 1988). IL-1 and other factors, such as platelet-derived growth factor and IFN-β, increase IL-6 mRNA accumulation in human fibroblasts (Walther et al., 1988). TNF-, LT-, and IL-1-mediated induction of IL-6 is at the transcriptional level (Walther et al., 1988). A transient increase of transcription rate declining within 6 h is observed upon TNF treatment, whereas a sustained increase in IL-6 gene transcription rate is observed up to 14 h in IL-1-treated cells (Walther et al., 1988). However, TNF and LT also induce an increase of IL-6 mRNA half-life, suggesting that both transcriptional activation and mRNA posttranscriptional stabilization are involved in the mechanism of TNF/LT-induced accumulation of IL-6 mRNA in fibroblasts (Akashi et al., 1990). IL-6 mRNA accumulation is also induced by TNF in other cell types (e.g., synoviocytes and keratinocytes) (Guerne et al., 1989; Trinchieri, unpublished observation). Interestingly, IL-6 is a potent inhibitor of TNF production by macrophages both in vitro and in vivo; inasmuch as TNF is a potent inducer of IL-6, the inhibition of TNF production by IL-6 can be viewed as the negative arm of a regulatory circuit (Aderka et al., 1989). TNF also induces accumulation of IL-β mRNA in fibroblasts, but probably not secretion of IL-1, suggesting that the effect of TNF on induction of IL-6 and other factors is not secondary to IL-1 production (Seelentag et al., 1989; Elias et al., 1989; Zucali et al., 1988).

TNF and IL-1 also induce the production of colony-stimulating factors from fibroblasts (Munker et al., 1986; Zucali et al., 1988) and from endothelial cells (Seelentag et al., 1987). The major types of CSF induced by TNF in fibroblasts have been identified as GM-CSF and G-CSF (Munker et al., 1986; Seelentag et al., 1989; Koeffler et al., 1988), whereas endothelial cells are induced to produce CSF-1, G-CSF, and GM-CSF (Seelentag et al., 1987). TNF induces G-CSF and GM-CSF mRNA accumulation by acting both at the transcriptional level (threefold increase in transcriptional rate) and at the posttranscriptional level (two-to sixteenfold increase in mRNA half-lives) (Koeffler et al., 1988). IL-1 also induces accumulation of G-CSF and GM-CSF transcripts, and in both fibroblasts and endothelial cells the combined effect of IL-1 and TNF was at least additive, suggesting that the two cytokines induce CSF production with different mechanisms (Seelentag et al., 1987, 1989).

Lu et al. (1988) showed that TNF enhances the production of CSF-1 and G-CSF from human monocytes and that TNF and IFN-γ are synergistic in this effect. Similarly, TNF and IFN-γ synergistically enhance production of GM-CSF and G-CSF by human lymphocytes, mostly $CD3^+$, $CD4^+$, $CD8^-$ T cells, stimulated by phytohemagglutinin (Lu et al., 1987, 1988). TNF was also shown to synergize with

IFN-γ in induction of Ly6 antigens on mouse T cells (Malek et al., 1989). TNF receptors are not expressed on fresh lymphocytes but are induced by mitogenic stimuli and by IL-2 (Owen-Schaub et al., 1989; Scheurich et al., 1987). Conversely, TNF can induce IL-2R (p55 chain) expression probably by inducing a NF-κB-like enhancer binding activity (Lowenthal et al., 1989). Induction of cytokines by TNF might also involve NK-κB induction. The mechanism of the synergism of TNF and IFN-γ in inducing CSF production by lymphocytes is not known. IFN-γ induces transcription activation of various genes acting as interferon-responsive enhancer elements different from κB (Reid et al., 1989), and it was shown not to induce NF-κB in B cells, even in conditions in which it enhances kappa chain gene transcription (Briskin et al., 1988). It is therefore possible that TNF and IFN-γ synergize on the induction of transcription of certain genes by acting on different enhancer elements.

The biologic relevance of the induction of CSF by TNF and IL-1 is confirmed by their ability to induce CSF in vivo; TNF and IL-1 injected intraperitoneally in mice induce appearance in the serum of a CSF able to induce CFU-GM with a peak at 3 h, preceding the peak of endotoxin-mediated induction of CSF by several hours (Vogel et al., 1987). It is therefore possible that TNF and/or IL-1 are the factors responsible for CSF production observed in mice following endotoxin injection. Combined injection of TNF and IL-1 at suboptimal doses resulted in an additive effect (Vogel et al., 1987). Production of CSF-1 and GM-CSF in lungs and spleens of TNF-treated mice was also demonstrated by Northern blot analysis of RNA extracted from these organs (Kauschansky et al., 1988).

V. IN VIVO EFFECTS OF TNF ON THE HEMATOPOIETIC SYSTEM

From the in vitro studies of the hematologic effect of TNF, it is possible to predict that several mechanisms may be simultaneously operative in vivo, with a final equilibrium depending on the effectiveness of the various mechanisms. In most studies in which TNF was administered in vivo in experimental animals, TNF was shown to alter blood cell kinetics and induce anemia (Tracey et al., 1988). Moldawer et al. (1989) showed that chronic TNF administration in rats induces anemia with approximately 30% decrease in total red blood cell (RBC) mass, with normal mean corpuscular hemoglobin content, and reticulocyte numbers. However, RBC survival was significantly shortened in TNF-treated animals and the incorporation of plasma ^{59}Fe into newly synthesized RBC was significantly reduced, suggesting that chronic TNF treatment produces anemia by reducing RBC synthesis and reducing the life span of circulating RBC (Moldawer et al., 1989). Akahane et al. (1987) showed that in the bone marrow of mice treated intravenously with TNF for up to 5 days, an almost complete disappearance of CFU-E and more than 90% suppression of BFU-E was observed, with an increase in the myeloid/erythroid ratio from 3.3 to 24.0. Contrasting results were obtained in normal mice treated with a single dose of TNF or nude mice inoculated with Chinese hamster ovary (CHO) cells expressing the human TNF gene. In the former model an inhibition of late-stage erythropoiesis was observed with a decrease in the number of CFU-E and circulating reticulocytes, whereas the BFU-E compartment was significantly stimulated in both the bone marrow and the spleen (Johnson et al., 1988). In the animal injected with the transfected CHO cells, similarly to the animals chronically treated with TNF, a profound anemia (hematocrit 27%) was observed, accompanied by a decrease in the number of both CFU-E and BFU-E in the bone marrow (Johnson et al., 1989). Anemia was associated with increased erythropoietin level, excluding an effect of TNF mediated through inhibition of erythropoietin production (Johnson et al., 1989). Ulich et al. (1988), did not detect anemia or alteration of RBC indices after daily intravenous injection of TNF for 1 week in rats except a slight reticulocytosis, unlike the previously described studies. In the bone marrow of the treated rats, a significant hyperplasia of late erythroid monoblasts was observed. The reason why in this latter study results so contrasting with those of the other studies were obtained is not clear, but in different experimental conditions, a predominance of either the enhancing effect of TNF on the proliferation of early hematopoietic cells and the induction of cytokines stimulating erythropoiesis, or the inhibitory effect of TNF on the proliferation of late erythroid cells and the activation of phagocytic cells regulating the RBC half-life, is possible.

The effect of TNF in vivo on the myeloid cells in the bone marrow is much less evident than that on erythroid cells. Chronic treatment of experimental animals with TNF resulted in a significant decrease of CFU-GM in the bone marrow in the study by Akahane et al. (1986) and a slight decrease of early myeloid cells in the study by Ulich et al. (1988), whereas Johnson et al. (1989) found no significant alteration in the number of CFU-GM or CFU-GEMM. Johnson et al. (1988) showed, however, that a single injection of TNF in mice induces in 3 days significant increase in the number of CFU-GM and CFU-GEMM in both bone marrow and spleen.

TNF treatment of rats induces lymphopenia and an initial neutropenia followed by a biphasic neutrophilia (Ulich et al., 1989a,b). The lymphopenia is not due to decreased lymphocyte recirculation (Ulich et al., 1989b) and might be dependent on cell death or, more likely, to transient binding of lymphocytes to TNF-activated endothelium (Bevilacqua et al., 1987). The hypothesis that TNF-induced lymphopenia is attributable to the transient adhesion to endothelium would explain the return to normal of circulating lymphocyte levels by 12 h (Ulich et al., 1989b). TNF-induced neutropenia reaches a maximum more rapidly and is shorter in duration than TNF-induced lymphopenia, suggesting difference in the molecules involved in the mechanism of adhesion of neutrophils and lymphocytes (Ulich et al., 1989b). Gamble et al. (1985) described two mechanisms of TNF-induced adhesion of neutrophils to endothelium: one induced rapidly depending on the effect of TNF on the neutrophils, and a second, requiring several hours, depending on TNF-mediated induction of adhesion molecules on endothelial cells. Because of the rapidity of the TNF-induced neutropenia, it is likely that the first mechanism is the most effective in vivo. TNF-induced neutrophilia is probably due to release of bone marrow neutrophils into circulation as well as to the demargination of neutrophils that have been transiently adherent to the endothelium (Ulich et al., 1989b). Consistent with this hypothesis is the synergistic effect of TNF and endotoxin to induce a dramatic loss of band and segmented neutrophils from the bone marrow (Ulich et al., 1989a). The broader second wave of neutrophilia is probably due to the release of endogenous IL-1 and other monokines induced by TNF (e.g., IL-6 and GM-CSF) (Ulich et al., 1989b).

TNF, similarly to IL-1, can accelerate restoration of hematopoiesis in animals compromised by sublethal doses of cytotoxic drugs or irradiation. Protection is obtained with a single dose or repeated injections. A single intraperitoneal injection of TNF, given 3 h after a lethal dose of irradiation that would kill 95% of mice in 30 days, protected in a dose-dependent manner up to 60% of the mice (Neta and Oppenheim, 1988). IL-1 alone was more effective than TNF on most mouse strains, but TNF was more effective than IL-1 in C3H/HeN mice, suggesting that the relative effectiveness of TNF and IL-1 depends on the genetic makeup of the host (Neta et al., 1988). When IL-1 and TNF are used together at suboptimal doses, they have a synergistic protective effect, suggesting that the two cytokines act through different radioprotective pathways (Neta et al., 1988). Slordal et al. (1989) showed that intravenous bolus administration of a single dose of murine TNF to BALB/c mice 20 h before sublethal total-body irradiation confers significant protection against radiation-induced neutropenia. TNF not only reduces the decline of neutrophils and total blood count after irradiation, but also accelerates the regeneration of hematopoietic precursors and the normalization of peripheral blood cell counts (Slordal et al., 1989).

Few detailed studies are available of hematologic alterations in patients treated with TNF. Moritz et al. (1989) reported a significant neutropenia in most patients with a peak at 30 min and return to normal or higher-than-normal values at 4 h. Creaven et al. (1989) showed a significant leukocytosis with increased immature forms at 1 to 2 days of treatment; leukocytosis resolved by day 3 or 4, even with continued drug administration. Interestingly, a monocytosis was found in most patients, possibly consistent with the differentiation effect to monocyte/macrophages demonstrated for TNF in vitro. The reported hematologic changes in patients treated with TNF are therefore remarkably similar to those described in experimental animals.

TNF and LT are also likely to play a role in the pathogenesis of diseases in which hematologic alterations are present. TNF is produced by certain leukemic cells, and in the case of hairy cell leukemia, it could be responsible for the suppression of normal hematopoiesis observed in the patients (Lindemann et al., 1989). Lymphocytes from severe aplastic anemia patients produce spontaneously and after in vitro stimulation high levels of TNF and IFN-γ (Hinterberger et al., 1989). The production of these cytokines is constitutive in the patients and unaffected by blood transfusion. Normalization of production of TNF-γ and TNF from patients' lymphocytes was observed to correlate with a clinical response to cyclosporin A (Hinterberger et al., 1989). These findings have been interpreted as possible evidence in favor of a pathogenic role of TNF overproduction in severe aplastic anemia (Hinterberger et al., 1989).

The in vivo effects of TNF on the hematopoietic system in experimental animals and in patients confirm that all or most of the in vitro observed effects of TNF also play a role in vivo, with different results depending on the balance among the different effects. In particular, the studies summarized above suggest that TNF in vivo stimulates early hematopoietic precursor cells, inhibits late precursor cells with a more significant effect on erythroid precursors, induces different cell types to produce CSF and other cytokines secondarily affecting the hematopoietic system, and affects leukocyte migration and adhesion to endothelium. These hematopoietic effects of TNF probably play a role in pathologic situations in which TNF is produced (e.g., toxic shock) (Vogel et al., 1988) and should be taken into account when therapeutic use of TNF is planned.

ACKNOWLEDGMENTS

The experimental work by the authors described in this review was supported, in part, by U.S. Public Health Science Grants CA-10815, CA-20833, CA-32898, and CA-40256. I would like to thank Mrs. Marion Kaplan for typing the manuscript.

REFERENCES

Aderka, D., Le, J., and Vilček, J. (1989). IL-6 inhibits lipopolysaccharide-induced tumor necrosis factor production in cultured human monocytes, U937 cells, and in mice, *J. Immunol., 143*: 3517.

Aggarwal, B. B., Eessalu, T. E., and Hass, P. E. (1985). Characterization of receptors for human tumor necrosis factor and their regulation by γ-interferon, *Nature (Lond.), 318*: 665.

Akahane, K., Hosoi, T., Urabe, A., Kawakami, M., and Takaku, F. (1987). Effects of recombinant human tumor necrosis factor (rTNF) on normal human and mouse hematopoietic progenitor cells, *Int. J. Cell Cloning, 5*: 16.

Akashi, M., Loussararian, A. H., Adelman, D. C., Saito, M., and Koeffler, H. P. (1990). Role of lymphotoxin in expression of interleukin 6 in human fibroblasts: stimulation and regulation, *J. Clin. Invest., 85*: 121.

Bachwich, P. S., Chensue, S. W., Larrick, J. W., and Kunkel, S. W. (1986). Tumor necrosis stimulates interleukin-1 and prostaglandin E_2 production in resting macrophages, *Biochem. Biophys. Res. Commun., 136*: 94.

Barber, K. E., Crosier, P. S., Gillis, S., and Watson, J. D. (1987). Human granulocyte-macrophage progenitors and their sensitivity to cytotoxins: analysis by limiting dilution, *Blood, 70*: 1773.

Beran, M., O'Brien, S., Andersson, B., McCredie, K. B., and Gutterman, J. U. (1988a). Tumor necrosis factor and human hematopoiesis. II. Inhibition and mode of action on normal and chronic myelogenous leukemia-derived granulocyte-macrophage progenitor cells, *Hematol. Pathol., 2*: 65.

Beran, M., O'Brien, S., Gutterman, J. U., and McCredie, K. B. (1988b). Tumor necrosis factor and human hematopoiesis. I. Kinetics and diversity of human bone marrow cell response to recombinant tumor necrosis factor alpha in short-term suspension cultures in vitro, *Hematol. Pathol., 2*: 31.

Bertani, A., Polentarutti, N., Sica, A., Rambaldi, A., Mantovani, A., and Colotta, F. (1989). Expression of c-jun Protooncogene in human myelomonocytic cells, *Blood, 74*: 1811.

Bevilacqua, M. P., Pober, J. S., Wheeler, M. E., Mendrick, D., Cotran, R. S., and Gimbrone, M. A. (1985). Interleukin-1 acts on cultured human vascular endothelium to increase the adhesion of polymorphonuclear leukocytes, monocytes, and related leukocyte cell lines, *J. Clin. Invest., 76*: 2003.

Breitman, T., Selonick, S., and Collins, S. (1980). Induction of differentiation of the human promyelocytic cell line (HL-60) by retinoic acid, *Proc. Natl. Acad. Sci. USA, 77*: 2936.

Briskin, M., Kuwabara, M. D., Sigman, D. S., and Wall, R. (1988). Induction of K transcription by interferon-γ without activation of NF-KB, *Science, 242*: 1036.

Broxmeyer, H. E., Williams, D. E., Lu, L., Cooper, S., Anderson, S. L., Beyer, G. S., Hoffman, R., and Rubin, B. Y. (1986). The suppressive influences of human tumor necrosis factors on bone marrow hematopoietic progenitor cells from normal donors and patients with leukemia: synergism of tumor necrosis factor and interferon-γ, *J. Immunol., 136*: 4487.

Cannistra, S. A., Groshek, P., and Griffin, J. D. (1988). Monocytes enhance gamma-interferon-induced inhibition of myeloid progenitor cell growth through secretion of tumor necrosis factor, *Exp. Hematol., 16*: 865.

Cassatella, M. A., Hartman, L., Perussia, B., and Trinchieri, G. (1989). Tumor necrosis factor and immune interferon synergistically induce cytochrome b_{-245} heavy chain gene expression and NADPH oxidase in human leukemic myeloid cells, *J. Clin. Invest., 83*: 1570.

Cassatella, M. A., Perussia, B., and Trinchieri, G. (1990). Tumor necrosis factor is a differentiation-inducing factor for hematopoietic cells, in: *Tumor Necrosis Factor: Structure, Mechanism of Action, Role in Disease and Therapy*. Bonavida, B., and Granger, G., eds., S. Karger, Basel, p. 114.

Caux, C., Saeland, S., Favre, C., Duvert, V., Mannoni, P., and Banchereau, J. (1990). TNF alpha strongly potentiates IL-3 and GM-CSF induced proliferation of human CD34$^+$ hematopoietic progenitor cells., *Blood 75*: 2292.

Celada, A., Klemsz, M. J., and Maki, R. A. (1989). Interferon-gamma activates multiple pathways to regulate the expression of the genes for major histocompatibility class II I-A beta, tumor necrosis factor and complement component C3 in mouse macrophage, *Eur. J. Immunol., 19*: 1103.

Chen, L., Novick, D., Rubinstein, M., and Revel, M. (1988). Recombinant interferon-beta 2 (interleukin-6) induces myeloid differentiation, *FEBS Lett., 239*: 299.

Clark, M. A., Chen, M. -J., Crooke, S. T., and Bomalaski, J. S. (1988). Tumour necrosis factor (cachectin) induces phospholipase A_2 activity and synthesis of a phospholipase A_2-activating protein in endothelial cells, *Biochem. J., 250*: 125.

Creaven, P. J., Brenner, D. E., Cowens, J. W., Huben, R. P., Wolf, R. M., Takita, H., Arbuck, S. G., Razack, M. S., and Proefrock, A. D. (1989). A phase I clinical trial of recombinant human tumor necrosis factor given daily for five days, *Cancer Chemother. Pharmacol., 23*: 186.

Cuturi, M. C., Murphy, M., Costa-Giomi, M. P., Weinmann, R., Perussia, B., and Trinchieri, G. (1987). Independent regulation of tumor necrosis factor and lymphotoxin production by human peripheral blood lymphocytes, *J. Exp. Med., 165*: 1581.

Cuturi, M. C., Anegón, I., Sherman, F., Loudon, R., Clark, S. C., Perussia, B., and Trinchieri, G. (1989). Production of hematopoietic colony-stimulating factors by human natural killer cells, *J. Exp. Med., 169*: 569.

Dayer, J. M., Beutler, B., and Cerami, A. (1985). Cachectin/tumor necrosis factor stimulates collagenase and prostaglandin E_2 production by human synovial cells and dermal fibroblasts, *J. Exp. Med., 162*: 2163.

Dayton, E., Perussia, B., and Trinchieri, G. (1983). Correlation between differentiation, expression of monocyte-specific antigens, and cytotoxic functions in human promyelocytic cell lines treated with leukocyte-conditioned medium, *J. Immunol., 130*: 1120.

Dayton, E. T., Matsumoto-Kobayashi, M., Perussia, B., and Trinchieri, G. (1985). Role of immune interferon in the monocytic differentiation of human promyelocytic cell lines induced by leukocyte conditioned medium, *Blood, 66*: 583.

DeBenedetti, F., Falk, L. A., Ellingsworth, L. R., Ruscetti, F. W., and Faltynek, C. R. (1990). Synergy between transforming growth factor-beta and tumor necrosis factor-alpha in the induction of monocytic differentiation of human leukemic cell lines, *Blood, 75*: 626.

Degliantoni, G., Murphy, M., Kobayashi, M., Francis, M. -K., Perussia, B., and Trinchieri, G. (1985a). Natural killer (NK) cell-derived hematopoietic colony-inhibiting activity and NK cytotoxic factor: relationship with tumor necrosis factor and synergism with immune interferon, *J. Exp. Med., 162*: 1512.

Degliantoni, G., Perussia, B., Mangioni, L., and Trinchieri, G. (1985b). Inhibition of bone marrow colony formation by human natural killer cells and by natural killer cell-derived colony-inhibiting activity, *J. Exp. Med., 161*: 1152.

DeTitto, E. H., Catterall, J. R., and Remington, J. S. (1986). Activity of recombinant tumor necrosis factor on *Toxoplasma gondii* and *Trypanosoma cruri*, *J. Immunol., 137*: 1342.

Digel, W., Stefanic, M., Schoniger, W., Buck, C., Raghavachar, A., Frickhofen, N., Heimpel, H., and Porzsolt, F. (1989). Tumor necrosis factor induces proliferation of neoplastic B cells from chronic lymphocytic leukemia, *Blood, 73*: 1242.

Duncombe, A. S., Heslop, H. E., Turner, M., Meager, A., Priest, R., Exley, T., and Brenner, M. K. (1989). Tumor necrosis factor mediates autocrine growth inhibition in a chronic leukemia, *J. Immunol., 143*: 3828.

Elias, J. A., Gustilo, K., Baeder, W., and Freundlich, B. (1987). Synergistic stimulation of fibroblast prostaglandin release by recombinant interleukin 1 and tumor necrosis factor, *J. Immunol., 138*: 3812.

Elias, J. A., Trinchieri, G., Beck, J. M., Simon, P. L., Sehgal, P. B., May, L. T., and Kern, J.

A. (1989). A synergistic interaction of IL-6 and IL-1 mediates the thymocyte-stimulating activity produced by recombinant IL-1-stimulated fibroblasts, *J. Immunol., 142*: 509.

Elias, L. (1988). Stimulation by tumor necrosis factor of HL-60 thymidine salvage pathway metabolism dissociated from proliferation, *J. Cell Physiol., 136*: 95.

Elias, L., Wogenrich, F., Wallace, J., and Longmire, J. (1980). Altered pattern of differentiation of proliferation of HL-60 promyelocytic leukemia cells in the presence of leucocyte conditioned medium, *Leukemia Res., 4*: 301.

Eliason, J. F., and Vassalli, P. (1988). Inhibition of hematopoiesis in murine marrow cell cultures by recombinant murine tumor necrosis factor alpha: evidence for long term effects on stromal cells, *Blood Cells, 14*: 339.

Evans, J. P. M., Mire-Sluis, A. R., Hoffbrand, A. V., and Wickremasinghe, R. G. (1990). Binding of G-CSF, GM-CSF, tumor necrosis factor-alpha and gamma-interferon to cell surface receptors on human myeloid leukemia cells triggers rapid tyrosine and serine phosphorylation of a 75 kd protein, *Blood, 75*: 88.

Ferrante, A., Nandoskar, M., Walz, A., Goh, D. H., and Kowando, J. C. (1988). Effect of tumor necrosis factor alpha and interleukin-1 alpha and beta on human neutrophil migration, respiratory burst and degranulation, *Int. Arch. Allergy Appl. Immunol., 86*: 82.

Gamble, J. R., Harlan, J. M., Klebanoff, S. J., and Vadas, M. A. (1985). Stimulation of the adherence of neutrophils to umbilical vein endothelium by human recombinant tumor necrosis factor, *Proc. Natl. Acad. Sci. USA, 82*: 8667.

Geissler, K., Tricot, G., Leemhuis, T., Walker, E., and Broxmeyer, H. E. (1989). Differentiation-inducing effect of recombinant human tumor necrosis factor α and γ-interferon in vitro on blast cells from patients with acute myeloid leukemia and myeloid blast crisis of chronic myeloid leukemia, *Cancer Res., 49*: 3057.

Griffin, G. E., Leung, K., Folks, T. M., Kunkel, S., and Nabel, G. J. (1989). Activation of HIV gene expression during monocyte differentiation by induction of NF-kappa B, *Nature, 339*: 70.

Guerne, P. A., Zuraw, B. L., Vaughan, J. H., Carson, D. A., and Lotz, M. (1989). Synovium as a source of interleukin 6 in vitro: contribution to local and systemic manifestation of arthritis, *J. Clin. Invest., 83*: 585.

Hansson, M., Beran, M., Andersson, B., and Kiessling, R. (1982). Inhibition of in vitro granulopoiesis by autologous and allogeneic human NK cells, *J. Immunol., 129*: 126.

Hemmi, H., Nakamura, T., Tamura, K., Shimizu, Y., Kato, S., Miki, T., Takahashi, N., Muramatsu, M., Numao, N., and Sugamura, K. (1987). Lymphotoxin: induction of terminal differentiation of the human myeloid leukemia cell lines HL-60 and THP-1, *J. Immunol., 138*: 664.

Herrmann, F., Gebauer, G., Lindenmann, A., Brach, M., and Mertelsmann, R. (1989). Interleukin-2 and interferon-gamma recruit different subsets of human peripheral blood monocytes to secrete interleukin-1 beta and tumour necrosis factor-alpha, *Clin. Exp. Immunol., 77*: 97.

Hinterberger, W., Adolf, G., Bettelheim, P., Geissler, K., Huber, C., Irschick, E., Kalhs, P., Koller, U., Lechner, K., and Meister, B. (1989). Lymphokine overproduction in severe aplastic anemia is not related to blood transfusion , *Blood, 74*: 2713.

Hoang, T., Levy, B., Onetto, N., Haman, A., and Rodriguez-Cimadevilla, J. C. (1989). Tumor necrosis factor alpha stimulates the growth of the clonogenic cells of acute myeloblastic leukemia in synergy with granulocyte/macrophage colony-stimulating factor, *J. Exp. Med., 170:* 15.

Hosoi, T., Takeda, K., and Konno, K. (1989). Synergism of prostaglandin E_2 plus TNF in induction of differentiation of human monocytoid leukemic U937 cells, *Anticancer Res.,* *9*: 615.

Johnson, C. S., Chang, M., and Furmanski, P. (1988). In vivo hematopoietic effects of tumor necrosis factor-alpha in normal and erythroleukemic mice: characterization and therapeutic applications, *Blood, 72*: 1875.

Johnson, R. A. Waddelow, T. A., Caro, J., Oliff, A., and Roodman, G. D. (1989). Chronic exposure to tumor necrosis factor in vivo preferentially inhibits erythropoiesis in nude mice, *Blood, 74*: 130.

Jongeneel, C. V., Shakhov, A. N., Nedospasov, S. A., and Cerottini, J. C. (1989). Molecular control of tissue specific expression at the mouse TNF locus, *Eur. J. Immunol., 19*: 549.

Kapp, A., Zeck-Kapp, G., and Bluhm, D. (1989). Human tumor necrosis factor is a potent activator of the oxidative metabolism in human polymorphonuclear neutrophilic granulocytes: comparison with human lymphotoxin, *J. Invest. Dermatol., 3*: 348.

Katakami, Y., Nakao, Y., Katakami, N., Koizumi, T., Ogawa, R., Yamada, H., Takai, Y., and Fujita, J. (1988). Cooperative effects of tumor necrosis factor-alpha and 1α, 25-dihydroxyvitamin D_3 on growth inhibition, differentiation, and c-myc reduction in human promyelocytic leukemia cell line HL-60, *Biochem. Biophys. Res. Comm., 152*: 1151.

Kaushansky, K., Broudy, V. C., Harlan, J. M., and Adamson, J. W. (1988). Tumor necrosis factor-alpha and tumor necrosis factor-beta (lymphotoxin) stimulate the production of granulocyte-macrophage colony-stimulating factor, macrophage colony-stimulating factor, and IL-1 in vivo, *J. Immunol., 141*: 3410.

Klebanoff, S. J., Vadas, J., Harlan, M., Sparks, L. H., Gamble, J. R., Agosti, J. M., and Waltersdorph, A. M. (1986). Stimulation of neutrophils by tumor necrosis factor, *J. Immunol., 136*: 4220.

Koeffler, H. P., Gasson, J., and Tobler, A. (1988). Transcriptional and posttranscriptional modulation of myeloid colony-stimulating factor expression by tumor necrosis factor and other agents, *Mol. Cell. Biol., 8*: 3432.

Kohase, M., Henriksen-Destefano, D., May, L. T., Vilček, J., and Sehgal, P. B. (1986). Induction of β_2 interferon by tumor necrosis factor: a homeostatic mechanism in the control of cell proliferation, *Cell, 45*: 659.

Krönke, M., Schluter, C., and Pfizenmaier, K. (1987). Tumor necrosis factor inhibits MYC expression in HL-60 cells at the level of mRNA transcription, *Cell Biol., 84*: 469.

Larrick, J. W., Graham, D., Toy, K., Lin, L. S., Senyk, G., and Fendly, B. M. (1987). Recombinant tumor necrosis factor causes activation of human granulocytes, *Blood, 69*: 640.

Lindemann, A., Ludwig, W. -D., Oster, W., Mertelsmann, R., and Herrmann, F. (1989). High-level secretion of tumor necrosis factor-alpha contributes to hematopoietic failure in hairy cell leukemia, *Blood, 73*: 880.

Lowenthal, J. W., Ballard, D. W., Bogerd, H., Bohnlein, E., and Greene, W. C. (1989). Tumor necrosis factor-α activation of the IL-2 receptor-α gene involves the induction of kB-specific DNA binding proteins, *J. Immunol., 142*: 3121.

Lu, L., Srour, E. F., Warren, D. J., Walker, D., Graham, C. D., Walker, E. B., Jansen, J., and Broxmeyer, H. E. (1987). Enhancement of release of granulocyte-and granulocyte-macrophage colony-stimulating factors from phytohemagglutin-stimulated sorted subsets of human T lymphocytes by recombinant human tumor necrosis factor-alpha, *J. Immunol., 141*: 201.

Lu, L., Walker, D., Graham, C. D., Waheed, A., Shadduck, R. K., and Broxmeyer, H. E. (1988). Enhancement of release from MHC class II antigen-positive monocytes of hematopoietic colony stimulating factors CSF-1 and G-CSF by recombinant human tumor necrosis factor-alpha: synergism with recombinant human interferon-gamma, *Blood, 72*: 34.

Malek, T. R., Danis, K. M., and Codias, E. K. (1989). Tumor necrosis factor synergistically acts with IFN-γ to regulate Ly6 A/E expression T lymphocytes, thymocytes, and bone marrow cells, *J. Immunol., 142*: 1929.

Metcalf, D. (1989). The molecular control of cell division, differentiation, commitment and maturation in hematopoietic cells, *Nature, 339*: 27.

Ming, W. J., Bersan, L., and Mantovani, A. (1987). Tumor necrosis factor is chemotactic for monocytes and polymorphonuclear leukocytes, *J. Immunol., 138*: 1469.

Moldawer, L. L., Marano, M. A., Wei, H., Fong, Y., Silen, M. L., Kuo, g., Manogue, K. R., Vlassara, H., Cohen, H., Cerami, A., and Lowry, S. F. (1989). Cachectin/tumor necrosis factor-alpha alters red blood cell kinetics and induces anemia in vivo, *FASEB J., 3*: 1637.

Moritz, T., Niederle, N., Baumann, J., May, D., Kurschel, E., Osieka, R., Kempeni, J., Schlick, E., and Schmidt, C. G. (1989). Phase I study of recombinant human tumor necrosis factor-alpha in advance malignant disease, *Cancer Immunol. Immunother., 29*: 144.

Mrowietz, U., Schroder, J. M., and Christophers, E. (1988). Recombinant human tumor necrosis alpha lacks chemotactic activity for human peripheral blood neutrophils and monocytes, *Biochem. Biophys. Res. Comm., 153*: 1223.

Mrowietz, U., Ternowitz, T., Schroder, J. M., and Christophers, E. (1989). Recombinant human tumor necrosis factor-beta lacks chemotactic activity for human peripheral blood neutrophils, monocytes, and T cells, *Scand. J. Immunol., 30*: 373.

Munker, R., and Koeffler, P. (1987). In vitro action of tumor necrosis factor on myeloid leukemia cells, *Blood, 69*: 1102.

Munker, R., Gasson, J., Ogawa, M., and Goeffler, H. P. (1986). Recombinant human TNF induces production of granulocyte-monocyte colony-stimulating factor, *Nature, 323*: 79.

Munker, R., DiPersio, J., and Koeffler, H. P. (1987). Tumor necrosis factor: receptors on hematopoietic cells, *Blood, 70*: 1730.

Murase, T., Hotta, T., Saito, H., and Ohno, R. (1987). Effect of recombinant human tumor necrosis factor on the colony growth of human leukemia progenitor cells and normal hematopoietic progenitor cells, *Blood, 69*: 467.

Murphy, M., Loudon, R., Kobayashi, M., and Trinchieri, G. (1986). Gamma interferon and lymphotoxin, released by activated T cells, synergize to inhibit granulocyte-monocyte colony formation, *J. Exp. Med., 164*: 263.

Murphy, M., Perussia, B., and Trinchieri, G. (1988). Effects of recombinant tumor necrosis factor, lymphotoxin and immune interferon on proliferation and differentiation of enriched hematopoietic precursor cells, *Exp. Hematol., 16*: 131.

Nagata, K., Tohda, S., Suzuki, T., and Nara, V. (1989). Effects of recombinant human tumor necrosis factor on the self-renewal capacity of leukemic blast progenitors in acute myeloblastic leukemia, *Leukemia, 3*: 626.

Nathan, C. F. (1989). Respiratory burst in adherent human neutrophils: triggering by colony-stimulating factors CSF-GM and CSF-G, *Blood, 73*: 301.

Neta, R., and Oppenheim, J. J. (1988). Cytokines in therapy of radiation injury, *Blood, 72*: 1093.

Neta, R., Oppenheim, J. J., and Douches, S. D. (1988). Interdependence of the radioprotective effects of human recombinant interleukin 1α, tumor necrosis factor α, granulocyte colony-stimulating factor, and murine recombinant granulocyte–macrophage colony-stimulating factor, *J. Immunol., 140*: 108.

Old, L. J. (1985). Tumor necrosis factor (TNF), *Science, 230*: 630.

Onozaki, K., Urawa, H., Tamatani, T., Iwamura, Y., Hashimoto, T., Baba, T., Suzuki, H., Yamada, M., Yamamoto, S., Oppenheim, J. J., and Matsushima, K. (1988). Synergistic interactions of interleukin 1, interferon-β, and tumor necrosis factor in terminally differentiating a mouse myeloid leukemic cell line (M1), *J. Immunol., 140*: 112.

Oster, W., Cicco, N. A., Klein, H., Hirano, T., Kishimoto, T., Lindenmann, A., Mertelsmann, R. H., and Herrmann, F. (1989). Participation of the cytokines interleukin 6, tumor necrosis factor-alpha, and interleukin 1-beta secreted by acute myelogenous leukemia blasts in autocrine and paracrine leukemia growth control, *J. Clin. Invest., 84*: 451.

Owen-Schaub, L. B., Crumb, W. L., Morin, G. I., and Grimm, E. A. (1989). Regulation of lymphocyte tumor necrosis factor receptors by IL-2, *J. Immunol., 143*: 2236.

Peetre, C., Gullberg, U., Nilsson, E., and Olsson, I. (1986). Effects of recombinant tumor necrosis factor on proliferation and differentiation of leukemic and normal hematopoietic cells in vitro: relationship to cell surface receptor, *J. Clin. Invest., 78*: 1694.

Pelus, L. M., Ottmann, O. G., and Nocka, K. H. (1988). Synergistic inhibition of human marrow granulocyte–macrophage progenitor cells by prostaglandin E and recombinant interferon-alpha-beta, and -gamma and an effect mediated by tumor necrosis factor, *J. Immunol., 140*: 479.

Perussia, B., Dayton, E., Fanning, V., Thiagarajan, P., Hoxie, J., and Trinchieri, G. (1983). Immune interferon and leukocyte-conditioned medium induce normal and leukemic myeloid cells to differentiate along the monocytic pathway, *J. Exp. Med., 158*: 2058.

Perussia, B., Kobayashi, M., Rossi, M. E., Anegón, I., and Trinchieri, G. (1987). Immune interferon enhances functional properties of human granulocytes: role of Fc receptors and effect of lymphotoxin, tumor necrosis factor, and granulocyte–macrophage colony-stimulating factor, *J. Immunol., 138*: 765.

Philip, R., and Epstein, L. B. (1986). Tumor necrosis factor as immunomodulator and mediator of monocyte cytotoxicity induced by itself, α-interferon, and interleukin-1, *Nature, 323*: 86.

Pierangeli, S. S., and Sonnenfeld, G. (1989). Effects of interferon-γ and tumor necrosis factor-α on macrophage enzyme levels, *J. Interferon. Res., 9*: 1.

Reid, L. E., Brasnett, A. H., Gilbert, C. S., Porter, A. C. G., Gewert, D. R., Stark, G. R., and Kerr, I. M. (1989). A single DNA response element can confer inducibility by both α- and γ-interferons, *Proc. Natl. Acad. Sci. USA, 86*: 840.

Ruggiero, V., Tavernier, J., Fiers, W., and Baglioni, C. (1986). Induction of the synthesis of tumor necrosis factor receptors by interferon γ, *J. Immunol., 136*: 2445.

Scheurich, P., Thoma, B., Ücer, U., and Pfizenmaier, K. (1987). Immunoregulatory activity of recombinant human tumor necrosis factor (TNF)-α: induction of TNF receptors on human T cells and TNF-α-mediated enhancement of T cell responses, *J. Immunol., 138*: 1786.

Schütze, S., Scheurich, P., Pfizenmaier, K., and Krönke, M. (1989). Tumor necrosis factor signal transduction: tissue specific serine phosphorylation of a 26-kDa cytosolic protein, *J. Biol. Chem., 264*: 3562.

Seelentag, W., Mermod, J. -J., Montesano, R., and Vassalli, P. (1987). Additive effects of interleukin 1 and tumour necrosis factor-alpha on the accumulation of the three granulocyte and macrophage colony-stimulating factor mRNAs in human endothelial cells, *EMBO J., 6*: 2261.

Seelentag, W., Mermod, J. -J., and Vassalli, P. (1989). Interleukin 1 and tumor necrosis factor-alpha additively increase the levels of granulocyte-macrophage and granulocyte colony-stimulating factor (CSF) in mRNA in human fibroblasts, *Eur. J. Immunol., 19*: 209.

Selinger, B., Killian, M., and Pfizenmaier, K. (1988). Distinct mechanisms of interferon-gamma and tumor necrosis factor-alpha action in oncogene-transformed mouse fibroblasts, *J. Cell Biochem., 38*: 205.

Shakhov, A. N., Collart, M. A., Vassalli, P., Nedospasov, S. A., and Jongeneel, C. V. (1990). kB-type enhancers are involved in lipopolysaccharide-mediated transcriptional activation of the tumor necrosis factor alpha gene in primary macrophages, *J. Exp. Med., 171*: 35.

Shalaby, M. R., Aggarwal, B. B., Rinderknecht, E., Svendersky, L. P., Finkle, B. S., and Palladino, M. A. J. (1985). Activation of human polymorphonuclear neutrophil functions by interferon-γ and tumor necrosis factor, *J. Immunol., 135*: 2069.

Sherry, B., and Cerami, A. (1988). Cachectin/tumor necrosis factor exerts endocrine, paracrine, and autocrine control of inflammatory response, *J. Cell Biol., 107*: 1269.

Slordal, L., Warren, D. J., and Moore, M. A. S. (1989). Effect of recombinant murine tumor necrosis factor on hematopoietic reconstitution in sublethally irradiated mice, *J. Immunol., 142*: 833.

Spies, T., Morton, C. C., Nedospasou, S. A., Fiers, W., Pious, D., and Strominger, J. L. (1986). Genes for the tumor necrosis factors and are linked to the major histocompatibility complex, *Proc. Natl. Acad. Sci. (USA), 83*: 8699.

Squinto, S. P., Doucet, J. P., Block, A. L., Morrow, S. L., and Davenport, W. D., Jr. (1989). Induction of macrophage-like differentiation of HL-60 leukemia cells by tumor necrosis factor-α: potential role of fos expression, *Mol. Endocrinol., 3*: 409.

Steffen, M., Cayre, Y., Manogue, K. R., and Moore, M. A. S. (1988). 1α, 25-dihydroxyvitamin D_3 transcriptionally regulates tumor necrosis factor mRNA during IL-60 differentiation, *Immunology, 63*: 43.

Sugarman, B. J., Aggarwal, B. B., Hass, P. E., Figari, I. S., Palladino, M. A., and Shepard, H. M. (1985). Recombinant human tumor necrosis factor-α: effects on proliferation of normal and transformed cells in vitro, *Science, 230*: 943.

Takeda, K., Iwamoto, S., Sugimoto, H., Takuma, T., Kawatani, N., Noda, M., Masaki, A., Morise, H., Arimura, H., and Konno, K. (1986). Identity of differentiation inducing factor and tumour necrosis factor, *Nature (London.), 323*: 338.

Takeda, K., Hosoi, T., Noda, M., Arimura, H., and Konno, K. (1988). Effect of fibroblast-derived differentiation inducing factor on the differentiation of human monocytoid and myeloid leukemia cell lines, *Biochem. Biophys. Res. Commun., 155*: 24.

Takuma, T., Takeda, K., and Konno, K. (1987). Synergism of tumor necrosis factor and interferon-gamma in induction of differentiation of human myeloblastic leukemic ML-1 cells, *Biochem. Biophys. Res. Comm., 145*: 514.

Tobler, A., Munker R., Heitjan, D., and Koeffler, P. (1987a). In vitro interaction of recombinant tumor necrosis factor alpha and all-*trans*-retinoic acid with normal and leukemic hematopoietic cells, *Blood, 70*: 1940.

Tobler, A., Johnston, D., and Koeffler, H. P. (1987b). Recombinant human tumor necrosis factor regulates c-myc expression in HL-60 cells at the level of transcription, *Blood, 70*: 200.

Tracey, K. J., Wei, H., Manogue, K. R., Fong, Y., Hesse, D. G., Nguyen, H. T., Kuo, G. C., Buetler, B., Cotran, R. S., Cerami, A., and Lowry, S. F. (1988). Cachectin/tumor necrosis factor induce cachexia, anemia and inflammation, *J. Exp. Med., 167*: 1211.

Trinchieri, G., Kobayashi, M., Rosen, M., Loudon, R., Murphy, M., and Perussia, B. (1986). Tumor necrosis factor and lymphotoxin induce differentiation of human myeloid cell lines in synergy with immune interferon, *J. Exp. Med., 164*: 1206.

Trinchieri, G., Murphy, M., and Perussia, B. (1987a). Regulation of hematopoiesis by T lymphocytes and natural killer cells, *CRC Crit. Rev. Oncol./Hematol., 7*: 219.

Trinchieri, G., Rosen, M., and Perussia, B. (1987b). Retinoic acid cooperates with tumor necrosis factor and immune interferon in inducing differentiation and growth inhibition of the human promyelocytic leukemic cell line HL-60, *Blood, 69*: 1218.

Trinchieri, G., Rosen, M., and Perussia, B. (1987c). Induction of differentiation of human myeloid cell lines by tumor necrosis factor in cooperation with 1α, 25-dihydroxy-vitamin D_3, *Cancer Res., 47*: 2236.

Tsujimoto, M., Yip, Y. K., and Vilček, J. (1986a). IFN enhances expression of cellular receptors for tumor necrosis factor, *J. Immunol., 136*: 2441.

Tsujimoto, M., Yokata, S., Vilček, J., and Weissman, C. (1986b). Tumor necrosis factor provokes superoxide anion generation from neutrophils, *Biochem. Biophys. Res. Comm., 137*: 1094.

Ulich, T. R., Castillo, J., Guo, K., and Souza, L. (1988). The hematologic effects of chronic administration of the monokines tumor necrosis factor, interleukin-1, and granulocyte-colony stimulating factor on bone marrow and circulation, *Am. J. Pathol., 134*: 149.

Ulich, T. R., Del Castillo, J., Ni, R., and Bikhazi, N. (1989a). Hematologic interaction of endotoxin tumor necrosis factor alpha (TNFalpha), Interleukin 1, and adrenal hormones and the hematologic effects of TNFalpha in *Corynebacterium parvum*-primed rats, *J. Leukocyte Biol., 45*: 546.

Ulich, T. R., Del Castillo, J., Ni, R., Bikhazi, N., and Calvin, L. (1989b). Mechanisms of tumor necrosis factor alpha-induced lymphopenia, neutropenia, and biphasic neutrophilia: a study of lymphocyte recirculation and hematologic interactions of TNF-α with endogenous mediators of leukocyte trafficking, *J. Leukocyte Biol., 45*: 155.

Vilček, J., Palombella, V. J., Henriksen-DeStefano, D., Swenson, C., Feinman, R., Hirai, M., and Tsujimoto, M. (1986). Fibroblast growth enhancing activity of tumor necrosis factor and its relationship to other polypeptide growth hormones, *J. Exp. Med., 163*: 632.

Vogel, S. N., Douches, S. D., Kaufman, E. N., and Neta, R. (1987). Induction of colony stimulating factor in vivo by recombinant interleukin 1α and recombinant tumor necrosis factor α, *J. Immunol., 138*: 2143.

Vogel, S. N., Kaufman, E. N., Tate, M. D., and Neta, R. (1988). Recombinant interleukin-1-α and recombinant tumor necrosis factor-α synergize in vivo to induce early endotoxin tolerance and associated hematopoietic changes, *Infect. Immun., 56*: 2650.

Walther, Z., May, L. T., and Sehgal, P. B. (1988). Transcriptional regulation of the interferon-β_2/B cell differentiation factor BSF-2/hepatocyte-stimulating factor gene in human fibroblasts by other cytokines, *J. Immunol., 140*: 974.

Williams, D. E., Cooper, S., and Broxmeyer, H. E. (1988). Effect of hematopoietic suppressor molecules on the in vitro proliferation of purified murine granulocyte-macrophage progenitor cells, *Cancer Res., 48*: 1548.

Yonemazu, M., Stephens, K. E., Ishizaka, A., Zheng, H., Hogue, R. S., Crowley, J. J., Hatherill, J. R., and Raffin, T. A. (1989). Effects of tumor necrosis factor on PMN chemotaxis, chemiluminescence and elastase activity, *J. Lab. Clin. Med., 114*: 674.

Zhang, Y., Lin, J. X., Yip, Y. K., and Vilček, J. (1988). Enhancement of cAMP levels and of protein kinase activity by tumor necrosis factor and interleukin 1 in human fibroblasts: role in the induction of interleukin 6, *Proc. Natl. Acad. Sci. USA, 85*: 6802.

Zoumbos, N. C., Djeu, J. Y., and Young, N. S. (1984). Interferon is the suppressor of hematopoiesis generated by stimulated lymphocytes in vitro, *J. Immunol., 133*: 769.

Zucali, J. R., Broxmeyer, H. E., Gross, M. A., and Dinarello, C. A. (1988). Recombinant human tumor necrosis factor alpha and beta stimulate fibroblasts to produce hemopoietic growth factors in vitro, *J. Immunol., 140*: 840.

14

TNF as Immunomodulatory Agent

BENJAMIN BONAVIDA
UCLA School of Medicine and the Jonsson Comprehensive Cancer Center, University of California, Los Angeles, California

I. INTRODUCTION

Tumor necrosis factor (TNF) is a multifunctional cytokine and a pleitropic molecule. It has been shown that TNF can selectively lyse certain transformed cells, stimulate the proliferation of normal and neoplastic cells, inhibit hemopoiesis, and act as a differentiation factor for certain leukemias. Further, TNF mediates severe inflammatory reactions, stimulates collagenase and prostaglandins, stimulates fibroblast and endothelial cells, regulates T- and B-cells immune responses, stimulates several cytokine from different normal cells and cell lines, and induces class I and class II MHC molecules (Old, 1985; Boch and March, 1987; Bonavida et al., 1988; Bonavida and Granger, 1990). Thus, among other functions, TNF-α is a potent immunoregulatory molecule.

Antigen-induced stimulation of T cells and B cells is usually manifested by proliferation and differentiation, resulting in the induction of T helper/T cytotoxic cells and immunoglobulin (Ig)-secreting B cells. The antigen-presenting MHC II-bearing cells (monocytes, Langherhans cells, B cells) play a central and pivotal role in the manifestation of both T- and B-cell responses. Direct cell–cell interactions and several soluble cytokine mediators act in concert and by a complex cascade of events result in the proliferation, differentiation, and auto regulation of the antigen-mediated immune response. Clearly, disturbances in the microenvironment of the immune response or dyregulation of cytokine induction and function could result in major changes in the immune response and can be accompanied by deleterious effects. To better understand the role played by each of the multiple cytokines produced during an immune response, experiments were designed both in vitro and in vivo to examine the direct effect and role played by each specific recombinant cytokine, or indirectly by the use of specific antibody to the cytokine in question and observe the outcome of the immune response. Based on this approach, several studies have examined the role by which TNF modulates an immune response. The following is a brief summary of the effects of TNF on T- and B-cell functions and other cells participating in the immune response and the role of TNF in cell-mediated cytotoxicity. Other chapters in the book cover in detail the role of TNF in inflammation, microbial infections, autoimmune disease, and tumor therapy.

II. EFFECT OF TNF ON T AND B LYMPHOCYTES

Scheurich et al. (1987) have investigated the effect of TNF-α on human peripheral blood T lymphocytes stimulated with anti-CD3 mAb crosslinked with antimouse Ig and cultured in the presence of IL-2 for up to 15 days. TNF-α receptor expression was minimal on resting T cells but steadily increased after mitogen stimulation and peaked at 6 days of culture and declined thereafter. The time course of TNF-α receptor expression was similar to that of high-affinity IL-2 receptor. The IFN-γ receptors were constitutively expressed on T cells and were not affected by mitogenic stimulation. Further, TNF-α enhanced the expression of class I MHC antigens on T cells with no change in the expression of class II MHC. TNF-α also enhanced the proliferation of activated cells when the cells expressed low IL-2 receptors. TNF-α induced IFN-γ production by T cells provided that IL-2 was present. It should be pointed out that the effects seen are usually at later stages of T-cell activation in long-term cultures and might reflect immunoregulatory effects of already activated T cells and not of resting or early activated T cells.

Pawelec et al. (1989) have examined CD4$^+$ and CD8$^+$ T-cell clones and demonstrated that CD4$^+$ T cells secrete TNF-α, although both cell types secreted equal amount of IFN-γ. Further, Cherwinski et al. (1988) have divided immune T-cell helper clones into TH1 and TH2 and demonstrated that the TH1 subset produced TNF-α and TNF-β, whereas TH2 produced TNF in lower quantity or not at all.

Initially, the direct effect of TNF-α on mitogen-stimulated murine thymocytes was studied by Dinarello et al. (1986) and there was no detectable enhancement of the proliferative response. The failure to detect a response might have been attributed to the lack of expression of TNF-α receptors on the cell surface and also upregulated the high-affinity IL-2 receptors in these cells. These findings prompted further examination of the direct effect of TNF in peripheral T-cells. Yokota et al. (1988) used purified human peripheral blood T cells and demonstrated that TNF-α augmented the proliferation of T cells, both CD4$^+$ and CD8$^+$ T cells, when stimulated by either immobilized monoclonal anti-CD3 antibodies or with antigen in the presence of paraformaldehyde-fixed monocytes. TNF-α-mediated enhancement of T-cell proliferation induced with immobilized anti-CD3 antibodies in the absence of exogenous IL-2. The ability of rTNF-α to enhance anti-CD3-mediated T-cell proliferation varied inversely with the concentration of lymphokines produced endogeneously in the cultures. However, the mechanism by which TNF-α enhances proliferation of mitogen-stimulated T cells is not clear. Thus TNF may induce IL-2-dependent T-cell growth. This hypothesis is compatible with the studies of Scheurich et al. (1987).

Further studies by Vine et al. (1988) indicated that TNF-α facilitated cell cycle entry form G0 into G1 of mitogen-activated T cells. Also, TNF-α up-regulated TNF-α receptor expression but did not stimulate IL-2 production. At the single T-cell level, TNF-α did not promote growth of IL-2 production of individual T cells stimulated by immobilized mitogens, although it enhanced the percentage of T cells that grew in response to immobilized mitogen and IL-2. Altogether, these results demonstrate a positive up-regulatory effect of TNF-α on T cells and suggest that TNF may play an important role in mitogen/antigen-induced T-cell responsiveness.

Studies done in the murine system demonstrated that murine TNF-α enhances the thymocyte proliferation in the presence of mitogens IL-1 or IL-2. By itself, TNF-α was not stimulatory. The response of TNF-α and IL-1 or IL-2 was synergistic (Ranges et al., 1988). The mechanism of TNF-α mediated enhancement of proliferation was not due to TNF-mediated activation of IL-1, IL-2, or IL-4 secretion by the thymocytes. Further studies are needed to sort out the underlying mechanisms of TNF-mediated effects on T cells and the role played by other cytokines in the overall response.

The effect of TNF-α on B cells was examined using highly purified B cells. Such cells respond to the mitogen-formalinized Cowan I stain *Staphylococcus aureus* (SA) and differentiate into Ig-secreting cells in the presence of IL-2. TNF-α alone added to SA-treated B cells has no effect on either proliferation or differentiation of the B cells into Ig-secreting cells. However, in the presence of IL-2, TNF-α augmented B-cell proliferation and differentiation (Jelinek and Lipsky 1987). A more detailed analysis of the TNF-α-mediated effect was made using a two-stage tissue culture system. When TNF-α was added in the presence of IL-2 during the initial phase of B- cell activation with SA, there was no noticeable increase of IL-2 receptor expression on the B cells. However, at the later stage in the presence of IL-2, activated B cells responded to TNF-α and there was a significant augmentation of proliferation and differentiation. Like activated T cells, activated B cells exhibit a marked increase in TNF-α receptor expression (Kehrl et al., 1987).

The foregoing studies showed significant effects of TNF on either purified T cells or B cells. However, the effect of exogenous TNF or endogenously produced TNF on the response by a mixed cell population was not evident. Studies by

Kashiwa et al. (1987) have examined the effect of TNF-α on PWM-induced B-cell maturation and differentiation. The PWM stimulated system was chosen, as it mimics antigen-induced stimulation in that all the three cell components, the T cells, B cells, and monocytes, are necessary and are involved in the overall T- and B-cell responses. In this system, both IgM- and IgG-secreting cells are activated, and further, it has been shown that the B-cell response by PWM is regulated by both macrophages and T cells or their products (Waldman and Broder, 1982). In these studies, the addition of rTNF-α at the initiation of cultured human peripheral blood lymphocytes and PWM resulted in a marked suppression of the generation of IgG and IgM plaque-forming cells (PFCs). As shown by others in subsequent studies, TNF-α had no effect on the viability or proliferation of T cells and B cells, thus ruling out a suppressive effect mediated by a cytostatic or cytotoxic of TNF on these cells.

The mechanism of TNF-mediated suppression of the PWM-induced response was examined (Kashiwa and Bonavida, 1990a,b). The suppressive effect was a late event in the pathway of B-cell maturation and differentiation as addition of TNF-α as late as 4 days after culture resulted in a significant decrease of Ig PFC. There was no detectable effect of TNF on mature B cells or on an Ig-secreting tumor B-cell line, thus ruling out a direct effect of TNF on B cells. However, the addition of TNF to T cells activated with mitogen in a two-step culture system resulted in a marked suppression of the B-cell response, indicating that TNF acted on the T helper cells or on the production of helper factors(s) controlling T-cell lymphokine secretion. Further, studies showed that TNF had no effect on T-cell-derived factors that act on PWM- or SAC-activated B cells and result in the secretion of helper factors with diminished B-cell differentiation factor (BCDF) activity, and this diminution was reversed by the addition of IFN-γ. Hence the addition of IFN-γ to TNF-suppressed cultures stored the response. The active role of INF-γ in the response was shown by anti-IFN-γ antibody added to T-helper factors and which resulted in diminished BCDF activity. Altogether, these results suggested that TNF-mediated suppression of PWM-stimulated cultures may be the result of selective inhibition of IFN-γ production by T cells, a necessary cytokine in the differentiation of B cells (Brunswick and Lake, 1985).

In contrast to the studies of Kashiwa et al. (1987), Kashiwa and Bonavida (1990a,b), Jelinek and Lipsky (1987) have reported that TNF-α enhanced the PWM response of B-cell differentiation into Ig-secreting cells. The latter investigators used T cells or macrophages. While the reason for these observed differences is not known, further studies using T-cell lines or clones are necessary to investigate the effect of TNF-α or TNF-β on the induction of IFN-γ and other cytokines.

The results by Kashiwa and Bonavida (1990a,b) suggest that during the PWN-induced response, endogeneously produced TNF may also regulate the B-cell response. This hypothesis was tested experimentally. First, the production of active

TNF in supernatants derived from PWM-stimulated human peripheral blood cells was determined. Using a sensitive radioimmunoassay, TNF was detected within 24 h of culture and reached peak levels at day 2 or 3 and the TNF level declined thereafter. The primary cellular source of TNF-α was plastic adherent monocytes. Based on the suppressive effect of exogenous TNF added to PWM cultures, the addition of anti-TNF monoclonal antibody to the culture resulted resulted in a significant increase in the Ig PFC response and the addition of anti-TNF antibody on day 2 or 3 of culture caused the maximum enhancement. These findings demonstrated that there was a good correlation between the kinetics of endogenous production of TNF and its down-regulatory activity.

TNF-β (also known as lymphotoxin, a T-cell product) was also examined for its effect on B cells. Kerhl et al. (1982) have shown that TNF-β used as a stimulus with SA-induced B-cell proliferation. Zola and Nikoloutsopoulos (1989) have examined the effect of TNF-β on activation, proliferation, and differentiation of human tonsil-derived B lymphocytes. Activation induced by anti IgM and IL-4 resulted in the expression of CD23 and up-regulation of MHC class II with minimal proliferation. TNF-β had no effect on the activation of resting B cells. However, TNF-β-augmented B-cell proliferation in the presence of BCGF or IL-2 confirmed the results of Kehrl et al. (1982) and Jelinek and Lipsky (1987). There were no changes in the differentiation status of the B cells as determined by various cell surface markers.

The administration of rhuTNF-α into mice at the same time as antigen (SRBC) enhanced the antibody response in a dose-dependent fashion. However, the response to a T-independent antigen was not affected by TNF-α (Ghiara et al., 1987). The differences in the effect of TNF-α seen varied with animal species, antigen use conditions (in vivo versus in vitro), and schedule and dose of TNF administered.

Recent studies by Gordon and Wofsy (1990) have examined the effect of TNF-α administered in vivo in mice on the subsequent response to antigens and mitogens. Mice were treated intraperitoneally with 10 μg of TNF-α on alternate days and at different times were tested for immune functions. Administration of TNF-α induced a progressive decline in splenic lymphocytes (CD4 and CD8) and an increase in splenic monocytes without altering the total number of cells. A marked inhibitory effect was seen in T-cell proliferation to PHA or Con A and the inhibition was apparent 1 day after a single injection of TNF-α. After 8 weeks the PHA response was reduced by 80% and the Con A response was abolished.

The B-cell response to LPS was not reduced initially, but after 4 weeks the response was reduced by 60%. The inhibitory response was due to the monocytes of treated mice. NK activity also declined in TNF-α-treated mice and was undetectable in 8-week treated mice. Similarly, the induction of cytotoxic allogenenic T cells was decreased in treated mice. The defect in T-cell response was paralleled by a decreased DTH response to soluble antigens. While in T-cell response was inhibited, the B-cell antibody response was not altered. These findings are reminiscent of the effect of PGE2 on the immune response, and it is possible that TNF-α-mediated secretion of PGE2 is responsible for the effects seen in vivo. Thus the effects in vivo are different from the effects in vitro.

Studies by Talmadge et al. (1987) examined the immunomodulatory activity of recombinant human and murine TNF-α in mice. Treatment of spleen cells with rHTNF did not alter the NK activity in vitro and intravenous injection of rHTNF 1 to 3 days before testing NK activity in vitro did not result in any augmentation of NK cytotoxicity. In the mixed lymphocyte reaction, recombinant human or mouse TNF-α augmented the proliferative response in a dose-dependent manner, and this increase required the presence of stimulator cells, as TNF had no effect on the responder cells. However, the CTL activity against a tumor cell was not affected by various doses of TNF. In vivo, the induction of cytotoxic cells to a tumor vaccine was significantly increased by TNF administration. In vitro macrophage-mediated cytotoxicity against tumor cell was augmented by 24-h treatment of thioglycollate-induced peritoneal macrophages by TNF. The same activation took place in vivo by TNF administration. Although these effects were observed, the exact mechanism by which TNF mediates these effects is not clear. Is TNF alone or TNF-induced cytokines responsible for the effects seen?

Although the role of endogeneous TNF-α production is important and plays a role in modulating the immune response as shown above, other cytokines may also be important as they play a role in regulating TNF production and activity. For example, IL-1 actions bear several similarities to TNF-mediated actions, and both agents have been shown to act synergistically/ Similarly, IL-6, which is also a pleiotropic molecule produced by macrophages, can act as an immunoregulatory molecule similar to IL-1, IL-6, and TNF-α. In addition, these cytokines regulate each others as well as their own production. Recombinant human IL-1 and TNF are capable of inducing their own production as well as each other's. IL-1 and TNF both induce IL-6 from monocytes, endothelial cells, smooth muscle cells, and B cells. TNF induction of IL-6 sets in motion the production of cytokines which act on T- and B-cell responses (Fiers et al., 1990). In contrast, IL-6 inhibits TNF production from monocytes; thus the induction of IL-6 by TNF may serve as a sort of feedback mechanism regulating TNF production (Aderka et al., 1990). TNF also stimulates the generation of GM-CSF (Munker et al., 1986), and GM-CSF has been shown to promote TNF production (Cannistra et al., 1988). Thus TNF regulates its own synthesis by both positive and negative feedback signals.

In vitro mixed lymphocyte cultures (MC) were used to determine the effect of TGB-β and TNF-α. TGF-β inhibits TNF-α production by monocytes (Espevik et al., 1987). The addition of TNF-α to TGF-β-treated cultures restored the CTL activity, and the addition of anti-TNF antibody inhibited the generation of CTL (Ranges et al., 1987). Thus TNF appears to have an immunostimulatory activity.

Economou et al. (1989) reported that IL-2 stimulates monocyte/macrophage to release TNF and TNF-α mRNA levels increased within 4 h of stimulation. IL-4 down-regulates TNF production and gene expression. Aderka et al. (1990) showed that IL-6 inhibited TNF production by monocytes and U937 cells; further IL-6 appears to antagonize the priming effects of GM-CSF or IFN-γ on TNF production. Thus since TNF induces IL-6 by monocytes, this induction of IL-6 may represent a negative-feedback regulatory signal for TNF production.

III. ACTIONS OF TNF ON MONOCYTE/MACROPHAGES, NK CELLS, AND NEUTROPHILS

The role of TNF-α in regulating macrophage activation was studied in severe combined immunodeficient mice (*Scid*), where both T- and B-cell functions are deleted (Bancroft et al., 1989). Spleen cells from Scid mice inoculated with heat-killed *Listeria* monocytogens (LM) secrete IFN-γ in a dose-dependent manner. The IFN-γ secretion was dependent on the presence of macrophages that do not produce IFN-γ. Both TNF-α and IFN-γ were tested in the supernatants of stimulated Scid cells. The kinetics of TNF production were rapid and plateaued at 20 h, whereas IFN-γ production was first detected at 18 h and plateaued at 48 h. This suggested that TNF-α may be responsible for the macrophage dependency of IFN-γ production by NK cells. This notion was corroborated by the addition of anti-TNF antibody, which abrogated IFN-γ production. Further, IFN-γ production was not seen with TNF-α alone but required the presence of LM. Thus these results demonstrated that macrophage interaction with antigen results in the production of TNF-α, which in turn activates NK cells to produce INF-γ. Also, both TNF and INF-γ activate macrophage Ia expression and tumoricidal activity.

While TNF-α is produced by NK cells and LGL (Degliantoni et al., 1986), studies by Ostensen et al. (1987) reported that TNF-α enhances NK cytolyic activity of human peripheral blood NK cells. Pretreatment of non adherent lymphocytes or purified CD16$^+$ cells with TNF-α for 18 h resulted in augmented NK cytotoxicity. The pretreament with both IL-2 and TNF-α further augmented the cytotoxicity additively or syngestically. The TNF-α treatment resulted in inducing IL-2 receptor expression by CD16$^+$ cells and the combination of IL-2 and TNF-α dramatically increased expression of the IL-2 receptor. These studies determined that TNF-α can act directly on NK cells, but the possible role of TNF-α-induced mediators from NK cells, such as IL-2 and IFN-γ, which might be responsible for the enhanced NK activity, was not ruled out.

Chouaib et al. (1989) studied the effect of TNF-α on IL-2-mediated differentiation of LGL into LAK cells. Pretreatment of LGL with TNF/IL-2 was sufficient to promote the IL-2/TNF-driven generation of LAK cytotoxicity without proliferation. This treatment also enhanced the level of IL-2 receptors. TNF was found in IL-2-treated LGL supernatants and anti-TNF antibody partially blocked the differentiation of LGL of LGL into LAK effector cells by IL-2. Thus TNF plays an important role in the sequential activation of LAK by IL-2.

Lympotoxin alone or in combination with retinoic acid induces functional and morphological differentiation of human myeloid leukemia cells (HL-60 and THP-1) into monocyte-like cells (Hemmi et al., 1987). These studies are corroborated by Trinchieri et al. (1986), who also showed TNF-mediated differentiation of myeloid cells into monocytes and synergy with IFN-γ. In contrast, NK cells or TNF-α inhibit formation of hemeatopoietic colonies (Degliantoni et al. 1986).

TNF has been shown to affect neutrophil functions such as neutrophil adherence to endothelial cells by increasing surface expression of the C3Bi receptor/adherence to endothelial cells by increasing surface expression of the C3Bi receptor/adherence glycoprotein and enhances ADCC against chicken red blood cells,. Klebanoff et al. (1988) reported that TNF-α was a weak stimulus of the neutrophil respiratory burst and degranulation. These effects were increased in the presence of unopsonized zymosan in the reaction mixture. The effect of TNF on granulocytes is rapid and appears to be independent of protein and nucleic acid synthesis. TNF does not act as an opsonin, but rather reacts with the neutrophil to increase its phagocytotic activity. This TNF-dependent phagocytosis is inhibited by mAb to the C3Bi receptors.

Shalaby et al. (1988) using highly purified TNF-α, showed that short treatment of PMN with TNF-α increased their ability to phagocytose latex beads and enhanced antibody directed cellular cytotoxicity against CRBC. In the presence of IFN-γ, a significant synergistic activity was observed.

IV. ROLE OF TNF-α IN NK-, NC-, AND MONOCYTE/MACROPHAGE-MEDIATED TUMOR CYTOTOXICITY

A. Role of LT and TNF in Natural-Killer-Cell-Mediated Cytotoxicity

Natural killer cells (NK) are a subcategory of peripheral blood leukocytes endowed with the ability to lyse certain sensitive target cells in the absence of presensitization. The mechanism of NK cytotoxicity has been the subject of numerous investigations. A stimulus secretion model was proposed which suggested that soluble cytotoxic factors were secreted following the NK target cell interaction and resulted in target cell lysis. Candidates for the putative mediator have been natural killer cytotoxic factor (NKCF), TNF-α, cytotoxic granules, and perforin.

TNF-α and perforin are cytotoxic to a variety of target cells, either NK sensitive or NK resistant, and are not species restricted. In contrast, NKCF is selectively cytotoxic to NK-sensistive targets and species specific. Several data accumulated to date suggest strongly that TNF-α and TNF-β are not candidates in the NK-CMC (Wright and Bonavida, 1987).

The target cell specificity of rTNF was found to be related to that of NKCF, with the exception of several NK-resistant cell lines that were lysed by rTNF in 20-h ^{51}Cr release assay. Antibody inhibition studies revealed that anti-TNF antibody mediated from partial to complete inhibition of lysis of U937 by unfrcationated supernatant containing NKCF. However, fractionation of such supernatant by chromatofocusing yielded two distinct peaks of cytotoxic activity. Anti-TNF antibody inhibited the acidic form of NKCF but not the neutral form. In the NK-CMC reaction, anti-TNF antibody did not yield consistent inhibition of NK-CMC reaction, anti-TNF antibody did not yield consistent inhibition of NK-CMC consistent with TNF-α not playing a major role in NK-CMC (Wright and Bonavida, 1987). These findings are not consistent with those of Degliantoni et al. (1986), who have reported complete inhibition of NKCF by anti-TNF antibody. However, their NKCF preparation was not characterization for the specific presence of NKCF activity and could have consisted primarily of TNF-α. Indeed, our findings with peripheral blood cells indicate that depending on the stimulus used and the donor, different NK-CF preparations are obtained with different proportions of TNF and NKCF activity (J. H. Chen et al., unpublished). Another line evidence was obtained on the role of NKCF and not TNF-α in NK-CMC. The NK-sensitive U937, also sensitive to TNF and NKCF, was used to derive variants following culture in NKCF- or TNF-α-containing media. After several weeks, the U9NR (NKCF variant) and U9TR (TNF variant) variant were tested for sensitivity to cytotoxicity by NKCF, TNF-α, and NK cells. The U9TR line was resistant to high concentrations of TNF and NKCF but was as sensitive as the parental U9 to NK-CMC. In contrast, the U9NR line was resistant to NKCF and TNF-α and wasalso resistant to NK-CMC. These results suggested strongly that TNF alone may not play a role in NK-CMC and that NKCF is probably the postulated factor. Further studies are needed to establish the biochemical as well as antigenic relationship between NKCF and TNF-α (Wright and Bonavida, in preparation).

Cytolysins and perforins have been implicated as cytotoxic mediators in both NK- and CTL-mediated reactions. These factors have been isolated from the granules of many types of cell lines or tumors and lyse target cells by forming pores in the membranes. They are not related to TNF-α or TNF-β. Their functional properties are not concordant with NK-CMC reactions as (1) they lyse nonselectively all kinds of targets cells, (2) lysis occurs within minutes as compared to 30 to 60 min for NK (3) lysis can take place at room temperature as compared to 37°C for NK-CMC, and (4) they form pores on the membrane whereas no pores are detected in NK-CMC reactions. Antibodies to perforin have shown partial inhibition of NK CMC (Millard et al., 1984; Podack et al., 1983, 1988).

B. Role of LT in CTL CMC

Several studies have been reported on the role of a cytolytic mediator in CTL-mediated cytotoxicity. However, the studies are controversial and not conclusive. CTL-mediated lysis is target specific and H-2 restricted, whereas lysis by LT and TNF is not. Further, the kinetics of lysis by CTL and LT are different and LT mediates its lytic effect in a long-term assay (18 to 48 h), whereas CTL killing can be observed as early as 1 h. The possibility that exogenous LT activity and LT internalization into the target by CTL exhibit different kinetics of lysis was analyzed by Schmid et al. (1985). These investigators have established a series of Lyt-2$^+$, nitrophenyl-specific T-cells that kill target cells in antigen-specific and H-2-restricted fashion in a 4-h assay. These lines also produced TNF-β that can lyse fibroblasts in 48 to 72 h. However, supernatants fluids from the Lyt-2$^+$ cell lines were shown to kill ^{51}Cr-labeled fibroblasts in a dose-dependent fashion during a 4-h assay when they were rapidly internalized via an osmotic procedure. These results suggest that TNF-β may act as a mediator for CTL lysis but the evidence is not conclusive and lysis of nonfibroblast target cells was not tested (Schmid et al., 1985).

The studies above with CTL and NK clearly indicate that TNF-α and LT do not play an active role in NK and CTL killing of target cells in a short-term assay, but do not rule out that these cells may secrete TNF-α or TNF-β upon stimulation by targets or other factors and mediate cytotoxic/cytostatic effect in a long-term assay. In any event, both NK- and CTL-mediated killing of target cells results in apoptosis. Apoptosis is a process whereby cells die in a controlled manner, in response to specific stimuli, apparently following an intrinsic program of cell death (Ken et al., 1972). In these instances, there is a series of striking similar morphological changes, particularly in the nucleus and nuclear DNA undergoes widespread change at intranucleosomal sites. The role of soluble mediators in NK and CTL must account for the induction of apoptosis either through triggering specific sites on the membrane of the targets or through the activation of endogenous endonucleases (Arends et al., 1990).

C. Role of TNF in Natural Cytotoxicity by Natural Cytotoxicity (NC) Cells

In the mouse system, two types of natural lymphocyte-mediated cytotoxicity have been described, NK and NC cells. These two types of natural cytotoxicity differ in many respects, such as target cell specificity, cell surface antigen expression, and kinetics of lysis. NK cells lyse target cells rapidly in 2 to 4 h, whereas NC kill target cells in longer periods (i.e., 18 h or longer). In a study by Ortaldo et al. (1985), these authors investigated the role of TNF-α in NC-mediated cytotoxicity of murine WEHI-164 target cells. These target cells were highly sensitive to TNF-α (both murine and human) and NC cytotoxicity was significantly blocked by rabbit antimouse TNF antibody. The same treatment had no effect on NK CMC. The NC cells appear to belong to myelomonocytic lineage, and like monocytes, produce TNF-α that is in part responsible for cytotoxicity. These results implied that NC mediate their cytotoxic activity by TNF-α.

D. Role of TNF in Macrophage-Mediated Cytotoxicity

Murine macrophages can be activated to express cytotoxicity toward a variety of tumor cells but cannot kill normal cells. Several reports indicate that macrophages can kill by different pathways, including TNF-α, IL-1, H_2O_2, NO, and cytolytic proteases. Decker et al. (1987) reported that TNF plays an important role in the killing of TNF-sensitive tumor cells by activated macrophages. However, killing of a large battery of TNF-resistant tumor cells by macrophages is mediated by TNF-independent mechanisms.

Higuchi et al. (1990) examined the cytotoxicity of activated macrophages against two target cells, one sensitive and the other resistant to TNF-α. The cytotoxicity against the TNF-sensitive line was abrogated by antibody to TNF-α. The lytic toxicity against the TNF-sensitive line was mediated by the production of NO_2^-/NO_3^- from *L*-arginine, as depletion of *L*-arginine from the culture medium inhibited cytotoxicity. These results showed that activated macrophages can express at least two cytolytic mechanisms independently of each other. However, the combination of TNF and NO resulted in synergistic cytotoxic activity.

While TNF-dependent macrophage cytotoxicity has been shown by many investigators by the use of anti-TNF antibody, such studies were interpreted as due to neutralization of TNF secreted by the macrophages. However, in many instance, the amount of secreted TNF could not account for lysis. Therefore, the role of cell-cell contact may be essential in many instances and the role of membrane TNF becomes a possibility. Studies by Decker et al. (1987) demonstrated that TNF-dependent lysis of tumor cells can be mediated by paraformaldehyde-fixed cells, which are unable to secrete TNF. The presence of TNF on the fixed macrophages was also shown by indirect radioimmunoassay. These results are important, as they demonstrate a role of membrane-bound TNF in cytotoxicity. Studies corroborating these findings were reported by Ichinore et al. (1988), who have shown that target cells are resistant to soluble TNF-α. They are killed in part by a TNF-dependent mechanism by monocytes bearing TNF-α on the membranes.

Whether cytotoxicity is mediated through the release of TNF from the fixed cells or through a signaling event is not clear. Kriegler et al. (1988) have reported a membrane-bound TNF of 26 kDa, a precursor of TNF that needs to be processed to 17 kDa in soluble form to be cytotoxic. It is possible that membrane-bound TNF can trigger the TNF receptor on the target cells and signal the target cells to induce programmed cell death, as anti-TNF receptor antibody has been shown to mimic the effect of TNF in inducing target cell lysis and DNA degradation (Espevik et al., 1990).

ACKNOWLEDGMENTS

This work was supported by DHHS Grant CA-43212 and in part by a grant from the Concern Foundation and the Bocron Foundation.

REFERENCES

Aderka, D., Reis, L., FL, and Lee, T. (1990). Interleukin-6: a cytokine induced by TNF, and once thought to mediate the antiviral action of TNF, inhibits TNF production in monocytes and U937 cells primed with GM-CSF, *Tumor Necrosis factor: Structure, Mechanism of Action, Role in Disease and Therapy* (B. Bonavida, and G. Granger, eds,), S. Karger, Basel, pp. 133–139.

Arends, M., Morris, R. G., and Wyllie, A. H. (1990). Apoptosis: the role of the endonuclease, *Am. J. Pathol., 136*: 593–609.

Bancroft, G. J., Sheehan, K. C. F., Schreiber, R. D., and Unanue, E. R. (1989). Tumor necrosis factor is involved in the T cell dependent pathway of macrophage activation in Scid mice, *J. Immunol., 143*: 127–130.

Beutler, B., Milsark, I. W., and Cerami, A. C. (1988). Passive immunization against cachectin/tumor necrosis factor protects mice from lethal effect of endotoxin, *Science, 229*: 869–871.

Bock, G., and March, J., eds. (1987). Tumor necrosis factor and related cytotoxins, Ciba Foundation Symposium 131: *Symposium on Tumor Necrosis Factor and Related Cytokines,* Ciba Foundation, London, Jan. 20–22, Wiley, Chichester, England.

Bonavida, B., and Granger, G., eds. (1990). *Tumor Necrosis Factor: Structure, Mechanism of Action, Role in Disease and Therapy,* S. Karger, Basel.

Bonavida, B., Gifford, G. E., and Kirchner, H., eds. (1988). *Tumor Necrosis Factor/Cachectin and Related Cytokines*, S. Karger, Basel.

Brunswick, M., and Lake, P. (1985). Obligatory role of gamma interferon in T cell replacing factor-dependent antigen specific on murine B cell response, *J. Exp. Med., 161*: 953–971.

Cannistra, S. A., Rambaldi, A., and Spriggs, D. R. (1988). Human granulocyte-macrophage colony stimulating factor induces expression of the tumor necrosis factor gene by the U937 cell line and by normal human monocytes, *J. Clin. Invest., 79*: 1720–1728.

Cherwinski, H. M., Schumacher, J. H., Brown, K. P., and Mosmann, T. R. (1988). Two types of mouse helper T cells clones. II. Further differences in lymphokine synthesis between TH_1 and TH_2 clones revealed by RNA hybridization, functionally monospecific bioassays, and monoclonal antibodies, *J. Exp. Med., 166*: 1229–1244.

Chouaib, S., Bertoglio, J., Blay, J. Y., Marchiol-Fournigault, C., and Fradelizi, D. (1989). Generation of lymphokine activates killer cells: synergy between tumor necrosis factor and interleukin 2, *Proc. Natl. Acad. Sci. USA, 85*: 6875–6879.

Decker, T., Lohmann-Matthes, M. C., and Gifford, G. (1987). Cell associated tumor necrosis factor (TNF) as a killing mechanism of activated cytotoxic macrophages, *J. Immonol., 138*: 957–960.

Degliantoni, G., Murphy, M., and Kobayashi, M. (1986). Natural killer (NK) cell derived hematopoietic colony inhibiting activity and NK cytotoxic factor relationship with tumor necrosis factor and synergism with immune interferon, *J. Exp. Med., 162*: 1512–1530.

Dinarello, C. A., Cannon, J. G., and Wolff, S. M. (1986). Tumor necrosis factor (cachectin) is an endogenous pyrogen and induces production of interleukin-1, *J. Exp. Med., 163*: 1433–1450.

Economu, J. S., McBride, S. H., Essner, R., Rhoaoles, K., Golub, S., Holmes, E. C., and Morton, D. C. (1989). tumor necrosis factor production by interleukin-2 activated macrophages in vitro and in vivo, *Immunology, 67*: 514-519.

Espevik, T., Figari, I. S., Ranges, G. E., and Palladino, M. A., (1987). Transforming growth factor-B1 (TGF-B1) and recombinant human tumor necrosis factor-α reciprocally regulate the generation of lymphokine-activated killer cell activity, *J. Immunol., 140*: 2312-2316.

Espevik, T., Brockhaus, M., Doetsche, H., Norestead, U., and Shalabey, R. (1990). Characterization of binding and biological effects of monoclonal antibodies against a human tumor mecrosis factor receptor, *J. Exp. Med., 171*: 415-426.

Fiers, W., Beyaert, R., and Bronkaert, P. (1990). In vitro and in vivo action of tumor necrosis factor, *Tumor Necrosis Factor: Structure, Mechanism of Action, Role in Disease and Therapy* (Bonavida, and G. Granger, eds.) S. Karger, Basel, pp. 77–81.

Ghiara, P., Borascki, D., Neucroni, L., Ghezzi, P., and Toglabue, A. (1987). Enhancement of in vivo immune response by tumor necrosis factor, *J. Immunol., 139*: 3676–3679.

Gordon, C., and Wofsy, D. (1990). Effects of recombinant murine tumor necrosis factor-α on immune function, *J. Immunol., 144*: 1753–1758.

Hemmi, H., Nakamura, T., and Tamua, K. (1987). Lymphotoxin: induction of terminal differentiation of the human myeloid leukemia cell lines; HL-60 and THP-1, *J. Immunol., 138*: 664.

Higuchi, M., Higashi, N., Taki, H., and Osawa, T. (1990). Cytolytic mechanisms of activated macrophages: tumor necrosis factor and *L*-arginine-dependent mechanisms act synergyistically as the major cytolytic mechanisms of activated macrophages, *J. Immunol., 144*: 1425-1431.

Jelinek, D. F., and Lipsky, P. E. (1987). Enhancement of human B cell proliferation and differentiation by tumor necrosis factor-α and interleukin-1, *J. Immunol., 139*: 2970–2976.

Kashiwa, H., and Bonavida, B. (1990a). Regulation of B cell activation and differentiation. II. Immunosuppressive role of endogenously produced TNFα in PWM stimulated polyclonal Ig PFC response (submitted).

Kashiwa, H., and Bonavida, B. (1990b). Regulation of B cell activation and differentiation. III. Restoration by interferon γ of TNF-β mediated suppression of human B cell differentiation into Ig producing cells (submitted).

Kashiwa, H., Wright, S. C., and Bonavida, B. (1987). Regulation of B cell activation and differentiation. I. Suppression of pokeweed mitogen induced B cell differentiation by tumor necrosis factor (TNF), *J. Immunol., 138*: 1383–1390.

Kehrl, J. H., Alvarez Mon, M., Delsinge, G. A., and Fauci, A. S. (1982). Lymphotoxin is an important T cell derived growth factor for human B cells, *Science, 238*: 1144–1146.

Kehrl, J. H., Miller, A., and Fauci, A. S. (1987). Effect of tumor necrosis factor-α on mitogen-activated human B cells, *J. Exp. Med., 166*: 786–791.

Ken, J. F. K., Wyllie, A. H., and Curie, A. P. (1972). Apoptosis: a basic biological phenomenon with wide ranging implications in tissue kinetics, *Br. J. Cancer, 26*: 239–257.

Klebanoff, S. J., Vadas, M. A., Harlan, J. M., et al. (1986). Stimulation of neutrophils by tumor necrosis factor, *J. Immunol., 136*: 4220-4225.

Kriegler, G., Perez, C., Defay, K., Albert, I., and Lu, S. D. (1988). A novel form of TNF/cachectin is a cell surface cytotoxic transmembrane protein: ramifications for the complex physiology of TNF, *Cell, 53*: 45-53.

Millard, P. J., Henkart, M. A., Reynolds, C. W., and Henkart, P. A. (1984). Purification and properties of cytoplasmic granules from cytotoxic rat LGL tumors, *J. Immunol., 123*: 3197.

Munker, R., Gasson, J., and Ogawa, M. (1986). Recombinant human TNF induces production of granulocyte monocyte colony stimulating factor, *Nature, 323*: 79-82.

Old, L. J. (1985). Tumor necrosis factor (TNF). *Science, 230*: 630.

Ortaldo, J. R., Mason, L. H., Mathieson, B. J., Liang, S. M., Flick, D. A., and Herberman, R. B. (1986). Mediation of mouse natural cytotoxic activity by tumor necrosis factor, *Nature 321*: 700-702.

Ostensen, M. E., Thiele, D. L., and Lipsky, P. E. (1987). Tumor necrosis factor-α enhances cytolytic activity of human natural killer cells, *J. Immunol., 138*: 4185-4191.

Pawelec, G., Sachandt, K., Rehlein, A., and Busch, F. W., (1989). Differential secretion of tumor necrosis factor α and granulocyte/macrophage colony stimulating factor but not interferon-γ from $CD4^+$ compared to $CD8^+$ human T cell clones, *Eur. J. Immunol., 19*: 197-200.

Podack, E. R., and Dennert, A. (1983). Assembly of two types of tubules with putative cytolytic function in cloned natural killer cells, *Nature, 302*: 442-445.

Podack, E. R., Olsen, K. J., Lowry, D. M., and Licktenfeld, M. (1988). Structure and function of perforin, *Gen. Top. Microbiol. Immunol., 140*: 11-21.

Ranges, G. E., Figari, I. S., Espevick, T., and Palladino, M. A. (1987). Inhibition of cytotoxic T cell development by transforming growth factor B and reversal by recombinant tumor necrosis factor, *J. Exp. Med., 166*: 991-998.

Ranges, G. E., Zlotnick, A., Espevick, T., and Dinarello, C. A. (1988). Tumor necrosis factor α/cachetin is a growth factor for thymocytes. Synergistic interactions with other cytokines, *J. Exp. Med., 167*: 1472-1478.

Scheurich, P., Thomas, B., and Ucer, (1987). Immunoregulatory activity of recombinant human tumor necrosis factor (TNF)-α: induction of TNF receptors on human T cells and TNF-α mediated enhancement of T cell responses, *J. Immunol., 138*: 1786-1790.

Schmid, D. S., Powell, M. B., Mahoney, K. A., and Ruddle, N. H. (1985). A comparison of lysis mediated by Lyt-2^+ TNF specific cytotoxic T lymphpocytes (CTL) lines with that mediated by rapidly internalized lymphotoxin-containing supernatant fluids: evidence for a role of soluble mediators in CTL mediated killing, *Cell. Immunol., 93*: 68-82.

Shalababy, M. R., Aggarwal, B. B., Rinderknecht, E., et al. (1985). Activation of human polymorphonuclear neutrophil functions by interferon and tumor necrosis factor, *J. Immunol., 135*: 2069-2073.

Talmadge, J. E., Phillips, H., Schneider, M. et al. (1987). Immunomodulatory properties of recombinant immune and human tumor necrosis factor, *Cancer Res., 4*: 544-550.

Trinchieri, G., Kobayahi, M., and Rosen, M. (1986). Tumor necrosis factor and lymphotoxin induce differentiation of human myeloid cells in synergy with immune interferon, *J. Exp. Med., 164*: 1206-1225.

Vine, J. B., Geppert, T. D., and Lipsky, P. E. (1988). T4 cell activation by immobilized PHA:

differential capacity to induce IL-2 responsiveness and Il-2 production, *J. Immunol., 141*: 2593-2600.

Waldmann, T. A., and Broder, S. (1982). Polyclonal B cell activators in the study of regulation of immunoglobulin synthesis in the human system, *Adv. Immunol., 32*: 1.

Wright, S. C., and Bonavida, B. (1987). Studies on the mechanism of natural killer cell-mediated cytotoxicity. IX. Functional comparison of human natural killer cytotoxic factors with recombinant lymphotoxin and tumor necrosis factor, *J. Immunol., 138*: 1791-1798.

Wright, S. C., and Bonavida, B. Studies on the mechanism of natural killer cell mediated cytotoxicity. X. Evidence for the role of NKCF in the NK lytic mechanism as U937 variant s resistant to TNFα are still NK sensitive in CMC reactions whereas variants resistant to NKCF are NK resistant (in preparation).

Yokota, S., Geppert, T. D., and Lipsky, P. E. (1988). Enhancement of antigen- and mitogen-induced human T lymphocyte proliferation by tumor necrosis factor-α, *J. Immunol., 140*: 531-536.

Zola, H., and Nikoloutsopoulos, A. (1989). Effect of recombinant human tumor necrosis factor β (TNF β) on activation, proliferation and differentiation of human B lymphocytes, *Immunoloyg, 67*: 231-236.

15

TNF and Viruses: Multiple Interrelationships

BERISH Y. RUBIN
Fordham University, Bronx, New York

I. INTRODUCTION

Tumor necrosis factor (TNF) and lymphotoxin (LT) were first described as antitumoral agents produced by macrophages and lymphocytes, respectively. The availability of substantial quantities of both of these reagents, as a result of recombinant DNA technology, has enabled the in-depth study of the biological properties of these proteins. TNF and LT bind to the same cell surface receptors and mediate a host of biological effects that are described in this book. This chapter examines the interactions between TNF and viruses, and discusses (1) viruses as inducers of TNF, (2) viruses as enhancers of the anticellular action of TNF, (3) TNF as an antiviral agent, and (4) the interaction between the human immunodeficiency virus (HIV) and TNF and the effect of TNF on the replication of this virus.

II. VIRUSES AS INDUCERS OF TNF

Observations suggesting that certain viral infections appear to destroy tumors in cancer patients prompted various investigators to attempt treating cancer patients with viruses (Moore, 1955; Southam, 1960; Cassell and Garrett, 1965). These initial studies revealed, in some cases, a partial antitumoral response. A study of the mechanism by which viral infections mediate this antitumoral response revealed that the viruses effect an augmentation of the antigenicity of tumor cells (Austin and Boone, 1979) and the production of interferon (IFN) (Stewart, 1979). In addition to containing IFN, culture supernatants of virally infected cells were found to contain a cytotoxic factor that was distinct from the interferons. To study this molecule, Aderka and co-workers (1986) examined the effect of monoclonal antibodies to TNF and LT on the anticellular activity of culture supernatants from peripheral blood mononuclear leukocytes infected with Sendai virus. These investigators observed that the cytotoxic activity was neutralized by antibody to TNF. Berent and co-workers (1986), using a cDNA probe for TNF, demonstrated that Sendai virus induces TNF mRNA production in peripheral blood mononuclear cells.

These observations prompted others to examine the TNF-inducing effect of additional viruses. These studies have revealed that a variety of viruses are capable of inducing either TNF or LT mRNA or protein. These include encephalomyocarditis virus (EMCV), adenovirus-2 (Ad-2), herpes simplex virus type II (HSV-2) (Wong and Goeddel, 1986), human T-lymphotropic virus type I (Tschachler et al., 1989), Newcastle disease virus (NDV) (Lorence et al., 1988; Lieberman et al., 1989), and HIV (Molina et al., 1989; Merrill et al., 1989; Roux-Lombard et al., 1989).

The ability of viruses to induce the production of TNF and the observed enhanced sensitivity of virally infected cells to the anticellular action of TNF (see Section III) suggest that TNF may play a role in the observed virally mediated antitumoral responses.

III. ENHANCEMENT OF THE TNF-MEDIATED CYTOCIDAL EFFECT IN VIRALLY INFECTED CELLS

The sensitivity of cells to the anticellular action of TNF or LT has been observed to be enhanced in cells treated with inhibitors of RNA and protein synthesis (Matthews and Watkins, 1978). Eifel and co-workers (1979), in their attempt to study the effect of a naturally mediated inhibition of protein synthesis on the anticellular action of LT, examined the anticellular action of LT on mouse L cells infected with vesicular stomatitis virus (VSV). These investigators observed that the simultaneous treatment of cells with LT and VSV for 6 h resulted in 100% cell lysis, whereas no significant toxicity was observed in cells treated for 6 h with either the LT or VSV alone. The ability of VSV to enhance the cytotoxic action of LT and TNF was confirmed by Aderka and co-workers (1985), who demonstrated that cells resistant to the anticellular action of these cytokines are sensitive if they are infected with this virus. This effect of viral infections on the anticellular action of TNF or LT has subsequently been reported to occur in cells infected with HSV (Koff and Fann, 1986; Paya et al., 1988), cytomegalovirus, Theiler's murine encephalomyelitis virus (Paya et al., 1988) and NDV (Lorence et al., 1988; Rood et al., 1990).

It has been suggested that TNF treatment of cells results in the production of protective protein(s) whose synthesis is blocked by inhibitors of RNA and protein synthesis (Wallach, 1984; Hahn et al., 1985). One such protein, the manganous superoxide dismutase, has been observed to play a critical role in cellular defense against the anticellular action of TNF (Wong and Goeddel, 1988; Wong ct al., 1989). As some viruses have been observed to inhibit RNA synthesis in their target cells, it seems reasonable to speculate that the ability of viruses to enhance the anticellular action of TNF might be the result of the ability of the viruses to block the production of the protective mechanism.

IV. TNF AS AN ANTIVIRAL AGENT

In 1986, Kohase and co-workers demonstrated that recombinant human TNF inhibits the replication of EMCV in aged human FS4 fibroblast cells and that this effect of TNF is neutralized by antibody to human interferon β (IFN-β). As these investigators were unable to demonstrate the presence of mRNA for IFN-β subtype 1 (IFN-β_1) but were able to detect mRNA coding for IFN-β subtype 2 (IFN-β_2), the authors concluded that the antiviral effect of TNF was mediated through the production of IFN-β_2. Shortly after the publishing of this report, there appeared two reports demonstrating that TNF and/or LT treatment of cells mediate an antiviral effect against VSV, EMCV, Ad-2, and HSV-2 (Mestan et al., 1986; Wong and Goeddel, 1986). These reports demonstrated that the presence of antibody to IFN-β either had no effect on the TNF-mediated antiviral effect (Wong and Goeddel, 1986) or only partially neutralized the antiviral action of TNF (Mestan et al., 1986). Both studies demonstrated the ability of TNF to induce the 2′, 5′-oligoadenylate synthetase, an enzyme induced in IFN-treated cells. Numerous reports have subsequently confirmed TNF's ability to induce an antiviral state; however, the role of IFN-β_2 in this effect was unclear (Ito and O'Malley, 1987; Arakawa et al., 1987; Van Damme et al., 1987b; Ruggiero et al., 1989a,b). The suggestion that IFN-β_2 was the intermediate in the TNF-mediated antiviral effect arose as a result of 1) Kohase and co-workers' ability to neutralize TNF's antiviral effect with antibody to IFN-β, (2) their ability to detect the presence of mRNA for IFN-β_2, (3) their inability to detect the presence of mRNA for IFN-β_1, and (4) the reports that demonstrated that IFN-β_2 exhibits an antiviral activity similar to that of IFN-β_1 (Zilberstein et al., 1986; Revel et al., 1986; Zilberstein et al., 1985). The antiviral activity of IFN-β_2 was, however, in 1982, already a matter of controversy (Content et al., 1982).

As gene sequence information became available for IFN-β_2 as well as other cytokines, it became apparent that this molecule was the same as molecules characterized by various laboratories and which had been assigned different names depending on the biological activity being studied by these investigators. Thus

IFN-β_2 was found to be homologous with a variety of molecules, including B-cell stimulatory factor 2 (BSF-2), 26-kDa protein, hybridoma/plasmacytoma growth factor (HPGF), hepatocyte stimulating factor (HSF), and interleukin-6 (IL-6) (Sehgal et al., 1987; Van Damme et al., 1987a; Gauldie et al., 1987; Tosato et al., 1988). This protein is now generally termed IL-6. Since recent information indicates the existence of only one IFN-β gene in the human species, IFN-β_1 is now designated simply IFN-β.

The availability of the purified recombinant form of the IL-6 molecule has allowed for a careful evaluation of its role in the TNF-mediated antiviral effect. It has been demonstrated that (1) purified recombinant IL-6 exhibits no antiviral activity; (2) the biological activity of IFN-β is neutralized by antibody to IFN-β, while the plasmacytoma growth factor (PCT-GF) activity of IL-6 is not neutralized by this antibody; (3) the PCT-GF activity of IL-6 is neutralized by antibody to IL -6, yet the biological activity of IFN-β is not neutralized by this antibody; (4) PCT-GF activity of IL-6 present in supernatants of TNF-treated cells is neutralized by antibody to IL-6 but not by antibody to IFN-β; and (5) the antiviral activity of TNF is neutralized by antibody to IFN-β and not by antibody to IL-6 (Reis et al., 1988). These results demonstrate that IL-6 lacks antiviral activity and that it is likely that it is IFN-β that is playing a role in the TNF-mediated antiviral effect. Despite the evidence suggesting that the TNF-mediated antiviral effect is mediated via IFN-β, Northern blot analysis performed on mRNA isolated from TNF-treated cells failed to reveal the presence of mRNA encoding IFN-β (Kohase et al., 1986). The recent availability of polymerase chain reaction technology has enabled a careful examination of the mRNAs present in TNF-treated cells. Jacobsen and co-workers (1989) and Reis and co-workers (1989), using this technology, have demonstrated that TNF treatment of cells induces the production of IFN-β mRNA. These findings, together with the demonstrated synergy between IFN-β and TNF in their antiviral actions, provide support for a role of IFN-β in the TNF-mediated antitumoral effect.

The ability of TNF to induce the 2′, 5′-oligoadenylate synthetase (Mestan et al., 1986; Wong and Goeddel, 1986) prompted an examination and comparison of the proteins induced in TNF-and IFN-treated cells. Beresini and co-workers (1988), employing two-dimensional gel electrophoresis, demonstrated that TNF treatment of cells results in an induction of four proteins that are also induced in response to IFN-γ. These proteins have molecular weights of 21,000, 25,000, 42,000, and 44,000 Dal (Beresini et al., 1988). Rubin and co-workers (1988), employing antibodies directed against several IFN-induced proteins, demonstrated that TNF treatment of human fibroblast cells results in the induction of three proteins whose syntheses are also observed to be induced in IFN-treated cells. The molecular weights of these proteins are 80,000, 67,000, and 56,000 Dal (80, 67, 56 kDa). An examination of the effect of the presence of antibodies to the IFNs on the TNF-mediated antiviral and protein-inducing effects revealed that the incubation of the TNF-treated cells in the presence of antibody to recombinant IFN-β reduces the antiviral efficacy of the TNF and blocks the ability of the TNF to induce the 80-kDa protein. Incubation with antibody to either IFN-α or IFN-γ failed to affect the TNF-mediated responses (Rubin et al., 1988). The inability of the antibody to IFN-β to block thc induction of thc 67-and 56-kDa proteins suggests that TNF induces these proteins via an IFN-independent mechanism. The residual antiviral state observed in TNF-treated cells that have been incubated in the presence of antibody to IFN-β may be the result of the continued synthesis of these TNF/IFN-induced proteins. Goetschy and co-workers (1989) recently reported that the gene encoding the IFN-induced 78-kDa protein, which is the human equivalent of the murine Mx gene, is also induced by TNF and its synthesis is dependent on protein synthesis. The dependence of this induction on protein synthesis is consistent with the observations of Rubin and co-workers (1988), as this human equivalent of the Mx gene is the same protein as the 80-kDa protein (Anderson et al., 1989), whose synthesis in TNF-treated cells is observed to be dependent on the induction of IFN-β.

V. TNF AND THE HUMAN IMMUNODEFICIENCY VIRUS (HIV)

The demonstrated ability of TNF to mediate an antiviral effect against a variety of viruses prompted Wong and co-workers (1988) to examine the effect of TNF on the infectivity and production of the human immunodeficiency virus. The authors reported that treatment of cells with TNF-α prior to and following HIV infection results in a reduction in the amount of P24 antigen expressed in the cells, thus suggesting that TNF pretreatment results in a reduced susceptibility of cells to HIV infection. This inhibitory effect of TNF was also reported to occur at the level of HIV mRNA and HIV production. This report was followed shortly thereafter by reports and cautionary notes from various laboratories, demonstrating that TNF enhances the infectivity and replication of HIV (Matsuyama et al., 1988, 1989; Ito et al., 1989; Folks et al., 1989; Michihiko et al., 1989; Okamoto et al., 1989). It was suggested that TNF administration in HIV-positive individuals might be detrimental since TNF treatment of HIV infected cells results in an enhanced replication of HIV and TNF's cytocidal activity is enhanced in virally infected cells (Matsuyama et al., 1989). Although there is no clear explanation for the discrepancy between the results of Wong et al. (1988) and others, the differences might reflect either the different cell types employed or the length of time following infection at which the data were collected.

Investigation of the molecular mechanism by which TNF enhances the replication of HIV has revealed that this effect is the result of the ability of TNF to cause the transcriptional activation of the HIV long terminal repeat (LTR) by inducing κB sequence binding protein(s) that bind the LTR (Osborn et al., 1989; Griffin et al., 1989; Duh et al., 1989; Banerjee et al., 1989).

The report of TNF's antiviral activity against HIV prompted the evaluation of the efficacy of TNF in patients with AIDS-related Kaposi's sarcoma (Aboulafia et al., 1989; Kahn et al., 1989). While intralesional injections of TNF resulted in a shrinkage of 94% of these lesions (Kahn et al., 1989), a once-weekly intravenous injection of 100 μg/m2 of TNF for 8 weeks failed to reduce the size of the Kaposi's lesions (Aboulafia et al., 1989). In the latter study, the serum HIV P24 antigen levels increased by more than 50% in three out of five patients. This increase may reflect either an increase in the rate of HIV replication or a release of P24 resulting from the increased sensitivity of HIV-infected cells to the cytocidal effects of TNF.

The recent report of Ito and co-workers (1990) demonstrating that TNF antagonizes the inhibitory effect of azidothymidine (AZT) on HIV replication in vitro further suggests that a cautious approach is warranted in studies employing TNF in the treatment of HIV-infected individuals.

The ability of HIV-infected cells to produce TNF and the ability of the TNF to enhance HIV production suggest that TNF may act in an autocrine manner in the induction of HIV expression. This hypothesis was evaluated and confirmed by Poli and co-workers (1990), who, while examining the effect of antibodies to TNF on the expression of HIV, observed the suppression of the constitutive and inducible levels of viral expression in chronically infected cells. As TNF can act in an autocrine manner to induce HIV expression and HIV-infected cells exhibit an enhanced sensitivity to the cytocidal effect of TNF, it is possible that TNF stimulates the replication and propagation of HIV in vivo and thereby is responsible in part or in full for the progression of the HIV infection from latency to active and efficient replication. If TNF were to play a role in this progression, circulating levels of TNF might be expected to increase with the severity of the disease. Examination of TNF titers in the sera of patients in fact reveals that while 100% of asymptomatic HIV-infected subjects and 84% of patients with lymphadenopathy syndrome have serum levels of TNF that are comparable to that of a control group, 100% of the AIDS patients and 55% of patients with AIDS-related complex (ARC) have elevated levels of TNF in their sera (Lahdevirta et al., 1988). A correlation between the progression of AIDS and serum levels of TNF was also reported in a study by Mintz and co-workers (1989) in which they demonstrate that 79% of patients with progressive encephalopathy were observed to have elevated levels of TNF in their sera, as compared with only 8% of patients without neurologic involvement. These elevated serum levels of TNF, which have been interpreted as being responsible for AIDS-related cachexia and myelin damage, may also reflect TNF's ability to enhance the progression of this disease.

REFERENCES

Aboulafia, D., Miles, S. A., Saks, S. R., and Mitsuyasu, R. T. (1989). Intravenous recombinant tumor necrosis factor in the treatment of AIDS-related Kaposi's sarcoma, *J. Acquired Immune Defic. Syndr.*, 2: 54.

Aderka, D., Novick, D., Hahn, T., Fischer, D. G., and Wallach, D. (1985). Increase of vulnerability to lymphotoxin in cells infected by vesicular stomatitis virus and its further augmentation by interferon, *Cell. Immunol.*, *92*: 218.

Aderka, D., Holtmann, H., Toker, L., Hahn, T., and Wallach, D. (1986). Tumor necrosis factor induction by Sendai virus, *J. Immunol.*, *136*: 2938.

Anderson, S. L., Smith, L. J., Lunn, R. M., Horisberger, M. A., and Rubin, B. Y. (1989). Characterization of an IFN-induced 80,000 dalton protein, *J. Interferon Res.*, *9*: S230.

Arakawa, T., Hsu, Y. R., Toth, E., and Stebbing, N. (1987). The antiviral activity of recombinant human tumor necrosis factor-alpha, *J. Interferon Res.*, *7*: 103.

Austin, F. C., and Boone, C. W. (1979). Virus augmentation of the antigenicity of tumor cell extracts, *Adv. Cancer Res.*,*30*: 301.

Banerjee, R., Karpen, S., Siekevitz, M., Lengyel, G., Bauer, J., and Acs, G. (1989). Tumor necrosis factor-alpha induces a kappa B sequence-specific DNA-binding protein in human hepatoblastoma HepG2 cells, *Hepatology*, *10*: 1008.

Berent, S. L., Torczynski, R. M., and Bollon, A. P. (1986). Sendai virus induces high levels of tumor necrosis factor mRNA in human peripheral blood leukocytes, *Nucleic Acids Res.*, *14*: 8997.

Beresini, M. H., Lempert, M. J., and Epstein, L. B. (1988). Overlapping polypeptide induction in human fibroblasts in response to treatment with interferon-alpha, interferon-gamma, interleukin 1 alpha, interleukin 1 beta, and tumor necrosis factor, *J. Immunol.*, *140*: 485.

Cassell, W. A., and Garrett, R. E. (1965). Newcastle disease virus as an antineoplastic agent, *Cancer*, *18*: 863.

Content, J., DeWit, L., Pierard, D., Derynck, R., DeClercq, E., and Fiers, W. (1982). Secretory proteins induced in human fibroblasts under conditions used for the production of interferon-β, *Proc. Natl. Acad. Sci. USA*, *79*: 2768.

Duh, E. J., Maury, W. J., Folks, T. M., Fauci, A. S., and Rabson, A. B. (1989). Tumor necrosis factor alpha activates human immunodeficiency virus type 1 through induction of nuclear factor binding to the NF-kappa B sites in the long terminal repeat, *Proc. Natl. Acad. Sci. USA*, *86*: 5974.

Eifel, P., Billingsley, A., and Lucas, Z. J. (1979). Rapid killing of viral-infected L cells by α-lymphotoxin, *Cell. Immunol.*, *47*: 197.

Folks, T. M., Clouse, K. A., Justement, J., Rabson, A., Duh, E., Kehrl, J. H., and Fauci, A. S. (1989). Tumor necrosis factor alpha induces expression of human immunodeficiency virus in a chronically infected T-cell clone, *Proc. Natl. Acad. Sci. USA*, *86*: 2365.

Gauldie, J., Richards, C., Harnish, D., Lansdorp, P., and Baumann, H. (1987). Interferon beta 2/B-cell stimulatory factor type 2 shares identity with monocyte-derived hepatocyte-stimulating factor and regulates the major acute phase protein response in liver cells, *Proc. Natl. Acad. Sci. USA*, *84*: 7251.

Goetschy, J. F., Zeller, H., Content, J., and Horisberger, M. A. (1989). Regulation of the interferon-inducible IFI-78K gene, the human equivalent of the murine Mx gene, by interferons, double-stranded RNA, certain cytokines, and viruses, *J. Virol.*, *63*: 2616.

Griffin, G. E., Leung, K., Folks, T. M., Kunkel, S., and Nabel, G. J. (1989). Activation of

HIV gene expression during monocyte differentiation by induction of NF-kappa B, *Nature*, *339*: 70.

Hahn, T., Toker, L., Budilovsky, S., Aderka, D., Eshhar, Z., and Wallach, D. (1985). Use of monoclonal antibodies to a human cytotoxin for its isolation and for examining the self-induction of resistance to this protein, *Proc. Natl. Acad. Sci. USA*, *82*: 3814.

Ito, M., and O'Malley, J. A. (1987). Antiviral effects of recombinant human tumor necrosis factor, *Lymphokine Res.*, *6*: 309.

Ito, M., Baba, M., Sato, A., Hirabayashi, K., Tanabe, F., Shigeta, S., and DeClercq, E. (1989). Tumor necrosis factor enhances replication of human immunodeficiency virus (HIV) in vitro, *Biochem. Biophys. Res. Commun.*, *158*: 307.

Ito, M., Baba, M., Mori, S., Hirabayashi, K., Sato, A., Shigeta, S., and DeClercq, E. (1990). Tumor necrosis factor antagonizes inhibitory effect of azidothymidine on human immunodeficiency virus (HIV) replication in vitro, *Biochem. Biophys. Res. Commun.*, *166*: 1095.

Jacobsen, H., Mestan, J., Mittnacht, S., and Dieffenbach, C. W. (1989). Beta interferon subtype 1 induction by tumor necrosis factor, *Mol. Cell. Biol.*, *9*: 3037.

Kahn, J. O., Kaplan, L. D., Volberding, P. A., Ziegler, J. L., Crowe, S., Saks, S. R., and Abrams, D. I. (1989). Intralesional recombinant tumor necrosis factor-alpha for AIDS-associated Kaposi's sarcoma: a randomized, double-blind trial, *J. Acquired Immune Defic. Syndr.*, 2: 217.

Koff, W. C., and Fann, A. V. (1986). Human tumor necrosis factor-alpha kills herpesvirus-infected but not normal cells, *Lymphokine Res.*, *5*: 215.

Kohase, M., Henriksen-DeStefano, D., May, L. T., Vilček, J., and Sehgal, P. B. (1986). Induction of beta 2-interferon by tumor necrosis factor: a homeostatic mechanism in the control of cell proliferation, *Cell*, *45*: 659.

Lahdevirta, J., Maury, C. P., Teppo, A. M., and Repo, H. (1988). Elevated levels of circulating cachectin/tumor necrosis factor in patients with acquired immunodeficiency syndrome, *Am. J. Med.*, *85*: 289.

Lieberman, A. P., Pitha, P. M., Shin, H. S., and Shin, M. L. (1989). Production of tumor necrosis factor and other cytokines by astrocytes stimulated with lipopolysaccharide or a neurotropic virus, *Proc. Natl. Acad. Sci. USA*, *86*: 6348.

Lorence, R. M., Rood, P. A., and Kelley, K. W. (1988). Newcastle disease virus as an antineoplastic agent: induction of tumor necrosis factor-alpha and augmentation of its cytotoxicity, *J. Natl. Cancer Inst.*, *80*: 1305.

Matsuyama, T., Hamamoto, Y., Okamoto, T., Shimotohno, K., Kobayashi, N., and Yamamoto, N. (1988). Tumour necrosis factor and HIV: a note of caution (Letter), *Lancet*, 2: 1364.

Matsuyama, T., Hamamoto, Y., Soma, G., Mizuno, D., Yamamoto, N., and Kobayashi, N. (1989). Cytocidal effect of tumor necrosis factor on cells chronically infected with the human immunodeficiency virus (HIV): enhancement of HIV replication, *J. Virol.*, *63*: 2504.

Matthews, N., and Watkins, J. F. (1978). Tumor-necrosis factor from the rabbit. I. Mode of action, specificity and physiological properties, *Br. J. Cancer*, *38*: 302.

Merrill, J. E., Koyanagi, Y., and Chen, I. S. (1989). Interleukin-1 and tumor necrosis factor alpha can be induced from mononuclear phagocytes by human immunodeficiency virus type 1 binding to the CD4 receptor, *J. Virol.*, *63*: 4404.

Mestan, J., Digel, W., Mittnacht, S., Hiller, H., Blohm, D., Moller, A., Jacobsen, H., and Kirchner, H. (1986). Antiviral effects of recombinant tumour necrosis factor in vitro, *Nature, 323*: 816.

Michihiko, S., Yamamoto, N., Shinozaki, F., Shimada, K., Soma, G., and Kobayashi, N. (1989). Augmentation of in-vitro HIV replication in peripheral blood mononuclear cells of AIDS and ARC patients by tumour necrosis factor (letter), *Lancet, 1*: 1206.

Mintz, M., Rapaport, R., Oleske, J. M., Connor, E. M., Koenigsberger, M. R., Denny, T., and Epstein, L. G. (1989). Elevated serum levels of tumor necrosis factor are associated with progressive encephalopathy in children with acquired immunodeficiency syndrome, *Am. J. Dis. Child., 143*: 771.

Molina, J. M., Scadden, D. T., Byrn, R., Dinarello, C. A., and Groopman, J. E. (1989). Production of tumor necrosis factor alpha and interleukin 1 beta by monocytic cells infected with human immunodeficiency virus, *J. Clin. Invest., 84*: 733.

Moore, A. E. (1955). Effect of viruses on tumors, *Annu. Rev. Microbiol.*, p. 393.

Okamoto, T., Matsuyama, T., Mori, S., Hamamoto, Y., Kobayashi, N., Yamamoto, N., Josephs, S. F., Wong-Staal, F., and Shimotohno, K. (1989). Augmentation of human immunodeficiency virus type 1 gene expression by tumor necrosis factor alpha, *AIDS Res. Human Retroviruses, 5*: 131.

Osborn, L., Kunkel, S., and Nabel, G. J. (1989). Tumor necrosis factor alpha and interleukin 1 stimulate the human immunodeficiency virus enhancer by activation of the nuclear factor kappa B, *Proc. Natl. Acad. Sci. USA, 86*: 2336.

Paya, C. V., Kenmotsu, N., Schoon, R. A., and Leibson, P. J. (1988). Tumor necrosis factor and lymphotoxin secretion by human natural killer cells leads to antiviral cytotoxicity, *J. Immunol., 141*: 1989.

Poli, G., Kinter, A., Justement, J. S., Kehrl, J. H., Bressler, P., Stanley, S., and Fauci, A. S. (1990). Tumor necrosis factor α functions in an autocrine manner in the induction of human immunodeficiency virus expression, *Proc. Natl. Acad. Sci. USA, 87*: 782.

Reis, L. F., Le, J. M., Hirano, T., Kishimoto, T., and Vilček, J. (1988). Antiviral action of tumor necrosis factor in human fibroblasts is not mediated by B-cell stimulatory factor 2/IFN-beta 2, and is inhibited by specific antibodies to IFN-beta, *J. Immunol., 140*: 1566.

Reis, L. F., Ho Lee, T., and Vilček, J. (1989). Tumor necrosis factor acts synergistically with autocrine interferon-beta and increases interferon-beta mRNA levels in human fibroblasts, *J. Biol. Chem., 264*: 16351.

Revel, M., Ruggieri, R., and Zilberstein, A. (1986). Expression of human IFN-beta$_2$ genes in rodent cells, *The Biology of the Interferon System 1985* (H. Schellekens and W. E. Stewart II, eds.), Elsevier, Amsterdam.

Rood, P. A., Lorence, R. M., and Kelley, K. W. (1990). Serum protease inhibitor abrogation of Newcastle disease virus enhancement of cytolysis by recombinant tumor necrosis factors alpha and beta, *J. Natl. Cancer Inst., 82*: 213.

Roux-Lombard, P., Modoux, C., Cruchaud, A., and Dayer, J. M. (1989). Purified blood monocytes from HIV 1-infected patients produce high levels of TNF alpha and IL-1, *Clin. Immunol. Immunopathol., 50*: 374.

Rubin, B. Y., Anderson, S. L., Lunn, R. M., Richardson, N. K., Hellermann, G. R., Smith, L. J., and Old, L. J. (1988). Tumor necrosis factor and IFN induce a common set of proteins, *J. Immunol., 141*: 1180.

Ruggiero, V., Antonelli, G., Conciatori, G., Gentile, M., Van Damme, J., and Dianzani, F.

(1989a). The in vitro antiviral activity of tumor necrosis factor (TNF) in WISH cells is mediated by IFN-beta induction, *Antiviral Res.*, *11*: 77.

Ruggiero, V., Antonelli, G., Gentile, M., Conciatori, G., and Dianzani, F. (1989b). Comparative study on the antiviral activity of tumor necrosis factor (TNF)-alpha, lymphotoxin/TNF-beta and IL-1 in WISH cells, *Immunol. Lett.*, *21*: 165.

Sehgal, P. B., May, L. T., Tamm, I., and Vilček, J. (1987). Human β_2 interferon and B-cell differentiation factor BSF-2 are identical, *Science*, *235*: 731.

Southam, C. M. (1960). Present status of oncolytic virus studies, *Trans. N.Y. Acad. Sci.*, 22: 687.

Stewart, W. E., II (1979). *The Interferon System*, Springer-Verlag, New York.

Tosato, G., Seamon, K. B., Goldman, N. D., Sehgal, P. B., May, L. T., Washington, G. C., Jones, K. D., and Pike, S. E. (1988). Monocyte-derived human B-cell growth factor identified as interferon-β_2 (BSF-2, IL-6), *Science*, *239*: 502.

Tschachler, E., Robert-Guroff, M., Gallo, R. C., and Reitz, M. S., Jr. (1989). Human T-lymphotropic virus I-infected T cells constitutively express lymphotoxin in vitro, *Blood*, *73*: 194.

Van Damme, J., Opdenakker, G., Simpson, R. J., Rubira, M. R., Cayphas, S., Vink, A., Billiau, A., and Van Snick, J. (1987a). Identification of the human 26-kD protein, interferon beta 2 (IFN-beta 2), as a B cell hybridoma/plasmacytoma growth factor induced by interleukin 1 and tumor necrosis factor, *J. Exp. Med.*, *165*: 914.

Van Damme, J., De Ley, M., Van Snick, J., Dinarello, C. A., and Billiau, A. (1987b). The role of interferon-beta 1 and the 26-kDa protein (interferon-beta 2) as mediators of the antiviral effect of interleukin 1 and tumor necrosis factor, *J. Immunol.*, *139*: 1867.

Wallach, D. (1984). Preparations of lymphotoxin induce resistance to their own cytotoxic effect, *J. Immunol.*, *132*: 2464.

Wong, G. H., and Goeddel, D. V. (1986). Tumour necrosis factors alpha and beta inhibit virus replication and synergize with interferons, *Nature*, *323*: 819.

Wong, G. H., and Goeddel, D. V. (1988). Induction of manganous superoxide dismutase by tumor necrosis factor: possible protective mechanism, *Science*, *242*: 941.

Wong, G. H., Krowka, J. F., Stites, D. P., and Goeddel, D. V. (1988). In vitro anti-human immunodeficiency virus activities of tumor necrosis factor-alpha and interferon-gamma, *J. Immunol.*, *140*: 120.

Wong, G. H., Elwell, J. H., Oberley, L. W., and Goeddel, C. V. (1989). Manganous superoxide dismutase is essential for cellular resistance to cytotoxicity of tumor necrosis factor, *Cell*, *58*: 923.

Zilberstein, A., Ruggieri, R., and Revel, M. (1985). Human interferon-beta$_2$: is it an interferon inducer? *The Interferon System*, Serono Symposia, Vol. 24 (G. B. Rossi and E. Dianzani, eds.), Raven Press, New York, p. 73.

Zilberstein, A., Ruggieri, R., Korn, J. N., and Revel, M. (1986). Structure and expression of cDNA and genes for human interferon-beta-2, a distinct species inducible by growth-stimulatory cytokines, *EMBO J.*, *5*: 2529.

16

Role of TNF in Resistance to Bacteria

EDWARD A. HAVELL
Trudeau Institute, Inc., Saranac Lake, New York

I. INTRODUCTION

By now the reader is no doubt aware of two well-studied in vivo effects caused by endogenously produced, or exogenously administered tumor necrosis factor (TNF). First, as its name implies, TNF is capable of causing intratumor hemorrhaging and necrosis of solid tumors (Carswell et al., 1975; Palladino et al., 1987; Havell and North, 1988). Second, TNF causes cachexia, a pathological state that is seen during overwhelming gram-negative bacterial infections, or which can be elicited by the parenteral injection of endotoxin (Beutler et al., 1986a; Beutler and Cerami, 1986). In contrast to the detrimental effects associated with the presence of TNF in the systemic circulation of the host during unrestricted bacterial proliferation and sepsis, there is a small, but growing body of evidence which indicates that small amounts of TNF produced locally within infected organs function in antibacterial resistance mechanisms. The purpose of this chapter is to present this evidence and to discuss possible roles for TNF in host defense against bacteria.

II. Historical Perspective on Bacteria- and Endotoxin-Induced TNF Production

For over 200 years, physicians have associated certain bacterial infections with either decreased incidences of certain types of malignancies or with "spontaneous regressions" of tumors (reviewed by Nauts, 1980). There are records of dramatic antitumor effects in patients in which pyogenic bacterial infections developed following surgery. Moreover, reductions in tumor mass, or the complete regression of malignant growths, were noticed following outbreaks of erysipelas in the area of solid tumors. Such observations led some physicians in the second half of the nineteenth century to attempt treating solid malignancies (generally sarcomas) by inoculating the erysipelas organism (*Streptococcus erysipelatis*, now called *S. pyogenes*) into tumors. This therapeutic approach resulted in a variety of outcomes, including complete, partial, or no tumor regressions, as well as frequent life-threatening infections caused by the injection of viable bacteria. Concerned for the safety of tumor-bearing patients injected with virulent bacteria, Dr. William B. Coley began injecting tumors with mixed culture filtrates (toxins) from broth cultures of *S. pyogenes* and *Bacillus prodigious* (now called *Serratia marcescens*) in the early 1890s (reviewed by Nauts, 1975). Coley (1894, 1896, 1897) reported a number of cases in which total tumor regression occurred following mixed toxin therapy. Because of the apparent safety of these preparations, this therapeutic approach gained a certain degree of acceptance within the medical community. The *Coley toxins* were made commercially available (Park Davis Preparation IX) and were used until the 1920s, when their use was generally supplanted by radiotherapy.

The injection of filtrates from broth cultures of different Gram-negative bacteria, including *S. marcescens*, also caused antitumor effects in rodents bearing solid tumors (Duran-Reynals, 1935; Fogg, 1936; Gratia and Linz, 1931; Shwartzman and Michailovsky, 1932; Shear, 1935). Generally, within hours of the injection of the culture filtrates into rodents bearing well-vascularized tumors, an intense reddening (intratumor hemorrhaging) of the center of the tumor was observed. Later, the cores of the tumors became necrotic. Shear (1943) reported that a purified preparation of polysaccharide isolated from the culture broth of *S. marcescens* when injected intraperitoneally (IP) into mice bearing a transplanted solid tumor (Sarcoma 37) caused tumor hemorrhagic necrosis. This investigator also observed that on occasion, the peripheral rim of tumor that normally survives the hemorrhagic reaction regressed completely. Some 20 years later, O'Malley et al. (1962) found that sera collected from mice shortly after the intravenous (IV) injection of a purified polysaccharide preparation isolated from the cell wall of *S. marcesens* when injected into Sarcoma 37-bearing mice caused hemorrhagic tumor necrosis. However, the experimental results of these investigators do not permit the determination of whether the "tumor-necrotizing activity" of these sera was due to residual polysaccharide, or to a polysaccharide-induced serum factor.

Carswell et al. (1975) clearly established that tumor-necrotizing activity appearing in sera of *M. bovis* (strain BCG)-infected mice shortly after the IV injection of endotoxin was due to an endotoxin-induced serum factor. These scientists named the factor responsible for the tumor-necrotizing activity of the post endotoxin serum *Tumor necrosis factor*. Carswell et al. (1975) also reported that TNF was cytotoxic for certain tumor cells in culture, and that macrophages appeared to be the source of this endotoxin-induced molecule. Since this time it has been established that TNF production in cultures of monocytes, macrophages, or macrophage cell lines can be induced by a variety of agents, including bacteria (Blanchard et al., 1987), endotoxin (Männel, 1980), virus (Aderka et al., 1986), phorbol myristate acetate (Pennica et al., 1984), interleukin-2 (Economou et al., 1989), or polyinosinic:polycytidylic acid (polyI:C) (Wong and Goedell, 1986). Moreover, TNF production is not limited to macrophages, for it has now been shown that T cells (Kobyashi et al., 1987; Steffen et al., 1988; Sung et al., 1988a), B cells (Sung et al., 1988b), natural killer (NK) cells (Cuturi et al., 1987), astrocytes (Lieberman et al., 1989), and muscle cells (Warner and Libby, 1989) can be induced to produce TNF-α.

III. EXOGENOUS TNF ENHANCES RESISTANCE TO BACTERIAL INFECTION

It has been known for some time that in addition to having the ability to elicit intratumor hemorrhagic necrosis, TNF-inducing agents, such as endotoxin, can have profound effects on the course of bacterial infections. Generally, when administered before infection, TNF-inducing agents enhance the resistance of the host to bacterial infection. In the mid-1950s, investigators reported that mice injected either with cell wall preparations of Gram-negative bacteria or endotoxin exhibited enhanced nonspecific resistance to bacterial infections. Rowley (1955) observed that mice injected IP or IV with crude cell wall preparations from either *Escherichia coli* or *Salmonella typhimurium* survived a normally lethal *E. coli* inoculum. Moreover, Rowley also reported that the ability of these cell wall preparations to confer protection against a lethal *E. coli* challenge was not diminished by boiling for 7 h. Dubos and Schaedler (1956) found that killed *Klebsiella pneumoniae* protected mice against *Staphylococcus aureus* infection, and that *Salmonella typhosa* endotoxin augmented the resistance of mice to *Mycobacterium tuberculosis.* Landy (1956) reported that different endotoxins protected mice against a lethal *S. typhosa* challenge. Generally, significant protection was afforded mice if they were injected with endotoxin 24 h before initiation of infection.

In addition to Gram-negative cell walls and endotoxin, other TNF-inducing agents were also found to enhance antibacterial resistance of mice if they were administered before initiation of infection. For example, Remington and Merigan (1970) reported that mice treated with the synthetic polyribonucleotide, polyI:C, survived a normally lethal *Listeria monocytogenes* inoculum. Recently, polyI:C has been shown to induce high titers of serum TNF and hemorrhagic tumor necrosis in mice bearing the SA-1 sarcoma (Havell and North, 1989). In Table 1 are presented the results of an experiment that compared the ability of endotoxin and polyI:C to confer protection to mice challenged with 10 LD_{50} of *Listeria.* It can be

TABLE 1 Protective Actions of TNF-Inducing Agents Against a Normally Lethal *Listeria monocytogenes* Infection

Treatment[a] 24 h prior to infection[b]	Number of mice surviving on day of infection					
	3	4	5	6	7	11
None	5/5	0/5				
PBS	5/5	0/5				
Endotoxin, 5 μg	5/5	5/5	5/5	5/5	5/5	5/5
PolyI:C, 5 μg	5/5	5/5	5/5	5/5	5/5	5/5

[a]Intravenous injection of agent in 0.2 mL of phosphate-buffered saline (PBS).
[b]One day after treatment, mice were injected intravenously with 10 LD_{50} of *L. monocytogenes.*

seen that mice injected intravenously with endotoxin (5 μg), or polyI:C (5 μg) 24 h before receiving this normally lethal *Listeria* inoculum survived the infection, whereas placebo (PBS)-treated mice died of overwhelming listeriosis by day 4 of infection.

In contrast to the protective effects that endotoxin or poly I:C have when given to mice prior to the injection of a lethal *Listeria* inoculum, their administration during a sublethal infection can result in the exacerbation of infection. Newborg and North (1979) reported that if endotoxin was given to mice at any time during the course of a sublethal immunizing *Listeria* infection, the numbers of bacteria, in the liver and spleen increased. The greatest infection-promoting effect of endotoxin occurred when it was administered at the end of the first day of infection. The administration of endotoxin at this time resulted in continued exponential bacterial growth until the death of the host. In Table 2 are presented the results of an experi-

TABLE 2 Infection-Promoting Actions of TNF-Inducing Agents

Treatment[a] 1 day after initiation of infection[b]	Number of mice surviving on day of infection			
	4	5	6	11
None	10/10	10/10	10/10	10/10
PBS	10/10	10/10	10/10	10/10
Endotoxin, 5 μg	10/10	0/10		
PolyI:C, 5 μg	10/10	3/10	0/10	

[a]Intravenous injection of agent in 0.2 mL of phosphate-buffered saline (PBS).
[b]Mice were injected with 0.1 LD_{50} of *L. monocytogenes.*

ment which show that the administration of endotoxin or poly I:C at the end of the first day of infection converts a normally sublethal *Listeria* infection into a lethal one.

Tumor necrosis serum (TNS) collected 2 h after the IV injection of endotoxin into mice infected for 14 days with *M. bovis* (BCG) was found not only to cause hemorrhagic tumor necrosis in mice bearing solid tumors (Carswell et al., 1975), but also to enhance resistance of mice to bacterial infection (Parent et al., 1980). Parent et al. (1987) reported that TNS-treated C3H/HeJ mice were protected against a subsequent challenge with either *K. pneumoniae* or *L. monocytogenes*. The C3H/HeJ strain of mice are highly refractory to endotoxin-induced effects (Coutinho et al., 1975; Ruco and Meltzer, 1978). In addition, it has been shown that C3H/HeJ macrophages do not produce endotoxin-induced TNF (Beutler et al., 1986b,c). Apparently, therefore, an endotoxin-induced factor present in TNS, rather than residual endotoxin itself, was responsible for the enhanced antibacterial resistance exhibited by the TNS-treated C3H/HeJ mice.

The genes for human TNF-α (Pennica et al., 1984; Shirai et al., 1985; Wang et al., 1985) and murine TNF-α (Fransen et al., 1985; Tavernier et al., 1987) have been cloned and expressed in *E. coli*. This has enabled the generation of sufficient quantities of recombinant (r) TNF proteins for use in clinical trials and in experimentation. Parant et al. (1987) were the first to report that like their aforementioned findings with TNS, treatment of C3H/HeJ mice with human rTNF resulted in enhanced nonspecific antibacterial resistance. These investigators observed that the IV injection of a dose of 3 μg of human rTNF administered 2 h before a normally lethal inoculum of *K. pneumoniae*, *L. monocytogenes*, or *Streptococcus pneumoniae* significantly enhanced the survival times of mice. Again, the use of C3H/HeJ strain of mice by these investigators excluded the possibility that endotoxin in the human rTNF preparation (which was produced in *E. coli*) mediated the observed protection afforded the treated mice. More recently, Cross et al. (1989) reported that transient protection against a lethal (10 LD_{50}) *E. coli* inoculum was afforded to C3H/HeJ mice which were treated immediately before infection with either murine rTNF (10 μg/kg) or murine rIL-lα (10^3 units). However, C3H/HeJ mice treated with both cytokines survived the normally lethal *E. coli* infection. This finding indicates that TNF and IL-lα can function synergistically to enhance host resistance to bacterial infection.

Experiments were also conducted in this laboratory (Havell, 1989) to assess whether pure preparations of murine rTNF would protect mice against a lethal *Listeria* infection and, if so, to determine the optimum time of treatment. Groups of mice were injected intravenously with 0.5 μg of murine rTNF either before (-24 h or -1 h) or after (+6 h) initiating a lethal (10 LD_{50}) *Listeria* infection. Control mice died by the fourth day of infection, whereas mice pretreated with murine rTNF had prolonged survival times. The greatest protection was afforded mice treated 1 h before infection, with 80% of these mice surviving the infection. Interestingly, murine rTNF had little or no effect on host survival time when it was given at the sixth hour of infection. These findings suggested that the prophylactic action of rTNF was due to an effect that was expressed very early during listeriosis. To determine the stage of infection at which the rTNF-mediated effect was expressed, *Listeria* growth was monitored at progressive times during the first day of infection in the livers and spleens of control mice and those treated with rTNF 1 h before infection. It was found that as early as 30 min after challenge, *Listeria* numbers in the livers and spleens of the rTNF-treated mice were two- and three-fold lower, respectively, than those of control mice. During the next 5.5 h, the rate of destruction of the bacteria in the livers of control mice and those treated with rTNF was the same. However, following this time, those bacteria surviving this initial killing event, believed to be mediated by resident liver macrophages (Newborg and North, 1980), proliferated at a slower rate than those in the livers of control mice. By the end of the first day of infection, *Listeria* numbers in the livers of the rTNF-treated mice were 10-fold lower than in control mice. These results establish that rTNF given immediately before infection causes two effects that result in significant reductions in organ-associated bacteria by the end of the first day of infection. One effect causes fewer bacteria to implant in the principal target organs (liver and spleen); the other causes a reduction in the bacterial growth rates in these organs. Because it was also found that rTNF was neither listeriostatic nor listericidal in vitro, it is almost certain that the in vivo anti-*Listeria* effects of rTNF occurs through host-mediated mechanisms.

IV. ENDOGENOUSLY PRODUCED TNF FUNCTIONS IN ANTIBACTERIAL RESISTANCE

A. TNF Production During *Listeria monocytogenes* Infections of Mice

Our interest in TNF and host resistance to bacteria actually began with the need to produce large amounts of tumor necrosis serum (TNF) for use in studies on endotoxin-induced (Havell et al., 1988; North and Havell, 1988) and polyI:C-induced (Havell and North, 1989) hemorrhagic necrosis and regression of the SA-1 sarcoma in mice. It has been known for some time that certain bacterial infections can dramatically alter the host's capacity to produce certain cytokines, including TNF. Bacteria, such as *Mycobacteria* or *Corynebacterium parvum* (now called *Propionibacterium acnes*), that evoke both hyperplasia of the reticuloendothelial system and strong T-cell-mediated immune responses, endow mice with an enhanced potential for the production of alpha/beta interferons (IFN-α/β) (Younger and Stinebring, 1965; Okamura et al., 1982) and TNF (Carswell et al., 1975; Green et al., 1977). Carswell et al. (1975) reported that *M. bovis* (BCG)-infected mice acquired a greatly enhanced capacity to produce serum TNF (TNS) in response to IV injection of endotoxin. These investigators found that peak amounts of endotoxin-induced serum TNF were produced by mice that had been infected for at least 14 days. Moreover, it was also reported that the greatest amounts of TNF appeared in the blood of these infected mice 2 h after the IV injection of endotoxin. Later, this same group (Green et al., 1977) reported that the IP injection of formalin-killed *P. acnes* also primed mice for endotoxin-induced serum TNF production. Maximum endotoxin-induced serum TNF production occurred 6 to 14 days after inoculation of *P. acnes*, which also correlated to the time when these mice exhibited maximum sensitivity to the toxic effects caused by endotoxin treatment.

Listeria monocytogenes is a Gram-positive, facultative intracellular bacterium which, like *M. bovis* (BCG) or *P. acnes*, evokes a strong T-cell-mediated immune response in mice (North, 1974). Within 1 day of the initiation of a sublethal *Listeria* infection, mice are not only primed for the production of IFN-α/β, but also acquire the capacity to produce endotoxin-induced gamma IFN (IFN-γ) (Nakane and Minagawa, 1985; Havell, 1986). Moreover, Ha et al. (1985) reported that *Listeria*-infected mice possessed an enhanced potential for the production of endotoxin-induced serum TNF. Based on these findings of Ha et al. (1985), experiments were undertaken in this laboratory to determine whether *Listeria*-infected mice could be employed in place of *P. acnes*-treated, or *M. bovis* (BCG)-infected mice as a source of high-titered endotoxin- and polyI:C-induced TNS. In Fig. 1 are presented the endotoxin- and polyI:C-induced TNF activities in sera collected at different times during a sublethal *Listeria* infection in mice. At the indicated times of infection, mice were injected with either endotoxin or polyI:C and the sera collected 2 h later and assayed for TNF cytotoxic activity on actinomycin-D-treated murine L929 fibroblasts. It can be seen that shortly after the IV injection of a sublethal immunizing *Listeria* inoculum (0.1 LD_{50}), mice acquire an enhanced capacity to produce TNF in response to injection with endotoxin or polyI:C. It is also evident from the results presented in Fig. 1 that a biphasic pattern for the enhanced production of TNF in response to stimulation with either agent occurs during listeriosis. The first peak of enhanced responsiveness for the production of TNF occurs 1 to 2 days following the initiation of infection, with infected mice producing ~100 times more endotoxin-induced serum TNF, and about 16 times more polyI:C-induced TNF than uninfected mice. The second peak of enhanced responsiveness for the production of TNF occurs on day 6 of infection—the time of peak anti-*Listeria* T-cell-mediated immunity (Havell et al., 1982). In addition to acquiring an enhanced capacity for TNF production, *Listeria*-infected mice were observed to develop an enhanced sensitivity to the toxic effects caused by the IV injection of endotoxin or polyI:C. While the results of these studies established that mice undergoing a sublethal *Listeria* infection were endowed with a greatly augmented potential for TNF production, the findings of other studies revealed that mice infected with a lethal

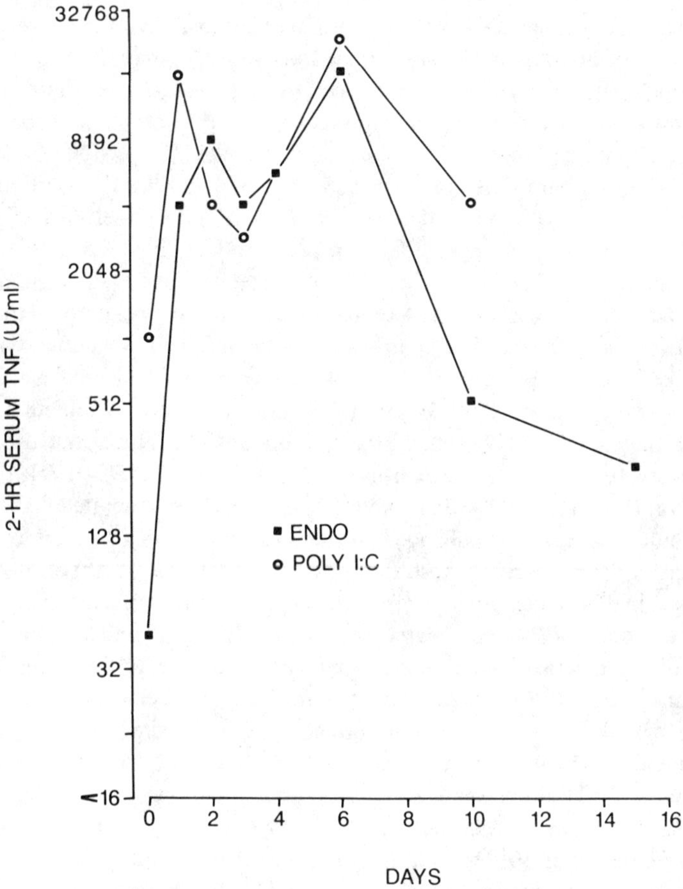

Figure 1 Mice were injected intravenously with 5×10^3 colony-forming units of *Listeria monocytogenes* (day 0). At the indicated times of infection, mice were injected intravenously with endotoxin (5 μg) or polyI:C (25 μg). Two hours later the mice were bled and the sera assayed for TNF cytotoxic activity on actinomycin D-treated murine L929 fibroblasts.

Listeria inoculum (10 LD_{50}) possessed an even greater potential for the production of TNF (Havell, unpublished observations).

In addition to the finding that *Listeria*-infected mice were primed for TNF production in response to endotoxin or polyI:C, it was found that during the course of a lethal *Listeria* infection TNF was present in the sera of mice that were not injected with a TNF-inducing agent (Havell, 1987). TNF was detected in the blood of mice within 24 h of the IV injection of a lethal *Listeria* inoculum. Thereafter, the amount of the TNF present in the blood increased concordantly with bacterial numbers in the liver and spleen and with the progression of morbidity. In contrast, at no time during a sublethal infection was TNF detected in the blood. However, TNF was found in the liver and spleen of the sublethally infected host (Havell, 1989). TNF assays of supernatants of organ homogenates prepared at progressive times of a sublethal infection revealed that low amounts of TNF were present in organs during the first 3 days of infection. It was found that the localized production of TNF in *Listeria*-infected organs increases and decreases concordantly with increases and decreases in the number of organ-associated bacteria. A similar correlation was made by Kindler et al. (1989) between the amount of TNF produced and bacterial numbers in the livers of mice infected with another facultative intracellular bacterium, *M. bovis* (BCG).

The collective results of studies showing that (1) mice given exogenous TNF exhibited enhanced resistance to *Listeria* infection (Section III), (2) small amounts of *Listeria*-induced TNF were present in infected organs of mice during the first 3 days of a sublethal infection, and (3) TNF causes a number of effects (reviewed in Section V) which conceivably could be of importance in host defense against bacteria suggested that the endogenously produced TNF localized within sites of infection might play a role in antibacterial resistance.

B. Endogenously Produced TNF Has Antibacterial Function

The response of mice to *L. monocytogenes* provides an excellent model for studying the possible roles of cytokines in nonspecific resistance to a Gram-positive, facultative intracellular parasite. Following the IV injection of a *Listeria inoculum,* 90% of the bacteria are cleared by the liver and the rest by the spleen (Newborg and North, 1980). During the first 6 h of infection, 80% of the bacteria locating in the liver are destroyed by resident liver macrophages (Kupffer cells). Those bacteria surviving this initial killing event grow exponentially for 2 to 3 days, after which their numbers begin to diminish due to development of specific anti-*Listeria* resistance. However, in mice injected with a lethal inoculum, the bacteria continue to proliferate exponentially until death of the host. Expression of anti-*Listeria* resistance is believed to be dependent on both the focusing of macrophages freshly recruited from the circulation into sites of infection and the activation of the bactericidal mechanisms of these cells (Mackaness, 1962; North, 1973). Macrophage activation is mediated by a newly generated population of specifically sensitized T cells, first detected in the spleen on the second day of the infection. It has been shown that peak numbers of *Listeria*-immune T cells are generated on, or around, the sixth day of infection, after which their numbers diminish as bacteria are eradicated from the organs (Havell et al., 1982). Following the resolution of a primary *Listeria* infection, mice possess a long-lived state of memory immunity. Anti-*Lis*-

teria memory immunity is associated with a small population of nonreplicating sensitized T cells, which enables the host to respond to a secondary *Listeria* infection in an accelerated manner (North and Deissler, 1975).

Experiments were carried out in this laboratory to determine whether endogenously produced TNF produced during a sublethal *Listeria* infection functions in antilisteria resistance. It was reasoned that if TNF plays a role in host defense against *Listeria*, the use of a specific anti-TNF antibody to block the action of the *Listeria*-induced TNF should result in the exacerbation of listeriosis. Indeed, this proved to be the case, for it was found that a sublethal infection was converted into a lethal one when mice were injected with an anti-TNF IgG at the end of the first day of infection (Havell, 1987). The anti-TNF IgG used in these experiments was raised in a rabbit against a pure preparation of murine rTNF and shown to neutralize the ability of natural murine TNF to destroy cultured murine L929 fibroblasts treated with actinomycin D (Havell, 1987). Table 3 shows the *Listeria* numbers present on day 3 of a *Listeria* infection in the livers and spleens of control mice and those treated with anti-rTNF IgG at the end of the first day of infection. Here it can be seen that giving the anti-rTNF IgG at 24 h of a sublethal *Listeria* infection results in a striking increase in the numbers of bacteria in the organs 48 h later. Nakane et al. (1988) also observed that anti-TNF antibody exacerbated murine listeriosis. Moreover, it was recently reported (Kindler et al., 1989) that anti-TNF antibody treatment decreases host resistance to *M. bovis* (BCG) infection.

The finding that anti-TNF IgG treatment of mice on the first day of a normally sublethal *Listeria* infection resulted in unrestricted bacterial proliferation and death of the host 2 to 3 days later indicated that endogenously produced TNF functions in

Table 3 *Listeria* Numbers in the Spleens and Livers of Control Mice and Anti-rTNF IgG-Treated Mice on the Third Day of Infection

	Log_{10} bacteria/organ[b]	
Host treatment[a] on day 1 of infection	Liver	Spleen
Control rabbit IgG	6.13 ± 0.32	6.14 ± 0.55
Rabbit anti-rTNFIgG	8.04 ± 0.36	7.71 ± 0.30

[a]Mice were injected intravenously with 5×10^3 colony-forming units of *L. monocytogenes*. One day later, groups of 5 mice were injected intravenously with control rabbit IgG, or rabbit anti-rTNFIgG (8×10^3 TNF neutralizing units). The amount (mg) of control rabbit IgG given was equivalent to that of the rabbit anti-rTNFIgG (mg). Two days later, individual livers and spleens were homogenized and serial 10-fold dilutions of the organ homogenates plated on trypticase so y agar.

[b]$\bar{X} \mp \text{SD}(n = 5)$.

an antibacterial resistance mechanism(s). In view of these findings and those mentioned earlier which showed that TNF was present in the *Listeria*-infected organs until the third day of infection, it was considered important to determine the effect of anti-TNF IgG on the course of infection when it was administered at different times (day 1, 3, or 5) of infection. Again, it was found that anti-TNF antibody given to mice on day 1 of infection resulted in increased numbers of bacteria in the liver and spleen and the eventual death of the host (Havell, 1989). In contrast, anti-TNF IgG administered on the third day of infection caused only a temporary increase in *Listeria* proliferation. Administration of the anti-TNF IgG on day 5 had virtually no effect on *Listeria* numbers in the liver and spleen. These findings indicate that *Listeria*-induced TNF functions in a resistance mechanism that is expressed early in infection.

C. *Listeria*-Induced TNF Functions in a T-Cell-Independent Resistance Mechanism

In *Listeria*-infected BALB/c athymic nude mice, *Listeria*-sensitized T cells are not generated, and a chronic state of infection develops (Heymer et al., 1976; Cheers and Waller, 1975; Newborg and North, 1980). Following the second day of infection, *Listeria* numbers in the liver and spleen persist at 1 to 5 $\times$ 10^5 bacteria per organ for several weeks. Athymic nude mice infected with *Listeria* for 1 day or 7 days were given anti-TNF IgG, and bacteria in the livers and spleens were enumerated at different times thereafter (Havell, 1989). *Listeria* numbers in the organs of the mice treated on the first day of infection increased exponentially until the death of the host. However, the administration of the antibody during the chronic phase of infection (day 7) had only a minor, short-term, enhancing effect on bacterial numbers, even though the *Listeria* numbers in the livers and spleens at the time of treatment were higher than on the first day of infection. These findings are therefore similar to those observed in T-cell-intact mice and indicate that TNF functions at an early stage of resistance, presumably independently of T cells. Similar conclusions were reached by Bancroft et al. (1989), who observed that the severity of *Listeria* infection in severe combined immunodeficiency (*scid*) mutant mice was greatly enhanced by treating these mice 24 h before infection with an anti-TNF monocolonal antibody.

D. Histology of Infected Livers of Mice Treated with Anti-TNF Antibody

A histological examination was made of the *Listeria*-infected livers of control mice and those which were treated on the first day of infection with anti-TNF IgG (Havell, 1989). It was found that the sites of infection in the livers of control mice on day 3 or 4 of infection consisted of large populations of mononuclear cells (granulomas) in which bacteria were difficult to find (Fig. 2A). In contrast, infec-

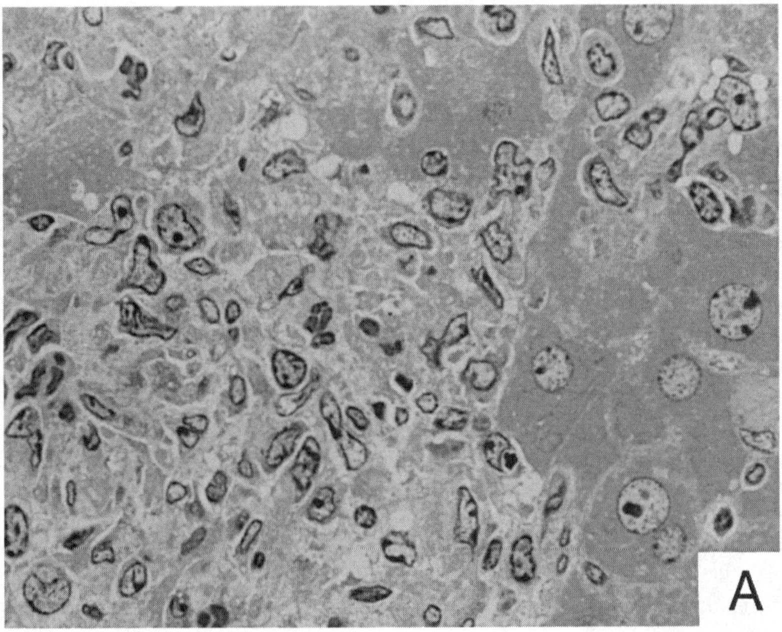

Figure 2A Histologic examination of *Listeria*-infected livers on day 3 of infection in mice (magnification x 1200). (This figure is reproduced with the permission of the *Journal of Immunology*.)

tious foci in the livers of the antibody-treated mice consisted of clusters of heavily infected hepatocytes with little, if any, involvement of host mononuclear cells (Fig. 2B). Thus, in anti-TNF IgG-treated mice, *Listeria* was free to multiply unchallenged in hepatocytes.

Kindler et al. (1989) also performed histological examinations of *M. bovis* (BCG)-infected livers from control mice and those treated with anti-TNF antibody. These investigators found that by the end of the first week of infection, the livers of control mice possessed a small number of granulomas, which consisted of clusters of small numbers of macrophages. Thereafter, the number and size of the granulomas increased over the next 2 week. It was found that treating mice with anti-TNF antibody on both days 7 and 14 of infection resulted in a 10-fold reduction in the number of granulomas present on day 21 of infection. The granulomas in the antibody-treated mice were ill-defined, lacking in macrophages and macrophage/epithelioid cells, but contained greater numbers of bacteria than were present in the fully differentiated granulomas in the livers of control mice. In addition,

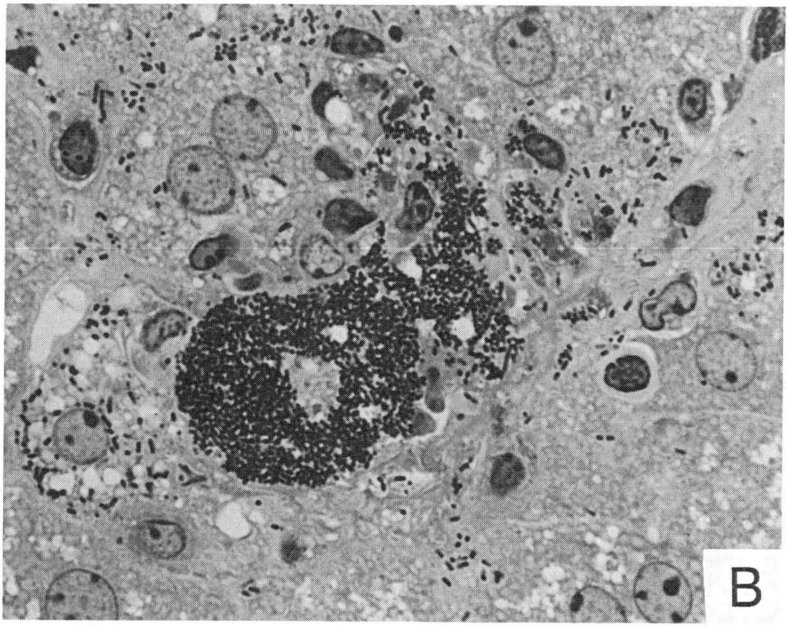

Figure 2B Histologic examination of *Listeria*-infected livers on day 3 of infection in mice treated with anti-rTNF IgG on day 1 of infection (magnification ×1200). (This figure reproduced with the permission of the *Journal of Immunology*.)

these investigators reported that TNF was present in the granulomas of control mice after the first week of infection and thereafter, the amounts of TNF increased. However, TNF was not detectable by immunofluorescent staining procedures performed on tissue sections of livers from the antibody-treated mice. Moreover, evidence was presented showing that exacerbation of *M. bovis* (BCG) infection in the antibody-treated mice was not due to adverse effects on macrophage function caused by anti-TNF antibody and complement. These collective findings led Kindler et al. (1989) to conclude that the localized production of TNF within sites of infection was necessary for the development of granulomas in which the bacteria are contained and eventually destroyed. Moreover, it was also concluded that the production of TNF in well-differentiated granulomas was essential for maintaining the integrity of these structures. This conclusion was based on a finding which showed that fully developed granulomas degenerated following anti-TNF antibody treatment of the host.

E. Role for TNF in the Expression of Antilisteria Memory Immunity

A long-lived state of immunologic memory follows the resolution of an immunizing *Listeria* infection in mice (North and Deissler, 1975). To determine whether *Listeria*-induced TNF functions in anti-*Listeria* memory immunity, anti-TNF antibody was administered to mice that had been given an immunizing *Listeria* inoculum 27 days earlier (Havell, 1989). One day after the administration of the antibody, mice were challenged with 10 LD_{50} of *Listeria* and the numbers of bacteria in the liver and spleen were determined at progressive times thereafter. It was found that whereas *Listeria* was rapidly eliminated from untreated immune mice, it increased in number in the organs of the antibody-treated mice. This finding indicated that TNF is involved in the expression of anti-*Listeria* memory immunity. It must also be mentioned that Nakane et al. (1988) reported that TNF, as well as IFN-γ, functions in host antibacterial resistance mechanism mounted against a secondary *Listeria* challenge.

V. POSSIBLE MODES OF ACTION OF TNF IN ANTIBACTERIAL RESISTANCE

A. Possible Involvement of TNF in Recruitment of Host Cells Having Bactericidal Function to Sites of Infection

Causal evidence of a role for TNF in host defense against bacteria comes primarily from studies showing that the administration of specific anti-TNF antibodies exacerbates bacterial infections (Havell, 1987; Nakane et al., 1988; Kindler et al., 1989; Havell, 1989; Bancroft et al., 1989). Through the use of anti-TNF antibody it was shown that during the course of a primary *Listeria* infection in mice, *Listeria*-induced TNF functions in an early T-cell-independent resistance mechanism(s). It was also found that when anti-TNF antibodies were administered to mice early in either *Listeria* or *M. bovis* (BCG) infections, granuloma formation in the livers was inhibited. The sites of infection in the livers of the antibody-treated mice consisted of great numbers of bacteria, and very few macrophages within, or around, these foci of infection. Thus a plausible function for TNF produced early in infection is in the recruitment of blood monocytes into infectious sites. In this regard it is known that TNF induces IL-1 synthesis in a variety of cell types (Dinarello et al., 1986; Le et al., 1987; Nawroth et al., 1987) and both of these cytokines have effects that not only increase the production of host cells having antibacterial function, but also serve to focus these cells at sites of inflammation. For example, TNF and IL-1 elicit the synthesis of colony-stimulating factors that promote the production of polymorphonuclear cells (PMNs) and monocytes (Morrisey et al., 1988; Munker et al., 1986), and IL-1 causes proliferation of antigen-activated T cells (Dinarello, 1984). TNF and IL-1 are also potent mediators of inflammation (Dinarello, 1984;

Movat et al., 1987) and induce the production of chemotactic factors that function to attract leukocytes (Matsushima et al., 1988). Furthermore, these two cytokines function synergistically in the elicitation of PMN emigration from blood to tissues (Sayers et al., 1988; Furie and McHugh, 1989). In regard to the latter effect, TNF and IL-1 are known to cause profound changes in vascular endothelial cells which lead to increased leukocyte adhesion (Gamble et al., 1985; Pohlman et al., 1986; Pober et al., 1986; Broudy et al., 1987). Such localized effects would serve to focus leukocytes at sites of bacterial implantation.

B. Effects of TNF on Host Cells Having Antibacterial Function

In addition to possible functions in recruiting host cells having antibacterial functions into inflammatory sites, TNF and/or TNF-induced cytokines are reported to enhance the antimicrobial functions of PMNs and macrophages. TNF enhances the ability of PMNs to kill *Legionella pneumophilia* (Blanchard et al. 1988) and activates the mycobicidal mechanisms of macrophages (Bermudez and Young, 1988). TNF has recently been reported to increase NK cell activity and is involved in processes which include NK cells to secrete INF-γ (Bancroft et al., 1989). IFNγ has been shown to mediate pleiotropic effects which would be important in nonspecific resistance mechanisms and in the generation and expression of specifically acquired T-cell-mediated immunity. Macrophages exhibit enhanced expression of class II major histocompatibility (MHC) antigens following treatment with IFN-γ (Steeg et al., 1982; Vogel et al., 1986). Moreover, TNF acts synergistically with IFNγ to augment Ia antigen (class II MHC) expression in macrophages (Chang and Lee, 1986). Increased class II MHC expression would serve to enhance the antigen-presenting function of these phagocytes in the generation of antibacterial immunity. Moreover, IFN-γ endows (primes) macrophages with an augmented potential for the destruction of tumor cells (Pace et al., 1983; Spitalny and Havell, 1984) and bacteria (Nathan et al., 1983; Schreiber et al., 1985; Kagaya et al., 1989). However, activation of the tumoricidal mechanisms of macrophages requires a "second signal," which can be provided by endotoxin (Pace et al., 1983), *Listeria* (Buchmeier and Schreiber, 1985), or polyI:C (Buchmeier and Schreiber, 1985). In regard to the nature of the stimulus provided by these agents, which triggers IFN-γ-primed macrophages to become fully activated, it has been found that TNF alone (Hori et al., 1987), or in combination with IL-1 (Chen et al., 1987), can affect the activation of the tumoricidal mechanisms of IFN-γ-treated macrophages. In view of the demonstrated abilities of endotoxin, *Listeria*, or polyI:C to induce the production of TNF, which in turn can elicit IL-1 synthesis, it is conceivable that TNF produced by IFN-γ-primed macrophages exposed to these agents functions in an autocrine manner to elicit the expression of the activated state. Macrophages treated with IFN-γ have been reported to posses an enhanced capacity to destroy *Listeria* (Schreiber et al., 1985). If TNF is required for the activation of the listericidal mechanism of IFN-γ-treated macrophages, it is possible that *Listeria*-induced macrophage TNF serves this function. Indeed, the results of experiments presented by Nakane et al. (1988, 1989) and Bancroft et al. (1989) indicate that endogenously produced TNF and IFN-γ are involved in the in vivo activation of the listericidal actions of macrophages. Moreover, it also has been shown that TNF and IFN-γ can function synergistically in augmenting macrophage killing of *Schistosoma mansoni* (Esparza et al., 1987) and enhancing PMN functions (Shalaby et al., 1985), which would be important in host resistance to infectious agents.

C. Possible Effects of TNF on Intracellular Bacterial Infections

Histological examination of livers from *Listeria*-infected mice treated with anti-TNF revealed that great numbers of bacteria were present in hepatocytes (Fig. 2b), whereas *Listeria* were absent in hepatocytes of control mice (Fig. 2a). These results suggest that a TNF-dependent mechanism prevents, or terminates, intracellular infection. It has been reported in this connection that murine fibroblasts are rendered susceptible to TNF-mediated lysis following infection with virus (Koff and Fann, 1986). If *Listeria* infection were also to render nonphagocytic cells sensitive to the cytolytic action of TNF, such an effect could result in the termination of intracellular infection. Bacteria released from lysed cells would then be vulnerable to host cells having listericidal functions. TNF and IFNγ have other actions that could serve to control, or terminate, intracellular bacterial infections. It has been shown that the intracellular multiplication of bacteria is inhibited in cells treated with these cytokines (Turco et al., 1984; Shermer-Avni et al., 1989). Moreover, IFN-γ proved cytotoxic for fibroblasts infected with *Chlamydia psittaci* (Byrne et al., 1989). In addition, IFN-γ was also found to indirectly cause the lysis of cells harboring intracellular bacteria through effects on host cells having cytolytic function (Klimpel et al., 1986; Kaufmann et al., 1986).

VI. CONCLUSIONS

It is now apparent that TNF produced during bacterial infections can be either beneficial or detrimental to the host. The production of amounts of TNF so large as to be detected in the systemic circulation is deleterious to the host. Such a situation occurs during overwhelming bacterial infections. In contrast, the presence of small amounts of TNF locally within infected tissues has now been shown to be essential in the development of resistance to infection with *L. monocytogenes* and *M. bovis* (BCG). Of interest is the fact that these facultative intracellular parasites also prime the host for TNF production. Since these bacteria lack endotoxin, the significance of priming the host for TNF production during infection may be to ensure that sufficient amounts of TNF are produced to generate a localized TNF-dependent resistance mechanism.

ACKNOWLEDGMENTS

The author would like to express his gratitude to Lynn Stiles, Joyce Reome, and Donald J. Auclair for their technical assistance in the performance of experiments conducted in this laboratory, and to Mary Durett for typing this manuscript. I would also like to express my appreciation to Dr. Robert J. North for his accomplished photomicroscopy. The work of the author presented in this chapter was supported by U.S. Public Health Service Grants AI-23544 and RR-50705 from the National Institutes of Health.

REFERENCES

Aderka, D., Holtmann, H., Toker, L., Hahn T., and Wallach, D. (1986). Tumor necrosis factor induction by sendai virus, *J.Immunol., 136*: 2938.

Bancroft, G. J., Sheehan, K. C., Schreiber, R. D., and Unanue, E. R. (1989). Tumor necrosis factor is involved in the T cell-independent pathway of macrophage activation in *scid* mice, *J. Immunol., 143*: 127.

Bermudez, L., and Young, L. S. (1988). Tumor necrosis alone or in combination with IL-2, but not IFNγ, is associated with macrophage killing of *Mycobacterium avium* complex, *J. Immunol., 140*: 3006.

Beutler, B., and Cerami, A. (1986). Cachectin and tumor necrosis factor as two sides of the same biological coin, *Nature (Lond.), 320*: 584.

Beutler, B., Greenwald, D., Hulmes, J. D., Chang, M., Pan, Y. -C. E., Mathison, J., Ulevitch, R., and Cerami, A. (1986a). Identity of tumor necrosis factor and the macrophage secreted factor cachetin, *Nature (Lond.), 316*: 552.

Beutler, B., Krochin, N., Milsark, I., Luedke, C., and Cerami, A. (1986b). Control of cachectin (tumor necrosis factor) synthesis: mechanisms of endotoxin resistance, *Science, 232*: 977.

Beutler, B., Tkacenko, V., Milsark, I., Krochin, N., and Cerami, A. (1986c). Effect of γ interferon on cachectin expression: reversal of the lps^d (endotoxin resistance) phenotype, *J. Exp. Med., 164*: 1791.

Blanchard, D. K., Djeu, J. Y., Klein, T. W., Friedman, H., and Stewart, W. E., II (1987). Induction of tumor necrosis factor by *Legionella pneumophilia, Infect. Immun., 55*: 433.

Blanchard, D. K., Djeu, J. Y., Klein, T. W., Friedman, H., and Stewart, W. E., II (1988). Protective effects of tumor necrosis factor in experimental *Legionella pneumophila* infections of mice via activation of PMN function, *J. Leukocyte Biol., 43*: 429.

Broudy, V. C., Harlan, J. M., and Adamson, J. W. (1987). Disparate effects of tumor necrosis factor-α/cachectin and tumor necrosis factor β/lymphotoxin on hematopoietic growth factor production and neutrophil adhesion molecule expression by cultured human endothelial cells, *J. Immunol., 138*: 4298.

Buchmeier, N. A., and Schreiber, R. D. (1985). Requirement of endogenous interferon-γ production for resolution of *Listeria monocytogenes* infection, *Proc. Natl. Acad. Sci. USA, 82*: 7404.

Byrne, G. I., Schobert, C. S., Williams, D. M., and Krueger, D. A. (1989). Characterization of gamma interferon-mediated cytotoxicity to chlamydia-infected fibroblast, *Infect. Immun., 57*: 870.

Carswell, E. A., Old, L. J., Kassel, R. L., Green, S., Fiore, N., and Williamson, B. (1975). An endotoxin-induced serum factor that causes necrosis of tumors, *Proc. Natl. Acad. Sci. USA, 72*: 3666.

Chang, R. J., and Lee, S. N. (1986). Effects of interferon-γ and tumor necrosis factor on the expression of an Ia antigen on a murine macrophage cell line, *J. Immunol., 137*: 2853.

Cheers, C., and Waller, R. (1975). Activated macrophages in congenitally athymic "nude" mice and in lethally irradiated mice, *J. Immunol., 115*: 844.

Chen, L., Suzuki, Y., and Wheelock, E. F. (1987). Interferon-γ synergizes with tumor necrosis factor and interleukin 1 and requires the presence of both monkines to induce antitumor cytotoxic activity in macrophages, *J. Immunol., 139*: 4096.

Coley, W. B. (1894). Treatment of inoperable malignant tumors with the toxins of erysipelas and *Bacillus prodigious*, *Trans. Am. Surg., 12*: 183.

Coley, W. B. (1896). The therapeutic value of the mixed toxins of erysipelas and *Bacillus prodigiosus* in the treatment of inoperable malignant tumors, *Am. J. Med. Sci., 112*: 251.

Coley, W. B. (1897). Spindle-celled sarcoma of the abdominal wall successfully treated by the mixed toxins of erysipelas and *Bacillus prodigiosus*, *Ann. Surg., 26*: 232.

Coutinho, A., Maller, G., and Gronowicz, E. (1975). Genetical control of B-cell responses. IV. Inheritance of the unresponsiveness to lipopolysaccharides, *J. Exp. Med., 142*: 253.

Cross, A. S., Sadoff, J. C., Kelly, N., Bernton, E., and Gemske, P. (1989). Pretreatment with recombinant murine tumor necrosis factor α/cachectin and murine interleukin 1 α protects mice from lethal bacterial infection, *J. Exp. Med., 169*: 2021.

Cuturi, M. C., Murphy, M., Costa-Giomi, M. P., Weinmann, R., Perussia, B., and Trincheri, G. (1987). Independent regulation of tumor necrosis factor and lymphotoxin production by human peripheral blood monocytes, *J. Exp. Med., 165*: 1581.

Dinarello, C. A. (1984). Interleukin-1. *Rev. Infect. Dis., 6*: 51.

Dinarello, C. A., Cannon, J. G., Wolff, S. M., Bernheim, H. A., Beutler, B., Cerami, A., Figari, I. S., Palladino, M. A., Jr., and O'Connor, J. V. (1986). Tumor necrosis factor (cachectin) is an endogenous pyrogen and induces production of interleukin 1, *J. Exp. Med., 163*: 1433.

Dubos, R. J., and Schaedler, R. W. (1956). Reversible changes in the susceptibility of mice to bacterial infections. I. Changes brought about by injection of pertussis vaccine of bacerial endotoxins, *J. Exp. Med., 104*: 53.

Duran-Reynals, F. (1935). Reaction of spontaneous mouse carcinomas to blood carried bacterial toxins, *Proc. Soc. Exp. Biol. Med., 32*: 1517.

Economou, J. S., McBride, W. H., Essner, R., Rhoades, K., Golub, S., Holmes, E. C., and Morton, D. L. (1989). Tumor necrosis factor production by IL-2 activated macrophages in vitro and in vivo, *Immunology, 67*: 514.

Esparza, I., Minnel, D, Ruppel, A., Falk, W., and Krammer, P. K. (1987). Interferon γ and lymphotoxin or tumor necrosis factor act synergistically to induce macrophage killing of tumor cells and shistosoma of *Schistosoma* manosoni, *J. Exp. Med., 166*: 589.

Fogg, L. C. (1936). Effect of certain bacterial products upon the growth of mouse tumor, *Public Health Rep.*, *51*: 56.

Fransen, L., Muller, R., Marmenout, A., Tavernier, J., Van der Heyden, J., Kawashima, E., Chollet, A., Tizard, R., Van Heuverswyn, H., Van Vliet, A., Ruysschaert, and Fiers, W. (1985). Molecular cloning of mouse tumor necrosis factor cDNA and its eukaryotic expression, *Nucleic Acids Res.*, *13*: 4417.

Furie, M. B., and McHugh, D. D. (1989). Migration of neutrophils across endothelial monolayer is stimulated by treatment of the monolayer with interleukin-1 or tumor necrosis factor-α, *J. Immunol.*, *143*: 3309.

Gamble, J. R., Harlan, J. M., Klebanoff, S. J., and Vadas, M. A. (1985). Stimulation of the adherence of neutrophils to umbilical vein endothelium by human recombinant tumor necrosis factor, *Proc. Natl. Acad. Sci. USA*, *82*: 8667.

Gratia, A., and Linz, R. (1931). Le phénomine de Shwartzman dans le sarcome du cobaye, *C. R. Soc. Biol.*, *108*: 427.

Green, S., Dobryansky, A., Chiasson, M. A., Carswell, E., Schwartz, M. K., and Old, L. J. (1977). *Corynebacterium parvum* as the priming agent in the production of tumor necrosis factor in the mouse, *J. Natl. Cancer Inst.*, *59*: 1519.

Ha, D. K. K., Leung, S. W., Fung, K. P., Choy, Y. M., and Lee, C. Y. (1985). Production of tumor necrosis factor in *Listeria monocytogenes*-infected animals, *Int. J. Immunopharmacol.*, *7*: 1.

Havell, E. A. (1986). Augmented induction of interferons during *Listeria monocytogenes* infection, *J. Infect. Dis.*, *153*: 960.

Havell, E. A. (1987). Production of tumor necrosis factor during murine listeriosis, *J. Immunol.*, *139*: 4225.

Havell, E. A. (1989). Evidence that tumor necrosis factor has an important role in antibacterial resistance, *J. Immunol.*, *143*: 2894.

Havell, E. A., Fiers, W., and North, R. J. (1988). The antitumor function of tumor necrosis factor (TNF). I. Therapeutic action of TNF against an established murine sarcoma is indirect, immunologically dependent, and limited by severe toxicity, *J. Exp. Med.*, *167*: 1067.

Havell, E. A., and North, R. J. (1989). Analysis of TNF involvement in hemorrhagic necrosis and regression induced by polyI:C or endotoxin, *The Biology of the Interferon System 1989* (Y. Kawade and S. Kobayashi, eds.), Kodansha Scientific, Tokyo, p. 247.

Havell, E. A., Spitalny, G. L., and Patel, P. J. (1982). enhanced production of murine interferon γ by T cells generated in response to bacterial infection, *J. Exp. Med.*, *156*: 112.

Heymer, B., Hof, H., Emmerling, P., and Finger, H. (1976). Morphology and time course of experimental listeriosis in nude mice, *Infect. Immun.*, *14*: 832.

Hori, K., Ehrke, M. J., Mace, K., and Mihich, E. (1987). Effect of recombinant tumor necrosis factor on tumoricidal activation of murine macrophages: synergism between tumor necrosis factor and γ-interferon, *Cancer Res.*, *47*: 5868.

Kagaya, K., Watanabe, K., and Fukazawa, Y. (1989). Capacity of recombinant gamma interferon to activate macrophages for *Salmonella*-killing activity, *Infect. Immun.*, *57*: 609.

Kaufmann, S. H. E., Hug, E., and Delibero, G. (1986). *Listeria monocytogenes*: reactive T lymphocyte clones with cytolytic activity against infected target cells, *J. Exp. Med.*, *164*: 363.

Kindler, V., Sappino, A. -P., Grau, G. E., Piquet, P. -F., and Vassalli, P. (1989). The inducing role of tumor necrosis factor in the development of bactericidal granulomas during BCG infection, *Cell, 56*: 731.

Klimpel, G. R., Niesel, D. W., and Klimpel, K. D. (1986). Natural cytotoxic effector cell activity against *Shigella flexneri*-infected Hela cells, *J. Immunol., 136*: 1081.

Kobayashi, Y., Asada, M., and Osawa, T. (1987). Production of lymphotoxin and tumor necrosis factor by a T cell-hybridoma, *Immunology, 60*: 213.

Koff, W. C., and Fann, A. V. (1986). Human necrosis factor alpha kills herpes virus-infected but not normal cells, *Lymphokine Res., 5*: 215.

Landy, M. (1956). Increased resistance following administration of bacterial lipopolysaccharides, *Ann. N.Y. Acad. Sci., 66*: 292.

Le, J., Weinstein, D., Gubler, U., and Vilček, J. (1987). Induction of membrane associated interleukin 1 by tumor necrosis factor in human fibroblasts, *J. Immunol., 138*: 2138.

Lieberman, A. P., Pitha, P. M., Shin, H. S., and Shin, M. L. (1989). Production of tumor necrosis factor and other cytokines by astrocytes stimulated with lipopolysaccharide or a neurotropic virus, *Proc. Natl. Acad. Sci. USA, 86*: 6348.

Mackaness, G. (1962). Cellular resistance to infection, *J. Exp. Med., 116*: 381.

Männel, D. E., Moore, R. N., and Mergenhagen, S. E. (1980). Macrophages as a source of tumoricidal activity (tumor-necrotizing factor), *Infect. Immun., 30*: 523.

Matsushima, K., Morishita, K., Yoshimura, T., Lavu, S., Kobayashi, Y., Lew, W., Appella, E., Kung, H. F., Leonard, E. J., and Oppenheim, J. J. (1988). Molecular cloning of a human monocyte-derived neutrophil chemotactic factor (MDNCF) and the induction of MDNCF mRNA by interleukin 1 and tumor necrosis factor, *J. Exp. Med., 167*: 1883.

Morrisey, P., Charrier, K., Bussler, L., and Alper, A. (1988). The influence of IL-1 treatment on the reconstitution of the hemopoeitic and immune systems after sublethal radiation, *J. Immunol., 140*: 4202.

Movat, H. Z., Burrowes, C. E., Cybalsky, M. I., and Dinarello, C. A. (1987). Acute inflammation and a Shwartzman-like reaction induced by interleukin-1 and tumor necrosis factor: synergistic action of the cytokines in the induction of inflammation and microvascular injury, *Am. J. Pathol., 129*: 463.

Munker, R., Gasson, J., Ogawa, M., and Koeffler, H. P. (1986). Recombinant human TNF induces production of granulocyte-monocyte colony stimulating factor, *Nature (Lond.)., 323*: 79.

Nakane, A., and Minagawa, T. (1985). Sequential production of alpha and beta interferons and gamma interferon in the circulation of *Listeria monocytogenes*-infected mice after stimulation with bacterial lipopolysaccharide, *Microbiol. Immunol., 29*: 659.

Nakane, A., Minagawa, T., and Kato, K. (1988). Endogenous tumor necrosis factor (cachectin) is essential to host resistance against *Listeria Monocytogenes* infection, *Infect. Immun., 56*: 2563.

Nakane, A., Minagawa, T., Kohanawa, M., Chen, Y., Sato, H., Moriyama, M., and Tsuroka, N. (1989). Interactions between endogenous gamma interferon and tumor necrosis factor in host resistance against primary and secondary *Listeria monocytogenes* infections, *Infect. Immun., 57*: 3371.

Nathan, C. F., Murray, H. W., Wiebe, M. E., and Rubin, B. Y. (1983). Identification of interferon-γ as the lymphokine that activates human macrophage oxidative metabolism and antimicrobial activity, *J. Exp. Med., 158*: 670.

Nauts, H. C. (1975). Beneficial effects of immunotherapy (bacterial toxins) on sarcoma of the soft tissues, other than lymphosarcoma, *Monograph 16*, Cancer Research Institute, New York, pp. 3-19.

Nauts, H. C. (1980). The beneficial effects of bacterial infections on host resistance to cancer, end results in 449 cases: a study and abstracts of reports in the World Medical Literature (1775-1980) and personal communications, *Monograph 8, 2nd ed.*, Cancer Research Institute, New York, pp. 3-26.

Nawroth, P. P., Bank, I., Handley, D., Cassimeris, J., Chess, L., and Stern, D. (1987). Tumor necrosis factor-α interacts with endothelial cell receptors to induce release of interleukin-1, *J. Exp. Med., 163*: 1363.

Newborg, M. F., and North, R. J. (1979). Suppressive effect of bacterial endotoxin on the expression of cell mediated anti-*Listeria* immunity, *Infect. Immun., 24*: 667.

Newborg, M., and North, R. J. (1980). On the mechanism of T cell-independent anti-*Listeria* resistance in nude mice, *J. Immunol., 124*: 571.

North, R. J. (1973). Cellular mediators of anti-*Listeria* immunity as an enlarged population of short-lived, replicating T cells, *J. Exp. Med., 138*: 342.

North, R. J. (1974). Cell mediated immunity and the response to infection, *Mechanisms of Cell-Mediated Immunity* (R. T. McCluskey and S. Cohen, eds.), Wiley, New York, pp. 185-219.

North, R. J., and Deissler, J. F. (1975). Nature of memory in T cell-mediated antibacterial immunity: cellular parameters that distinguish between the active immune response and a state of memory, *Infect. Immun., 12*: 761.

North, R. J., and Havell, E. A. (1988). The antitumor function of tumor necrosis factor (TNF). 2. Analysis of the role of endogenous TNF in endotoxin-induced hemorrhagic necrosis of an established sarcoma, *J. Exp. Med., 167*: 1086.

Okamura, H., Kawaguchi, K., Shoji, K., and Kawade, Y. (1982). High-level induction of gamma interferon with various mitogens in mice pretreated with *Propionibacterium acnes*, *Infect. Immun., 38*: 440.

O'Malley, W. E., Achinstein, B., and Shear, M. J. (1962). Action of bacterial polysaccharide on tumors. II. Damage of sarcoma 37 by serum of mice treated with *Serratia marcescens* polysaccharide, and induced tolerance, *J. Natl. Cancer Inst., 29*: 1169.

Pace, J. L., Russell, S. w., Torres, B. A., Johnson, H. J., and Gray, P. G. (1983). Recombinant mouse γ interferon induces the priming step in macrophage activation for tumor cell killing, *J. Immunol., 130*: 2011.

Palladino, M. A., Jr., Shalaby, M. R., Kramer, S. M., Ferraiolo, B. L., Baughman, R. A., Deleo, A. H., Crose, D., Marfino, B., Aggarwal, B. B., Figari, I. S., Liggitt, D., and Patton, J. S. (1987). Characterization of the antitumor activities of human tumor necrosis factor-α and the comparison with other cytokines: induction of tumor specific immunity, *J. Immunol., 138*: 4023.

Parant, M., Parant, F., and Chedid, L. (1980). Enhancement of resistance to infections by endotoxin-induced serum factor from *Mycobacterium bovis* BCG-infected mice, *Infect. Immun., 28*: 654.

Parant, M., Parant, F., Vinit, M. -A., and Chedid, L. (1987). Action protectrice du tumor necrosis factor (TNF) obtenu par recombinaison génétique l' infection expérimentale bactérienne ou fongique, *C. R. Acad. Sci. Paris, 304*: 1.

Pennica, D., Nedwin, G. E., Hayfleck, S. S., Seeburg, D. H., Derynek, R., Palladino, M.a.,

Kohr, W. J., Aggarwal, B. B., and Goeddel, D. V. (1984). Human tumor necrosis factor: precursor structure, expression and homology to lymphotoxin, *Nature (Lond.), 312*: 724.

Pober, J. S., Gimbrone, M. A., Lapierre, L. A., Mendrick, D. L., Fiers, W., Rothelein, R., and Springer, T. A. (1986). Overlapping patterns of activation of human endothelial cells by interleukin-1, tumor necrosis factor, and immune interferon, *J. Immunol., 137*: 1893.

Pohlman, T. H., Stanness, K. A., Beatty, P. G., Ochs, H. D., and Harlan, J. M. (1986). An endothelial cell surface factor(s) induced in vitro by lipopolysaccharide, interleukin-1 and tumor necrosis factor-α increases neutrophil adherence by a CDW18-dependent mechanism, *J. Immunol., 136*: 4548.

Remington, J. S., and Merigan, T. C. (1970). Synthetic polyanions protect mice against intracellular bacterial infection, *Nature (Lond.), 226*: 361.

Rowley, D. (1955). Stimulation of natural immunity to *Escherichia coli* infections: observations on mice, *Lancet, 268*(1): 232.

Ruco, L. P., and Metlzer, M. S. (1978). Macrophage activation for tumor cytotoxicity: tumoricidal activity by macrophages form C3H/HeJ mice requires at least two activation stimuli, *Cell. Immunol., 41*: 35.

Sayers, J. J., Wiltrout, T. A., Bull, C. A., Denn, A. C., Pilaro, A. M., and Lokesh, B. (1988). Effect of cytokines on polymorphonuclear neutrophil infiltration by IL-1 and tumor necrosis factor, *J. Immunol., 141*: 1670.

Schreiber, R. D., Hicks, L. J., Celada, A., Buchmeier, N. A., and Gray, P. W. (1985). Monoclonal antibodies to murine γ-interferon which differentially modulate macrophage activation and antiviral activity. *J. Immunol., 134*: 1609.

Shalaby, M. R., Aggarwahl, B. B., Rindertnecht, E., Svedersky, L. P., Finkel, B., and Pallidino, M. A. (1985). Activation of human polymorphonuclear neutorphil functions by interferon-gamma and tumor necrosis factors, *J. Immunol., 135*: 2069.

Shear, M. J. (1935). Studies on the chemical treatment of tumors. II. The effect of disturbances in fluid exchange on transplanted mouse tumors, *Am. J. Cancer, 25*: 66.

Shear, M. J. (1943). Chemical treatment of tumors. V. Isolation of the hemorrhage-producing fraction from *Serratia marcescens (Bacillus prodigiosus)* culture filtrate, *J. Natl. Cancer Inst., 4*: 81.

Shermer-Avni, Y., Wallach, D., and Sarov, I. (1989). Reversion of the antichlamydial effect of tumor necrosis factor by tryptophan and antibodies to beta interferon, *Infect. Immun., 57*: 3484.

Shirai, T., Yamaguchi, H., Ito, H., Todd, C. W., and Wallace, R. B. (1985). Cloning and expression of the gene for human tumor necrosis factor, *Nature (Lond.), 313*: 803.

Shwarzman, G., and Michailovsky, N. (1932). Phenomenon of local skin reactivity to bacterial filtrates in the treatment of mouse sarcoma 180, *Proc. Soc. Exp. Biol. Med., 29*: 737.

Spitalny, G. L., and Havell, E. A. (1984). Monoclonal antibody to MuIFNγ inhibits lymphokine-induced antiviral and macrophage tumoricidal activities, *J. Exp. Med., 159*: 1560.

Steeg, D. S., Moore, R. N., Johnson, H. J., and Oppenheim, J. J. (1982). Regulation of macrophage Ia antigen expression by a lymphokine with immune interferon activity, *J. Exp. Med., 156*: 1780.

Steffen, M., Ottman, O. G., and Moore, M. A. S. (1988). Simultaneous production of tumor necrosis factor-α and lymphotoxin by normal T cells after induction with IL-2 and anti-T3, *J. Immunol., 140*: 2621.

Sung, S. S., Bjorndahl, J. M., Wang, C. Y., Kao, H. T., and Fu, S. M. (1988a). Production of tumor necrosis factor/cachectin by human T cell lines and peripheral blood T lymphocytes stimulated by phorbol myristate acetate and anti-CD3 antibody, *J. Exp. Med., 167*: 937.

Sung, S. S., Jung, L. K. L., Walters, J. A., Chen, W., Wang, C. Y., and Fu, S. M. (1988b). Production of tumor necrosis factor/cachetin by human B cells and tonsillar B cells, *J. Exp. Med., 168*: 1539.

Tavernier, J., Fransen, L., Marmenout, A., Van der Heyden, J., Mueller, R., Ruysschaert, M. R., Van Vliet, A., Bauvdem, R., and Fiers, W. (1987). Isolation and expression of the genes coding for mouse and human tumor necrosis factor (TNF) and biological properties of recombinant TNF, *Lymphokines,* Vol. 13 (D. R. Webb and D. V. Goeddel, eds), Academic Press, New York, pp. 181–198.

Turco, J., Thompson, H. A., and Winkler, H. H., (1984). Interferon-γ inhibits growth of *Coxiella burnetti* in mouse fibroblasts, *Infect. Immun., 45*: 781.

Vogel, S. N., Havell, E. A., and Spitalny, G. L. (1986). Monoclonal antibody -mediated inhibition of interferon-γ-induced macrophage antiviral resistance and surface antigen expression, *J. Immunol., 136*: 2917.

Wang, A . M., Creasey, A. A., Laduer, M. B., Lin, L. S., Strickler, J., Van Ardsdell, J. N., Yamamoto, R., and Mark, D. F. (1985). Molecular cloning of the complementary DNA for human tumor necrosis factor, *Science (Washington, D.C.), 228*: 149.

Warner, S. J. C., and Libby, P. (1989). Human vascular smooth muscle cell target for and source of tumor necrosis factor, *J. Immunol., 142*: 100.

Wong, G. H. W., and Goeddel, D. V. (1986). Tumor necrosis factors α and β inhibit virus replication and synergize with interferons, *Nature (Lond.), 323*: 819.

Younger, J. S., and Stinebring, W. R. (1965). Interferon appearance stimulated by endotoxin, bacteria, or viruses in mice pretreated with *Escherichia coli,* endotoxin or infected with *Mycobacterium tuberculosis, Nature (Lond.), 208*: 456.

17

Roles of TNF in Malaria and Other Parasitic Infections

I. A. CLARK and W. B. COWDEN
Zoology Department and John Curtin School of Medical Research, Australian National University, Canberra, Australia

I. THE NATURE OF PARASITIC INFECTIONS

Infectious agents range considerably in size, from viruses, through rickettsias, bacteria, and protozoa, to multicellular organisms. Although all of these can fairly be said to parasitize the host, only the protozoa and larger organisms are deemed parasites, and thus to cause parasitic diseases. When viewed alongside those preceding it, in this chapter we illustrate that the size of the invading organism seems to bear little relevance to determining the cytokine response elicited in the host. As will be seen, there is now a considerable literature on TNF* and what are called parasitic infections, just as for those caused by smaller organisms such as viruses and bacteria.

In terms of morbidity and mortality, malaria, caused by a protozoan parasite, is undoubtedly the major human infectious disease, irrespective of the size of the causative agent. As such it has generated the largest literature within parasitology, and this, plus the small amount of research as yet done on TNF and parasites other than malaria, will be reflected in the prominence given to malaria in this review.

---

*Since the role of TNF-β is essentially uninvestigated in the context of parasitic disease, the term *TNF* throughout this chapter is to be taken as TNF-α. TNF-β data are given once only, in Section VI.A.2.

II. MALARIA: THE ORIGINAL LINK BETWEEN TNF AND INFECTIOUS DISEASE

As well as being a worthy subject of research in its own right, malaria is a useful model for investigating the mechanisms underlying systemic infectious diseases in general. It is an intriguing disease. The infectious agent is restricted to the host's erythrocytes, yet somehow causes systemic multiorgan pathology, damaging cells and tissues with which it has no direct contact. What is most remarkable is that this disease, caused by a protozoan, cannot, except by demonstrating the presence of the infectious agent, reliably be separated from the syndromes caused by certain viruses, bacteria, or rickettsias. This suggests common pathways of pathophysiology.

The link between TNF and malaria preceded, by some years, its associations with other infectious diseases, and would not have been countenanced had not the organism been large and easy to see on a simple blood smear. We needed to explain how various macrophage activators, such as BCG and *Corynebacterium parvum*, long known to protect against certain viruses and bacteria, could also protect against certain mouse malarias. In the process, necrosis of parasites occurred inside circulating red cells, as happens in natural recovery from these parasites (reviewed by Clark et al., 1987d). Evidently, a soluble factor was involved, and the only plausible one at the time, linking pretreatment with BCG or *C. parvum* with subsequent necrosis of a rapidly dividing cell, was TNF, described not long before at the Sloan-Kettering Memorial Institute in New York (Carswell et al., 1975).

At the time lipopolysaccharide (LPS) was the only known trigger for TNF release, so we proposed that some product of the malarial parasite, functionally similar to LPS, could induce macrophages in malaria-infected individuals to release a range of mediators, including TNF (Clark, 1978). It was also argued (Clark, 1978; Clark et al., 1981) that these macrophage products were largely responsible for both intraerythrocytic necrosis of the parasites and, when produced excessively, caused the host pathology, including the fever, hypoglycemia, bone marrow depression, coagulopathy, hypergammaglobulinemia, hypotension, and rise in acute phase reactants seen in malaria. We also proposed that this was the origin of these same changes in gram-negative septicemia (Clark et al., 1981). In these earlier studies malaria was found to prime mice for TNF production as effectively as did *C. parvum*, and crude TNF inhibited mouse malaria in vivo. This observation was soon confirmed, in a closely related model, by Taverne et al. (1981). Equally, crude TNF appeared to inhibit *Plasmodium falciparum* in vitro (Haidaris et al., 1983). Not surprisingly, the poorly defined materials and assays available at the time tempered enthusiasm among other malariologists, and interest remained limited until the advent of recombinant TNF (rTNF).

III. PROTECTIVE EFFECTS OF TNF AGAINST MALARIA PARASITES

A. Activity Against Blood Forms

Once it became possible to test rTNF against malaria parasites in vitro, it was soon shown to lack direct toxicity against *Plasmodium falciparum* (Jensen et al., 1987) or *P. yoelii* (Taverne et al., 1987). Nevertheless, in vivo activity could be demonstrated (Taverne et al., 1987; Clark et al., 1987a). This required the earlier proposals to be modified to include a TNF-dependent final mediator, and the candidate currently most favored is lipid peroxidation products generated within plasma. TNF sensitizes leukocytes to secrete reactive oxygen species, to which, in vivo, malaria parasites are extremely vulnerable (reviewed by Clark et al., 1989a). Under these conditions a range of products of lipid peroxidation, to which *P. falciparum* is very susceptible (Clark et al., 1987b), are produced (Buffinton et al., 1988). This is consistent with a recent report by Rockett et al., (1988) that the antimalarial activity of serum containing endogenous TNF was entirely removed by depleting it of its lipoprotein fraction. Another intriguing prospect is that metabolic products of prostaglandins, which are induced by TNF, could help inhibit parasite growth in vivo. This possibility arises from the recent demonstration by Ohnishi et al. (1989) that oligomeric prostaglandin derivatives inhibit growth of *Plasmodium chabaudi* and *Plasmodium vinckei* in BALB/c mice.

Recent data from our laboratory implies a role for activated macrophages if TNF is to generate the mediator that is toxic to malaria parasites. As shown in Table 1, serum collected from *C. parvum*-primed mice 2 h after they had received r-human TNF was toxic to *P. falciparum* in vitro, but serum from normal mice similarly treated was not. Further information consistent with TNF, requiring collaboration with some host factor, such as degree of macrophage activation, comes from the

Table 1. Macrophage Dependence of the Antiparasite Effect of TNF

Treatment	% Inhibition of *P. falciparum* in vitro (2.4% mouse serum v/v)
C. parvum[a]	0
TNF[b]	0
C. parvum + TNF[c]	82

Source: G. A. Butcher and I. A. Clark, unpublished data.

[a]Mice were given 1 mg of *C. parvum* iv only and bled on day 11.

[b]Mice were given 10 μg of TNF iv only and bled 2 h later.

[c]Mice were given 1 mg of *C. parvum* iv followed by 10 μg of TNF on day 11 and bled 2 h later.

studies of Stevenson and Ghadirian (1989). These authors found that exogenous TNF altered the course and outcome of *P.chabaudi* (AS strain) infection in the A/J, but not C57 B1/6, strain of syngeneic mice.

While it is evident, therefore, that TNF can initiate a chain of events (probably involving free radicals) that can inhibit malaria parasites, it is by no means established that this operates in vivo. Cavacini et al. (1989) have analyzed *P. chabaudi* infection in P/J mice. These animals proved to have poorly activated macrophages during the course of infection, as evidenced by negligible chemiluminescence and capacity to kill tumor cells in vitro, but they cleared the parasite as well as did control mice. This implies that the resolution of this infection, shown earlier by this group to be antibody-independent and yet require T lymphocytes (reviewed in Cavacini et al., 1989), may occur without the involvement of macrophages. Possible explanations yet to be explored include release of TNF-β from activated T cells, and TNF-α embedded in the membrane of cytotoxic T lymphocytes (Liu et al., 1989). The former seems more plausible, since the end product of the immune response is parasite necrosis inside circulating red cells, and red cells do not carry the H-2 antigens required for recognition by cytotoxic T cells. Equally, the nonoxidative cytotoxic effects of neutrophils against malaria parasites (Kharazami et al., 1984) or the antiparasitic effects of endogenous nitric oxide (reviewed by Griffith and Randall, 1989) are not excluded by these data. It is also possible that these non-macrophage pathways operate at the low parasitemias observed by Cavacini et al. (1989), but that at higher parasite loads, when the mice are sick and measurable TNF is circulating, the TNF/oxidant mechanisms could come into play.

B. Activity Against Liver Forms

The hepatic stage (or sporozoite) of the malaria parasite precedes the blood form in the organism's life cycle and is antigenically quite distinct from it. Earlier attempts to understand the host response to sporozoites were focused on antibodies, but in recent years cytokines, including γ-interferon (Ferreira et al., 1986) and TNF (Schofield et al., 1987), have been shown to protect hepatocytes in vitro, and mice, against malarial sporozoites. Another school of thought holds that cytotoxic T lymphocytes are the direct effector cells, selectively eliminating sporozoite-infected hepatocytes on contact (Hoffman et al., 1989). This activity is cell dependent and not detected in culture supernatants, implying a contact-dependent process not mediated by soluble factors. One involvement of TNF in this process could be through its capacity to enhance surface expression of class I HLA antigens (Collins et al., 1986) since these antigens form part of the structure recognized on target cell surfaces by cytotoxic T lymphocytes. Furthermore, recent studies on the nature of contact killing of target cells by cytotoxic T lymphocytes, involving TNF detection by indirect immunofluorescence and immunoelectron microscopy and using TNF-specific antibodies to inhibit cytotoxicity, implicate this monokine in the killing process (Liu et al., 1989). TNF was demonstrated to be an integral membrane protein, so would not be expected to appear in culture supernatants. These studies suggest that the two current approaches to understanding the immunity to malarial sporozoites, and thus to develop a vaccine, may be more closely related than is as yet acknowledged.

The activity of TNF against each of these stages of the life cycle of the malaria parasite in the vertebrate host needs closer scrutiny before its role can be properly defined. In particular, in vivo use of neutralizing antibody to TNF, and the use of in situ hybridization to determine the tissue localization, should prove fruitful. There is ample precedent to suggest that the eventual outcome will reveal the involvement of several cytokines, acting in concert. One plausible mediator of these TNF-induced effects is C-reactive protein, a hepatocyte product that protects these cells against liver forms of *P. falciparum* and *P. yoelii* (Pied et al., 1989). C-reactive protein is induced in humans by both exogenous TNF (Selby et al., 1987) and malaria infections (Naik and Voller, 1984). IL-6, which is induced by TNF (Brouckaert et al., 1989) and directly involved in generating C-reactive protein (Morrone et al., 1988), is found to be raised in both human (Kern et al., 1989) and mouse (Grau et al., 1989a) malarial serum. A role for nitric oxide (reviewed by Griffith and Randall, 1989) in these events can also not be discounted.

IV. CONSEQUENCES OF EXCESSIVE TNF PRODUCTION IN MALARIA

A. Reproducing Malarial Illness and Pathology with rTNF

With the advent of rTNF it became possible to test our prediction that this cytokine has a central role in the disease produced by malaria infection. Accordingly, we compared tissue damage and metabolic changes in mice severely ill from *P. vinckei* infection with the changes seen in others given a single injection of r human TNF. Since only infected mice could be expected to release TNF systemically, we gave TNF to mice with early, nonclinical, malarial infections. These animals proved to be much more sensitive to TNF than were normal mice, and amounts harmless to controls reproduced the pulmonary neutrophil margination, hypoglycemia, high serum lactate, and liver injury seen in terminally ill mice (Clark et al., 1987c). As will be discussed later, no leukocyte accumulations were evident in cerebral blood vessels. These observations were extended to include fetal death (Clark and Chaudhri, 1988a) and dyserythropoiesis and erythrophagocytosis (Clark and Chaudhri, 1988b). We have since found that interleukin-1 synergizes strongly with TNF to produce all of these changes (unpublished data).

Other studies appearing at this time (and undertaken for reasons unassociated with malaria) reinforce just how closely TNF toxicity parallels the pathology seen in this disease. The changes produced in dogs provide a good example (Tracey et al., 1987). As with mice, leukocytes accumulated in pulmonary blood vessels, and lactate levels increased. Additionally, hypotension, hemorrhagic lesions, adrenal medullary necrosis, and acute renal tubular necrosis were recorded. All of these changes, including the hepatomegaly TNF administration produces in rats (Feingold et al., 1988), as well as those reproduced with TNF in mice, can occur in severe human malaria (reviewed by Kitchen, 1949; Phillips and Warrell, 1986).

Even more striking parallels with clinical malaria are seen in tumor patients given parenteral TNF, in whom fatigue, fever, chills, headache, thrombocytopenia, anorexia, hypotension, myalgia, nausea, vomiting, and diarrhea are routinely recorded (e.g. Spriggs et al., 1988; Jakubowski et al., 1989). These changes are worse with higher doses. Even the more esoteric biochemical changes recorded in malaria, such as hypertriglyceridemia (Onongbu and Onyeneke, 1983) and low serum iron (Phillips et al., 1986), are observed in patients to whom TNF has been administered (Creagen et al., 1988; Jakubowski et al., 1989; Michie et al., 1988). In addition, the clotting cascade may be activated in both TNF recipients (Bauer et al., 1989) and malaria patients (Pukrittayakamee et al., 1989; Section V.E), and as discussed in Section V.D.2, altered mental states can be induced. Also, the labial herpes often seen in malaria may be reproduced by infusing TNF into tumor patients (Diehl et al., 1988; Tanneberger et al., 1988), implying a role for TNF in malarial immunosuppression. Remarkably, this array of changes is often induced by doses of rTNF too small to cause a detectable rise in serum TNF (noted by Jakubowski et al., 1989; Wiedenmann et al., 1989), so it is not surprising that patients with clinical falciparum malaria, in whose serum high levels of TNF can be detected (see below), may often exhibit this constellation of changes in a severe and protracted form. As discussed later (Section V.D.2), this implies that sequestered parasitized red cells may be less important, and cytokines per se more important, in the pathogenesis of the pathology of falciparum malaria than currently supposed.

The mechanism of these TNF-induced changes is yet to be deduced in many cases. One interesting new development is the incrimination of nitric oxide generated from L-arginine by endothelial cells in TNF-induced hypotension (reviewed by Griffith and Randall, 1989), implying a similar mechanism for the hypotension of malaria.

B. Increased Serum TNF in Animal and Human Malaria

However closely injected TNF might reproduce the illness, tissue damage, and biochemical changes seen in malaria, the link remains tenuous unless TNF can be detected in the host's serum and shown to correlate with disease outcome. This has been reported for the diseases caused by two rodent malarial parasites, one of which causes cerebral malaria (Grau et al., 1987b) and another that leads to a more systemic illness (Clark and Chaudhri, 1988b; Fig. 1). Several groups have screened banks of sera from a range of acute human infections for TNF and found it in-

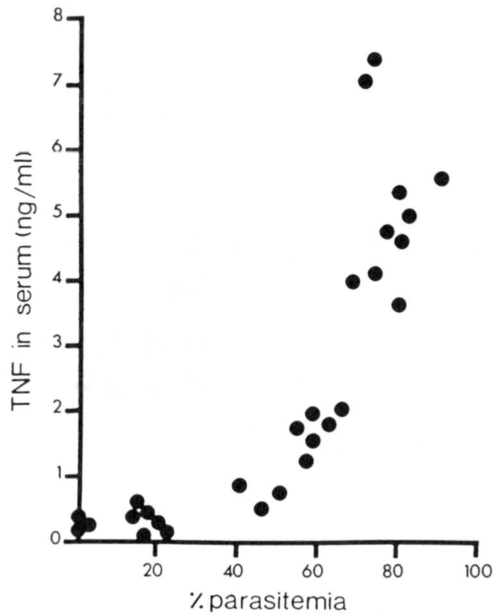

Figure 1 Serum TNF levels throughout the course of infection in individual *P. vinckei*-infected mice. (Reproduced, with permission, from *British Journal of Haematology.*)

creased in those with malaria (Scuderi et al., 1986; Teppo and Maury, 1987; van der Meer et al., 1988). Others have now reported more systematic studies. For example, Grau et al. (1989b) examined a group of 65 Malawian children and found that serum TNF at time of admission correlated with high parasite load, hypoglycemia, severity of disease (as measured by a prognostic index), and mortality (Fig. 2). Nevertheless, serum TNF levels varied greatly, with a wide overlap of concentrations in the various categories. As discussed in Section V.A, this highlights a problem inherent in studying malaria in tropical countries, where variations in host tolerance, derived from previous malarial exposure, make interpretation of data difficult. Conversely, the clearer patterns discerned by Kern et al. (1989), who used the same assay as Grau et al. (1989b) to measure serum TNF, but in a group of nonimmune Europeans who had not traveled to tropical areas before, probably reflects their lack of previous exposure. Patients with complicated malaria [combined organ dysfunction, hypotension, thrombocytopenia, the highest parasite densities (Fig. 3), and the longest durations between onset of clinical symptoms and

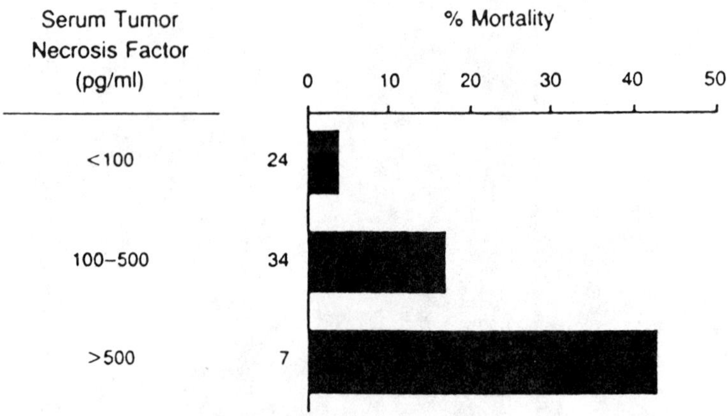

Figure 2 Relationship between serum level of TNF at time of admission to hospital and outcome of disease in children with falciparum malaria. (Reproduced, with permission, from *New England Journal of Medicine*, vol. 320, p. 1586, 1989.)

diagnosis; $n = 18$] had significantly higher TNF values than those in whom malaria ran a more benign course ($n = 22$; $p < 0.001$).

In another African study, plasma TNF levels were raised in 59% of Gambian children with acute malaria (Kwiatkowski et al., 1989). Again variation was present, conceivably attributable to contrasts in previous malarial history or the different assay employed. Increased TNF production was confirmed by measuring the in

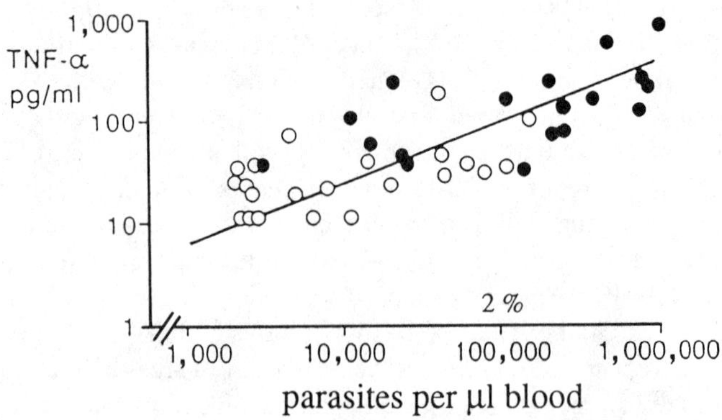

Figure 3 TNF concentrations in relation to number of parasitized red cells in 18 complicated (●) and 22 uncomplicated (○) cases of malaria. (Reproduced, with permission, from *American Journal of Medicine*.)

vitro output by peripheral blood mononuclear cells from malaria patients, which was significantly higher than that from controls. As discussed in the next section, a particularly valuable contribution by this study was the information that schizogony, the process whereby red cells containing mature organisms burst to release the next generation of young parasites, also releases a trigger for TNF production.

In a recent study of malarial patients in the Solomon Islands, involving 44 semi-immune adults living in an endemic area, our group found that serum TNF levels correlated directly with both fever and parasite density (Butcher et al., 1990). The same assay as that used by Grau et al., (1989b) and Kern et al. (1989) was employed. Inevitably, serum levels of TNF and other cytokines are crude indicators of the changes that occur during malaria, since they measure only the net outcome of production, binding to cell receptors, excretion, and neutralization by inhibitors in serum. The tools are now becoming available to enable each of these aspects to be addressed, so a much more precise picture of events will probably be pieced together over the next few years.

C. Malaria Parasites as a Trigger for TNF Release

When malaria parasites divide synchronously, so that a shower of merozoites (newly budded parasites) is released into the plasma at regular intervals (schizogony), the illness in the host waxes and wanes in phase with this process, with a lag time of several hours (Golgi, 1889). Thus it has long been assumed (reviewed by Maegraith, 1948) that release of parasite products at schizogony somehow causes host illness and pathology. With these precedents in mind we predicted that these products would prove to be the trigger for TNF in malaria (Clark et al., 1981; Clark, 1982a,b). The alternative argument, put forward by Phillips and Warrell (1986) and Warrell (1987), is that any endotoxemia-like changes in malaria (implying TNF-inducible changes, because of the close associations between endotoxemia and TNF) were not a part of malaria itself, but the consequences of secondary gram-negative septicemia.

The first experimental evidence that malarial products might trigger TNF release came from Hotez et al. (1984), who reported that lysed malaria parasites would induce release of a functionally defined macrophage product. This later proved to be TNF. More recently, Bate et al.(1988) found that soluble antigenic material from several murine malarias would trigger in vitro release of TNF. Polyclonal antibody raised to these *P. yoelii* antigens prevented this material, but not endotoxin, from inducing TNF. Conversely, a monoclonal antibody against the KDO antigen of endotoxin blocked the induction of TNF by LPS, but not by malaria antigens (Playfair et al., 1990). Thus contaminant endotoxin is most unlikely to have triggered the TNF release these authors measured. This work was repeated in vivo (Bate et al. 1989). Subsequently, analogous antigens from *P. falciparum*, in conditions that excluded any contaminating endotoxin, were shown to induce TNF

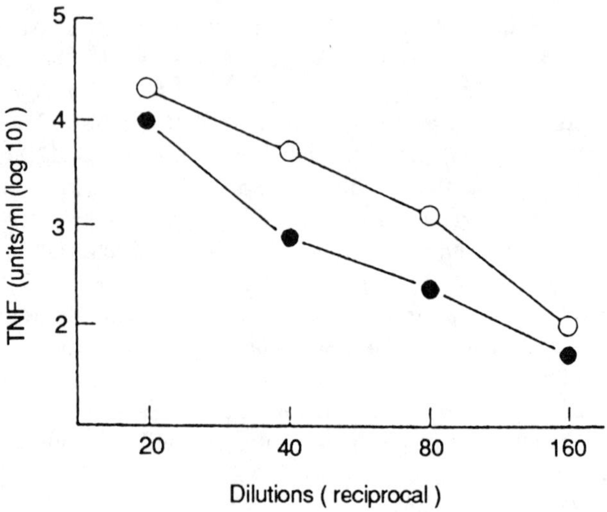

Figure 4 TNF secretion by human blood monocytes stimulated by heat-stable soluble antigens of *P. falciparum* in the presence (●) or absence (○) of polymyxin B. Much of the reduction of TNF in the presence of polymyxin B may be due to malarial antigens reactive to this antibiotic. (Jakobsen et al., 1988; reproduced, with permission, from *Parasite Immunology*.)

release from human monocytes (Taverne et al., 1990; Fig. 4). As before, antisera specific to soluble, heat-stable human malaria antigens prevented this material, but not endotoxin, from including TNF. Picot et al. (1990) obtained similar results, using polymyxin B rather than antibody specific to malarial antigens to deal with the question of possible endotoxin contamination. They reported that the optimal ratio for TNF production was one to three parasitized erythrocytes per macrophage. Finally, the circle seems complete with the demonstration (Kwiatkowski et al., 1989) that human peripheral blood mononuclear cells, co-cultured with *P. falciparum*-infected red cells, release TNF, on cue, a short time after schizogony (Fig. 5). Thus in a perfectly synchronous infection we should expect a brief pulse of TNF detectable soon after schizogony, and negligible amounts for the rest of the cycle. Its toxic effects would persist for an appreciable time (Waage et al., 1989), producing cycles of illness with the timing originally observed a century ago by Golgi.

This synchrony of schizogony and manifestations of illness (which includes the onset of even the most severe symptoms; Kitchen, 1949) would not occur were endotoxin from secondary septicemia the main trigger for TNF in malaria, as is inherent in the proposals of Phillips and Warrell (1986) and Warrell (1987). These authors were no doubt influenced by having found *Limulus* lysate positivity in

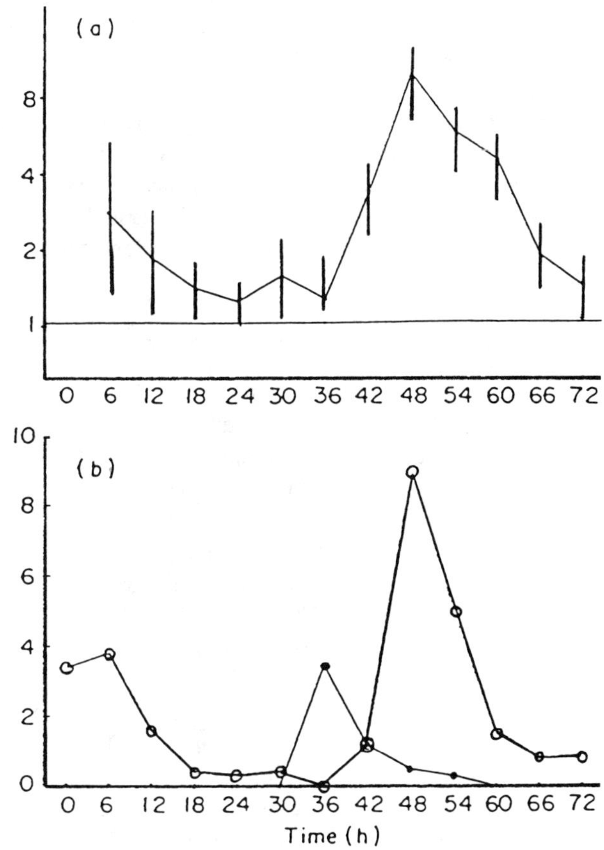

Figure 5 TNF production (a) in co-cultures of mononuclear cells and parasitized erythrocytes. Results in panel (a) are expressed as the rate of TNF secretion in the parasitized, compared to unparasitized red cells. Standard error bars are shown. Time course (b) of the development of the numbers of schizonts (●), expressed as percent parasitemia, falls abruptly just before TNF production begins to rise in panel (a). The emergence of new merozoites (○) follows schizont rupture. (Reproduced, with permission, from *Clinical and Experimental Immunology*.)

plasma from two-thirds of a group of cerebral malaria patients (Usawattanakul et al., 1985). Once thought specific for endotoxin, this assay is now known to respond to a wide variety of materials, including, notably, soluble antigens released from *P. falciparum* (Jakobsen et al., 1988). Tubbs (1980) probably detected these same antigens. There are, nevertheless, grounds for predicting that concurrent sepsis should exacerbate malaria, since endotoxin and TNF have been shown to synergize strongly in vivo (Rothstein and Schreiber, 1988). These authors found that very small doses of endotoxin, too small to be harmful alone, were extremely toxic when administered together with a small dose of TNF.

D. Confirmation with Neutralizing Antibody In Vivo

One sure way to test if a cytokine has an essential role in a disease process is to see if a neutralizing antibody directed against it, when administered early in the course of the disease, alters its character. A group at the University of Geneva has focused on this approach. They reported several years ago that the IgG fraction of a rabbit polyclonal antibody raised against mouse TNF would prevent mice infected with *P. berghei* (ANKA strain) from developing the signs and histological changes of cerebral malaria (Grau et al., 1987b). Subsequent experiments showed that administering polyconal anti-IL-3 and anti-γ GM-CSF together (but not separately) prevented both the occurrence of the neurological syndrome and the rise in serum TNF. This combined treatment also reduced macrophage accumulation in the spleen (Grau et al., 1988a). Monoclonal antibody against IFN-γ also abolished the rise in serum TNF and the cerebral malaria, but did not affect the distribution of tissue macrophages (Grau et al., 1989c). From these results has emerged a model of a sequential cytokine cascade, involving cell recruitment and activation as well as effector function, in the mouse model of cerebral malaria (Grau et al., 1989d). This is discussed further in SectionV.D. The in vivo use of neutralizing antibodies, sometimes giving several together to overcome the functional duplication inherent in cytokine activity, is sure to expand as sufficient quantities become available.

V. ASPECTS OF MALARIA OPENED TO FURTHER RESEARCH BY THE TNF THEORY OF THE DISEASE

A. Tolerance to Malaria

Any theory that seeks to explain the origin of illness and pathology in malaria must accommodate malarial tolerance, a phenomenon commonly seen after repeated attacks of malaria, in the majority of children in hyperendemic areas (e.g. Wilson et al., 1950). These children are evidently quite healthy, yet carry a parasite load up to thousands of times greater than that sufficient to cause severe illness in a previously uninfected person. It is generally agreed that if the biological basis of this absence of illness and pathology were understood, the reasons for their presence in others would be clearer. We have suggested before (Clark et al., 1987d, 1989b) that this might be an example of acquired tolerance to TNF, as reported in animals (Fraker et al., 1988) and human beings (Hersch et al., 1987). Another mechanism of malarial tolerance, again involving TNF, has been proposed by Taverne et al. (1990). Antibodies they raised against certain malarial antigens could prevent this material from triggering TNF release. As these authors point out, such antibodies circulating after one infection could limit the capacity of a subsequent infection to generate TNF, and hence to cause illness and pathology. Both of these mechanisms, which could coexist, are amenable to further testing. As Playfair et al. (1990) have recently noted, the second of these possibilities could be harnessed to develop an antidisease, as distinct from antiparasite, vaccine. This concept of vaccinating to block a parasite product, rather than to inhibit parasite growth, has long been in routine use in tetanus and diphtheria, so there is no immediate reason why it should not also succeed in malaria.

B. Malarial Hypoglycemia

Hypoglycemia, often with a preceding hyperglycemia, has been recognized in human malaria since at least the 1920s (Peterson, 1926) and is now agreed to be an important complication in falciparum malaria, producing symptoms that can be confused with cerebral malaria (reviewed by Phillips, 1989). Early attempts to rationalize it were based on the idea of consumption of host glucose by the parasite. Clark et al. (1981) argued that a monokine, termed glucocorticoid antagonizing factor (GAF) by Moore et al. (1978) and shown by them to block hepatic gluconeogenesis in endotoxic mice, was responsible. Subsequently, White et al. (1987) and Taylor et al. (1988) reported biochemical changes consistent with blocked hepatic gluconeogenesis in young malaria patients who were hypoglycemic. Before long the term GAF became obsolete, since its function proved to be one of the many activities shared by IL-1 (Hill et al., 1986) and TNF (McCallum et al., 1987). Meanwhile, we had shown that a small dose of TNF would induce hypoglycemia in mice with subclinical malarial infection (Clark et al., 1987c) and serum TNF levels were later shown to correlate with hypoglycemia in children with severe falciparum malaria (Grau et al., 1989a). We have observed this same relationship in *P. vinckei*-infected mice (Fig. 6).

Subsequently, Hill et al. (1989) demonstrated that the IL-6 induced by IL-1 and TNF (Brouckaert et al., 1989), and not these monokines themselves, is what actually blocks hepatic gluconeogenesis. Like TNF, IL-6 has now been shown to correlate with the severity of illness in falciparum malaria (Kern et al., 1989). It also correlated with TNF levels in these studies, so it seems a reasonable prediction that IL-6, like TNF, will prove to correlate with malarial hypoglycemia. This can be expected to occur only when liver glycogen is depleted, thus creating a need for gluconeogenesis, with its attendant susceptibility to IL-6. This is consistent with

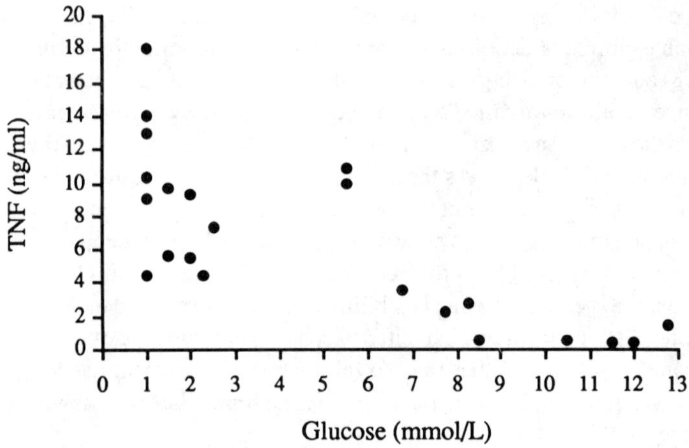

Figure 6 Relationship between serum TNF levels and blood glucose levels in individual *P. vinckei*-infected mice (linear $r = 0.751$, $p = 0.0001$).

the observation that children (whose livers are more readily depleted of glycogen; Pagliara et al., 1973) are more prone to malarial hypoglycemia than are adults (reviewed by Phillips, 1989). It is also in keeping with the depleted liver glycogen found by White et al. (1983) in most of a group of hypoglycemic malaria patients they studied in Thailand. The tools used in the molecular biological studies of Hill and McCallum (1990), and such reagents as neutralizing antibody to IL-6, therefore appear to warrant being applied to malarial hypoglycemia.

C. Malarial Hypergammaglobulinemia

The serum of malarial patients, particularly after repeated attacks, contains large amounts of gamma globulin (Turner and Voller, 1966). For some time this has been attributed to a malarial mitogen, active for lymphocytes, found both in serum of patients (Strickland, 1978) and in supernatants from cultured parasites (Greenwood et al., 1979). But lymphocyte proliferation alone is insufficient for Ig production: maturation of the B cells has also to be explained. One of the earlier names for IL-6 was B-cell stimulatory factor 2 (BSF-2), which was characterized and cloned on its ability to induce activated B cells to mature into immunoglobulin-producing cells (reviewed by Kishimoto and Hirano, 1988). Thus the recent report that serum TNF and IL-6 levels are increased in malaria (Kern et al., 1989) allows a more thorough investigation of the origins of malarial hypergammaglobulinemia. Much of this Ig is not directed against malaria antigens but is specific for various autoantigens (Kataaha et al., 1984). As well as inducing the IL-6 to bring about B-cell maturation, chronically surging TNF levels could, by increasing surface expression of HLA antigens (Collins et al., 1986), cause self to be recognized by antigen-presenting cells. There is precedent in other diseases for high serum IL-6 to be associated with hypergammaglobulinemia (Yoshizaki et al., 1989) and autoantibody production (Hirano et al., 1987).

D. Cerebral Malaria

Cerebral dysfunction is the most common serious manifestation of falciparum malaria. It may take virtually any clinical form, up to and including unrousable coma (reviewed by Kitchen, 1949), and its pathogenesis is undoubtedly the most contentious topic in the malaria literature. The traditional view of the pathogenesis of this condition is that blood flow through cerebral vessels is impaired by the adhesion of parasitized red cells (Clark and Tomlinson, 1949; Macpherson et al., 1985). This condition is modeled, although imperfectly, in *P. berghei* (ANKA strain) infections in certain strains of mice. As discussed below, this model has at least allowed cerebral malaria to be examined from the cytokine viewpoint.

1. *Mouse Cerebral Malaria*

As noted above, *P. berghei* ANKA produces distinctive cerebral lesions in mice. Mackey et al. (1980) and Rest (1982) described the associated histological changes, which include adhesion of monocytes to cerebral vessel endothelium and injury to adjacent vessel walls, with resultant edema and petechial hemorrhage. In contrast to human cerebral malaria, there is no suggestion that parasitized red cells adhere to the walls of cerebral or other blood vessels, or that they are more concentrated here than in the rest of the circulation. The first indication that the syndrome was host-mediated came from Finley et al. (1982), who reported that these lesions did not occur in nu/nu mice. This implied the involvement of some T-cell-dependent response in its pathogenesis, and CD4-positive lymphocytes have since been incriminated (Grau et al., 1986).

As reviewed in Section II, our laboratory proposed some time ago that monokines were responsible for much of the pathology seen in malaria (Clark et al., 1981). This concept, including the involvement of TNF, was expanded by Rest (1983) to encompass the cerebral pathology seen in mice infected with *P. berghei* ANKA. Section IV.D summarizes the studies in which neutralizing antibodies to mouse TNF (Grau et al., 1987b), IL-3 and GM-CSF (Grau et al., 1988a), and IFN-γ (Grau et al., 1989c) were used in vivo to establish the argument that a T-cell-dependent cytokine cascade, culminating in TNF release, orchestrates the onset of cerebral pathology in *P. berghei* ANKA-infected mice (Grau et al., 1989d). Notably, all three treatments reduced serum TNF levels and also leukocyte adherence to cerebral vascular endothelium, a process likely to be mediated, at least in part, by the intracellular adhesion molecule-1 (ICAM-1). TNF normally induces expression of this and other molecules on endothelial cells (reviewed by Cotran, 1987) but not in the presence of cyclosporin A (Kahn and Barton, 1989). This is consistent with the observation that cyclosporin A, at a dose too low to influence B-cell function or parasite growth, prevents cerebral malaria in this infection (Grau et al., 1987a). This group has also correlated serum TNF with presence of cerebral pathology (Grau et al., 1987b; reviewed by Grau et al., 1989a) and describe having reproduced the plugging of cerebral vessels with leukocytes, as seen in mouse cerebral malaria, by administering TNF to normal CBA mice (Grau et al., 1989a).

Our experience with TNF in mouse malarias is at variance with these observations. We consistently find that injected TNF produces a syndrome that is unlike that seen in *P. berghei* ANKA infections, and precisely as seen in *P. vinckei*-infected mice (Clark et al., 1987c; Table 2). TNF infusions, given over a range of times and doses, induce midzonal liver necrosis, neutrophil adherence in pulmonary vessels, and hypoglycemia, none of which, in our experience, do not accompany *P. berghei* ANKA cerebral malaria, but are invariably present in *P. vinckei* infections (Table 2). Again, as seen in terminal *P. vinckei* infections (Fig. 7), cerebral vessels have remained clear of adherent leukocytes over a range of TNF regimens. The reasons for this discrepancy may become clear when details of the TNF treatment outlined in Grau et al. (1989a) are published.

Furthermore, on comparing serum TNF levels across a range of mouse malarias, we have found that the highest endogenous levels occur in those infections exhibiting the pathology that can be reproduced by injecting this cytokine—that is, in terminal *P. vinckei* infections (Fig. 8). In our hands serum TNF levels have simply reflected parasite densities. *P. berghei* ANKA-infected mice exhibit monocyte adherence and cerebral sysmptoms at 10–30% parasitemia, at which point we find that they have the lowest serum TNF level of any mice ill with malaria. In contrast, circulating levels of TNF are highest with *P. vinckei* (Fig. 8), but monocytes do not adhere, and cerebral symptoms and pathology do not occur (Table 2). For these reasons we suggest that the cerebral pathology seen in mice infected with *P. berghei* ANKA is governed by TNF produced locally within the cerebral blood vessels, and not by systemic levels of this cytokine. It seems likely that some local event, as yet undefined, attracts circulating monocytes to adhere to cerebral endothelium in *P. berghei* ANKA infections, but not those caused by (for example) *P. vinckei.* Alternatively, synergy between TNF and some as yet uninvestigated cytokine that circulates at a higher level in *P. berghei* ANKA than in *P. vinckei* infections, the combination having a predilection for cerebral vessels, has to be considered. Since neutralizing antibody to IFN-γ prevents development of the cerebral lesions in *P. berghei* ANKA infections (Grau et al., 1989c), and IFN-γ induces adhesion of monocytes to cultured endothelial cells (Mentzer et al., 1986; Nickoloff et al., 1988), this cytokine possibly plays a more important local role in this syndrome than is currently realized. The ability of IFN-γ and/or TNF to increase adhesion of lymphocytes to cerebral microvascular cells (Hughes et al., 1988) may have relevance here. Further work on this model of cerebral malaria is likely to

Table 2 TNF Toxicity Mimics *P. vinckei*, But Not *P. berghei* ANKA, Pathology

	Serum TNF	Leukocytes in brain vessels	Evan's Blue permeability to brain	Brain hemorr-hage	Cerebral clinical signs	Hypo-glycemic	Midzonal liver necrosis
TNF toxicity[a]	+++	–	–	–	–	+	+
Terminal *P. vinckei*	+++	–	–	–	–	+	+
Terminal *P. berghei* (ANKA)	+	+	+	+	+	–	–

[a]2 μg human rTNF, in osmostic pumps, for 5 days; 5 μg of TNF iv per day for 2 days, or 7.5 μg of TNF iv per day for 2 days, given to mice carrying a low-density infection of *P. vinckei* or *P. chabaudi*.

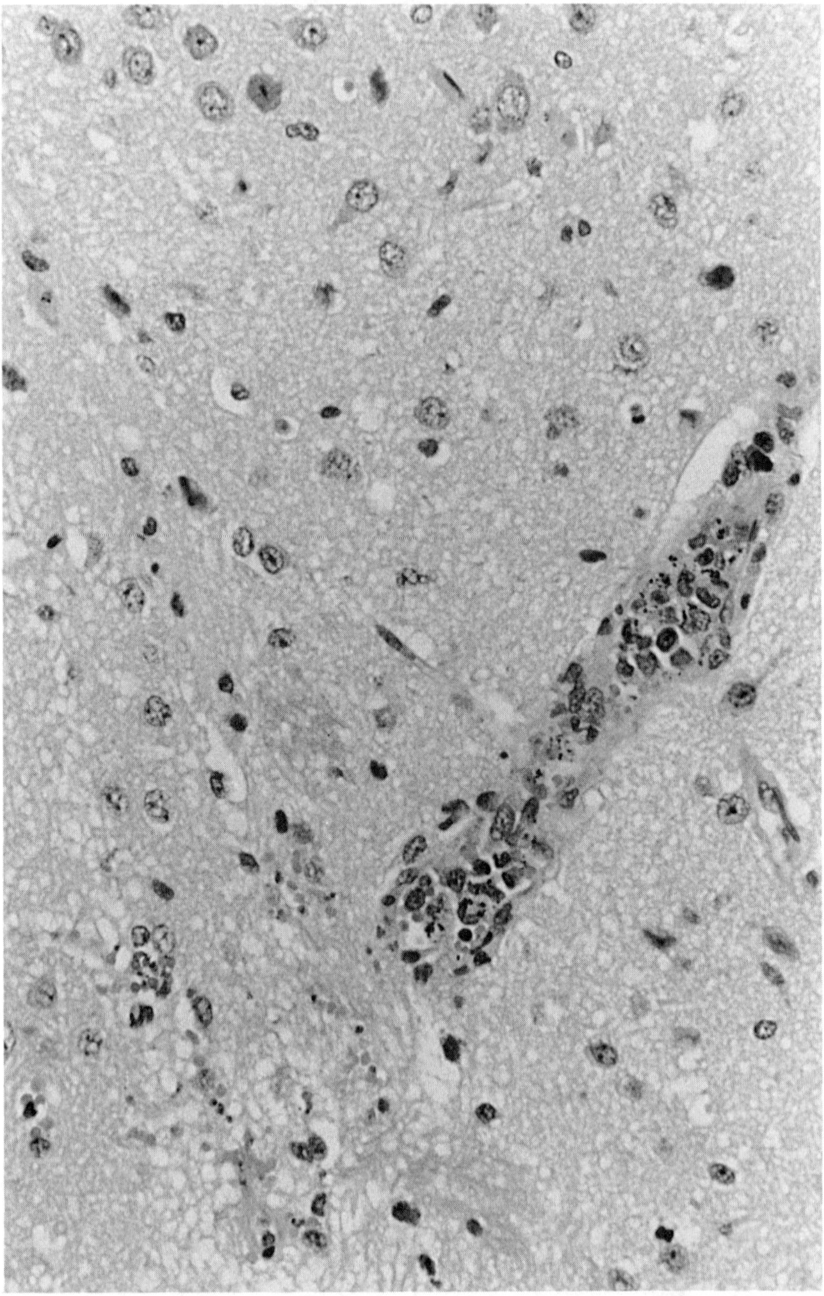

(a)

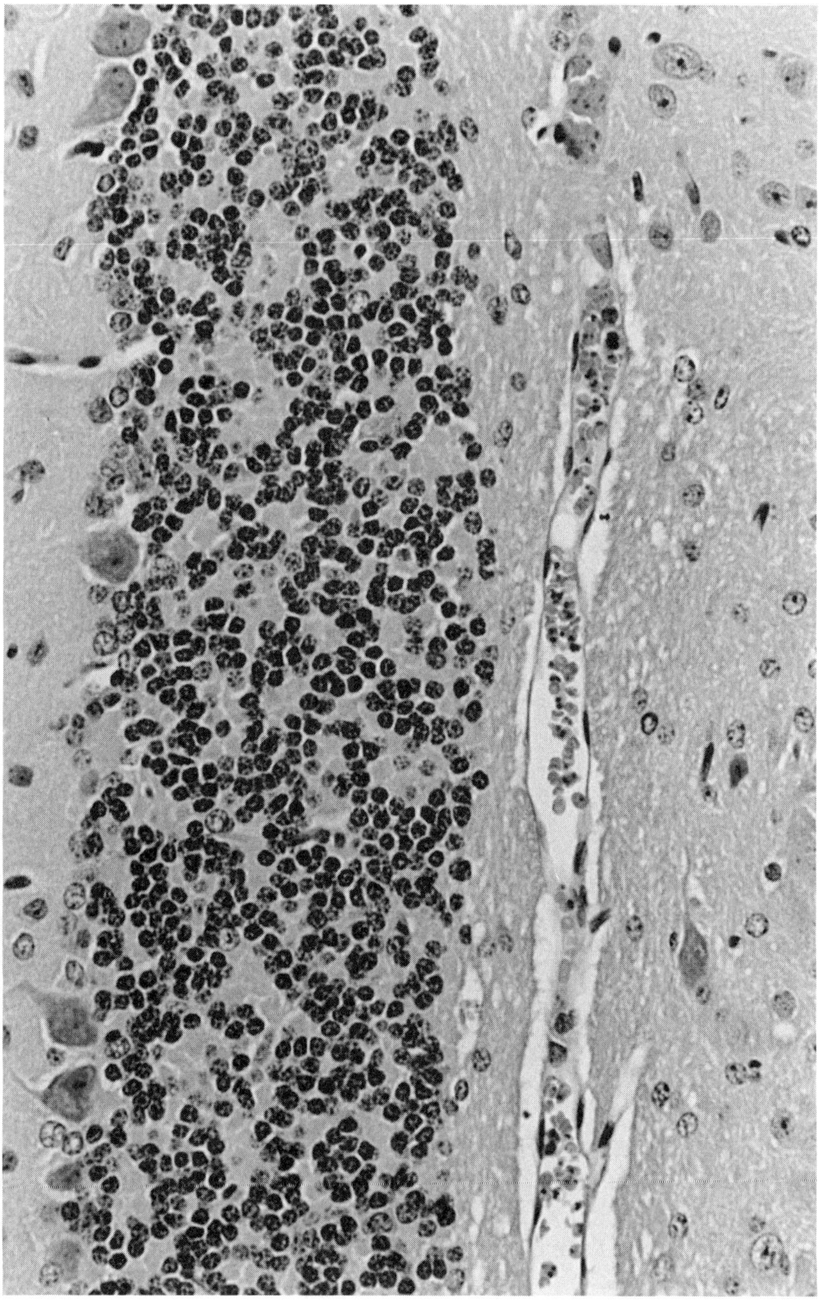

(b)

Figure 7 Cerebral blood vessels of mice terminally ill with (a) *P. berghei* (ANKA strain) and (b) *P. vinckei*. Adherent monocytes are present in (a) and absent in (b), which (see Fig. 8) has the higher serum TNF levels.

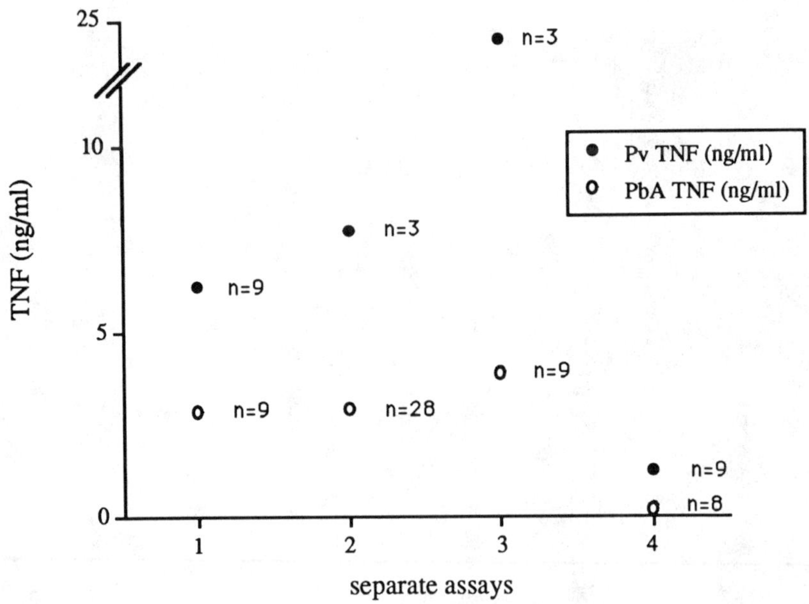

Figure 8 Four separate assays, some months apart, in which terminal *P. vinckei* and *P. berghei* (ANKA strain) sera were tested at the same time. Despite variations in assay sensitivities, TNF levels in *P. vinckei* sera were consistently higher than those in *P. berghei* (ANKA strain) sera.

focus on the site of production of cytokines and induction of adhesion molecules within the cerebral vessels, as well as systemic levels of cytokines other than TNF.

As further circumstantial evidence to favor local cerebral cytokine production in this model, we note that mouse cerebral malaria typically occurs in the absence of obvious systemic involvement, whereas in the human disease cerebral symptoms are usually the culmination of a period of multiorgan, systemic, TNF-inducible pathology. This implies that cerebrally sequestered monocytes may supply most of the functionally important TNF in *P. berghei* ANKA infections, whereas it is produced systemically in the human disease.

2. *Human Cerebral Malaria*

a. Sequestration of Parasitized Red Cells. Red cells containing mature P. falciparum parasites are absent from the circulating blood because they adhere to the inner wall of the smaller blood vessels, particularly the postcapillary venules. This process is referred to as sequestration, and it may cause small vessels to appear as if they were "packed" or "plugged" with parasitized red cells. If this adhesion concentrates in a particular organ, it is reasonable to assume, as has been done for decades, that flow will be obstructed, the supply of nutrients and oxygen will be diminished, and function will suffer accordingly. This has become the conventional view of cerebral malaria (reviewed by Warrell, 1987) and indeed has been extended to explain degenerative changes seen in bone marrow in these patients (see Section V.F). There has never, however, been undisputed evidence that this "plugging" phenomenon is invariably present in cerebral malaria, and it has never been explained how sequestration can be intense in a range of organs in *Aotus trivigatus* monkeys infected with *P. falciparum* without causing pathologic changes in the adjacent tissue (Jervis et al., 1972). Macpherson et al. (1985) reported sequestration in all 7 of their cerebral malaria cases, and only in 2 of 6 controls, but Kean and Smith (1944), reviewing 12 cases of cerebral malaria, noted that none of the brains showed vessels "plugged" with parasitized red cells. In contrast, of the 16 brains with "plugged" vessels in their series of 100 cases, none came from patients with cerebral malaria. Similarly, Toro and Roman (1978) reported parasite accumulations in cerebral blood vessels in only 4 of their 19 cases of cerebral malaria, although they were present in all 19 brains described by Oo et al. (1987). Differences in the definition of cerebral malaria could account for some of these contrasts, but clearly the matter is far from resolved.

To be tenable as the essential cause of cerebral malaria, a theory based simply on parasites plugging blood vessels has to explain how malaria-tolerant children, who are heavily infected but seemingly normal (Section V.A), manage to keep their high parasite loads sequestered in parts of the vascular tree where they do not cause harm. Equally, it has to be assumed that those patients who develope cerebral symptoms have in some way caused parasitized red cells to sequester preferentially in the smaller cerebral vessels, since parasite counts have been shown not to differ significantly between patients with cerebral malaria and severe noncerebral malaria (e.g., Olweny et al., 1986). Macpherson et al. (1985) suggested endothelial pseudopodia served this function, while others, adopting a molecular approach, have incriminated such adhesion molecules as thrombospondin, CD36, and ICAM-1 (reviewed by Miller, 1989; Howard and Gilladoga, 1989). TNF is reported to increase production of both thrombospondin (Dunn et al., 1989) and ICAM-1 (Rothlein et al., 1988) by human endothelial cells, and the binding to these cells of erythrocytes parasitized by certain (but not all) strains of *P. falciparum* (Berendt et al., 1989), which these authors showed operates through ICAM-1. Thus the involvement of these molecules is consistent with adhesiveness of red cells increasing during clinical malaria, when TNF is circulating (Section IV.B). Of course, this theory of cerebral malaria requires preferential sequestration in the brain; we are no further ahead if such up-regulation of adhesion molecules, or the particular adhesiveness of a certain strain of *P. falciparum*, occurs throughout the vasculature rather than selectivity on endothelial cells in cerebral vessels. This question has yet to be addressed experimentally.

Another concern in implying that effective sequestration requires cytokines is to reconcile this with the adhesion of parasitized red cells in malaria-tolerant children, which evidently is no less avid than the adhesion in ill patients, since mature parasites are equally rare in the peripheral blood of both groups. Since their heavy parasite load is not making them ill, it seems most unlikely (Section V.A) that TNF or a functionally similar cytokine has much influence on events within their circulation. Thus red cell sequestration in these children has to be argued to operate through a different but equally efficient mechanism, one that restricts parasites to locations where they do not impede blood flow significantly. It is conceivable that cytokines preferentially up-regulate adhesion molecules in capillaries and small venules (particularly in the brain, for this process to cause cerebral malaria), and that sequestration in malaria-tolerant children, intense even without cytokines, is restricted to larger-diameter vessels.

The main dilemma with a mechanism of cerebral malaria that relies solely on blood flow being hindered is to reconcile it with the stroke literature and explain why nearly all patients who recover from cerebral malaria have no residual neurological deficit (Warrell et al., 1982), implying negligible cellular damage. Studies on the pathogenesis of strokes have indicated that cerebral infarction, and subsequent long-term loss of function, can occur if perfusion pressure to any part of the brain is 15 to 20 mmHg or less for a period of 20 to 30 min (reviewed by Adams, 1989). This would be compounded by the systemic hypotension that often accompanies cerebral malaria and was seen in over half of the cases studied by Macpherson et al, (1985). Thus it would be most surprising if a simple oligemic coma, perhaps lasting for several days (Kitchen, 1949), could routinely resolve with rapid and full return of neurological function. As proposed recently (Wyler, 1988; Clark et al., 1989b), this aspect of cerebral malaria is less of a difficulty when the direct effects of TNF on cerebral function (Section V.D.2.c) are taken into account. This also applies to the findings of Warrell et al. (1988), who found that cerebral blood flow and cerebral vascular resistance did not alter significantly when comatose malarial patients regained consciousness in response to treatment.

b. Serum TNF Levels in Human Cerebral Malaria. To date three groups have published TNF levels in serum from *P. falciparum*-infected patients showing various manifestations of disease, including cerebral malaria. As noted in Section IV.B, Grau et al. (1989b) found that high-serum TNF correlated with various disease parameters, but the data presented do not allow a conclusion to be drawn on whether those with cerebral symptoms had different TNF levels from the rest of their patients. Kern et al. (1989) found a strong correlation between multiple system dysfunction and serum TNF levels, whether or not cerebral malaria was one of the complications observed. Elevated serum TNF was associated with cerebral malaria in all 12 patients who developed this complication, but all except 2 of them had other complications as well. Hence the multiplicity of system involvement, rather than cerebral malaria alone, was associated with raised TNF levels. Similarly, in the studies of Kwiatkowski et al. (1989), those with cerebral symptoms did not have TNF levels that stood out from the values recorded for other patients with severe malaria. This is consistent with the outcome of clinical trials with rTNF, which produced a range of changes, including, at times, altered mental states (Section IV.A). These trials, combined with results of Kern et al. (1989), are consistent with cerebral malaria being part of TNF-induced multiorgan pathology with variable involvement rather than being singled out in the way that is possible with hypoglycemia (Grau et al., 1989b: Section V.B).

c. Direct Neurological Effects of TNF. Over the past few years TNF has been given to tumor patients in numerous clinical trials, providing an opportunity to examine the toxic effects of this cytokine in humans. As discussed in Section IV.A, a malaria-like syndrome is produced. The clinical picture is mild when compared to that seen in falciparum malaria, in keeping with the low doses given and the minimal serum TNF levels attained. These levels are much lower (Jakubowski et al., 1989; Wiedenmann et al., 1989) than those recorded in clinical malaria (Kern et al., 1989; Grau et al., 1989b) and sepsis (Waage et al., 1987; Girardin et al., 1988). The changes induced include severe headaches and altered mental states, typically the extreme lethargy that so often ushers in cerebral malaria (Spriggs et al., 1988; Sherman et al., 1988; Steinmetz et al., 1988). In some patients these changes can be severe enough to be dose-limiting. This type of alteration is also seen in patients receiving infusions of IL-2, a cytokine that induces TNF in patients (Mier et al., 1988). In one IL-2 study, 15 of 44 patients developed behavioral changes sufficiently severe to warrant acute intervention, and 22 had severe cognitive defects (Denicoff et al., 1987). We presume that if the TNF or IL-2 doses had been increased, such as to attain serum TNF levels seen in acute falciparum malaria and sepsis, all of the side effects, including those affecting the central nervous system, would have been correspondingly more severe, even though sequestered parasitized red cells were, of course, absent. As occurs in cerebral malaria, sepsis, and the coma associated with other acute systemic infections, the altered neurological function returned to normal once treatment with IL-2 or TNF ceased (Sherman et al., 1988; Spriggs et al., 1988).

The origin of these neurological effects of TNF has not yet been established. As in so many cytokine-induced effects, an interreactive network of mediators is undoubtedly also involved in the brain (reviewed by Bocci, 1988). TNF and IL-1 are implicated in the mechanism of slow-wave sleep (Shoham et al., 1987) and also act directly on the CNS to cause anorexia (Plata-Salaman et al., 1988), so there are precedents for these cytokines having direct, inhibitory effects on the brain. The influence of cytokines on neurophysiology is as yet little investigated. Recent studies by Ellison et al. (1990) have been directed at the effects of IL-2 infusion on the function of the cerebral vasculature in rats. Using a cranial window, they documented impaired ability of the pial arterioles to respond to vasomotor stimuli. Serum TNF was increased in these animals. As these authors note, this defect could compromise the ability of cerebral microvessels to regulate blood flow. Such studies could pave the way for a similar approach to cerebral malaria.

In summary, there is no doubt that parasitized red cells often adhere in the small blood vessels in brains of cerebral malaria patients, but their importance in the pathogenesis of this condition is not resolved. Even if this adherence can be shown to act more strongly in the brain (perhaps via TNF and the adhesion molecules it induces) so that parasitized red cells congregate especially in the cerebral vessels, and thus cause coma through cerebral ischemia, it is still most awkward to explain why residual neurological deficits are so rare on recovery. Proposing a direct effect of TNF, as seen in immunotherapy trials, removes this problem. This could act in part by reducing the vasomotor response of cerebral vessels (Ellison et al., 1990). The functional consequences of this reduction could be exacerbated if adhering red cells were obstructing the flow, but be physiologically manageable in vivax malaria, where these obstructions are lacking. In short, cytokines such as TNF may initiate cerebral malaria, and the condition may become fatal if appreciable sequestration or erythrocyte rosetting (Wahlgren et al., 1989) is concentrated in cerebral vessels. It should also be noted that Kern et al. (1989) reported much lower cytokine levels in vivax rather than falciparum malaria. This in itself, rather than the absence of adhering parasitized red cells in this infection, could go much of the way to explain why cerebral symptoms are much rarer in those infected with *P. vivax*.

E. Malarial Coagulopathy

Following older autopsy reports of thrombosis in falciparum malaria, Dennis et al. (1967) undertook a systematic study of coagulation pathways in this disease. They concluded that clotting factors were depleted, and provided evidence of decreased plasminogen activation. On these grounds they proposed that intravascular coagulation was an important contributor to the pathogenesis of severe malaria. Despite confirmatory reports in patients (Jaroonvesama, 1972; Edwards, 1980) and in monkeys (O'Leary et al., 1971) infected with *P. falciparum*, other authors found the phenomenon to be of little functional significance (Vreeken and Cremer-Goote, 1978; Phillips et al., 1986). The general consensus at present is that the coagulation cascade is indeed activated but does not often contribute to disease outcome (Pukrittanyakamee et al., 1989). These authors found that increased consumption of antithrombin III, indicating increased thrombin formation, was a sensitive indicator of disease severity.

Since there is now appreciable evidence that serum TNF increases as malarial illness worsens (Section IV.B), it is instructive to examine the influence that this could have on coagulation indices during the infection. The first detailed investigation of TNF and clotting was by Nawroth and Stern (1986), who reported that the procoagulant activity of endothelial cells was enhanced when they were cultured in the presence of TNF. More recently, Bauer et al. (1989) conducted a study of clotting pathways in 23 cancer patients receiving TNF infusions. Enhanced cleavage of prothrombin (forming thrombin) was documented by showing increases in plasma levels of F_{1+2} and protein C activation peptide. Decreased antithrombin levels implied increased throbin generation and raised plasma concentrations of fibrinopeptide A indicated increased proteolysis, by thrombin, of fibrinogen to fibrin and thus of clot formation. Although the activation of the coagulation cascade in malaria has not yet been studied in this detail, the most recent information (Pukrittanyakamee et al., 1989) is consistent with these changes shown to be induced by TNF.

Clotting is a dynamic process, influenced by the rate of fibrin degradation (by plasmin) as well as by its formation. Plasmin generation is controlled by serine proteases termed *plasminogen activators*, which are controlled, in turn, by two plasminogen activator inhibitors, PAI-1 and PAI-2. TNF has been reported to stimulate transcription of the genes for both PAI-1 and PAI-2 (Medcalf et al., 1988), and this in vitro evidence of increased protein production has now been confirmed in vivo (van Hinsbergh et al., 1988). This would lead to decreased plasminogen activation, as documented in malarial patients by Dennis et al. (1967).

In summary, both malaria and TNF infusion increase fibrin formation and decrease its rate of removal. Since both serum TNF (Kern et al., 1989) and activation of coagulation (Pukrittanyakamee et al., 1989) increase in parallel with disease severity in falciparum malaria, further studies on a possible causal link seem warranted. As a cautionary tale it should be noted that even though thrombocytopenia is common in human malaria (Dennis et al., 1967) and TNF infusion into tumor patients induces thrombocytopenia (Spriggs et al., 1988), Grau et al. (1988b) were unable to prevent platelet counts falling in *P. berghei* (ANKA strain)-infected mice by pretreating them with polyclonal anti-TNF antibody. Model differences may account for this outcome.

F. Dyserythropoiesis and Erythrophagocytosis

Anemia is synonymous with malaria. Because the parasite inhabits the red cell, which it must burst in order to propagate, the obvious initial conclusion was that this process was central to the fall in hematocrit seen in this disease. As reviewed in Clark and Tomlinson (1949), it was soon realized that the fall in erythrocyte numbers is out of proportion to the number of red cells parasitized and that other factors must contribute to this process. Phagocytosis of unparasitized red cells was recorded long ago in monkey (Taliaferro and Cannon, 1936) and human (Clark and Tomlinson, 1949) malaria, and for decades was regarded as sufficient explanation for this discrepancy. More recently, others have found dyserythropoiesis in the bone marrow of patients with falciparum malaria (Srichaikul et al., 1967; Abdalla et al., 1980; Dörmer et al., 1983) and stressed its contribution to malarial anemia.

Seeking an explanation for these changes, Wickramasinghe et al. (1987) conducted a light and electron microscopy study of bone marrow from patients with cerebral malaria. They saw an analogy with the Macpherson et al. (1985) concept of cerebral malaria and concluded that sequestration of parasitized red cells was probably causing the bone marrow dysfunction by restricting blood flow and thus inducing hypoxic changes. This explanation proved inadequate, however, when dyserythropoiesis and erythrophagocytosis were observed (Wickramasinghe et al., 1989) in vivax malaria, in which the microvasculature is not obstructed by parasitized red cells.

Following the lead of Shah et al. (1978) in their studies of endotoxicity, we proposed that TNF might be the cause of the bone narrow depression seen in malaria (Clark et al., 1981). Subsequently Sassa et al. (1983) reported than an undefined monokine, later identified as TNF (Beutler et al., 1985), would inhibit the growth and differentiation of erythroid progenitor cells in vitro. Several years later, when rTNF became available, it was shown to inhibit proliferation of hemopoietic cells in culture (Peetre et al., 1986). The following year we found that among the changes rTNF could induce prematurely in malaria-infected mice were dyserythropoiesis and erythrophagocytosis (Clark and Chaudhri, 1988b). We commonly observed phagocytosis of erythroblasts, a phenomenon also reported by Wickramasinghe et al. (1987, 1989) in human malaria. Subsequent experiments by Johnson et al. (1989) showed that erthropoiesis was inhibited in nude mice in which were grafted cells expressing the human TNF gene. The decreased erythrocyte synthesis and reduced erythrocyte life span found in these studies are consistent with the dyserythropoiesis and erythrophagocytosis discussed above.

A definitive series of experiments on the role of TNF in malarial anemia were conducted by Miller et al. (1989), who compared erythropoiesis in infected and normal mice receiving continuous TNF infusions via implanted osmotic pumps. In both groups of mice they observed a reduction in erythroid progenitor cells and a reduced incorporation of ^{59}Fe into erythrocytes. When malaria-infected mice were given neutralizing antiserum raised against mouse TNF, both erythropoiesis and ^{59}Fe incorporation were increased significantly.

A further compelling, though indirect argument for a central role for cytokines such as TNF in malarial anemia can be derived by making species comparisons. Mice are innately much more tolerant to both malaria and TNF (Clark et al., 1987c) than are human subjects, and also, evidently, to whatever it is that causes malarial anemia: patients can become anemic with a parasite load less than one thousandth of that required for onset of anemia in mice (Phillips et al., 1986). These authors also note that patients with concomitant sepsis have a more severe malarial anemia, an observation consistent with the synergistic activity of LPS and TNF (Rothstein and Schreiber, 1988). Furthermore, Phillips et al. (1986) found anemia to be worse in patients with severe complicated malaria, and it is these that have the highest serum TNF levels (Kern et al., 1989; Grau et al., 1989b). The low serum iron and high serum ferritin recorded by Phillips et al. (1986) in anemic malaria patients also could be expected to accompany TNF-induced anemia, since TNF infusion has been found to reduce serum iron concentrations in tumor patients (Michie et al., 1988), and TNF induces expression of the gene for ferritin heavy-chain production (Torti et al., 1988).

G. Fetal Death in Malaria

A high incidence of intrauterine death, abortion, and premature labor occurs in falciparum malaria. Torpin (1941), for instance, recorded a 60% fetal mortality in his series of patients. The sinusoids of the placenta are found to be crowded with parasitized red cells, and placental pathology, including perivillous fibroid deposits and thickening of the basal lamina of the trophoblast, are seen (Walter et al., 1982). Quinine treatment has been suggested and discarded as a cause of these changes (reviewed by Warrell, 1987). There is at present no consensus on what causes fetal death in malaria, but current evidence, in experimental malaria as well as the broader literature, points to an involvement of TNF.

If an overproduction of monokines, particularly TNF, did indeed cause the illness and tissue damage seen in endotoxicity and malaria (Clark et al., 1981; Clark, 1982a), it seemed reasonable that TNF might initiate the fetal death seen in both endotoxicity (Zahl and Bjerkines, 1943) and malaria. Accordingly, we injected a small dose of human TNF into 16-day pregnant mice. These animals had been made sensitive to this cytokine by either low load infection with *P. vinckei* or by intravenous extract of *Coxiella burneti* given 10 days earlier. Some fetal death occurred with a TNF dose as low as 1.5 μg, per mouse, and the lowest amount to cause the loss of all fetuses was 4 μg (Clark and Chaudhri, 1988a). This dose was insufficient to cause more than a transient illness in the female mice. Some fetuses were expelled alive, but most were dead. Others were dead in utero, with detached placental disks. *P. vinckei* infections were then initiated in other pregnant mice, and timed so that when malaria would be expected to soon make them ill (about 70% of their red cells containing parasites) 16 to 17 days of their 21-day gestational period had elapsed. When the first signs of impending abortion were evident, these mice were bled for serum TNF assays, and dissected. As shown in Table 3, almost all of the fetuses were dead, and serum TNF levels had reached 1.6 ng/ml. TNF was not detectable in unparasitized mice, or others with lower parasite loads, when they were at the same stage of pregnancy (Table 3).

Evidence that implicates TNF in the onset of human infection-induced preterm labor has since come from several sources. Whereas normal human third-trimester amniotic fluid has been shown to contain, on average, 0.9 ng TNF/ml (Jäättelä et al., 1988), considerably higher levels have been recorded in pregnancies complicated by infection and subsequent preterm onset of labor (Casey et al., 1988; Romero et al., 1989). We can find no information on whether the malarial antigens that can trigger TNF release, or TNF itself, can cross into the amniotic fluid. However, the outcome of our mouse malaria experiments (Clark and Chaudhri, 1988a), combined with the foregoing studies on patients, make it reasonable to predict that the fetal loss seen in pregnancies complicated by malaria are causally associated with high levels of circulating TNF. From the work of Grau et al. (1989b) and Kern et al. (1989) TNF can be expected to be elevated in the plasma of these women.

TNF could cause fetal death in several ways. One possibility is through IL-6-induced inhibition of hepatic gluconeogenesis (Section V.B), and thus maternal hypoglycemia, to which the fetus is very susceptible (reviewed by Phillips, 1989). It is also feasible that the fetus may be harmed by TNF retarding growth of the trophoblast, as has been suggested to occur in sepsis by Hunt et al. (1989) on the basis of their finding that TNF was highly inhibitory to DNA synthesis by trophoblast cells. Another possibility, not mutually exclusive of the others, is that TNF may operate through its capacity to induce release of prostaglandins (which

Table 3. TNF in Malaria-Induced Abortion in Mice

(a) TNF-induced abortion

Experiment number	Parasitemia	*n*	TNF dose (μg)	Outcome[a]
1	1–5	7	5	40/47
2	1–15	5	4–5	21/26
3	15–20	4	1.5–2.5	13/25

[a]Proportion of fetuses found dead in utero or expelled 24 h after injection of TNF.

(b) Endogenous plasma TNF levels at time of malaria-induced abortion

Day of pregnancy	Number of mice	Parasitemia %	Plasma TNF levels (ng/ml)	Condition of fetuses
16	8	0	0	All alive
16	6	20–30	0	All alive
17	7	0	0	All alive
17	14[b]	68–87	1.6 ± 0.9	95/97 dead

Source: Clark and Chaudhri, 1988a. Reproduced with permission from *American Journal of Tropical Medicine and Hygiene*.

[b]These mice were bled for TNF assay when the first signs of impending abortion were evident.

Table 4. Indomethacin Delays TNF-Induced Fetal Death in Mice Carrying a Low Density of *P. vinckei*

Group	Number of Mice	Treatment	Time post TNF injection (h)
			2 4 6 8 10 12 14 16 18 20 22 24 →
1	15	60 mg/kg indomethacin + 7.5 μg rTNF	→ Abortion (at 20–24 h)
2	10	Olive oil + 7.5 μg rTNF	→ Abortion (at 8–12 h)
3	5	Indomethacin + saline	→ Remained well and showed no change

Source: S. Andrews, B.Sc. Honours Thesis, Australian National University, 1988.

mediate myometrial contractions) from a number of cell types, including those of the intrauterine tissues (Casey et al., 1989; Romero et al., 1989). This is consistent with our group's findings that a single injection of indomethacin delayed the fetal loss caused by exogenous TNF (Table 4). All of these principles are open to further testing, in other infectious diseases associated with both abortion and the likelihood of TNF generation, as well as in malaria. Listeriosis and brucellosis are obvious examples.

As Jäättelä et al. (1988) discuss, TNF could well have various physiological functions in normal pregnancy and labor, just as it does in the normal immune response. As in much of the other pathology caused by this cytokine, the fetal death associated with TNF may therefore be viewed as another example of a cytokine, above normal limits, exceeding its physiological functions and causing pathology.

VI. TNF AND NONMALARIAL PARASITES

Compared to the attention given to TNF and malaria, interest in TNF and other parasitic infections is in its infancy. A few groups have become interested in the possibility of an antiparasitic role for this cytokine in protozoan diseases other than malaria, and still fewer, as yet, are examining whether TNF has a role in protection against larger parasitic organisms. This work is reviewed below.

A. Protective Effects of TNF Against Parasites

1. *Protozoans Other Than* Plasmodium *sp.*

The first group to examine whether TNF might have a role in host resistance against protozoans other than malaria (De Titto et al., 1986), found that recombinant human TNF inhibited in vitro intracellular multiplication of blood forms of *Trypanosoma cruzi*, a South American flagellate, in murine macrophages. Extracellular *T. cruzi* and intracellular *Toxoplasma gondii* were unaffected, as were *T. cruzi* inside human fibroblasts. This group subsequently showed that TNF would protect mice against either of these parasites (Black et al., 1989), a finding that parallels the outcome of experiments with malaria (Section III.A). As also found earlier with malaria (Section IV.A), mice infected with either *T. cruzi* or *T. gondii* were much more sensitive to the effects of TNF than were normal mice. The in vivo activity against *T. gondii* was soon confirmed by Chang et al. (1990), who reported that IL-1, alone or in synergy with TNF, would also protect mice. Furthermore, *T. gondii* proved to prime mice to an endotoxin-induced increase in TNF, as does *P. vinckei* (Clark et al., 1981).

The central question still unanswered is whether material from *T. cruzi* or *T. gondii* can trigger TNF release from macrophages, as Bate et al. (1988, 1989) and Taverne et al. (1990) have documented for *Plasmodium* sp. The closest approach to this problem has been by Hotez et al. (1984), who found that a lysate of *Trypanosoma brucei*, an African species, would cause macrophages to release a mediator with the capacity to suppress lipoprotein lipase in preadipocytes. This activity was later ascribed to TNF. The nature of the TNF trigger in *T. brucei* warrants careful reexamination, rigorously excluding the effects of contaminant endotoxin, as the malaria workers (e.g., Taverne et al. 1990) have done, and using an antibody-based assay for cytokine detection. This approach could be expanded to include other trypanosomes and *T. gondii*. Should the answers prove as clear-cut as for malaria (Section IV.C), the case for involvement of TNF and other cytokines in host resistance to these genera of parasites will have been strengthened considerably.

A more direct approach is to see if passively administered anti-TNF neutralizing antibody influences the course of the infection. This has recently been done by Titus et al. (1989), who found that mice given anti-TNF had exacerbated lesions of cutaneous leishmaniasis (caused by *Leishmania major*), and more parasites within those lesions. Liew et al. (1990) have recently developed these arguments further. It is not yet known whether the trigger for the TNF neutralized by these antibodies was of *Leishmania* origin, but this seems a reasonable prediction and warrants investigation. These authors also reported that treating infected mice with exogenous TNF reduced lesion size and parasite content.

The more pathogenic *Leishmania* parasite, *L. donovani*, which causes visceral leishmaniasis (Kala-azar), appears to have evolved mechanisms that ensure its survival within macrophages. One possibility is an impaired capacity for *L. donovani*–

infected macrophages to generate TNF, as Descoteaux and Matlashewski (1989) have recently demonstrated. This was argued at the level of selectively reduced gene expression, and shown not to be a general impairment of all signal transduction pathways in infected cells.

The other protozoan organism investigated in this context is *Entamoeba histolytica*, a human gut parasite that causes invasive amebiasis in tropical countries. In combination with IFN-γ, TNF has been shown to endow murine macrophages (Denis and Chadee, 1989a) and human neutrophils (Denis and Chadee, 1989b) with the capacity to kill *E. histolytica* trophozoites in vitro. In the case of macrophages, colony-stimulating factor-1 was synergistic with the other cytokines.

2. *Multicellular Parasites*

The possible involvement of TNF in protection against these more complex parasites has been even less closely studied. Dammoneville et al. (1988) have reported that TNFβ, and to a lesser extent TNFα, can, in the presence of IFN-γ, instruct normal platelets to kill larvae of *Schistosoma mansoni*. *S. mansoni* antigens were able to induce $CD4^+$ T cells to release these cytokines. In addition, a role for TNF in the phenomenon of host-induced expulsion of adult nematodes from the small intestine has recently been reasoned by Smith (1989) using the model *Nippostrongylus brasiliensis* in the rat.

B. TNF and Pathology of Nonmalarial Parasite Infections

Again, this field has been reasoned through, but little studied. Clark (1978) and Wright et al. (1988) have outlined the case of TNF involvement in babesiosis, largely because *Babesia* sp. sensitizes animals to endotoxin, and bovine babesiosis has striking parallels to human malaria. Similarly, *Babesia rhodaini* produces a syndrome in mice that is indistinguishable, apart from the absence of malarial pigment, to that caused by *P. vinckei*. To our knowledge the only experimental information linking TNF and *Babesia* sp. is a report that *Babesia microti*, like *P. vinckei*, primes mice for endotoxin-induced release of TNF (Wood and Clark, 1984). It has also been pointed out that the innate tolerance of a host species to endotoxicity correlates with the load of *Babesia* sp. parasites required to cause onset of clinical illness (Clark, 1982b). This relationship must exist if the mediators of endotoxicity (of which TNF is the key component) play a central role in the pathogenesis of illness in babesiosis, as suggested earlier (Clark, 1978).

This same relationship between parasite load at the time of illness and innate sensitivity to endotoxicity was noted to exist for African trypanosomes and its various host species (Clark, 1978). Thus our group predicted that these parasites, along with those that cause malaria and babesiosis, generate host illness by inducing host macrophages to release a range of mediators, including TNF (Clark, 1978). Several years later, when investigating the origins of the lipoprotein lipase suppression associated with *Trypanosoma brucei* infections, Kawakami and Cerami (1981) found it to be mediated by a macrophage product that later proved to be identical to TNF (Beutler et al., 1985). This group subsequently found this monokine, then defined only by its capacity to inhibit enzymes associated with lipid metabolism, to be triggered, in vitro, by a lysate of *T. brucei* (Hotez et al., 1984). They argued a role for this mediator in the cachexia of African tryopanosomiasis. Thus the time seems ripe to use the developments that have taken place in malaria and TNF to investigate further the host injury caused by *Trypanosoma* sp.

Despite the capacity of *L. donovani* to impair the ability of the macrophages it infects to produce TNF (Descoteaux and Matlashewski, 1989), the output of this cytokine in Kala-azar patients, at least in terms of serum levels (Scuderi et al., 1986), is increased. Conceivably, this arises from the large increase in macrophage numbers that occurs in this disease (reviewed by Maegraith, 1976). Indirect evidence consistent with TNF being involved in the origins of Kala-azar comes from its close clinical similarity to certain forms of malaria, from which it be distinguished only with care (Kitchen, 1949).

Ovington (1987) and Smith (1989) appear to be the first authors to draw attention to how many of the pathophysiological changes that occur in the host during nematode infection could reasonably be explained by invoking cytokines, particularly TNF and IFN-γ. As reviewed by these authors, these changes include anorexia, cachexia, altered protein, carbohydrate and lipid metabolism, increased prostaglandin production, and the presence of acute phase proteins in the serum. There seems little doubt that knowledge of these aspects of the effects of parasite nematodes on the host is set to expand.

VII. SUMMARY

Comprehension of the involvement of cytokines in the host response against invading parasites, to the detriment of the parasite and (in larger doses) to the host, is expanding rapidly. Most of these studies, largely for historic reasons and availability, have been done with TNF rather than the other mediators. As is emerging in other fields, study of interleukin-1 alone, and synergistically with TNF and IFN-γ, warrants further exploration in parasitic diseases. There may well be a similar story for TNF-β, waiting to unfold.

It is appropriate here to show deference to earlier malariologists, back to the nineteenth century, whose observations and reasoning were evidently accurate when they attributed malarial illness and pathology (including cerebral malaria) to a malarial toxin (reviewed by Clark and Tomlinson, 1949). The only additional insight required of present-day workers has been to see the malaria parasite not as a source of a direct toxin, but of molecules, harmless in themselves, that can act as a trigger for toxic products of host origin. As a final twist, low concentrations of these host-derived "toxins" are not only harmless, but necessary for normal biological functions. They are deleterious only when overproduced.

ACKNOWLEDGMENTS

Our laboratory is supported by the malaria component of the UNDP/World Bank/WHO Special Programme for Research and Training in Tropical Diseases, the National Health and Medical Research Council of Australia, and Peptide Technology Ltd., Sydney. We are also indebted to Peptide Technology Ltd. for supply of anti-TNF antibodies, and to the Asahi Chemical Company, Tokyo, for supplies of human rTNF. We thank Kylie Place for invaluable technical support.

REFERENCES

Abdalla, S., Weatherall, D.J., Wickramasinghe, S. N., and Hughes, M. (1980). The anaemia of *P. falciparum* malaria, *Br. J. Haematol., 46*: 171.

Adams, J. H. (1989). Cerebral infarction: its pathogenesis and interpretation, *J. Pathol., 157*: 281.

Bate, C. A. W., Taverne, J., and Playfair, J. H. L. (1988). Malarial parasites induce TNF production by macrophages, *Immunology, 64*: 227.

Bate, C. A. W. Taverne, J., and Playfair, J. H. L. (1989). Soluble malarial antigens are toxic and induce the production of tumor necrosis factor in vivo, *Immunology, 66*: 600.

Bauer, K. A., Cate, H. T., Barzeger, S., Spriggs, D. R., Sherman, M. L., and Rosenberg, R. D. (1989). Tumor necrosis factor infusions have a procoagulant effect on the hemostatic mechanisms of humans, *Blood, 74*: 165.

Berendt, A. R., Simmons, D. L., Tansey, J., Newbold, C. I., and Marsh, K. (1989). Intercellular adhesion molecule-1 is an endothelial cell adhesion receptor for *Plasmodium falciparum, Nature, 341*: 57.

Beutler, B., Greenwald, D., Hulmes, J. D., Chang, M., Pan, Y. -C., Mathison, J., Ulevitch, R., and Cerami, A. (1985). Identity of tumor necrosis factor and the macrophage-secreted factor cachectin, *Nature, 31*: 552.

Black, C M., Israelski, D. M., Suzuki, Y., and Remington, J. S. (1989). Effect of recombinant tumor necrosis factor on acute infection in mice with *Toxoplasma gondii* or *Trypanosoma cruzi, Immunology, 68*: 570.

Bocci, V. (1988). Central nervous system toxicity of interferons and other cytokines, *J. Biol. Regul. Homeostatic Agents,* 2: 107.

Brouckaert, P., Spriggs, D. R., Demetri, G., Kufe, D. W., and Fiers, W. (1989). Circulating interleukin 6 during a continuous infusion of tumor necrosis factor and interferon-γ, *J. Exp. Med., 169*: 2257.

Buffinton, G. D., Hunt, N. H., Cowden, W. B., and Clark, I. A. (1988). Detection of short-chain carbonyl products of lipid peroxidation from malaria parasite (*Plasmodium vinckei*)-infected red blood cells exposed to oxidative stress, *Biochem. J., 249*: 63.

Butcher, G. A., Garland, T., Ajdukiewicz, A. B., and Clark, I. A. (1990). Plasma TNF associated with malaria in patients in the Solomon Islands, *Trans. R. Soc. Trop. Med. Hyg. 84*: 658.

Carswell, E. A., Old, L. J., Kassel, R. L., Green, S., Fiore, N., and Williamson, B. (1975). An endotoxin-induced serum factor that causes necrosis of tumors, *Proc. Natl. Acad. Sci. USA, 72*: 3666.

Casey, M. L., Cox, S. M., Beutler, B., Milewich, L., and MacDonald, P. C. (1988). Cachectin/tumor necrosis factor-α formation in human decidua, *J. Clin. Invest., 83*: 430.

Cavacini, L. A, Guidotti, M., Parke, L. A., Melancon-Kaplan, J., and Weidanz, W. P. (1989). Reassessment of the role of splenic leukocyte oxidative activity and macrophage activation in expression of immunity to malaria, *Infect. Immun., 57*: 3677.

Chang, H. R., Grau, G. E., and Perchere, J. C. (1990). Role of TNF and IL-1 in infections with *Toxoplasma gondii, Immunology, 69*: 33.

Clark, H. C., and Tomlinson, W. J. (1949). The pathologic anatomy of malaria, *Malariology*, Vol. 2, (M. F. Boyd, ed.), W. B. Saunders, Philadelphia, p. 874.

Clark, I. A. (1978). Does endotoxin cause both the disease and parasite death in acute malaria and babesiosis? *Lancet, ii*: 75.

Clark, I. A., Virelizier, J. L., Carswell, E. A. and Wood, P. R. (1981). Possible importance of macrophage-derived mediators in acute malaria, *Infect. Immun., 32*: 1058.

Clark, I. A. (1982a). Suggested importance of monokines in pathophysiology of endotoxin shock and malaria, *Klin. Wochenschr., 60*: 756.

Clark, I. A. (1982b). Correlation between susceptibility to malaria and babesia parasites and to endotoxin, *Trans. R. soc. Trop. Med. Hyg., 76*: 4.

Clark, I. A., and Chaudhri, G. (1988a). Tumor necrosis factor in malaria-induced abortion, *Am. J. Trop. Med. Hyg., 39*: 246.

Clark, I. A., and Chaudhri, G. (1988b). Tumor necrosis factor may contribute to the anaemia of malaria by causing dyserythropoiesis and erythrophagocytosis, *Brit. J. Haematol., 70*: 99.

Clark, I. A., Hunt, N. H., Butcher, G. A., and Cowden, W. B. (1987a). Inhibition of murine malaria (*Plasmodium chabaudi*) *in vivo* by recombinant interferon-γ or tumor necrosis factor, and its enhancement by butylated hydroxyanisole, *J. Immunol., 139*: 3493.

Clark, I. A., Butcher, G. A., Buffinton, G. D., Hunt, N. H., and Cowden, W. B. (1987b). Toxicity of certain products of lipid peroxidation to the human malaria parasite *Plasmodium falciparum, Biochem. Pharmacol., 36*: 543.

Clark, I. A., Cowden, W. B., Butcher, G. A., and Hunt, N. H., (1987c). Possible roles of tumor necrosis factor in the pathology of malaria, *Am. J. Pathol., 129*: 192.

Clark, I. A., Hunt, N. H., and Cowden, W. B. (1987d). Immunopathology of malaria, *Immune Responses in Parasitic Infections* (E. J. L. Soulsby, ed.), CRC Press, Boca Raton, Fla., p. 1.

Clark, I. A., Chaudhri, G., and Cowden, W. B. (1989a). Some roles of free radicals in malaria, *Free Radical Biol. Med., 6:* 315.

Clark, I. A., Chaudhri, G., and Cowden, W. B. (1989b). Roles of tumour necrosis factor in the illness and pathology of malaria, *Trans. R. Soc. Trop. Med. Hyg., 83*: 436.

Collins, T., Lapierre, L. A., Fiers, W., Strominger, J. L., and Pober, J. S. (1986). Recombinant human tumor necrosis factor increases mRNA levels and surface expression of HLA-A,B antigens in vascular endothelial cells and dermal fibroblasts *in vitro, Proc. Natl Acad. Sci. USA, 83*: 446.

Cotran, R. S. (1987). New roles of the endothelium in inflammation and immunity, *Am. J. Pathol., 129*: 407.

Creagan, E. T., Kovach, J. S., Moertel, C. G., Frytak, S., and Kvols, L. K. (1988). A phase 1 clinical trial of recombinant human tumor necrosis factor, *Cancer, 62*: 2467.

Dammoneville, M., Wietzerbin, J., Pancre, V., Delanoye, A., Capron, A., and Auriault, C. (1988). Recombinant tumor necrosis factors mediate platelet cytotoxicity to *Schistosoma mansoni* larvae, *J. Immunol., 140*: 3962.

Denicoff, K. D., Rubinow, D. R., Papa, M. Z., Simpson, C., Seipp, C. A., Lotze, M. T., Chang, A. E., Rosenstein, D., and Rosenberg, S. A. (1987). The neuropsychiatric effects of treatment with interleukin-2 and lymphokine-activated killer cells, *Ann. Intern. Med., 107*: 293.

Denis, M., and Chadee, K. (1989a). Cytokine activation of murine macrophages for in vitro killing of *Entamoeba histolytica* trophozoites, *Infect. Immun., 57*: 1750.

Denis, M., and Chadee, K. (1989b). Human neutrophils activated by interferon-γ and tumour necrosis factor-α kill *Entamoeba histolytica* in vitro, *J. Leukoctyte Biol., 46*: 270.

Dennis, L. H., Eichelberger, J. W., Inman, M. M., and Conrad, M. E. (1967). Depletion of coagulation factors in drug-resistant *Plasmodium falciparum* malaria, *Blood, 29*: 713.

Descoteaux, A., and Matlashewski, G. (1989). *c-fos* and tumor necrosis factor gene expression in *Leishmania donovani*-infected macrophages, *Mol. Cell. Biol., 9*: 5223.

De Titto, E. H., Caterall, J. R., and Remington, J. S. (1986). Activity of recombinant tumor necrosis factor on *Toxoplasma gondii* and *Trypanosoma cruzi, J. Immunol., 137*: 1342.

Diehl, V., Pfreundschuh, M., Steinmetz, H. T., and Schaadt., M. (1988). Phase 1 studies of recombinant human tumor necrosis factor in patients with malignant disease, *Tumor Necrosis Factor/Cachectin and Related Cytokines* (B. Bonavida, G. E. Gifford, H. Kirchner, and L. J. Old, eds.), S. Karger, Basel, p. 183.

Dörmer, P., Dietrich, M., Kern, P., and Horstmann, R. D. (1983). Ineffective erythropoiesis in acute human *P. falciparum* malaria, *Blut, 46*: 279.

Dunn, S. M., Hillman, A. J., Stomski, F., Jin, B., Lucas, C. M., Boyd, A. W., Krissansen, G. W., and Burns, G. F. (1989). Leukocyte adhesion molecules involved in inflammation, *Transplant. Proc., 21*: 31.

Edwards, I. R. (1980). Malaria with disseminated intravascular coagulation and peripheral tissue necrosis successfully treated with streptokinase, *Br. Med. J., 1*: 1252.

Ellison, M. D., Krieg, R. J., and Merchant, R. E. (1990). Cerebral vasomotor responses after recombinant interleukin-2 infusion,*Cancer Res., 50*: 4377..

Feingold, K. R., Soued, M., and Grunfeld, C. (1988). Tumor necrosis factor stimulates DNA synthesis in the liver of intact rats, *Biochem. Biophys. Res. Commun., 153*: 576.

Ferreira, A., Schofield, L., Enea, V., Schellekens, H., van der Meide, P., Collins, W. E., Nussenzweig, R. S., and Nussenzweig, V. (1986). Inhibition of development of exoerythrocytic forms of malaria parasites by γ-interferon, *Science, 232*: 881.

Finley, R. W., Mackey, L. J., and Lambert, P. -H. (1982). Virulent *P. berghei* malaria: prolonged survival and decreased cerebral pathology in cell-deficient nude mice, *J. Immunol., 129*: 2213.

Fraker, D. L., Stovroff, M. C., Merino, M. J., and Norton, J. A. (1988). Tolerance to tumor necrosis in rats and the relationship to endotoxin tolerance and toxicity, *J. Exp. Med., 168*: 95.

Girardin, E., Grau, G. E., Dayer, J. -M., Roux-Lombard, P., and Lambert, P-H. (1988). Tumor necrosis factor and interleukin-1 in the serum of children with severe infectious purpura, *N. Engl. J. Med., 319*: 397.

Golgi, C. (1889). Reprinted in: B. H. Kean, K. E. Mott, and A. J. Russell, eds. (1978). *Tropical Medicine and Parasitology Classic Investigations,* Vol. 1 Cornell University Press, Ithaca, N.Y., p. 26.

Grau, G. E., Piquet, P. F., Engers, H. D., Louis, J. A., Vassalli, P., and Lambert, P. H. (1986). $L3T4^{+}$ T lymphocytes play a major role in the pathogenesis of murine cerebral malaria, *J. Immunol., 137*: 2348.

Grau, G. E., Gretener, D., and Lambert, P. H. (1987a). Prevention of murine cerebral malaria by low-dose cyclosporin A, *Immunology, 61*: 521.

Grau, G. E., Fajardo, L. F., Piquet, P. F., Allet, B., Lambert, P. H., and Vassali, P. (1987b). Tumor necrosis factor (cachectin) as an essential mediator in murine cerebral malaria, *Science, 237*: 1210.

Grau, G. E., Kindler, V., Piquet, P. F., Lambert, P. H., and Vassalli, P. (1988a). Prevention of experimental cerebral malaria by anticytokine antibodies: interleukin 3 and granulocyte macrophage colony-stimulating factor are intermediates in increased tumor necrosis factor production and macrophage accumulation, *J. Exp. Med., 168*: 1499.

Grau, G. E., Piquet, P. F., Gretener, D., Vesin, C., and Lambert, P. H. (1988b). Immunopathology of thrombocytopenia in experimental malaria, *Immunology, 65*: 501.

Grau, g. E., Piquet, P. F., Vassalli, P., and Lambert, P. -H. (1989). Tumor necrosis factor and other cytokines in cerebral malaria: experimental and clinical data, *Immunol. Rev., 112*: 49.

Grau, G. E., Taylor, T. E., Molyneux, M. E., Wirima, J. J., Vassali, P., Hommel, M., and Lambert, P. -H. (1989b). Tumor necrosis factor and disease severity in children with falciparum malaria, *N. Engl. J. Med., 320*: 1586.

Grau, G. E., Heremans, H., Piquet, P. F., Piontaire, P., Lambert, P. H., Billiau, a., and Vassalli, P. (1989c). Monoclonal antibody against interferon γ can prevent experimental cerebral malaria and its associated overproduction of tumor necrosis factor, *Proc. Natl. Acad. Sci. USA, 86*: 5572.

Grau, G. E., Kindler, V., Piquet, P. F., Lambert, P. H., and Vassalli, P. (1989d). Involvement of tumor necrosis factor and other cytokines in immune-mediated vascular pathology, *Int. Arch. Allergy Appl. Immunol., 88*: 34.

Greenwood, B. M., Oduloju, A. J., and Platts-Mills, T. A. E. (1979). Partial characterization of a malaria mitogen, *Trans. R. Soc. Trop. Med. Hyg., 73*: 178.

Griffith, T., and Randall, M. (1989). Nitric oxide comes of age, *Lancet, ii*: 875.

Haidaris, c. G., Haynes, J. D., Meltzer, M. S., and Allison, A. C. (1983). Serum containing tumor necrosis factor is cytotoxic for the human malarial parasite *Plasmodium falciparum, Infect. Immun., 42*: 385.

Hersh, E. M., Schwartz, J., and Scuderi, P. (1987). Phase 1 study of tumor necrosis factor (TNF) administered by continuous intravenous infusion to cancer patients, *Immunobiology, 175*: 94.

Hill, M. R. Stith, R. D., and McCallum, R. E. (1989). Mechanism of action of interferon-β2 interlukin-6 on induction of hepatic liver enzymes. *Ann. N.Y. Acad. Sci., 557*: 502.

Hill, M. R., Stith, R. D., and McCallum, R. E. (1986). Interleukin-1: a regulatory role in glucorticoid-regulated hepatic metabolism, *J. Immunol., 137*: 858.

Hirano, T., Taga, T., Yasukawa, K., Nakajima, N., Takatsuki, F., Shimizu, M., Murashima,

A., Tsunasawa, S., Sakiyama, F., and Kishimoto, T. (1987). Human B-cell differentiation factor defined by an anti-peptide antibody and its possible role in autoantibody production, *Proc. Natl Acad. Sci. USA, 84*: 228.

Hoffman, S. L., Isenberger, D., Long, G. W., Sedegah, M., Szarfman, A., Waters, L., Hollingdale, M. R., van der Meide, P. H., Finbloom, D. S., and Ballou, W. R. (1989). Sporozoite vaccine induces genetically restricted T cell elimination of malaria from hepatocytes, *Science, 244*: 1078.

Hotez, P. J., Le Trang, N., Fairlamb, A. H., and Cerami, A. (1984). Lipoprotein lipase suppression in 3T3-LI cells by a haemoprotozoan-induced mediator from peritoneal exudate cells, *Parasite Immunol., 6*: 203.

Howard, R. J., and Gilladoga, A. D. (1989). Molecular studies related to the pathogenesis of cerebral malaria, *Blood, 74*: 2603.

Hughes, C. C. W., Male, D. K., and Lantos, P. L. (1988). Adhesion of lymphocytes to cerebral microvascular cells: effects of interferon-γ, tumour necrosis factor and interleukin-1, *Immunology, 64*: 677.

Hunt, J. S., Soares, M. J., Lei, M. -G., Smith, R. N., Wheaton, D., Atherton, R. A., and Morrison, D. C. (1989). Products of lipopolysacharide-activated macrophages (tumor necrosis factor-α, transforming growth factor-β) but not lipopolysaccharide modify DNA synthesis by rat trophoblast cells exhibiting the 80-kDa lipopolysaccharide binding protein, *J. Immunol., 143*: 1606.

Jäättelä, M., Kuusela, P., and Saksela, E. (1988). Demonstration of tumor necrosis factor in human amniotic fluids and supernatants of placental and decidual tissues, *Lab. Invest., 58*: 48.

Jakobsen, P. H., Baek, L., and Jepsen, S. (1988). Demonstration of soluble *Plasmodium falciparum* antigens reactive with *Limulus* amoebocyte lysate and polymyxin B, *Parasite Immunol., 10*: 593.

Jakubowski, A. A., Casper, E. S., Gabrilove, J. L., Templeton, M. A., Sherwin, S. A., and Oettgen, H. F. (1989). Phase 1 trial of intramuscularly administered tumor necrosis factor in patients with advanced cancer, *J. Clin. Oncol., 7*: 298.

Jaroonvesama, N. (1972). Intravascular coagulation in falciparum malaria, *Lancet, i*: 221.

Jensen, J. B., Vande Waa, J. A., and Karadsheh, A. J. (1987). Tumor necrosis factor does not induce *Plasmodium falciparum* crisis forms, *Infect. Immun., 55*: 1722.

Jervis, R. H., Sprinz, H., Johnson, A. J., and Wellde, B. T. (1972). Experimental infection with *Plasmodium falciparum* in *Aotus* monkeys, *Am. J. Trop. Med. Hyg., 21*: 272.

Johnson, R. A., Waddelow, T. A., Caro, J., Oliff, A., and Roodman, G. D. (1989). Chronic exposure to tumor necrosis factor in vivo preferentially inhibits erythropoiesis in nude mice, *Blood, 74*: 130.

Kahn, J., and Barton, R. W. (1989). Selective suppression of TNF-induced ICAM-1 expression by cyclosporin A (CsA), *J. Leukocyte Biol., 46*: 340.

Kataaha, P. K., Facer, C. A., Mortazavi-Milani, S. M., Stierle, H., and Holborow, E. J. (1984). Stimulation of autoantibody production in normal blood lymphocytes by malaria culture supernatants, *Parasite Immunol., 6*: 481.

Kawakami, M., and Cerami, A. (1981). Studies of endotoxin-induced decrease in lipoprotein lipase activity, *J. Exp. Med., 154*: 631.

Kean, B. H., and Smith, J. A. (1944). Death due to estivo-autumnal malaria: a résumé of one hundred autopsy cases, 1925–1942, *Am. J. Med., 24*: 317.

Kern, P., Hemmer, C. J., Van Damme, J., Gruss, H. -J., and Dietrich, M. (1989). Elevated tumour necrosis factor alpha and interleukin-6 serum levels as markers for complicated *Plasmodium falciparum* malaria, *Am. J. Med., 87*: 139.

Kharazami, A., Jepson, S., and Valerius, N. H. (1984). Polymorphonuclear leukocytes defective in oxidative metabolism inhibit in vitro growth of *Plasmodium falciparum*: evidence against an oxygen dependent mechanism, *Scand. J. Immunol., 20*: 93.

Kishimoto, T. and Hirano, T. (1988). Molecular regulation of B lymphocytes response, *Annu. Rev. Immunol., 6*: 485.

Kitchen, S. F. (1949). Falciparum malaria, *Malariology,* Vol. II (M. F. Boyd, ed.), W. B. Saunders, Philadelphia, p. 995.

Kwiatkowski, D., Cannon, J. G., Manogue, K. R., Cerami, A., Dinarello, C. A., and Greenwood, B. M. (1989). Tumor necrosis factor production in falciparum malaria and its association with schizont rupture, *Clin. Exp. Immunol., 77*: 361.

Liew, F. Y., Parkinson, C., Millot, S., Severn, A., and Carrier, M. (1990). Tumour necrosis factor (TNFα) in leishmaniasis, *Immunology, 69*: 570.

Liu, C. -C., Detmers, P. A., Jiang, S., and Young, J. D. -E. (1989). Identification and characterization of a membrane-bound cytotoxin of murine cytolytic lymphocytes that is related to tumor necrosis factor/cachectin, *Proc. Natl Acad. Sci. USA, 86*: 3286.

Mackey, L. J., Hochmann, A., June, C. H., Contras, C. E., and Lambert, P. -H. (1980). Immunopathological aspects of *Plasmodium berghei* infection in five strains of mice, *Clin. Exp. Immunol., 42*: 412.

Macpherson, G. G., Warrell, M. J., White, N. J., Looareesuwan, S., and Warrell, D. A. (1985). Human cerebral malaria: a quantitative ultrastructural analysis of parasitized erythrocyte sequestration, *Am. J. Pathol., 119*: 385.

Maegraith, B. (1948). *Pathological Processes in Malaria and Blackwater Fever*, Blackwell, Oxford, p. 345.

Maegraith, B. (1976). *Adams and Maegraith: Clinical Tropical Diseases*, 6th ed., Blackwell, Oxford, p. 176.

McCallum R. E., Stith, R. D., and Hill, M. R. (1987). Inhibited steroid induction of PEPCK in hepatoma cells treated with IL-1 and TNF, *J. Leukocyte Biol., 42*: 545.

Medcalf, R. L., Kruithof, E. K. O., and Schleuning, W. -D. (1988). Plasminogen activator inhibitor 1 and 2 are tumor necrosis factor/cachectin-responsive genes, *J. Exp. Med., 168*: 751.

Mentzer, S. J., Faller, D. V., and Burakoff, S. J. (1986). Interferon-γ induction of LFA-1 mediated homotypic adhesion of human monocytes. *J. Immunol., 137*: 108.

Michie, H. R., Spriggs, D. R., Manogue, K. R., Sherman, M. L., Revhaug, A., O'Dwyer, S. T., Arthur, K., Dinarello, C. A., Cerami, A., Wolf, S. M., Kufe, D. W., and Wilmore, D. W. (1988). Tumor necrosis factor and endotoxin induce similar metabolic responses in human beings, *Surgery, 104*: 280.

Mier, J. W., Vachino, G., Van der Meer, J. W. M., Numerof, R. P., Adams, S., Cannon, J. G., Bernheim, H. A., Atkins, M. B., Parkinson, D. R., and Dinarello, C. A. (1988). Induction of circulating tumor necrosis factor (TNF-α) as the mechanism of the febrile response to interleukin-2 (IL-2) in cancer patients, *J. Clin. Cancer, 8*: 426.

Miller, K. L., Silverman, P. H., Kullgren, B., and Mahlmann, L. J. (1989). Tumor necrosis factor alpha and the anemia associated with murine malaria, *Infect. Immun., 57*: 1542.

Miller, L. H. (1989). Binding of infected red cells, *Nature, 341*: 18.

Moore, R. N., Goodrum, K. J., Couch, R., and Berry, L. T. (1978). Factors affecting macrophages function: glucocorticoid antagonizing factor, *J. Reticuloendothel. Soc., 23*: 321.

Morrone, G., Ciliberto, G., Oliviero, S., Arcone, R., Dente, L., Content, J., and Cortese, R. (1988). Recombinant interleukin 6 regulates the transcriptional activation of a set of human acute phase genes, *J. Biol. Chem., 263*: 12554.

Naik, P., and Voller, A. (1984). Serum C-reactive protein levels and falciparum malaria, *Trans. R. Soc. Trop. Med. Hyg., 78*: 812.

Nawroth, P. P., and Stern, D. M. (1986). Modulation of endothelial cell hemostatic properties by tumor necrosis factor, *J. Exp. Med., 163*: 740.

Nickoloff, B. J., Reusch, M. K., Bensch, K., and Karasek, M. A. (1988). Preferential binding of monocytes and Leu 2^+ T lymphocytes to interferon-γ treated cultured skin endothelial cells and ceratinocytes, *Arch. Dermatol. Res., 28*; 235.

Ohnishi, S. T., Ohnishi, N., Oda, Y., and Katsuoka, M. (1989). Prostaglandin derivatives inhibit the growth of malarial parasites in mice, *Cell Biochem. Funct., 7*: 105.

O'Leary, D. S., Barr, C. F., Wellde, B. T., and Conrad, M. E. (1971). Experimental infection with *Plasmodium falciparum* in *Aotus* monkeys, *Am. J. Trop. Med. Hyg., 21*: 282.

Olweny, C. L. M., Chauhan, S. S., Simooya, O. O., Bulsara, M. K., Njelsani, E. K., and Van Thuc, H. (1986). Adult cerebral malaria in Zambia: preliminary report of clinical findings and treatment response, *J. Trop. Med. Hyg., 89*: 123.

Onongbu, I. C., and Onyeneke, E. C. (1983). Plasma lipid changes in human malaria, *Tropenmed. Parasitol., 34*: 193.

Oo, M. M., Aikawa, M., Than, T., Aye, T. M., Myint, P. T., Igarashi, I., and Schoene, W. C. (1987). Human cerebral malaria: a pathological study, J. Neuropathol. Exp. Neurol., 46*: 223.*

Ovington, K. S. (1987). *Nippostrongylus brasiliensis*: physiological and metabolic responses of rats to primary infection, *Exp. Parasitol., 63*: 10.

Pagliara, A. S., Karl, I. E., Haywood, M., and Kipris, D. M. (1973). Hypoglycemia in infancy and childhood, *J. Pediatr., 82*: 365.

Pectre, C., Cullberg, U., Nilsson, E., and Olsson, I. (1986). Effects of recombinant tumor necrosis factor on proliferation and differentation of leukemic and normal hemopoietic cells in vitro, *J. Clin. Invest., 78*: 1694.

Peterson, W. F. (1926). Blood sugar during the crisis of malaria fever, *Proc. Soc. Exp. Biol. Med., 23*: 753.

Phillips, R. E. (1989). Hypoglycaemia is an important complication of falciparum malaria, *Q. J. Med., 71*: 477.

Phillips, R. E., and Warrell, D. A. (1986). The pathophysiology of severe falciparum malaria, *Parasitol. Today,* 2: 271.

Phillips, R. E., Looareesuwan, S., Warrell, D. A., Lee, S. H., Karbwang, J., Warrell, M. J., White, N. J., Swasdichau, C., and Weatherall, D. J. (1986). The importance of anaemia in cerebral and uncomplicated falciparum malaria: role of complications, dyserythropoiesis and iron sequestration, *Q. J. Med., 58: 305.*

Picot, S., Peyron, F., Vuillez, J. P., Barbe, G., Marsh, K., and Ambroise-Thomas, P. (1990). Tumor necrosis factor production by human macrophages stimulated in vitro by *Plasmodium falciparum, Infect. Immun., 58*: 214.

Pied, S., Nussler, A., Pontet, M., Miltgen, F., Matile, H., Lambert, P. H., and Mazier, D.

(1989). C-reactive protein protects against preerythrocytic stages of malaria, *Infect. Immun., 57*: 278.

Plata-Salaman, C. R., Oomura, Y., and Kai, Y. (1988). Tumor necrosis factor and interleukin-1B: suppression of food intake by direct action in the central nervous system, *Brain Res., 448*: 106.

Playfair, J. H. L., Taverne, J., Bate, C. A. W., and de Souza, J. B. (1990). The malaria vaccine: anti-parasite or anti-disease? *Immunol. Today, 11*: 25.

Pukrittayakamee, S., White, N. J., Clemens, R., Chittamas, A., Karges, H. E., Desakorn, V., Looareesuwan, S., and Bunnag, D. (1989). Activation of the coagulation cascade in falciparum malaria, *Trans. R. Soc. Trop. Med. Hyg., 83*: 762.

Rest, J. R. (1982). Cerebral malaria in inbred mice. 1. A new model and its pathology, *Trans. R. Soc. Trop. Hyg., 76*: 410.

Rest, J. R. (1983). Pathogenesis of cerebral malaria in golden hamsters and inbred mice, *Contrib. Microbiol. Immunol., 7*: 139.

Rockett, K. A., Targett, G. A. T., and Playfair, J. H. L. (1988). Killing of blood-stage *Plasmodium falciparum*, by lipid peroxides from tumor necrosis serum, *Infect. Immun., 56*: 3180.

Romero, R., Manogue, K. R., Mitchell, M. D., Wu, Y. K., Oyarzun, E., Hobbins, J. C., and Cerami, A. (1989). Infection and labour. IV. Cachectin-tumor necrosis factor in the amniotic fluid of women with intraamniotic infection and preterm labor, *Am. J. Obstet. Gynecol., 161*: 336.

Rothlein, R., Czajkowski, M., O'Neill, M. M., Marlin, S. D., Mainolfi, E., and Merluzzi, V. J. (1988). Induction of intercellular adhesion molecule 1 on primary and continuous cell lines by proinflammatory cytokines, *J. Immunol., 141*: 1665.

Rothstein, J. L., and Schreiber, H. (1988). Synergy between tumor necrosis factor and bacterial products causes hemorrhagic necrosis and lethal shock in normal mice, *Proc. Natl. Acad. Sci. USA, 85*: 607.

Sassa, S., Kawakami, M., and Cerami, A. (1983). Inhibition of the growth and differentiation of erythroid precursor cells by an endotoxin-induced mediator from peritoneal macrophages, *Proc. Natl Acad. Sci. USA, 80*: 1717.

Schofield, L., Ferreira, A., Nussenzweig, V., and Nussenzweig, R. A. (1987). Antimalarial activity of tumor necrosis factor and gamma-interferon, *Fed. Proc., 46*: 760.

Scuderi, P., Lam, K. S., Ryan, K. J., Petersen, E., Salmon, S. E., Sterling, K. E., Finley, P. R., Ray, C. G., and Slymen, D. J. (1986). Raised serum levels of tumor necrosis factor in parasitic infections, *Lancet, ii*: 1364.

Selby, P., Hobbs, S., Viner, C., Jackson, E., Jones, A., Newell, D. D., Calvert, A. H., McElwain, T., Fearon, K., Humphreys, J., and Shiga, T. (1987). Tumour necrosis factor in man: clinical and biological observations, *Br. J. Cancer, 56*: 803.

Shah, R. G., Green, S., and Moore, M. A. S. (1978). Colony stimulating and inhibiting activities in mouse serum after *Corynebacterium parvum*-endotoxin induced treatment, *J. Reticuloendothel. Soc., 23*: 29.

Sherman, M. L., Spriggs, D. R., Arthur, K. A., Imamura, K., Frei, E. F., and Kufe, D. W. (1988). Recombinant human tumor necrosis factor administered as a five-day continuous infusion in cancer patients: phase 1 toxicity and effects on lipid metabolism, *J. Clin. Oncol., 6*: 344.

Shoham, S., Davenne, D., Cady, A. B., Dinarello, C. A., and Krueger, J. M. (1987). Recombinant tumor necrosis factor and interleukin 1 enhance slow-wave sleep, *Am. J. Phys.*, *253*: R142.

Smith, N. C. (1989). The role of free oxygen radicals in the expulsion of primary infections of *Nippostrongylus brasiliensis, Parasitol. Res.*, *75*: 423.

Spriggs, D. R., Sherman, M. L., Michie, H., Arthur, K. A., Imamura, K., Wilmore, D., Frei, E., and Kufe, D. W. (1988). Recombinant human tumor necrosis factor administered as a 24-hour intravenous infusion: a phase 1 and pharmacologic study, *J. Natl. Cancer Inst.*, *80*: 1039.

Srichaikui, T., Panikbutr, N., and Jeumtrakul, P. (1967). Bone marrow changes in human malaria, *Annal. Trop. Med. Parasitol.*, *8*: 40.

Steinmetz, T., Schaadt, M., Gahl, R., Schenk, V., Diehl, V., and Pfreundschug, M. (1988). Phase 1 study of 24-hour continuous intravenous infusion of recombinant human tumor necrosis factor, *J. Biol. Response Modif.*, *7*: 417.

Stevenson, M. M., and Ghadirian, E. (1989). Human recombinant tumor necrosis factor alpha protects susceptible A/J mice against lethal *Plasmodium chabaudi* AS infection, *Infect. Immun.*, *57*: 3936.

Strickland, G. T. (1978). Lymphocyte mitogenic factor in sera from patients with falciparum malaria, *Tropenmed. Parasitol.*, *29*: 198.

Taliaferro, W. H., and Cannon, P. R. (1936). The cellular reactions during primary infections and super-infections of *Plasmodium brasilianum* in Panamanian monkeys, *J. Infect. Dis.*, *59*: 72.

Tanneberger, St., Lenk, H., Muller, U., Ebert, J., and Shiga, T. (1988). Human pharmacoiogical investigation of a human recombinant tumor necrosis factor preparation, *Tumor Necrosis Factor/Cachectin and Related Cytokines* (B. Bonavida, G. E. Gifford, H. Kirchner, and L. J. Old, eds.) S. Karger, Basel, p. 205.

Taverne, J., Dockrell, H. M., and Playfair, J. H. L. (1981). Endotoxin-induced serum factor kills malarial parasites in vitro, *Infect. Immun.*, *33*: 83.

Taverne, J., Tavernier, J., Fiers, W., and Playfair, J. H. L. (1987). Recombinant tumor necrosis factor inhibits malaria parasites in vivo but not in vitro, *Clin. Exp. Immunol.*, *67*: 1.

Taverne, J., Bate, C. A. W., Sarker, D. A., Maeger, A., Rook, G. A. W., and Playfair, J. H. L. (1990). Human and murine macrophages produce TNF in response to soluble antigens of *Plasmodium falciparum, Parasite Immunol.*, *12*: 33.

Taylor, T. E., Molyneux, M. E., Wirima, J. J., Fletcher, K. A., and Morris, K. (1988). Blood glucose levels in Malawian children before and during the administration of intravenous quinine for severe falciparum malaria, *N. Engl. J. Med.*, *319*: 1040.

Teppo, A. M., and Maury, C. P. J. (1987). Radioimmunoassay of tumor necrosis factor in serum, *Clin. Chem.*, *33*: 2024.

Titus, R. G., Sherry, B., and Cerami, A. (1989). Tumor necrosis factor plays a protective role in experimental murine cutaneous leishmaniasis, *J. Exp. Med.*, *170*: 2097.

Toro, G., and Roman, G. (1978). Cerebral malaria: disseminated vasculomyelinopathy, *Arch. Neurol.*, *35*: 271.

Torpin, R. A. (1941). Malaria in pregnancy, *Am. J. Obstet. Gynecol.*, *41*: 882.

Torti, S. V., Kwak, E. L., Miller, S. C., Miller, L. L., Reingold, G. M., Myambo, K. B., Young, A. P., and Torti, F. M. (1988). The molecular cloning and characterisation of murine ferritin heavy chain, a tumor necrosis factor-inducible gene, *J. Biol. Chem., 263*: 12683.

Tracey, K. J., Lowry, S. F., Fahey, T. J., Albert, J. D., Fong, Y., Hesse, D., Beutler, B., Manogue, K. R., Calvano, S., Cerami, A., and Shires, G. T. (1987). Cachectin/tumor necrosis factor induces lethal shock and stress hormone response in the dog, *Surg. Gynecol. Obstet., 164:* 415.

Tubbs, H. (1980). Endotoxin in human and murine malaria, *Trans. R. Soc. Trop. Med. Hyg., 74*: 121.

Turner, M. W., and Voller, A. (1966). Studies on immunoglobulins of Nigerians. 1. The immunoglobulin levels of a Nigerian population, *J. Trop. Med. Hyg., 69*: 99.

Usawattanakul, W., Tharavanij, S., Warrell, D. A., Looareesuwan, S., White, N. J., Supavej, S., and Soikratoke, S. (1985). Factors contributing to the development of cerebral malaria. II. Endotoxin, *Clin. Exp. Immunol., 61*:562.

van der Meer, J. W. M., Endres, S., Lonneman, G., Cannon, J. G., Ikejima, T., Okusawa, S., Gelfand, J. A., and Dinarello, C. A. (1988). Concentrations of immunoreactive human tumor necrosis factor alpha produced by human mononuclear cells in vitro, *J. Leukocyte Biol., 43*: 216.

van Hinsbergh, V. W. M., Kooistra, T., van der Berg, E. A., Princen, H. M. G., Fiers, W., and Emeis, J. J. (1988). Tumor necrosis factor increases the production of plasminogen activator inhibitor in human endothelial cells in vitro and in rats in vivo, *Blood, 72*: 1467.

Vreeken, J., and Cremer-Goote, Th. M. (1978). Haemostatic defect in nonimmune patients with falciparum malaria: no evidence of diffuse intravascular coagulation, *Br. Med. J., 2*: 533.

Waage, A., Halstensen, A., and Espevik, T. (1987). Association between tumour necrosis factor in serum and fatal outcome in patients with meningococcal disease, *Lancet, i*: 355.

Waage, A., Bratzaeg, P., Haltensen, A., Kierulf, P., and Espevik, T. (1989). The complex pattern of cytokines in serum from patients with meningococcal septic shock: association between interleukin 6, interleukin 1 and fatal shock, *J. Exp. Med., 169*: 333.

Wahlgren, M., Carlson, J., Udonsangpetch, R., and Perlman, P. (1989). Why do *Plasmodium falciparum*-infected erythrocytes form spontaneous erythrocyte rosettes? *Parasitol. Today, 5*: 183.

Walter, P. R., Garin, Y., and Blot, P. (1982). Placental pathologic changes in malaria: a histologic and ultrastructural study, *Am. J. Pathol., 109*: 330.

Warrell, D. A. (1987). Pathophysiology of severe falciparum malaria in man, *Parasitology, 94* (Suppl.): 53.

Warrell, D. A., Looareesuwan, S., Warrell, M. J., Kasemsarn, P., Intaraprasert, R., Bunnag, D., and Harinasuta, T. (1982). Dexamethasone proves deleterious in cerebral malaria: a double-blind trial in 100 comatose patients, *N. Engl. J. Med., 306*: 313.

Warrell, D. A., Veall, N., Chathavanich, P., Karbwang, J., White, N. J., Looareesuwan, S., Phillips, R. E., and Pongpaew, P. (1988). Cerebral anaerobic glycolysis and reduced cerebral oxygen transport in human cerebral malaria, *Lancet, ii:* 534.

Wiedenmann, B., Reichardt, D., Rath, U., Theilman., L., Shüle, B., Ho, A. D., Schlick, E., Kempeni, J., Hunstein, W., and Kommerell, B. (1989). Phase 1 trial of intravenous continuous infusion of tumour necrosis factor in advanced metastatic carcinomas, *J. Cancer Res. Clin. Oncol., 115*: 189.

White, N. J., Warrell, D. A., Chanthavanich, P., Looareesuwan, S., Warrell, M. J., Krishna,

S., Williamson, D. H., and Turner, R. C. (1983). Severe hypoglycemia and hyperinsulinemia in falciparum malaria, *N. Engl. J. Med., 309*: 61.

White, N. J., Marsh, K., Turner, R. C., Miller, K. D., Berry, C. D., Williamson, D. H., and Brown, J., (1987). Hypoglycaemia in African children with severe malaria, *Lancet, i*: 708.

Wickramasinghe, S. N., Phillips, R. E., Looareesuwan, S., Warrell, D. A., and Hughes, M. (1987). The bone marrow in human cerebral malaria: parasite sequestration within sinusoids, *Br. J. Haematol., 66*: 295.

Wickramasinghe, S. N., Looareesuwan, S., Nagachinta, B., and White N. J. (1989). Dyserythropoiesis and ineffective erythropoiesis in *Plasmodium vivax* malaria, *Br. J. Haematol., 72*: 91.

Wilson, D. B., Garnham, P. C. C., and Swellengrebel, N. H. (1950). A review of hyperendemic malaria, *Trop. Dis. Bull., 47*: 591.

Wood, P. R., and Clark, I. A. (1984). Macrophages from *Babesia* and malaria infected mice primed for monokine release, *Parasite Immunol., 6*: 309.

Wright, I. G., Goodger, B. V., and Clark, I. A. (1988). Immunopathology of *Babesia bovis* and *Plasmodium falciparum* infections, *Parasital. Today, 4*: 214.

Wyler, D. J. (1988). Steroids are out in the treatment of cerebral malaria: what's next?, *J. Infect. Dis., 158*: 320.

Yoshizaki, Y., Matsuda, T., Nishimoto, N., Kuritani, T., Taiho, L., Aozasa, K., Nakahata, T., Kawai, H., Tagoh, H., Komori, T., Kishimoto, S., Hirano, T., and Kishimoto, T. (1989). Pathogenic significance of interleukin-6 (IL-6/BSF-2) in Castleman's disease, *Blood, 74*: 1360.

Zahl, P. A., and Bjerkines, C. (1943). Induction of decidua-placental hemorrhage in mice by the endotoxins of gram-negative bacteria, *Proc. Soc. Exp. Med. Biol., 34*: 329.

18

TNF in Autoimmune Diseases, Graft-Versus-Host Reactions, and Pulmonary Fibrosis

PIERRE VASSALLI, GEORGES E. GRAU, and PIERRE-FRANÇOIS PIGUET
University of Geneva, Geneva, Switzerland

I. INTRODUCTION

Considering its enormously pleiotropic range of action, and in particular its role as a powerful mediator of inflammation and inducer of tissue damage, it may not be surprising that TNF has been found to be involved in autoimmunity. The protective mechanisms of humoral and cellular immunity are frequently accompanied by the appearance of inflammatory reactions, which may facilitate the elimination of the antigen but which also create lesions, sometimes sufficiently harmful to lead to severe or even lethal tissue damage; this is the very basis of the concept of immunopathology. In the case of immune reactions in which the antigen is a component of the host itself (i.e., in the so-called autoimmune diseases or in diseases involving at some stage an autoimmune mechanism), the severity of local damage may be expected to be worsened in tissues that are not only the site of an inflammatory reaction triggered by the immune response, but also the very target of this response. TNF is an essential mediator, through a number of pathways, in a variety of inflammatory reactions, some of them mediated by T cells (Grau et al., 1987; Kindler et al., 1989). It is also a potentially damaging and cytotoxic agent, one of its sources of local release being T lymphocytes stimulated by the antigen they recognize. Therefore, its involvement in autoimmune disorders seems all the more likely.

With these rather simple considerations in mind, it may seem very surprising that in the diseases whose autoimmune basis is most firmly established, namely systemic lupus erythematosus (SLE) and insulin-dependent diabetes mellitus (IDDM), an essential pathogenic role has been attributed to a genetically determined status of *low TNF producer.* The observation of local TNF synthesis in the lesions of these two diseases—that is, renal glomeruli that are progressively destroyed as the result of deposition of circulating immune complexes in SLE, and insulitis, in which the β cells of the Langerhans islets are the direct targets of autoimmunity in IDDM—is compatible with a role of TNF in the production or progression of the local damage. However, the contrasting observation that systemic injections of TNF in mice starting before clinical evidence of these diseases prevents or retards their appearance and early death (Jacob and McDevitt, 1988; Satoh et al., 1989; Jacob et al., 1990a) indicates, together with other evidence, that the main relationship between TNF and autoimmunity may be at a more general, still poorly understood level.

Aside from these two paradigms of autoimmunity, there are a number of other diseases in which at least an autoimmune component is suspected, even though the target antigenic determinant has not always been clarified. It is probably a common occurrence that foreign substance, either by molecular mimicry (because it resembles a molecule of the host) or by different types of association to a host tissue, or even a self component rendered antigenic as the result of denaturation, elicits a reaction directed to host tissues. In this chapter we consider the little which is presently known about the involvement of TNF in these lesions and diseases. It will describe also two conditions in which involvement of TNF has been more directly studied and found to be decisive. One concerns an immune response directed against the host but elicited by a grafted foreign tissue containing T lymphocytes; this is the *graft-versus-host reaction* (GVHR), mainly observed in humans after bone marrow transplantation. The other condition is that of a peculiar pulmonary lesion eventually leading to extensive lung fibrosis, the bleomycin-induced pneumopathy, in which the immune response of the host after bleomycin exposure (in humans as the result of cancer chemotherapy) is required for the elicitation of the local disease; a pulmonary disease similarly involving TNF and fibrosis but without evidence of autoimmunity (i.e., silicosis), will also be considered. With the latter exception, in all the diseases mentioned above, from SLE to bleomycin pneumopathy, the nature of the lesions observed, and not only their localization, is very different, and this appears to reflect the differences in pathways for the action of TNF in a given disease or pathological situation.

II. TNF ACTIONS ON IMMUNE RESPONSES

Before reviewing the possible relationship between TNF and autoimmunity, it may be useful to consider that TNF may not only act as an effector of the consequences of an immune response, but also as a potential modifier of the immune response itself.* There are relatively few available data, which concern the effects of TNF on normal immune responses in the mouse, not to speak of humans, or on the in vitro behavior of stimulated T lymphocytes. Furthermore, the interpretation of some of these data is complicated by the variety of protocols used to explore in vivo the possible involvement of TNF at the level of a normal immune response. A single injection of TNF (less than 1 μg/mouse) at the time of immunization has been reported to increase moderately the number of antibody-producing cells observed in the spleen 5 days after immunization with heterologous erthrocytes, but to have no effect in the case of a thymus independent antigen (Ghiara et al., 1987). A dose-dependent, moderate enhancement of the humoral response to a single injection of TNF has been observed, while repeated injections did not modify the humoral response to the other antigens (Gordon et al., 1989). Since TNF is a potent inducer of interleukin-6, which, among other effects, promotes the maturation of plasma cells, an increase of antibody formation by TNF might indeed be expected; it should, however, affect all types of antigen. Injection of neutralizing anti-TNF antibody at the time of immunization might be a more accurate way to assess a possible role of TNF in an immune response. Using this approach, we did not observe any significant effect on the IgM or IgG antibody levels in primary or secondary responses to sheep erthrocytes. As indicated below, we also did not observe a significant effect of anti-TNF antibody treatment on the humoral response to bovine type II collagen. As for T lymphocytes' function or proliferation, TNF used in vitro has been reported to act as a comitogen in a thymocyte proliferation assay (Ranges et al., 1988), and perhaps more significantly, to increase the proliferation of mature T and B lymphocytes (Sugarman et al., 1985; Yokota 1988; Kehrl et al., 1987; Shalaby et al., 1988). Resting T cells do not appear to have receptors for TNF, but high-affinity TNF receptors appear on T lymphocytes after primary activation in vitro; in this case, TNF, among other effects on T lymphocytes (e.g., increased production of IFN-γ), increases the expression of high-affinity IL-2 receptors, thus leading to an enhanced proliferation response in the presence of IL-2 (Scheurich et al., 1987). The activity of NK cells appears also to be enhanced in vitro in the presence of TNF (Ostensen et al., 1987). If these effects are of significant importance in vivo, one would expect to observe some modifications of T-cell responses in mice having blocking levels of anti-TNF antibody in circulating blood. However, the injection of anti-TNF antibody had no effect on the proliferation response of parental T lymphocytes in the spleen of lethally irradiated semiallogeneic hosts, contrasting with a marked decrease of the epidermal and intestinal lesions of this GVHR, as discussed below (Piguet et al., 1987). Repeated injections of anti-TNF antibody in the peritoneal cavity of mice rejecting allogenic tumor cells growing intraperitoneally

**Editors' note*: For a more detailed discussion of the actions of TNF on immune responses, see Chapter 14.

had at best a limited effect on the generation of cytotoxic antitumor T cells, since there was only a small or inconsistent effect on the time at which complete rejection of the tumor cells occurred (B. Cuenod and D. Guy-Grand, personal communication).

In contrast, using repeated injections of TNF, an experimental protocol which, as mentioned, has a marked preventive effect on the appearance of some spontaneous autoimmune diseases of mice, Gordon and Wofsy (1990) observed a progressive diminution of CD4 and CD8 T lymphocytes, as well as a marked reduction of the response of T and B cells to mitogens in vitro, and of NK activity. In vivo, the generation of cytotoxic T lymphocytes to an allogeneic target was decreased, as well as DTH responsiveness (but not humoral responses). This decrease in T-cell function correlated neither with the decreased number of T cells of normal animals, nor with a direct alteration of their function since the lymphocytes of TNF treated mice responded normally to mitogens. These observations suggest that the basal production of TNF in the organism may modulate cellular immune responses, with a high level depressing the responses and a low level presumably having the opposite effect. This last addition to the long list of TNF effects may be of critical importance to assess the role of TNF in autoimmunity, in which the same specific immune reaction is constantly taking place, and where, as discussed below, people who are low TNF producers may be more at risk.

In this chapter the term *TNF* refers to TNF-α; there is very little information on the role of lymphotoxin or TNF-β in the conditions discussed, because it has not been widely explored.

III. AUTOIMMUNE DISEASES

A. SLE and Related Autoimmune Disorders

Since there is much more information concerning the implication of TNF in the murine models resembling SLE than in the human disease, the observations made in mice will be reported first.

1. *Murine Hereditary Autoimmune Diseases Related to SLE*

In two strains of mice in which the progressive appearance of autoantibodies characteristic of SLE is associated with a high incidence of early death by renal failure, namely the MRL-lpr/lpr and the (NZB $\times$ NZW)F1 mice, there is a spontaneous release of TNF by cells which, in mice of nonsusceptible strains, do not release TNF in the absence of stimulation. In MRL-lpr/lpr mice, a striking constitutive high level of TNF mRNA expression has been found in the abnormal subpopulation of $CD4^-$ and $CD8^-$ lymphocytes that accumulate in the lymphoid organs (Murray and Martens, 1989); this is associated with an increased amount of IFN-γ mRNA, but not of mRNAs for IL-2, IL-4, IL-5, and IL-6, suggesting that this is not the result of some kind of general activation process in these cells. Aside from these very peculiar cells, whose exact nature and role in the disease are incompletely understood, freshly isolated and unstimulated renal glomeruli of these mice spontaneously release TNF (and IL-1β) in vitro when signs of lupus nephritis become evident (Boswell et al., 1988); glomerular macrophages and mesangial cells, which are rather prominent in murine autoimmune nephritis, may represent the local source of this release (Boswell et al., 1988). In support of this possibility, it has been observed that Kupffer cells isolated from the livers of these mice also spontaneously release TNF in vitro, a property that appears at 6 weeks of age and progressively augments with time. These livers progressively show signs of activation of Kupffer cells and of local macrophages (Magilavy and Rothstein, 1988), as well as infiltration by NK cells (Magilavy et al., 1987). Comparable results of detectable TNF mRNA level in the renal cortex, increasing with age and when signs of glomerular disease become conspicuous, have been obtained with (NZB × NZW)F1 mice (Brennan et al., 1989a), the autoimmune features of which evolve somewhat more slowly than those of MRL-1pr/1pr mice. All these observations led to the suggestion that an increased local release of TNF could play an important role in the severity and rapidity of evolution of the glomerular lesions (Brennan et al., 1989a). Injections of 1FN-γ to (NZB × NZW) F1 mice accelerate the development of glomerulonephritis (Jacob et al., 1987). Since in numerous conditions a synergism has been observed between IFN-γ and TNF, in part perhaps because IFN-γ increases the level of TNF receptors on various cells (Aggarwal et al., 1985), several groups of investigators injected various doses of TNF over a period of several months into (NZB × NZW)F1 mice, expecting to observe an acceleration of the renal disease. The results obtained were in fact more complex, since they went in opposite directions, depending on the dose of TNF used, and thus were not compatible with a simple, one-sided role for TNF in the pathogenesis of the disease.

With very low doses of TNF (0.2 μg) injected three times a week for 2 to 4 months, Brennan et al. (1989a) observed a marked increase in the mortality from renal disease, provided that the injections were started at 4 months rather than at 2 months of age; injections between 2 and 4 months of age were without effect. Since the manifestations of autoimmunity and the level of circulating immune complexes are low before 4 months in these mice, it appears that this regimen of low doses of TNF mainly aggravates a local injury when it has already started. This would be in keeping with the idea that the enhanced local release of TNF observed in these mice and in the MRL-lp/lpr mice acts as an aggravating rather than as a triggering factor. It must be noted, however, that in view of the short half-life (a few minutes) of recombinant TNF in the serum when administered in vivo and of the very small amount of TNF injected, its effective time of action with this protocol is probably very brief. One would therefore expect that higher amounts of exogenous TNF may lead to further acceleration of these lesions. However, when the three-weekly schedule of injection described above was raised to 2 μg per injection, Brennan et al. (1989a) did not find further aggravation, but rather no detectable modification of the course of the renal disease when compared to that of untreated mice. Using a similar schedule of intraperitoneal injections with 10 μg of TNF (a closely comparable amount, when judged by specific activity in a bioassay, performed by the same supplier of recombinant TNF), Jacob and McDevitt (1988) observed in fact a striking improvement in the treated mice, with injections started at 4 months of age and lasting 3 months. This improvement was still very remarkable long after the cessation of the treatment, since at 11 months 90% of the TNF injected mice were alive and only 15 to 20% of the control; 30% of the treated mice were still alive at 15 months, all controls being dead at 12 months. A beneficial effect of chronic TNF injections on renal disease was confirmed by Gordon et al. (1989), with the additional interesting observation that this treatment has no effect on the level of circulating autoantibody.

Another important finding was made in the study of Jacob and McDevitt (1988): Peritoneal exudate cells of NZW mice, stimulated in various ways, release very little TNF when compared to similar cells of NZB or BALB/c mice, with an intermediate production by F1 mouse cells. This last observation suggests that an altered expression of the TNF gene could be of essential importance for the development of the autoimmune disease, since the genome of the NZW parent contributes critically, in some unknown way, to the occurrence and severity of nephritis in F1 mice, compared to the mild autoimmune reactions observed in the NZB parent.

The existence of a genetic alteration responsible for lowering TNF release in (NZW × NZB)F1 mice is in apparent contrast with the observation of increased TNF release in the damaged glomeruli of these F1 mice, and with aggravating effect obtained by the chronic administration of very low doses of TNF when the renal disease has begun, as described above. This contradiction may be resolved, at least in part, if an increased exposure to TNF results in a decreased T-cell responsiveness (Gordon and Wofsy, 1990), as reported in the introduction to this chapter, and if a lower general capacity to produce TNF has the opposite effect. The improvement of renal disease resulting from chronic TNF treatment is not accompanied by a decrease in the level of circulating immune complexes (Gordon et al., 1989), whose progressive glomerular deposition is usually considered as the event responsible for the renal damage leading to premature death by renal failure. In the hypothesis of a link between a decreased capacity to release TNF, T-cell responsiveness and glomerular disease, one would have to postulate that cellular immunity is also involved in some way in the local damage. Repeated injections of TNF may thus act by decreasing a local reaction of cellular immunity, as it decreases DTH and other T-cell reactions in normal mice. In this case there would be no contradiction between a local harmful effect of TNF, whose increased glomerular production might be involved in some way in renal damage, and a protective effect observed in the same conditions in *high TNF producers*, which would act at a completely different level. No attempts at suppressing or decreasing TNF activity by repeated injections of anti-TNF antibody, started at different times, have yet been made in (NZB × NZW)F1 or NZB mice; experiments of this type may shed some light on the interpretation of the complex role of TNF in autoimmune diseases.

The TNF gene is located within the major histocompatibility complex, and there exists a strong association between various MHC class II haplotypes and autoimmune disorders. This suggests that the inherited variations in the level of TNF gene expression described by Jacob and Devitt (1988) may be related to allelic variations in the promoter region of the gene, perhaps related to MHC polymorphism. This led these authors to explore, by the study of restriction fragment length polymorphorism (RFLP), possible polymorphism of the TNF gene in various mouse strains. Using a DNA fragment derived from exon 4 of the TNF gene, a different RFLP pattern was found in NZB and NZW mice; however, there were no clear relationship in these RFLP patterns and that of other strains either displaying autoimmune features or not. A more extensive study of RFLP of the TNF gene in a large variety of normal (inbred or wild type) and autoimmune mice led other authors to the conclusion that since the same allele is inherited in most varieties of mice, genetic evidence linking variations of the TNF gene and autoimmune diseases in mice was in fact lacking (Richter et al., 1989). It is nevertheless clear that this type of approach rests heavily on the availability of adequate markers of polymorphism in the region of the DNA studied. Recently, a repetitive simple tandem motif (microsatellite) present in the promoter region of the TNF gene has been used as a polymorphic marker. This allowed us to conclude that the TNF allele thus detected in NZW mice (which themselves have no autoimmune features) is distinct from that found in all other haplotypes explored (Jongeneel et al., 1990). Further exploration of this sort, indicating that there is a variety of TNF alleles, will reveal if there are indeed alleles associated with regulatory diversity in TNF expression, and if there is a correlation between the presence of these alleles and an increased susceptibility to autoimmunity, as suggested by the disease observed in the (NZB × NZW)F1 compared to the mild autoimmune features of their NZB parents.

2. *Human SLE*

There is relatively little information concerning the possible involvement of TNF in human SLE. The TNF blood level, detected by a radioimmunoassay, is very low is SLE patients and not different from that of normal subjects; in a few patients with SLE presenting an infection, an increase in TNF blood level was found, which was, however, in the range of that found in similarly infected patients not presenting SLE (Maury and Teppo, 1989). Thus SLE patients could not be classified as low TNF producers by this very crude approach. In view of the association between SLE and other autoimmune diseases in humans and of the observations in mice reported in the preceding section, a systematic study of a possible correlation between MHC class II haplotypes and TNF production was carried out in a large number of patients with SLE and in healthy individuals using in vitro mitogenic stimulation of blood mononuclear cells to trigger TNF release. A striking correlation was found in healthy subjects between the HLA-DR2 and DQW haplotypes and low TNF production on one hand, and DR3 and DR4 haplotypes and high TNF production on the other. The same correlation was found in SLE patients, but a point of essential importance emerged: There is a correlation between MHC class II haplocytes (and thus the level of TNF release in vitro) and the clinical form of the disease. DR2, DQW-1-positive SLE patients have a high incidence of nephritis; in contrast, DR3- and DR4-positive SLE patients are not not predisposed to nephritis (Jacob et al., 1990a). Thus these results suggest not only the existence of a relationship between MHC class II haplocytes and the level of TNF production to a given stimulus, but also that this relation influences the clinical form of the disease in patients with SLE. The resemblance of these observations to those made in NZB and (NZB × NZW)F1 mice is striking in view of the possibility that the introduction of the "low responder" TNF gene of the NZW mice into F1 mice may be one of the factors transforming the mild autoimmunity of NZB mice into a severe disease ending in renal failure. More extensive studies, especially studies exploring possible links between the course of the disease and allelic variations of the TNF gene, as discussed for the mouse, are required to understand the possible role played, in SLE and other human autoimmune disorders, by the inherited ability to produce more or less TNF.

2. Autoimmune Diabetes (IDDM)

The mechanism leading to pancreatic B-cell destruction in insulin-dependent diabetes mellitus (IDDM) have received much attention, especially since the discovery of two animal mutants that develop a genetically transmitted autoimmune diabetes bearing a striking resemblance to human IDDM, the BB rats, and the nonobese diabetic (NOD) mice. The existence of an insulitis characterized by a mononuclear cell infiltration of the Langerhans islets led to study the possibility that lymphokines released by stimulated T lymphocytes or by activated macrophages may be instrumental in the destruction of the islet beta cells, or in the perpetuation and exacerbation of the autoimmune stimulation leading to this insulitis. It has indeed been observed that cultures of human islet cells in the presence of interferon-γ and TNF induced the expression of MHC class II antigens on islet beta cells (while interferon-γ alone, or in association with IL-1, was ineffective) (Pujol-Borrell et al., 1987). Thus local production of TNF, which has been demonstrated in the insulitis of NOD mice (Held et al., 1990), may contribute to local antigen presentation on MHC class II molecules by cells that are normally devoid of antigen presentation capacity, a mechanism believed to be of potential importance in autoimmunity. In addition, different in vitro studies concluded that some lymphokines have a direct but slow cytotoxic effect on pancreatic beta cells, as judged by tests of chromium release or by a decreased capacity to release insulin: TNF seems to act synergistically in this respect with interferon-γ and/or IL-1, while having little effect alone (Mandrup-Poulsen et al., 1987; Pukel et al., 1988; Campbell et al., 1988).

In vivo investigations have therefore been performed on BB rats and NOD mice to explore the role of cytokines in this type of disease. Observations involving TNF in the pathogenesis of IDDM, although in a way apparently bearing little relationship to a possible local toxic effect of TNF on beta cells, have stemmed from two directions:

1. The observation that injections of an immunomodulator agent derived from a streptococcal preparation inhibits the development of diabetes in BB rats (Satoh et al., 1988) and NOD mice (Toyota et al., 1986). Since this preparation induced in vivo the production of various cytokines, the idea that the disease could be decreased or suppressed by injections of cytokines arose, and among the cytokines used, only injections of TNF modified the disease, and their effect was indeed protective (Satoh et al., 1989).
2. Application to the NOD mice of a treatment of repeated injection of TNF comparable to that found to have a protective effect on the nephritis of (NZB × NZW)F1 mice. Again, this treatment was found to have protective effects on the progression of the autoimmune diabetes (Jacob et al., 1990b) while the schedules of injection and doses of TNF used were slightly different in these two studies, starting at 4 (Satoh et al., 1989) or 8 or 9 weeks of age (Jacob et al., 1990b) and lasting 3 months (Jacob et al., 1990b) or more (Satoh et al., 1989), results, as judged by the decrease in incidence of diabetes and prevention of insulitis on histologic sections were rather comparable. However, the protective effect was significant but not total, unlike the prevention observed after injections of the streptococcal-derived immunomodulator agent (Toyota et al., 1986). This difference may be attributed to a more uniform release of TNF in the latter situation and/or to a contributing effect of other cytokines. In the last respect, Jacob et al. (1990b) found that repeated injections of IL-1 also have a marked protective effect on the evolution of diabetes in NOD mice.

In these two studies, another observation was made, which relates to the level of TNF production by cells of NOD mice compared to those of other strains, when submitted to identical stimuli. The peritoneal exudate cells of various strains of mice were stimulated in different ways, and those of NOD mice showed the lowest induction of TNF mRNA (Satoh et al., 1989) and the lowest release of TNF, about 3 to 5 times less than cells from SWR mice, which have the same genetic origin than NOD mice, but are not diabetes-prone. The same was also true of IL-1 release (Jacob et al., 1990b). Blood release of TNF obtained with various inducing agents was also lowest, among the strains tested, in NOD mice (Satoh et al., 1989).

Thus all of these observations are very similar to those discussed above concerning the lupus-like nephritis of autoimmune mice, with the only difference that

IL-1 released by stimulated macrophages appears also to be decreased in NOD mice compared to the other normal or autoimmune strains tested; this may be relevant to the observation of a protective effect of IL-1 injections made only in NOD mice (Jacob et al., 1990b). At the present stage, the tentative conclusions that have been reached concerning the different modes of action of TNF in autoimmune nephritis also apply to autoimmune diabetes, with, however, one important contradiction that remains to be solved: in human, IDDM is most commonly associated with the MHC haplocytes DR3 and DR4, which have been correlated, as mentioned above, to the condition of high TNF production (Jacob et al., 1990b).

C. Rheumatoid Arthritis and Experimental Autoimmune Arthritis

1. Rheumatoid Arthritis in Humans

TNF in culture induces the proliferation of fibroblasts (Sugarman et al., 1985; Vilček et al., 1986) and their release of prostaglandin E_2 and collagenase (Dayer et al., 1985); it also promotes cartilage and bone resorption (Bertolini et al., 1986; Saklatvala et al., 1985). This led to explore its presence and that of IL-1, which shares some of these properties (Saklatvala, 1986; Pettipher et al., 1986), in the synovial fluid and tissue of patients with rheumatoid arthritis. This inflammatory disease, which is suspected to have an autoimmune component, is characterized by the proliferation of synovial cells accompanied with cartilage and bone erosion. Using radioimmunoassays, TNF has been found in the synovial fluids in a variable percentage (in the range 25 to 50%) of patients with rheumatoid arthritis, and also in arthritis of other origins, classified as *reactive arthritis*, but it has not been detected in the synovial fluids obtained during arthroscopy performed for knee pain in some patients (Hopkins and Meager, 1988). When tested, TNF-β has not been detected. Synovial fluid TNF does not appear to be specifically related to rheumatoid arthritis; it may simply reflect a local inflammatory reaction, although not all studies found a good correlation between TNF levels and the abundance of leukocytes in synovial fluids (Saxne et al., 1988). The source of synovial fluid TNF may be both synovial tissue and mononuclear cells present in the synovial fluid (Yocum et al., 1989); by in situ hybridization on synovial cells, TNF mRNA is detectable mostly in monocytes and macrophages (Firestein et al., 1990). IL-1 or an IL-1-like factor has also been detected in the synovial fluid (Fontana et al., 1982; Brennan et al., 1989b) but its presence, at least in some cases, may be secondary to that of TNF, since anti-TNF antibody in synovial cell cultures prevents the release of IL-1 in the culture supernatant (Brennan et al., 1989b). Finally, when tested, IFN-γ has also been detected in the synovial fluids of patients with rheumatoid arthritis (Yocum et al., 1989), and in some patients, probably with the most active disease, TNF and IFN-γ have been reported to be detectable in the blood (Saxne et al., 1988).

In conclusion TNF may not play a more specific role in rheumatoid arthritis than in many other forms of inflammation, would it not be for some of its effects on chondrocytes and their possible more specific link to chronic joint disease. There are at least two peculiar effects exerted by TNF on chondrocytes: cartilage resorption and the release of GM-CSF. Like IL-1, TNF can stimulate resorption of human articular cartilage; cultures of chondrocytes exposed to TNF are stimulated to produce plasminogen activators of the urokine and tissue-type, and IL-1 exerts a synergistic effect (Campbell et al., 1990): plasminogen activators are the only neutral proteases released in these stimulated cultures, and it is thus conceivable that they may play an important role in TNF (and IL-1)-mediated cartilage destruction (Campbell et al., 1990). The recent observation that TNF, known, like IL-1, to induce the synthesis of GM-CSF by endothelial cells and fibroblasts (Munker et al., 1986; Seelentag et al., 1987; Koeffler et al., 1987; Seelentag et al., 1989), has the same effect on chondrocytes (Campbell et al., manuscript submitted) probably explains the presence of GM-CSF in synovial fluids (Xu et al., 1989). This is a potential source of perpetuation of the local inflammation, since among other effects, GM-CSF attracts and activates neutrophils (Gasson et al., 1984; Weisbart et al., 1985); furthermore, there is evidence that local GM-CSF may contribute to the increased expression of MHC class II antigen on synovial macrophages (Alvaro-Garcia et al., 1989).

2. *Spontaneous and Experimental Autoimmune Arthritis in Mice*

About 75% of 5 to 6-month-old females of the MRL-lpr/lpr strain spontaneously develop an arthritis with many similarities to human rheumatoid arthritis, including the presence of circulating IgM rheumatoid factor (Hang et al., 1982). Surprisingly, while so much attention has been given to the renal disease of these and other autoimmune mice, no experimental study attempting to explore the local synthesis of TNF and the effects of exogenous TNF injection has been published to date.

There are models of experimental arthritis, in particular adjuvant and collagen-induced arthritis, which also bear strong resemblance to human rhematoid arthritis and whose susceptibility is similarly linked to the MHC (for a review, see Stuart et al., 1988). There are no reports exploring the role of TNF in these models. In preliminary experiments using type II collagen arthritis in mice, we have observed that the development of the arthritis, assessed by footpad swelling and histologic study, is almost totally prevented by anti-TNF antibody treatment administered shortly after immunization; at this time, small amount of TNF mRNA is detectable in whole foodpad mRNAs, but signs of arthritis are only mild, sometimes barely detectable. In contrast, this treatment has little influence when started at the time of full-blown arthritis, suggesting that it does not act merely by neutralization of TNF accumulating in inflamed joints, or that such neutralization occurs too late, when a possible self-perpetuating chain of inflammatory events has already been established in the joints (TNF mRNA is, however, not detectable in whole footpads mRNAs at this stage of severe disease). Thus TNF seems involved at least in the early events of arthritis. An interesting observation is that the anti-TNF antibody treatment, even when almost fully protective of the disease, does not modify the serum titer of anticollagen antibodies occurring after immunization. It thus appears that cell-mediated immune mechanisms, not anticollagen antibodies, play a decisive role in the establishment of the arthritis, by mechanisms that remain to be studied; these observations further emphasize the complexity of TNF involvement in immune and inflammatory reactions.

IV. TNF AND GRAFT-VERSUS-HOST REACTION

The graft-versus-host reaction (GVHR) is a disease resulting from the transfer into a severely immuno-compromised host of allogeneic immunocompetent T cells. In the absence of an immune response of the host, these cells react against the histocompatibility antigens of the host. In humans it usually occurs after bone marrow transplantation, of which it is a major complication since GVHR is a potentially lethal disease. There are several experimental forms of the disease, with different clinical forms and rapidity of evolution, depending on differences in MHC class I and/or class II, or of minor histocompatability differences between donor and host (Kornhold and Sprent, 1978), and depending also on the number of allogeneic parental T lymphocytes transferred. However, in general the disease evolves in two phases. The acute phase is characterized by widespread focal areas of cell necrosis (the form of necrosis called *apoptosis*) occurring in epithelial tissues, most conspicuously in the skin and intestine. The chronic phase, which ends in cachexia and death, is accompanied by severe hematopoietic defects, sclerosis in various tissues, and complete atrophy of the lymphoid organs (Rappaport et al., 1979). In the variety of tissue alterations induced by GVHR in humans or mouse (for a review, see Rappaport et al., 1979), many bear resemblance with lesions observed in some diseases considered to have autoimmune features: in the skin, lichen planus and scleroderma; in the gut, coeliac disease; in the lung, fibrosing alveolitis (Piguet et al., 1989b); in the liver, primary biliary cirrhosis (Satoh et al., 1989); and so on. Injection of large numbers of parental T lymphocytes into F1 mice may mimic an autoimmune disease of the lupus type (Rolink et al., 1983). The pathogenesis of this variety of lesions is very incompletely understood, and there is not even agreement whether donor T lymphocytes are indeed the main direct effectors of all these various clinical and histological aspects of the reaction (Gale, 1985; Ferrara et al., 1989; Parkman, 1989).

The role of TNF in GVHR has been studied in a mouse model in which, after lethal irradiation, semiallogeneic recipients are injected with parental bone marrow cells mixed with selected amounts of parental peripheral T lymphocytes (Piguet et al., 1987). When only T-cell-depleted parental bone marrow cells are injected, no morbidity, no lethality, and no pathology are observed in the following weeks or months. In contrast, in the following 2 to 3 weeks after the transfer of bone-marrow containing foreign T cells, an acute disease develops, clinically evident because of weight loss and hair ruffling, followed more or less rapidly by death of some of the animals. The main lesions, in mice sacrificed 15 to17 days after induction of the disease, are found in the gut and in the skin, and are made of isolated epithelial and epidermal cell necrosis accompanied by an intraepithelial lymphocytic infiltration with some degree of mononuclear cell accumulation in the gut lamina propria and the dermis; in the lung, lesions of alveolitis are observed (Piguet et al., 1987, 1989b). The presence of TNF mRNA within these various lesions, explored by Northern blotting, is most clearly observed in the lung (Piguet et al., 1989b) (perhaps because in the situation of an air-filled organ in which mononuclear cells accumulate in the interstitium, an increase in TNF mRNA is easier to detect than in the very heterogeneous mRNAs obtained from solid tissues). TNF mRNA is related to the occurrence of GVHR, since it is not observed in mice injected with T-depleted bone marrow cells. There is no detectable TNF activity in the blood during the evolution of these lesions. A definitive answer on the role of TNF in the pathogenesis of these acute lesions of GVHR has been obtained by injecting an anti-TNF or an irrelevant control antibody 1 week of induction of the disease, before the occurrence of clinical symptoms. At sacrifice, on day 15 to 17, the anti-TNF antibody treatment almost completely prevents the epidermal and intestinal lesions (Piguet et al., 1987) but has only a moderate effect on the pulmonary lesions (Piguet et al., 1989b). It is thus clear that a local release of TNF plays a decisive role in the pathogenesis of the lesions observed in the skin and the gut.

There are several ways, not necessarily mutually exclusive, to interpret the role of TNF in this GVHR. Epidermal and intestinal necrosis could result from a local release of TNF, by activated macrophages or stimulated T cells. There is evidence that TNF is directly and rapidly toxic for some epithelial cells, such as thyroid cells (Taverne et al., 1987); however, TNF receptors have not been detected on the surface of enterocytes (J. Wietzerbin, personal communication). Furthermore, the anti-TNF antibody treatment prevents not only the necrosis of isolated epidermal cells and enterocytes, but also the local mononuclear cell infiltration. It seems conceivable that an important effect of local TNF release rests in its known capacity to induce, on the membranes of the endothelial cells of the venules, the appearance of cell adherence molecules such as ICAM, ELAM, and VCAM (for a review, see Kishimoto et al., 1989), which lead to the adherence, on the surface of these stimulated endothelial cells, of leukocytes, polymorphonuclears, and lymphocytes, respectively, and then promote tissue infiltration by inflammatory cells. The effect of anti-TNF treatment could in part be explained by the interruption, at its very beginning, of the effect of this progressively autoamplifying loop, triggered by the release of TNF by stimulated T lymphocytes. Stimulated T lymphocytes infiltrating the epithelial cell layer could contribute to the necrosis of isolated epithelial cells, by the release of TNF, and/or by other mechanisms of cytotoxicity. In the gut, most of the infiltrating intraepithelial cells have been shown to be donor $CD8^+$ T cells, which may damage host epithelial cells by "conventional" cytotoxicity mechanisms, but it must be stressed that there is strong evidence for immunologically nonspecific mechanisms in epithelial lesions, since fetal gut grafts of donor phenotype present in mice undergoing GVHR show the same type of intestinal damage as the host gut (Guy-Grand and Vassalli, 1986). Another interpretation of the anti-TNF antibody treatment, which would make the role of TNF in GVHR perhaps more trivial, is that this treatment directly interferes with recirculation of donor lymphocytes, since it has recently been observed that stimulated lymphocytes can bear a membrane form of TNF (Kinkhabwala et al., 1990). However, if this were indeed a major mechanism of protection from tissue damage, anti-TNF antibody would be expected to completely prevent further evolution of the GVHR, in particular its chronicity and lethality, in contrast to what is observed. Furthermore, the proliferation response in the spleen of lethally irradiated mice 5 days after injection of allogeneic lymphocytes is not modified by anti-TNF antibody treatment (Piguet et al., 1987).

The chronic phase of the GVHR has been little explored so far, and with respect to TNF, it can only be mentioned that this phase is characterized by the appearance of sclerosis in various places, most conspicuously as areas of scleroderma; sclerosis is a known consequence of prolonged TNF released in small amounts, as discussed below. As just mentioned, weekly injections of anti-TNF antibody during the course of GVHR certainly retard or in some cases may even prevent the occurrence of mortality, but does not completely suppress it (Piguet et al., 1987). The lesions observed in the treated mice in the chronic phase of the disease have not yet been explored.

Treatment with anti-TNF antibody has also been effective in some but not all GVH assays. It must be stressed that the pathogenic mechanisms involved in these assays are not clearly understood and may be very different from those of lesions resulting from the systemic disease. In the classical GVH assay of spleen enlargement 10 days after the injection of parental cells into newborn mice, anti-TNF antibody treatment prevents the appearance of splenomegaly (Shalaby et al., 1989). On the other hand, we have observed that this treatment has little or no effect in the popliteal GVH assay; in this case, injection of parental T lymphocytes into the footpad of semiallogeneic recipients results in a lymphoproliferative response in the draining lymph node, made principally of host cells (Piguet et al., 1977).

The very limited information available of TNF in humans in GVHR, or in the opposite situation of graft rejection indicates that TNF is released in these conditions. In GVHR, a correlation has been observed between the severity of the disease and the blood level of TNF detected by an ELISA (Irle et al., 1988); in kidney graft rejection, TNF has been detected in the blood of the renal veins (Maury and Teppo, 1987).

V. TNF AND PULMONARY FIBROSIS

As mentioned above, TNF is known to stimulate fibroblast division in vitro (Vilcek et al., 1986). In vivo, slow subcutaneous perfusion of low doses of TNF during one week leads to the formation of subcutaneous mass made of fibroblasts and collagen with an accumulation of small neovessels (Piguet e al., 1990a). There are disease suspected to have an autoimmune basis and in which an essential feature is excessive fibroblast proliferation and collagen deposition, such as scleroderma. While a possible role for TNF has been considered in this disease (Le Roy et al., 1989), clinical data exploring this hypothesis are not available at the present time.

In two forms of pulmonary disease characterized by progressive and extensive sclerosis, bleomycin-induced pneumopathy, and silicosis, there is strong evidence, on the basis of experimental models, for a critical role of TNF in the induction of the fibrotic reaction (Piget et al., 1989a, 1990b). Bleomycin pneumopathy, a complication of the use of bleomycin in cancer chemotherapy, can also be seen in rodents after systemic or intratracheal injection of this drug (Adamson and Bowden, 1979). While the mechanisms leading to the toxic reaction and some of its consequences are not known (alvelolar epithelial cells are the main site where the drug accumulates early after injection), pulmonary fibrosis appears to be the end result of an autoimmune process, since it does not occur, or only to a small extent, in athymic mice (Schrier et al., 1983), and it is prevented by depletion of T lymphocytes (Piguet et al., 1989a). In contrast, silicosis probably acts primarily on lungs macrophages, and there appears to be no autoimmune component, at least in its experimental form in mice, since the lesions of athymic and euthymic mice show only little difference (Hubbard, 1989). However, since the evidence indicating a role for TNF in the pulmonary fibrosis is identical in both experimental conditions, silicosis is also treated in this section.

A single intratracheal instillation of bleomycin into susceptible strains of mice induces necrosis of alveolar epithelial and endothelial cells, followed by the growth of fibroblasts and collagen deposition. This is accompanied by the lasting appearance of TNF mRNA in lung RNA extracts, evident only 5 days after instillation; IL-1 mRNA is not detectable (Piguet et al., 1989a). Similarly, after a single intratracheal instillation of silica, there is, within a week or so, appearance of TNF mRNA in lung RNA extracts, lasting for at least 4 months, but no appearance of IL-1 mRNA and no significant variations in the level of TGF-β mRNA (accumulation of this cytokine has been reported in the bleomycin-induced pneumopathy (Khalil et al., 1989); in situ hybridization for TNF mRNA shows its presence within the silicotic nodules (piguet et al., 1990b). In both experimental conditions, intravenous injection of anti-TNF antibody starting at the time of instillation markedly decreases the lesions and the level of collagen deposition as determined by a hydroxyproline assay; conversely, perfusion of low amounts of TNF for 1 week, not leading by itself to detectable pulmonary damage and increased collagen deposition, results into a significant increase in lung collagen and hydroxyproline content (Piguet et al., 1990b). Thus it seems clear that lung injuries leading to persistent increased local production of TNF are followed by lung fibrosis. Whether in this condition TNF acts alone in a rather direct way or in conjunction with other cytokines (such as TGF-β), perhaps involving a complex chain of mediators, remains to be determined; the main source of TNF release in the lung, possibly different in the two diseases discussed, should also be clarified.

On the basis of these observations, it is reasonable to speculate that TNF may have some role in the extensive fibrosis of diffuse interstitial pneumonitis in humans (Colby and Churg, 1986), a disease with several potentially different initiating mechanisms, one being a prolonged immune complex alveolitis. Use of anti-TNF antibody has indeed been shown to prevent experimental immune complex alveolitis (Warren et al., 1989); the triggering factors of TNF release in this condition may be the binding of the immune complexes to monocytes and polymorphonuclear leukocytes through their Fc receptors, since it has been shown that cross-linking of monocyte Fc receptors can induce TNF release (Debets et al., 1990).

VI. CONCLUSIONS

Perhaps the most striking conclusions that can be drawn from the various observations reported in this chapter relate to the various disguises that can be assumed by TNF action. Some of these disguises are reflected by the very contrasting pathological aspects in which local TNF release is involved as the result of a variety of initial mechanisms of tissue damage. However, another essential aspect of TNF implication, which may govern the severity and rapidly of progression of these local lesions where an autoimmune reaction is permanently at play, is probably at a more general level: it appears that there is a genetic capacity to a given individual to be a "low" or "high" TNF producer, but contrary to what might have been expected, it is the low TNF producer status that may favor the progression of autoimmune lesions, at least in SLE and autoimmune diabetes. Study of the relationship between TNF and autoimmunity thus reveals that, in considering the various involvements of TNF in health and disease, some of the present perplexity might be attenuated by the recognition that the distinction between damage and protection, "bad" or "good," is an erroneously finalistic approach, as is the case in immunopathology in general. The consequences of "local" and "occasional" TNF release should be balanced with those of general release and "constitutive" capacity to produce TNF; the effects of TNF production should not be reduced to a mere distinction between "organ" and "systemic" pathology, no more than to a simplistic pathogenic concept of "too much versus too little" TNF.

REFERENCES

Adamson, I. Y. R., and Bowden, D. H. (1979). Bleomycin-induced injury and metaplasia of alveolar type 2 cells, *Am. J. Pathol., 96*: 531.

Aggarwal, B. B., Eessalu, T. E., and Hass, P. E., (1985). Characterization of receptors for human tumour necrosis factor and their regulation by γ-interferon, *Nature, 318: 665.*

Alvaro-Gracia, J. M., Zvaifler, M. J., and Firestein, G. S. (1989). Cytokines in chronic inflammatory arthritis. IV. Granulocyte/macrophage colony-stimulating factor-mediated induction of class II MHC antigen on human monocytes: a possible role in rheumatoid arthritis, *J. Exp. Med., 170*: 865.

Bertolini, D. R., Nedwin, G. E., Bringman, T. S., Smith, D. D., and Mundy, G. R. (1986). Stimulation of bone resorption and inhibition of bone formation in vitro by human tumour necrosis factors, *Nature, 319*: 516.

Boswell, J. M., Yui, M. A., Burt, D. W., and Kelley, V. E. (1988). Increased tumor necrosis factor and IL-1-beta gene expression in the kidneys of mice with lupus nephritis, *J. Immunol., 141*: 3050.

Brennan, D. C., Yui, M. A., Wuthrich, R. P., and Kelley, V. E. (1989a). Tumor necrosis factor and Il-1 in New Zealand black/white mice: enhanced gene expression and acceleration of renal injury, *J. Immunol., 143*: 3470.

Brennan, F. M., Chantry, D., Jackson, A., Maini, R., and Feldmann M. (1989b). Inhibitory effect of TNFα antibodies on synovial cell interleukin-1 production in rheumatoid arthritis, *Lancet, ii* (8657): 244.

Campbell, I. L., Iscaro, A., and Harrison, L. C. (1988). IFN-γ and tumor necrosis factor-α: cytotoxicity to murine islets of Langerhans, J. Immunol., 141*: 2325.*

Campbell, I. K., Piccoli, D. S., Roberts, M. J., Muirden, K. D., and Hamilton, J. A. (1990). The effect of tumor necrosis factors α and β on the resorption of human articular cartilage and on the production of plasminogen activator by human articular chondrocytes, *Arthritis Rheum., 33*: 542.

Colby, T. V., and Churg, A. C. (1986). Patterns of pulmonary fibrosis, *Pathol. Annu., 21*: 277.

Dayer, J. M., Beutler, B., and Cerami, A. (1985). Cachectin/tumor necrosis factor stimulates collagenase and prostaglandin E_2 production by human synovial cells and dermal fibroblasts, *J. Exp. Med., 162*: 2163.

Debets, J. M. H., Van de Winkel, J. G. J., Ceuppens, J. L., Dieteren, I. E. M., and Buurman, W. A. (1990). Cross-linking of both Fc-γ RI and Fc-γ RII induces secretion of tumor necrosis factor by human monocytes, requiring high affinity Fc-Fc-γ-R interactions: functional activation of Fc-γ-RII by treatment with proteases or neuraminidase, *J. Immunol., 144*: 1304.

Ferrara, J. L. M., Guillen, F. J., van Dijken, P. J., Marion, A., Murphy, G. F., and Burakoff, S. J. (1989). Evidence that large granular lymphocytes of donor origin mediate acute graft versus host disease, *Transplantation, 47*: 50.

Firestein, G. S., Alvaro-Gracia, J., and Maki, R. (1990). Quantitative analysis of cytokine gene expression in rheumatoid arthritis, *J. Immunol., 144*: 3347.

Fontana, A., Hentgartner, H., Weber, E., Fehr, K., Grob, P. J., and Cohen, G. (1982). Interleukin-1 activity in synovial fluid of patients with rheumatoid arthritis, *Rheumatol. Int.,* 2: 49.

Gale, R. P. (1985). Graft-versus-host disease, *Immunol. Rev. 88*: 193.

Gasson, J. C., Weisbart, R. H., Kaufman, S. E., Clark, S. C., Hewick, R. M., Wong, G. G., and Golde, D. W. (1984). Purified human granulocyte-macrophage colony-stimulating factor: direct action on neutrophils, *Science, 226*: 1339.

Ghiara, P., Boraschi, D., Nencioni, L., Ghezzi, P., and Tagliabue, A. (1987). Enhancement of in vivo immune response by tumor necrosis factor, *J. Immunol., 139*: 3676.

Gordon, C., and Wofsy, D. (1990). Effects of recombinant murine tumor necrosis factor-α on immune function, *J. Immunol., 144*: 1753.

Gordon, C., Ranges, G. E., Greenspan, J. S., and Wofsy, D. (1989). Chronic therapy with recombinant tumor necrosis factor-α in autoimmune NZB/NZW F1 mice, *Clin. Immunol. Immunopathol., 52*: 241.

Grau, G. E., Fajardo, L. F., Piguet, P. F., Allet, B., Lambert, P. H., and Vassalli, P. (1987). Tumor necrosis factor (cachectin) as an essential mediator in murine cerebral malaria, *Science, 237*: 1210.

Guy-Grand, D., and Vassalli, P. (1986). Gut injury in mouse graft-versus-host reaction: study of its occurence and mechanisms, *J. Clin. Invest., 77*: 1584.

Hang, L. M., Theofilopoulos, A. N., and Dixon, F. J. (1982). A spontaneous rheumatoid arthritis-like disease in MRL/1 mice, *J. Exp. Med., 155*: 1690.

Held, W., MacDonald, H. R., Weissman, I. L., Hess, M. W., and Mueller, C. (1990). Genes encoding tumor necrosis factor α and granzyme A are expressed during development of autoimmune diabetes, *Proc. Natl. Acad. Sci. USA, 87*: 2239.

Helfgott, S. M., Dynesisus-Trentham, R., Brahn, E., and Trentham, D. E. (1985). An arthritogenic lymphokine in the rat, *J. Exp. Med., 162*: 1531.

Hopkins, S. J., and Meager, A. (1988). Cytokines in synovial fluid. II. The presence of tumour necrosis factor and interferon, *Clin. Exp. Immunol., 73*: 88.

Hubbard, A. K. (1989). Role for T lymphocytes in silica-induced pulmonary inflammation, *Lab. Invest., 61*: 46.

Irle, C., Salamin, A. F., Bagucilupo, A., Chapuis, B., Gratwohl, A. Hows, J., Piguet, P. F., and Grau, G. E. (1988). Serum TNF levels during graft versus host disease after bone marrow transplantation, *Bone Marrow Transplant., 3*: 127.

Jacob, C. O., and McDevitt, H. O. (1988). Tumour necrosis factor-α in murine autoimmune "lupus" nephritis, *Nature, 331*: 356.

Jacob, C. O., van der Meide, P. H., and McDevitt, H. O. (1987). In vivo treatment of (NZB × NZW)F1 lupus-like nephritis with monoclonal antibody to γ interferon, *J. Exp. Med., 166*: 798.

Jacob C. O., Aiso, S., Michie S. A., McDevitt, H. O., and Acha-Orbea, H. (1990a). Prevention of diabetes in nonobese diabetic mice by tumor necrosis factor (TNF): similarities between TNF-α and interleukin 1, *Proc. Natl. Acad. Sci. USA, 87*: 968.

Jacob, C. O., Fronek, A., Lewis, G. D., Koo, M., Hansen, J. A., and McDevitt, H. O. (1990b). Heritable major histocompatibility complex class II-associated differences in production of tumor necrosis factor α: relevance to genetic predisposition to systemic lupus erythematosus, *Proc. Natl. Acad. Sci. USA, 87*: 1233.

Jongeneel, C. V., Acha-Orbea, H., and Blankenstein, T. (1990). A polymorphic microsatellite in the tumor necrosis factor-α promoter identifies an allele unique to the NZW mouse strain, *J. Exp. Med., 171*: 2141.

Kehrl, J. H., Miller, A., and Fauci, A. S. (1987). Effect of tumor necrosis factor alpha on mitogen-activated human B cells, *J. Exp. Med., 166*: 786.

Khalil, N., Bereznay, O., Sporn, M., and Greenberg, A. H. (1989). Macrophage production of transforming growth factor β and fibroblast collagen synthesis in chronic pulmonary inflammation, *J. Exp. Med., 170*: 727.

Kindler, V., Sappino, A. P., Grau, G. E., Piguet, P. F., and Vassalli P. (1989). The inducing role of tumor necrosis factor in the development of bactericidal granulomas during BCG infection: a focal autoamplifying process of tissue organisation, *Cell, 56*: 731.

Kinkhabwala, M., Sehajpal, P., Skolnik, E., Smith, D., Sharma, V. K., Vlassara, H., Cerami A., and Suthanthiran, M. (1990). A novel addition to the T cell repertory: cell surface expression of tumor necrosis factor/cachectin by activated normal human T cells, *J. Exp. Med., 171*, 941.

Kishimoto, T. K., Larson, R. S., Corbi, A. L., Dustin, M. L., Staunton, D. E., and Springer, T. A. (1989). The leukocyte integrins, *Adv. Immunol., 46*: 149.

Koeffler, H. P., Gasson, J., Ranyard, J., Souza, L., Shepard, M., and Munker, R. (1987). Recombinant human TNFα stimulates production of granulocyte colony-stimulating factor, *Blood, 70*: 55.

Korngold, R., and Sprent, J. (1978). Lethal-graft-versus-host disease after bone marrow transplantation across minor histocompatibility barriers in mice: prevention by removing mature T cells from the marrow, *J. Exp. Med., 148*: 1687.

LeRoy, E. C., Smith, E. A., Kahaleh, M. B., Trojanowska, M., and Silver, R. M. (1989). A strategy for determining the pathogenesis of systemic sclerosis, *Arthritis Rheum., 32*: 817.

Magilavy, D. B., and Rothstein, J. L. (1988). Spontaneous production of tumor necrosis factor α by Kupffer cells of MRL/lpr mice, *J. Exp. Med., 168*: 789.

Magilavy, D. B., Steinberg, A. D., and Latta, S. L. (1987). High hepatic natural killer cell activity in murine lupus, *J. Exp. Med., 166*: 271.

Mandrup-Poulsen, T., Bendtzen, K., Dinarello, C. D., and Nerup J. (1987). Human tumor necrosis factor potentiates human interleukin 1-mediated rat pancreatic β-cell cytotoxicity, *J. Immunol., 139*: 4077.

Maury, C. P. J., and Teppo, A. M. (1987). Raised serum levels of cachectin/tumor necrosis factor α in renal allograft rejection, *J. Exp. Med., 166*: 1132.

Maury, C. P. J., and Teppo, A. M. (1989). Tumor necrosis factor in the serum of patients with systemic lupus erythematosus, *Arthritis Rheum., 32*: 146.

Munker, R., Gasson, J., Ogawa, M., and Koeffler, H. P. (1986). Recombinant human TNF induces production of granulocyte-monocyte colony-stimulating factor, *Nature, 323*: 79.

Murray, L., and Martens, C. (1989). The abnormal T lymphocytes in lpr mice transcribe interferon-γ and tumor necrosis factor-α genes spontaneously in vivo, *Eur. J. Immunol., 19*: 563.

Ostensen, M. E., Thiele, D. L., and Lipsky, P. E. (1987). Tumor necrosis factor-α enhances cytolytic activity of human natural killer cells, *J. Immunol., 138*: 4185.

Parkman, R. (1989). Graft-versus-host disease: an alternative hypothesis, *Immunol. Today, 10*: 362.

Pettipher, E. R., Higgs, G. A., and Henderson, B. (1986). Interleukin 1 induces leukocyte infiltration and cartilage proteoglycan degradation in the synovial joint, *Proc. Natl. Acad. Sci. USA, 83*: 8749.

Piguet, P. F., Dewey, H. K., and Vassalli, P. (1977). Origin and nature of the cells participating in the popliteal graft versus host reaction in mouse and rat, *Cell. Immunol., 31*: 242.

Piguet, P. F., Grau, G. E., Allet, B., and Vassalli, P. (1987). Tumor necrosis factor/cachectin is an effector of skin and gut lesions of the acute phase of graft-vs.-host disease, *J. Exp. Med., 166*: 1280.

Piguet, P. F., Collart, M. A., Grau, G. E., Kapanci, Y., and Vassalli, P. (1989a). Tumor necrosis factor/cachectin plays a key role in bleomycin-induced pneumopathy and fibrosis, *J. Exp. Med., 170*: 655.

Piguet, P. F., Grau, G. E., Collart, M. A., Vassalli, P., and Kapanci, Y. (1989b). Pneumopathies of the graft-versus-host reaction: alveolitis associated with an increased level of tumor necrosis factor mRNA and chronic interstitial pneumonitis, *Lab. Invest., 56*: 731.

Piguet, P. F., Grau, G. E., and Vassalli, P. (1990a). Subcutaneous perfusion of tumor necrosis factor induces local proliferation of fibroblasts, capillaries, and epidermal cells, or massive tissue necrosis, *Am. J. Pathol., 136*: 103.

Piguet, P. F., Collart, M. A., Grau, G. E., Sappino, A. P., and Vassalli, P. (1990b). Requirement of tumour necrosis factor for development of silica-induced pulmonary fibrosis, *Nature, 344*: 245.

Pujol-Borrell, R., Todd, I., Doshi, M., Bottazzo, G. G., Sutton, R., Gray, D., Adolf, G. R., and Feldmann, M. (1987). HLA class II induction in human islet cells by interferon-γ plus tumour necrosis factor or lymphotoxin, *Nature, 326*: 304.

Pukel, C., Baquerizo, H., and Rabinovitch, A. (1988). Destruction of rat islet cell monolayers by cytokines: synergistic interactions of interferon-γ, tumor necrosis factor, lymphotoxin, and interleukin 1, *Diabetes, 37*: 133.

Ranges, G. E., Zlotnik, A., Espevik, T., Dinarello, C. A., Cerami, A., and Palladino, M. A., Jr. (1988). Tumor necrosis factor alpha/cachectin is a growth factor for thymocytes: synergistic interactions with other cytokines, *J. Exp. Med., 167*: 1472.

Rappaport, H., Khall, H., Halle-Pannenko, O., Pritchard, L., Dantchev, D., and Mathe, G. (1979). Histopathological sequence of events in adult mice undergoing lethal graft-versus-host-reaction developed across H-2 and/or non H-2 histocompatibility barriers, *Am. J. Pathol., 96*: 121.

Richter, G., Qin, Z., Diamantstein, T., and Blankenstein, T. (1989). Analysis of restriciton fragment length polymorphism in lymphokine genes of normal and autoimmune mice, *J. Exp. Med., 170*: 1439.

Rolink, A. G., Pals, S. T., and Gleichmann, E. (1983). Allosuppressor and allohelper T cells in acute and chronic graft versus host disease. II. F1 recipients carrying mutations at H-2K and/or I-A, *J. Exp. Med., 157*: 755.

Saitoh, T., Fujiwara, M., Nomoto, M., Kamimura, T., Ishiara, K., and Asakura, H. (1989). Histologic studies on the hepatic lesions induced by graft versus host reaction in MHC class I disparate hosts compared with primary biliary cirrhosis, *Am. J. Pathol., 135*: 301.

Saklatvala, J. (1986). Tumour necrosis factor α stimulates resorption and inhibits synthesis of proteoglycan in cartilage, *Nature, 322*: 547.

Saklatvala, J., Sarsfield, S. J., and Townsend, Y. (1985). Pig interleukin 1: purification of two immunologically different leukocyte proteins that cause cartilage resorption, lymphocyte activation, and fever, *J. Exp. Med., 162*: 1208.

Satoh, J., Shintani, S., Oya, K., Tanaka, S. -I., Nobunaga, T., Toyota, T., and Goto, Y. (1988). Treatment with strepococcal preparation (OK-432) suppresses anti-islet autoimmunity and prevents diabetes in BB rats, *Diabetes, 37*: 1188.

Satoh, J., Seino, H., Abo, T., Tanaka, S.-I., Shintani, S., Ohta, S., Tamura, K., Sawai, T., Nobunaga, T., Oteki, T., Kumagai, K., and Toyota, T. (1989). Recombinant human tumor necrosis factor α suppresses autoimmune diabetes in nonobese diabetic mice, *J. Clin. Invest., 84*: 1345.

Saxne, T., Palladino, M. A., Heinegard, D., Talal, N., and Wollheim, F. A. (1988). Detection of tumor necrosis factor α but not tumor necrosis factor β in rheumatoid arthritis synovial fluid and serum, *Arthritis Rheum., 31*: 1041.

Scheurich, P., Thoma, B., Ucer, U., and Pfizenmaier, K. (1987). Immunoregulatory activity of recombinant human tumor necrosis factor (TNF)-α: induction of TNF receptors on human T cells and TNF-α-mediated enhancement of T cell responses, *J. Immunol., 138*: 1786.

Schrier, D. J., Phan, S. H., and McGary, M. (1983). The effects of the nude (nu/nu) mutation on bleomycin-induced pulmonary fibrosis, *Am. Rev. Respir. Dis., 127*: 614.

Seelentag, W. K., Mermod, J. -J., Montesano, R., and Vassalli, P. (1987). Additive effects of interleukin 1 and tumour necrosis factor-α on the accumulation of the three granulocyte and macrophage colony-stimulating factor mRNAs in human endothelial cells, *EMBO J., 6*: 2261.

Seelentag, W., Mermod, J. -J., and Vassalli, P. (1989). Interleukin 1 and tumor necrosis factor-α additively increase the levels of granulocyte-macrophage and granulocyte colony-stimulating factor (CSF) mRNA in human fibroblasts, *Eur. J. Immunol., 19*: 209.

Shalaby, M. R., Espevik, T., Rice, G. C., Ammann, A. J., Figari, I. S., Ranges, G. E., and Palladino, M. A. (1988). The involvement of human tumor necrosis factors-alpha and beta in the mixed lymphocyte reaction, *J. Immunol., 141*: 499.

Shalaby, M. R., Fendly, B., Sheehan, K. C., Schreiber, R. D., and Ammann, A. J. (1989). Prevention of the graft-versus-host reaction in newborn mice by antibodies to tumor necrosis factor-alpha, *Transplantation, 47*: 1057.

Stuart, J. M., Watson, W. C., and Kang, A. H. (1988). Collagen autoimmunity and arthritis, *FASEB J., 2*: 2950.

Sugarman, B. J., Aggarwal, B. B., Hass, P. E., Figari, I. S., Palladino, M. A., and Shepard, M. H. (1985). Recombinant human tumor necrosis factor-alpha: effects on proliferation of normal and transformed cells in vitro, *Science, 230*: 943.

Taverne, J., Rayner, D. C., van der Meide, P. H., Lydyard, P. M., Bidey, S. P., and Cooke, A. (1987). Cytotoxicity of tumor necrosis factor for thyroid epithelial cells and its regulation by interferon-gamma, *Eur. J. Immunol., 17*: 1855.

Toyota, T., Satoh, J., Oya, K., Shintani, S., and Okano, T. (1986). Streptococcal preparation (OK-432) inhibits development of type I diabetes in NOD mice, *Diabetes, 35*: 496.

Trentham, D. E., Dynesisus, R. A., and David, J. R. (1978). Passive transfer by cells of type II collagen-induced arthritis in rats, *J. Clin. Invest., 62*: 359.

Vilček, J., Palombella, V. J., Henriksen-DeStefano, d., Swenson, C., Feinman, R., Hirai, M., and Tsujimoto, M. (1986). Fibroblast growth enhancing activity of tumor necrosis factor and its relationship to other polypeptide growth factors, *J. Exp. Med., 163*: 132.

Warren, J. S., Yabroff, K. R., Remick, D. G., Kunkel, s. L., Chensue, S. W., Kunkel, R. G., Johnson, K. J., and Ward, P. A. (1989). Tumor necrosis factor participates in the pathogenesis of acute immune complex alveolitis in the rat, *J. Clin. Invest., 84*: 1873.

Weisbart, R. H., Golde, D. W., Clark, s. C., Wong, G. G., and Gasson, J. C. (1985). Human granulocyte-macrophage colony-stimulating factor is a neutrophil activator, *Nature, 314:*: 361.

Xu, W. D., Firestein, G. S., Taetle, R., Kaushansky, K., and Zvaifler, N. J. (1989). Cytokines in chronic inflammatory arthritis. II. Granulocyte–macrophage colony-stimulating factor in rheumatoid synovial effusions, *J. Clin. Invest., 83*: 876.

Yocum, D. E., Esparza, L., Dubry, S., Benjamin, J. B., Volz, R., and Scuderi, P. (1989). Characteristics of tumor necrosis factor production in rheumatoid arthritis, *Cell. Immunol., 122*: 131.

Yokota, S., Geppert, T. D., and Lipsky, P. E. (1988). Enhancement of antigen and mitogen induced human T lymphocyte proliferation by tumor necrosis factor-alpha, *J. Immunol., 140*: 531.

19

Pleiotropic Effects of TNF in Infection and Neoplasia: Beneficial, Inflammatory, Catabolic, or Injurious

KEVIN J. TRACEY
New York Hospital–Cornell University Medical Center, New York, New York

ANTHONY CERAMI
Rockefeller University, New York, New York

I. INTRODUCTION

Tumor necrosis factor α/cachectin (TNF) is an important mediator of diseases caused by infection, inflammation, or neoplasia. Depending on its concentration in tissues, and the presence of other mediators that influence its biological effects, the net effect of TNF produced in disease states may ultimately benefit or injure the host (Fig. 1). Although cytokine mediators are normally produced during infection or invasion and act in concert with the immune system to protect the host, it has become clear that the acute overproduction of TNF may be catastrophic, mediating shock, tissue injury, and death; moreover, when produced chronically it mediates anorexia, increased catabolism, weight loss, and death from the complications of protein-calorie deprivation. Here we summarize the results of our own studies and those of many others investigating the role of TNF as a mediator of the deleterious effects of acute and chronic disease. The implications of this work, performed primarily during the last 5 years, are discussed in terms of both disease pathogenesis and the anticipated development of future therapies.

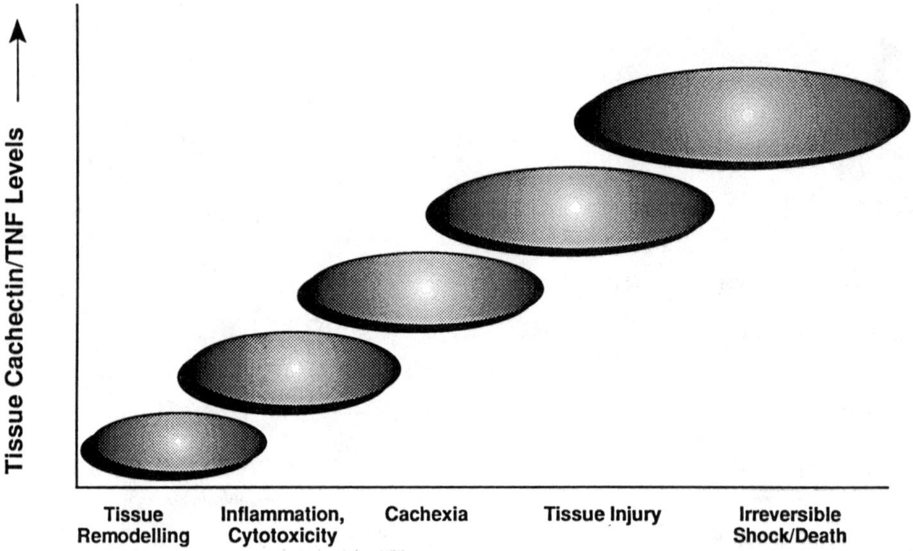

Figure 1 Net biological effects of cachectin/TNF according to tissue levels. Very low quantities of TNF produced in tissues mediate beneficial effects in the coordination of tissue remodeling, inflammation, and wound healing; chronic exposure toTNF mediates cachexia and increased catabolism (as occurs in chronic infection or cancer); and the acute release of large quantities of TNF (as occurs in overwhelming septicemia) triggers potentially catastrophic shock and tissue injury. [Reprinted from Tracey et al. (1989).]

II. MECHANISMS OF TNF ACTION RELATED TO WASTING AND CACHEXIA

A. Historical Perspective

Chronic disease in mammals characteristically induces a lethal wasting diathesis: termed *cachexia* (from the Greek meaning "to have it bad"), the afflicted host develops weight loss, weakness, anorexia, and net catabolism of body protein and lipid. This state of accelerated catabolism and wasting differs from the "normal" host metabolic response to simple food deprivation; under the latter condition the host develops an adaptive metabolic response that ultimately conserves protein and mobilizes lipid, whereas the cachectic host becomes progressively depleted of both lipid and protein (Brennan, 1977; Morrison, 1975). The weakened and depleted victim of cachexia then succumbs to the effects of undernourishment even though the invasive pathogenic or neoplastic burden may be quite small. Although early investigators presumed that the invading cells acted to usurp the energy supplies of the host, studies of parasite-associated cachexia in *Trypanosomiasis*-infected rabbits suggested that cachexia is actually mediated by a host-derived factor produced during the immune response to the disease (Rouzer and Cerami, 1980). This mediator was purified as a secretory protein from endotoxin-activated murine macrophages (cell line RAW.264.7) by Beutler et al. (1985) and named "Cachectin" for its presumed role as a catabolic mediator. The NH2-terminal sequence was subsequently noted to be strongly homologous to human TNF (Beutler et al., 1985), a molecule previously described (Carswell et al., 1975) as a mediator of the necrosis of certain transplantable tumors and cell lines. The molecular cloning of the corresponding genes confirmed that cachectin and TNF are identical (Caput et al., 1986). With the availability of recombinant human cachectin/TNF (Tracey et al., 1986) it was possible to initiate studies of its biological effects as a pathogenic mediator. (Reviewed in Tracey et al., 1989.)

B. Anorexia and Weight Loss

TNF was found to be a mediator of anorexia and weight loss from studies performed by injecting rats intraperitoneally twice daily with the cytokine (Tracey et al., 1988). TNF-treated rats consumed less food and developed cachexia with net losses of whole-body protein and lipid. This pattern of TNF-induced body compartment losses differed from that observed in partially starved pair-fed controls which became depleted of lipid but tended to retain protein. It has been teleologically reasoned that preferential sparing of protein is an adaptive response that preserves mobility and function during food shortages in nature, but these responses are overridden by TNF-induced anorexia and wasting. One as yet unexplained observation from these studies of TNF-induced cachexia was the development of tolerance to the anorexigenic and weight-losing effects of TNF (Tracey et al., 1988). Socher and co-workers also noted this desensitization in mice injected repeatedly with TNF for days (Socher et al., 1988). The tachyphylactic state could be studied by progressively doubling the daily dose of TNF; in this way the anorectic state could be maintained by giving large doses that would normally be lethal to the non-tolerized animal (Tracey et al., 1988). Subsequently, Norton and colleagues (Fraker et al., 1988) investigated the mechanisms underlying this tachyphylaxis and concluded that the development of tolerance was not secondary to either circulating inhibitors or increased clearance of TNF from the serum compartment. Interestingly, tolerance to the anorectic effects did not develop during 5 days of continuous intravenous infusion of TNF both in rats and humans (Michie et al., 1989), or in mice bearing genetically engineered tumors that continuously secrete h-TNF (Oliff et al., 1987). The development of tolerance to TNF during intermittent but not continuous modes of administration may have important implications in both chronic cachexia and endotoxin tolerization, but to date the biology of this tachyphalactic state remains undefined. While mediating a decrease of body weight, TNF also induces a net increase of whole-body water content (Tracey et al., 1988; Michie et al., 1989), which may be due in part to a direct reduction of skeletal muscle cell transmembrane potentials and a resultant sequestration of intracellular sodium (Tracey et al., 1986). Finally, these studies provided the first evidence that monoclonal TNF antibodies could attenuate the development of anorexia and weight loss during cachectic wasting, potentially offering a novel approach to the treatment of cachexia (Tracey et al., 1988).

C. Protein Loss

A hallmark of the cachectic state is a net depletion of whole-body protein that adversely affects mobility, respiratory musculature function, and mortality. Protein depletion is observed following chronic administration of rh-TNF to experimental animals or human subjects, as evidenced by whole-body nitrogen deficits, decreases of carcass protein, and net release of amino acids from skeletal muscle (Tracey et al., 1988; Starnes et al., 1988; Fraker et al., 1989; Warren et al., 1987; Flores et al., 1989). Flores and colleagues (Flores et al., 1989) found that infusing TNF stimulated increased rates of skeletal muscle and liver proteolysis. They theorized that these effects contributed to the net losses of protein observed in inflammation and cancer. The cellular mechanisms underlying these in vivo effects have been studied using both myocyte cultures and isolated skeletal muscle organ preparations in vitro. Incubation of L-6 myoblasts with TNF leads to a sudden release of lactate into the medium and a rapid depletion of intracellular glycogen as the cells revert to a state of net catabolism (Lee et al., 1987). Chronic exposure in vivo to TNF mediated a decrease of skeletal muscle protein content in part by a coordinate decrease of the transcription of genes encoding the myofibrillar proteins, myosin light chain, and actin (Fong et al., 1989). Moldawer and co-workers suggested that the proteolytic effects of TNF on skeletal muscle observed in vivo are not mediated by a direct effect on the myocyte, however, since addition of this cytokine to skeletal muscle organ cultures did not induce accelerated protein breakdown (Moldawer et al., 1987). In one study using very low doses of TNF, Michie and co-workers (Michie et al., 1989) found that the magnitude of nitrogen loss following continuous TNF infusion was similar to pair-fed controls, suggesting that higher TNF levels are to trigger increased proteolysis. As noted above, the mode of administration (episodic injection versus continuous infusion) may ultimately impact on its metabolic effects. it is clear that TNF acts to induce a mediator(s) of proteolysis in vivo, but to date the identity of this factor(s) is unknown.

D. Lipid Loss

TNF directly mediates the catabolism of high-energy lipid reserves stored in adipocytes. When exposed to TNF, lipid-laden adipocytes become catabolic and depleted of triglyceride, and subsequently revert to a fibroblast-like morphology depleted of triglyceride, and subsequently revert to a fibroblast-like morphology (Torti et al., 1985). This catabolic state results in part from a TNF-mediated suppression of the transcription of several key lipogenic enzymes (Torti et al., 1985). Moreover, TNF suppresses the expression of lipoprotein lipase (Beutler et al., 1985), a membrane-associated enzyme that normally serves to mediate the uptake of circulating lipid from the circulation. Its suppression effectively prevents adipocyte uptake of exogenous lipid. As predicted by these cellular events, the administration of TNF to both animals and humans confirmed that it promotes the net depletion of lipid and the mobilization of stored fat (Tracey et al., 1988; Starnes et al., 1988). Humans given intravenous TNF develop increased serum levels of circulating triglyceride and enhanced rates of whole-body turnover of glycerol and free fatty acid indicating that this cytokine in vivo stimulates of whole-body lipolysis and fat utilization (Starnes et al., 1988).

E. Liver Responses

The classical manifestations of cachexia include increased levels of serum triglycerides and acute-phase proteins and decreases in serum albumin. The net effects of TNF on hepatocyte cellular function and gene expression contribute in several ways to the development of these characteristic responses. For instance, in contrast to its lipogenesis-suppressing effect in adipocytes, TNF stimulates hepatic lipogenesis (Feingold and Grunfeld, 1987), and the combined effects of increased hepatic lipid production and decreased peripheral clearance probably mediate the accumulation of triglycerides in the plasma compartment of the cachectic host. Recently, Grunfeld and co-workers found that hypertriglyceridemia and increased hepatic lipogenesis persisted even after animals had become tolerant to the anorectic effects of TNF (Grunfeld et al., 1989), suggesting that the hepatocyte does not readily adapt to the tachyphylactic effects of TNF. Total liver weight, DNA content, and total protein are increased in animals chronically exposed to TNF (Tracey et al., 1988; Fong et al., 1989), and these changes are associated with both increased acute-phase protein biosynthesis (Perlmutter et al., 1986) and the specific downregulation of albumin biosynthesis (Perlmutter et al., 1986; Brenner et al., 1990). TNF is capable of stimulating transcription by increasing binding of nuclear factor to the NF-κB site (Duh et al., 1989), but whether this or some other regulatory mechanism is involved in the transcriptional events leading to increased acute-phase protein biosynthesis is unknown. Warren and his colleagues found that TNF mediates increased hepatocyte uptake of amino acids via glucagon-dependent pathways, a mechanism that might facilitate substrate uptake during the increased demands of lipogenesis, ureagenesis, and acute-phase protein synthesis that are integral to the development of cachexia (Warren et al., 1988; Warren et al., 1987).

F. Central Nervous System (CNS) Responses

The first study reporting the CNS effects of TNF revealed it to be a potent pyrogen that mediates a biphasic fever curve (Dinarello et al., 1986). Following intravenous administration of rh-TNF to rabbits an early temperature increase is the result of a direct effect of TNF on the hypothalamus; the development of a subsequent fever spike is due to increasing levels of another pyrogenic cytokine, interleukin-1 (IL-1), which is induced by TNF (Dinarello et al., 1986). The pyrogenic effects of TNF have been confirmed in other experimental animals and humans (Hesse et al., 1988; Kettelhut and Goldberg, 1988; Starnes et al., 1988), and these studies indicate that TNF-mediated increases of core temperature are associated with a net increase of whole-body metabolic rate. TNF is also a potent anorexigenic agent that apparently acts by a direct effect on the hypothalamic feeding centers: injection of minute quantities of TNF directly into the cerebral ventricles induced anorexia and an altered responsiveness of hypothalamic glucose-sensitive neurons (Plata-Salaman et al., 1988). Pituitary endocrine function is also altered by TNF: ACTH release is increased, but secretion of thyrotropin is inhibited (Michie et al., 1988; Pang et al., 1989). These CNS effects of TNF have important implications for the metabolic manifestations of several diseases, including the cachexia invariably associated with HIV infection (AIDS).

Since brain-derived astrocytes can be stimulated with lipopolysaccharide or a neurotropic virus to produce TNF (Lieberman et al., 1989), and elevated serum TNF levels correlate to the severity of brain involvement in children with AIDS (Mintz et al., 1989), it is plausible to suggest that local TNF production in brain might contribute to the anorexia of AIDS. A recent study addressed the net effects of TNF produced continuously in the CNS by implanting nude mice intracerebrally with a CHO cell line that had been genetically engineered to secrete human TNF continuously (Tracey et al., 1990). The predominate effect of brain-derived TNF was anorexia, which progressed to death by starvation within 2 weeks; this differed markedly from the effects observed when the TNF-secreting cells were implanted in skeletal muscle. Although tumors located in either site produced similarly elevated levels of circulating cachectin/TNF, the animals with peripherally produced TNF developed classical cachexia with losses of protein and lipid over 6 to 8 weeks, but animals with CNS-produced TNF exhibited only lipid losses, which were indistinguishable from starved controls. The importance of the paracrine effects of TNF was also evidenced by the growth of hair in brain tumor-bearing but not intramuscular tumor-bearing animals (Tracey et al., 1990). Although the mechanisms underlying this hypertrichosis are unknown at present, it is interesting to note that increased hair growth has been noted in some patients with anorexia nervosa (Boyar, 1980) or cancer cachexia (Hegedus and Schorr, 1972). These studies indicate that the predominate effect of intracerebrally produced TNF is anorexia, and that the site of locally produced TNF (e.g., CNS) may exert a profound influence on whole-body metabolism. Moreover, the circulating blood levels are not predictive of the net metabolic effects of TNF produced in tissues.

G. Anemia

Another hallmark of cachexia is anemia, caused by a net depletion of red blood cell mass that is independent of the associated protein-calorie deficit. TNF-induced cachexia is also associated with the development of anemia (Tracey et al., 1988) mediated by a reduction of red blood cell (RBC) life span, reduced incorporation of iron into newly synthesized RBCs, and increased RBC destruction (Moldawer et al., 1989). The depletion of red blood cell mass cannot be attributed to protein-calorie deprivation alone, since anemia is not observed in controls that are pair-fed the quantity of food consumed the previous day by the TNF-injected animals (Tracey et al., 1988). Given the importance of understanding the role of TNF as a modulator of erythropoiesis in health and disease, it is not surprising that several groups have employed in vitro assays to study these effects, but these studies have yielded conflicting results as to its regulatory effects on stem cells. TNF has been found to stimulate hematopoietic growth factor release from endothelial cells (Broudy et al., 1986) but also to directly inhibit erythroid differentiation (Peetre et al., 1986). Nonetheless, the available animal studies suggest that the net effect of chronically overproduced TNF is anemia (Tracey et al., 1988; Moldawer et al., 1989; Johnson et al., 1989), an observation that perhaps offers some insight into the mechanisms underlying development of the anemia associated with chronic inflammation or infection.

H. Summary of TNF-Induced Cachexia

TNF produced locally or systemically is capable of inducing a state of cachexia (Table 1). As a catabolic factor TNF induces energy mobilization from peripheral tissue by direct cellular effects in adipocytes and myocytes, and indirectly by stimulating the release of the glucose counterregulatory "catabolic" hormones (Tracey et al., 1987). TNF-mediated CNS effects amplify the associated increases of energy expenditure, oxygen consumption, and body temperature, but simultaneously lead to a suppression of food intake that worsens the protein-calorie deficit and hastens the development of weight loss, weakness, and wasting. Moreover, during TNF-induced cachexia the normally adaptive, protein-conserving responses to starvation are lost, and both lipid and protein compartments become depleted. If the cachectic state is not reversed, the afflicted host inevitably succumbs to the complications of malnutrition and organ failure. This brief summary does not address the complex cascade of other endogenous mediators that are induced by TNF and subsequently amplify and propagate its net metabolic effects (an abbreviated list of TNF-inducible factors is given in Table 2). For example, one such TNF-inducible cytokine, IL-1, is pyrogenic, anorexigenic, and capable of increasing the

Table 1 Pleiotropic Biological Effects of TNF in the Mediation of Cachexia

Tissue	Biological effect
Central nervous system	Fever
	Anorexia
	ACTH release
	TSH suppression
Muscle	Amino acid efflux
	Increased protein catabolism (via unidentified secondary mediator)
	Lactate efflux
	Glycogen degradation
	Decreased lipogenesis via decreased synthesis of lipogenic enzymes
	Efflux of free fatty acid and triglyceride
Liver	Increased lipogenesis
	Stimulation of glucagon-mediated amino acid transport
	Decreased albumin and increased acute-phase protein biosynthesis
Systemic	Hypertriglyceridemia
	Increased serum lactate
	Anemia
	Increased whole-body water
	Increased resting energy expenditure

sensitivity of host tissues to the toxic and catabolic effects of TNF (Waage and Espevik, 1988). Lipopolysaccharide also synergistically influences the effects of TNF and amplifies its toxicity during gram-negative infection (Rothstein and Schreiber, 1988). Thus the net effects of TNF depend on the quantity produced, the presence of other factors in the cellular milieu, and the site of production in tissues.

I. Role of TNF in Cancer-Associated Cachexia

The poor nutritional status of many patients with cancer precludes the use of aggressive and potentially lifesaving surgical and chemotherapeutic strategies. Worse yet, many victims of cancer succumb not to the direct effects of their increasing tumor burden, but rather to the complications of cachexia-induced malnu-

Table 2 Abridged List of Factors Induced by Cachectin/TNF

Cytokines	IL-1 IL-6 GM-CSF TGF-β MDNCF
Eicosanoids	Prostaglandins Leukotrienes Platelet-activating factor
Hormones	Corticotropin/cortisol Epinephrine Norepinephrine Glucagon
Cell surface proteins	Endothelial procoagulant factors ICAM ELAM HLA-A and HLA-B MHC antigens CR3
Miscellaneous	Superoxide radicals Collagenases and elastases Neurophil degranulation

Source: Modified from Tracey et al. (1989).

trition and wasting. Recently, animal models have been studied in an effort to develop a better understanding of TNF in the pathogenesis of cancer-associated cachexia. Using a rat sarcoma model, Stovroff and co-workers (1989a,b) found that tumor-infiltrating macrophages produced TNF, and that the development of cachexia correlated with increasing TNF production. Sherry and colleagues (1989) used murine TNF antibodies to partially reverse the anorexia and weight-loss of tumor-associated cachexia in mice. Interestingly, however, antibody administration prevented neither the increases in serum acute-phase protein levels, nor the development of anemia, suggesting either that the antibody was unable to neutralize the endogenously produced TNF completely, or that other factors are involved in the direct mediation of these effects. Studies of serum TNF levels in patients with cancer have yielded conflicting results: Although peripheral blood monocytes from cancer patients produced more TNF than normals (Aderka et al., 1985), and

Balkwill and colleagues found increased serum TNF levels (Balkwill et al., 1987), the latter observation was not confirmed by other investigators (Socher et al., 1988b). As emphasized by recent studies addressing the whole-body metabolic effects of locally produced TNF (Tracey et al., 1990), it is likely that the net biological effects of TNF may be independent of the predominate serum levels and may rather be dependent on the paracrine effects of the cytokine. While much work remains before the complete picture of TNF's role in cancer-associated cachexia is clear, the data available suggest that it may occupy a pivotal role as a trigger to many (if not all) of the complex metabolic responses that contribute to the development of debilitating anorexia, increased catabolism, and weight loss.

J. Role of TNF in AIDS

Cachexia invariably afflicts the HIV-infected patient, and in nearly all cases, hastens their demise. HIV is capable of stimulating monocytes to produce TNF (Merrill et al., 1989), and the cytokine has been detected in serum samples obtained from AIDS patients (Lahdevirta et al., 1988). In addition to the potential role of TNF as a mediator of AIDS-associated cachexia (by the mechanisms outlined above), recent evidence has implicated TNF in the activation of the latent phase of HIV infection. During the protracted subclinical latent phase, the virus lies dormant in host cells, but conversion to the active phase of AIDS is associated with fulminating viremia and rapid progression of the disease and associated cachexia. In a model of latent HIV infection using a chronically infected T-cell line, Folks and colleagues (Folks al., 1989) found that TNF induced the long terminal repeat and increased HIV expression in these cells. It appears that this upregulation of viral expression occurs by the activation of the specific nuclear factor NF-κB (Duh et al., 1989), thus providing a link between cytokine production and viral activation. Others have suggested that TNF possesses antiviral function that may be useful in the therapy of AIDS, but no antiviral effects were found in one clinical study of TNF therapy in HIV-infected patients (Aboulafia et al., 1989). To date, no consensus has emerged on the relative roles of TNF as either beneficial or detrimental in HIV infection or AIDS-associated cachexia.

III. TNF IN SEPTIC SHOCK SYNDROME

A. TNF as a Mediator of Lethal Shock and Tissue Injury

Septic shock syndrome is a catastrophic consequence of invasive infection that in the United States may account for up to 150,000 deaths per year. Despite major advances in antibiotic therapy and intensive care, the mortality of septic shock syndrome remains excessive and varies from 20 to 90%, depending on the age of the patient and the coexistence of pulmonary complications. The characteristics of septic shock syndrome include the development of hypotension, dehydration, hemorrhagic necrosis of vital organs, and death. In 1944, Franke and colleagues identified the activity of gram-negative lipopolysaccharide in the mediation of lethal endotoxic shock and organ injury (Franke, 1944). Forty years later, experiments utilizing the infusion of rh-cachectin/TNF revealed that the activity of this LPS-inducible cytokine directly accounts for the development of lethal shock and tissue injury in a manner that was indistinguishable from septic shock syndrome (Tracey et al., 1986). These early studies, performed first in rats (Tracey et al., 1986) and subsequently in dogs (Tracey et al., 1987), indicated that the appearance of TNF in serum was capable of triggering a cascade of metabolic events that culminate in irreversible shock, dehydration, suppression of cardiac function, and hemorrhagic necrosis of vital tissues. Necropsy of animals succumbing to TNF-induced shock revealed evidence of ischemic necrosis in the bowel, acute renal tubular necrosis, and pulmonary edema. Congestion of capillaries by adherent leukocytes contributed to the ischemic and inflammatory tissue changes. Hemorrhagic adrenal necrosis was observed in dogs, which also developed extremely marked elevations of circulating catecholamines, cortisol, and glucagon Tracey et al., 1987). More recently, Natanson et al. reported that a 30-min infusion of TNF induces a complex series of cardiovascular changes that persist for 7 to 10 days and are remarkably similar to those produced by bacteria (Natanson et al., 1989).

B. Mechanism of TNF-Mediated Shock and Tissue Injury

Some of the multiple biological activities of TNF that have been implicated in the development of shock and tissue injury are summarized in Table 3. Hemorrhagic necrosis and underperfusion of vital organs occurs in part from a suppression of myocardial function (Tracey et al., 1987; Natanson et al., 1989) and from thrombosis in capillaries mediated by increased endothelial procoagulant activity (Nawroth and Stern, 1986; Bevilacqua et al., 1986). Moreover, TNF induces the expression of a cell surface tissue factor that promotes coagulation by generating thrombin, decreasing thrombomodulin, and decreasing activated protein C. The net effect of these endothelial changes is an increased propensity for clot formation in the capillary beds of vital tissues. Taylor and co-workers (Taylor et al., 1987) found that these lethal TNF-induced coagulopathic changes could be reversed by the infusion of exogenous protein C, thus affording protection to baboons given *E. coli* infusion. In addition to altering endothelial surface coagulability, TNF also induces the expression of the endothelial activating antigens ICAM and ELAM (Pober et al., 1986a,b; Pober, 1988; Cotran et al., 1986). The expression of these molecules increases leukocyte adhesion to the endothelial surface, and once thus marginated, TNF directly mediates superoxide radical production by both neutrophil and endothelial cells (Nathan, 1987; Matsubara and Ziff, 1986). The net effects of local stasis, margination, and superoxide radical production contribute to the development of hemorrhagic necrosis and tissue injury.

Table 3 Pleiotropic Biological Effects of TNF in the Development of Lethal Shock and Tissue Injury

Tissue	Biological effect
Endothelium	Hemmorhagic tissue necrosis from increased procoagulant activity and suppression of cofactor activity for anticoagulant protein C
	PAF and IL-1 biosynthesis
	Leukocyte margination via increased ICAMs and ELAMs
	Superoxide radical production
	Capillary leak syndrome
	Nitrous oxide production
Cardiovascular	Hypotension and suppressed cardiac function
	Dehydration and decreased pulmonary capillary wedge pressure
	Lactic acidosis
Pulmonary	Respiratory failure
	Adult respiratory distress syndrome
	Hypoxia
	Pulmonary edema
Renal	Acute tubular necrosis
	Polyuria followed by anuria
	Glycosuria
Gastrointestinal	Focal and segmental bowel ischemia
	Pancreatitis
	Diarrhea
Central nervous system	Fever
	Anorexia
	Sympathetic discharge
	Headache
	Mental status changes

Hypotension induced by TNF occurs via a complex series of cardiovascular changes that includes decreased myocardial function, intravascular dehydration, and loss of peripheral vasoconstriction (Tracey et al., 1987; Natanson et al., 1989). Capillary leak syndrome, an extravasation of plasma water and albumin during septic shock syndrome, may be mediated by a TNF-induced separation of endothelial tight junctions (Stolpen et al., 1986) and possibly by endothelial cell cytotoxicity (Sato et al., 1986). The induction of IL-1 and IL-2 by TNF have also been implicated in the development of systemic fluid leak (Rosenstein et al., 1986). Eicosanoid mediators induced by TNF, particularly platelet-activating factor (PAF), appear to play a role in the mediation of TNF-induced hypotension and shock. Endothelial cell and leukocyte biosynthesis of PAF is triggered by TNF (Camussi et al., 1987), and PAF in turn induces hypotension, pulmonary edema, (Bessin et al., 1983; Mojorad et al., 1983), and TNF-induced bowel necrosis (Tracey et al., 1986; Sun and Hsueh, 1988). Excessive nitric oxide formation has recently been implicated in the development of TNF-induced hypotension, since the NO inhibitor N^9-methyl-*L*-arginine reversed the decreases of blood pressure mediated by infusing TNF (Kilbourn et al., 1990). Finally, pretreatment of experimental animals with the cyclooxygenase inhibitor ibuprofen abolishes some of the toxic cardiovascular and metabolic changes induced by TNF (Evans et al., 1989; Kettelhut et al., 1987), suggesting that these eicosanoids also act as secondary mediators of these effects.

C. Anti-TNF Antibody Prevents Septic Shock

Understanding TNF's role as a pivotal mediator of shock and lethal tissue injury has important implications for the therapy of septic shock syndrome. The effects of a neutralizing murine monoclonal TNF antibody (mAb) have recently been studied in a model of clinically relevant gram-negative septic shock syndrome, established by infusing an LD_{100} dose of live *E. coli* in baboons (Tracey et al., 1987). Baboons were studied in pairs; experimental animals were passively immunized against TNF either 1 or 2 h before bacterial infusion; controls received only carrier vehicle at similar times. An antibiotic was administered to all animals that survived for more than 10 h. The controls developed lethal septic shock syndrome and uniformly succumbed to the effects of hemorrhagic tissue necrosis and organ injury within hours. Anti-TNF mAb prevented the development of shock in all cases, and when administered 2 h before bacteria, completely protected against death (Tracey et al., 1987). Moreover, since all animals remained bacteremic for up to 8 h, these findings suggested that (1) lethality in septic shock syndrome was dissociable from the presence of circulating bacteria, and was actually dependent on the effects of TNF itself, and (2) that septic shock syndrome represents another example of immune-system overresponsiveness, where an overproduction of a pivotal mediator is capable of causing the demise of the host. Subsequently, Hinshaw and co-workers (1989) reported that the pathophysiology and lethality of gram-negative sepsis could be reversed by administering anti-TNF monoclonal antibody even after bacterial infusion. Moreover, similar protective effects of anti-TNF antibodies have been observed in animals given intravenous lipopolysaccharide (Beutler et al., 1985c; Mathison et al., 1988) or infected with cerebral malaria (Grau et al., 1987).

The protective effect of anti-TNF is probably due in part to the neutralization of acutely elevated circulating TNF levels that are capable of triggering shock (Tracey et al., 1986), but recent evidence indicates that these antibodies also attenuate the serum production of IL-1 and IL-6 (Fong et al., 1989). The recent availability of sensitive and specific assays for these cytokines prompted us to measure these levels in frozen serum specimens from the baboons described above (Tracey et al., 1987). Bacteremia in controls led to progressive increases in TNF, IL-1, and IL-6, but despite similar levels of bacteremia, animals protected against TNF did not develop increased IL-1 or IL-6 (Fong et al., 1989). Since IL-6 potentiates the lethality of TNF (Waage and Espevik, 1988), these data suggest that lethality in septic shock syndrome is the net result of both the direct effects of TNF and the complex cascade of secondary humoral mediators that it triggers. A TNF-binding protein(s) has recently been isolated (Seckinger et al., 1989; Engelmann et al., 1989) that may block the activity of the cytokine by interfering with the interaction of the ligand with its receptor; it has been suggested that this "anticytokine" may provide a mechanism whereby the host can protect itself from the toxic effects of TNF. The results of ongoing clinical trials are not yet available, but it is hoped that anti-TNF therapy will prove useful in the future clinical management of septic shock syndrome.

IV. TNF AS A MEDIATOR OF BENEFICIAL HOST RESPONSES

Although understanding the pathogenic effects of TNF in disease may facilitate the development of novel therapies, most assuredly the TNF gene has not been conserved throughout mammalian evolution in order to fulfill a role as a mediator of host toxicity. A growing body of evidence now supports the theory that when TNF is produced in lesser quantities and in a timely fashion, it mediates a variety of beneficial responses that enhance host defense mechanisms against pathogens, accelerate wound healing, and modulate the remodeling of senescent tissues. Fahey and co-investigators (Fahey et al., 1990) have recently found that TNF is produced locally in wound chambers during the normal "inflammatory" phase of wound healing, where it probably acts as a mediator of capillary ingrowth and angiogenesis and as an inducer of other growth factors, including TGF-β, PDGF, and IL-6 (Folkmann and Klagsburg, 1987, 1988; Zhang et al., 1988).

The paradoxical properties of TNF as a destructive and rebuilding mediator are ideally suited to a proposed role in the mediation of normal tissue remodeling (Vlassara et al., 1988). As a growth factor TNF is capable of stimulating the proliferation of fibroblasts and mesenchymal cells (Ranges et al., 1988; Sugarman et al., 1985; Kirstein et al., 1986), and as a cytotoxic mediator it also induces the biosynthesis of collagenases, eicosanoids, and superoxide radicals. Long-lived tissue proteins tend over time to accumulate glucose-derived protein cross-links termed *advanced glycosylation end products* (AGE) (Brownlee et al., 1988). Macrophages bear receptors that recognize these modified proteins, and receptor–ligand interaction induces TNF and IL-1 biosynthesis (Vlassara et al., 1988). Thus the AGE-mediated induction of TNF and IL-1 in senescent tissues may signal the macrophage clearance of old proteins and lead to cytokine-mediated rejuvenation of tissue matrices. In addition, cytokines may contribute to the pathogenesis of disease states characterized by an imbalance of this system with an increased accumulation of AGE-modified proteins (e.g., diabetes mellitus or old age) and the resultant abnormal proliferative and destructive effects in tissues (Vlassara et al., 1988).

The role of TNF as a mediator of increased host defense against infection has been studied in bacterial, fungal, and parasitic infection. It has been found to enhance antifungal activity in polymorphonuclear leukocytes (Djeu et al., 1986) and eosinophil toxicity to parasites (Silberstein and David, 1986). Pretreatment of mice with TNF conferred protection against lethal intraperitoneal infection with *E. coli*, suggesting a role in host defenses against bacterial infection (Cross et al., 1989). Titus and colleagues (1989) found that the ability of mice to resist cutaneous infection with *L. major* correlated directly with their capacity to produce TNF following parasitic challenge, and moreover, treatment of infected mice with TNF led to shortened period of infection. Finally, a single dose of TNF administered to rats protected them against the lethality of experimentally induced peritonitis (Sheppard et al., 1989). These and other data lend plausibility to the theory that timely production of this cytokine (in the appropriate doses) may ultimately improve immunological responsiveness and benefit the mammalian host.

V. PERSPECTIVE

TNF produced during injury, infection, inflammation, or neoplasia ultimately mediates beneficial or injurious effects. These net effects depend in part on the doses produced, the site of tissue production, and the presence of other cytokines in the cellular milieu. When very low quantities are produced in senescent or wounded tissues, TNF may participate in normal tissue remodeling and wound healing, but the release of larger quantities mediates inflammation and tissue destruction. Although tolerance may develop, chronic exposure to TNF is capable of triggering a state of increased catabolism and lethal cachexia. The acute release of large amounts of TNF into the systemic circulation is capable of triggering a catastrophic state of lethal shock and tissue injury. This pleiotropic cytokine is also capable of conferring protection against some pathogens and of inducing a complex humoral cascade of other cytokines. These observations suggest that ultimately the development of future therapies based on the mechanisms of TNF function will be designed to amplify or inhibit these effects in disease.

REFERENCES

Aboulafia, D., Miles, S. A., Saks, S. R., and Mitsuyasu, R. T. (1989). Intravenous recombinant tumor necrosis factor in the treatment of AIDS-related Kaposi's sarcoma, *J. Acquired Immune Defic. Syndr.*, 2: 54.

Aderka, D., Fisher, S., Levo, Y., Holtmann, H., Hahn, T., and Wallach, D. (1985). Cachectin/tumour-necrosis-factor production by cancer patients [letter], *Lancet*, 2: 1190.

Baskwill, F., Osborne, R., Burke, F., Naylor, S., Talbot, D., Durbin, H., Tavernier, J., and Fiers, W. (1987). Evidence for tumour necrosis factor/cachectin production in cancer, *Lancet*, 2: 1229.

Bessin, P., Bonnet, J., Apffel, D., Soulard, C., Desgroux, I., Pelas, I., and Benveniste, J. (1983). Acute circulatory collapse caused by platelet-activating factor in dogs, *Eur. J. Pharmacol.*, *86*: 403.

Beutler, B., Greenwald, D., Hulmes, J. D., Chang, M., Pan, Y. C., Mathison, J., Ulevitch, R., and Cerami, A. (1985a). Identity of tumour necrosis factor and the macrophage-secreted factor cachectin, *Nature*, *316*: 552.

Beutler, B., Mahoney, J., Le Trang, N., Pekala, P., and Cerami, A. (1985b). Purification of cachectin, a lipoprotein lipase-suppressing hormone secreted by endotoxin-induced RAW 264.7 cells, *J. Exp. Med.*, *161*: 984.

Beutler, B., Milsark, I. W., and Cerami, A. C. (1985c). Passive immunization against cachectin/tumor necrosis factor protects mice from lethal effect of endotoxin, *Science*, *229*: 869.

Bevilacqua, M. P., Pober, J. S., Majeau, G. R., Fiers, W., Cotran, R. S., and Gimbrone, M. A., Jr. (1986). Recombinant tumor necrosis factor induces procoagulant activity in culturesd human vascular entothelium: characterization and comparison with the actions of interleukin 1, *Proc. Natl. Acad. Sci. USA*, *83*: 4533.

Boyar, R. M. (1980). Anorexia nervosa, *Principles of Internal Medicine* (K. J. Isselbacher, R. D. Adams, E. Braunwald, R. G. Petersdorf, and J. D. Wilson, eds.), McGraw-Hill, New York, pp. 416–418.

Brennan, M. F. (1977). Uncomplicated starvation versus cancer cachexia, *Cancer Res.*, *37*: 2359.

Brenner, D. A., Buck, M., Feitelberg, S. P., and Chojkier, M. (1990). Tumor necrosis factor-alpha inhibits albumin gene expression in a murine model of cachexia, *J. Clin. Invest.*, *85*: 248.

Broudy, V. C., Harlan, J. M., and Adamson, J. W. (1987). Disparate effects of tumor necrosis factor-alpha/cachectin and tumor necrosis factor-beta/lymphotoxin on hematopoietic growth factor production and neutrophil adhesion molecule expression by cultured human endothelial cells, *J. Immunol.*, *138*: 4298.

Brownlee, M., Cerami, A., and Vlassara, H. (1988). Advanced glycosylation end products in tissue and the biochemical basis of diabetic complications, *N. Eng. J. Med.*, *318*: 1315.

Camussi, G., Bussolino, F., Salvidio, G., and Baglioni, E. (1987). Tumor necrosis factor/cachectin stimulates peritoneal macrophages, polymorphonuclear neutrophils, and vascular endothelial cells to synthesize and release platelet-activating factor, *J. Exp. Med.*, *166*: 1390.

Caput, D., Beutler, B., Hartog, K., Thayer, R., Brown Shimer, S., and Cerami, A. (1986). Identification of a common nucleotide sequence in the 3′-untranslated region of mRNA molecules specifying inflammatory mediators, *Proc. Natl. Acad. Sci. USA*, *83*: 1670.

Carswell, E. A., Old, L. J., Kassel, R. L., Green, S., Fiore, N., and Williamson, B. (1975). An endotoxin-induced serum factor that causes necrosis of tumors, *Proc. Natl. Acad. Sci. USA*, *72*: 3666.

Cotran, R. S., Gimbrone, M. A., Jr., Vevilacqua, M. P., Mendrick, D. L., and Pober, J. S. (1986). Induction and detection of a human endothelial activation antigen in vivo, *J. Exp. Med.*, *164*: 661.

Cross, A. S., Sadoff, J. C., Kelly, N., Bernton, E., and Gemski, P. (1989). Pretreatment with recombinant murine tumor necrosis factor-alpha/cachectin and murine interleukin 1-alpha protects mice from lethal bacterial infection, *J. Exp. Med.*, *169*: 2021.

Dinarello, C. A., Cannon, J. G., Wolff, S. M., Bernheim, H. A., Beutler, B., Cerami, A., Figari, I. S., Palladino, M. A., Jr., and OConnor, J. V. (1986). Tumor necrosis factor (cachectin) is an endogenous pyrogen and induces production of interleukin 1, *J. Exp. Med.*, *163*: 1433.

Djeu, J. Y., Blanchard, D. K., Halkias, D., and Friedman, H. (1986). Growth inhibition of *Candida albicans* by human polymorphonuclear neutrophils: activation by interferon-gamma and tumor necrosis factor, *J. Immunol.*, *137*: 2980.

Duh, E. J., Maury, W. J., Folks, T. M., Fauci, A. S., and Rabson, A. B. (1989). Tumor necrosis factor alpha activates human immunodeficiency virus type 1 through induction of nuclear factor binding to the NF-kappa B sites in the long terminal repeat, *Proc. Natl. Acad. Sci. USA*, *86*: 5974.

Engelmann, H., Aderka, D., Rubinstein, M., Rotman, D., and Wallach, D. (1989). A tumor necrosis factor-binding protein purified to homogeneity from human urine protects cells from tumor necrosis factor toxicity, *J. Biol. Chem.*, *264*: 11974.

Evans, D. A., Jacobs, D. O., Revhaug, A., and Wilmore, D. W. (1989). The effects of tumor necrosis factor and their selective inhibition by ibuprofen, *Ann. Surg.*, *209*: 312.

Fahey, T. J., III, Sherry, B., Tracey, K. J., Van Deventer, S. J. H., Jones, W. G., Jr., Minei, J. P., Morgello, S., Shires, G. T., and Cerami, A. (1990). Cytokine production in a model of wound healing: the appearance of MIP-1, MIP-2, cachectin/TNF, and IL-1, *Cytokine* (in press).

Feingold, K. R., and Grunfeld, C. (1987). Tumor necrosis factor-alpha stimulates hepatic lipogenesis in the rat in vivo, *J. Clin. Invest.*, *80*: 184.

Flores, E. A., Bistrian, B. R., Pomposelli, J. J., Dinarello, C. A., Blackburn, G. L., and Istfan, N. W. (1989). Infusion of tumor necrosis factor/cachectin promotes muscle catabolism in the rat: a synergistic effect with interleukin 1, *J. Clin. Invest.*, *83*: 1614.

Folkmann, J., and Klagsburg, M. (1988). Angiogenic factors, *Science*, *235*: 442.

Folkmann, J., and Klagsburg, M. (1987). A family of angiogenic peptides, *Nature*, *329*: 671.

Folks, T. M., Clouse, K. A., Justement, J., Rabson, A, Duh, E., Kehrl, J. H., and Fauci, A. S. (1989). Tumor necrosis factor alpha induces expression of human immunodeficiency virus in a chroniccally infected T-cell clone, *Proc. Natl. Acad. Sci. USA*, *86*: 2365.

Fong, Y., Moldawer, L. L., Marano, M. A., Wei, H., Barber, A., Manogue, K. R., Tracey, K. J., Kuo, G. C., Fischman, D. A., Cerami, A., and Lowry, S. F. (19891a). Chronic cachectin/TNF or IL-1 alpha induces cachexia with redistribution of body proteins, *Am. J. Physiol.*, *256*: R659.

Fong, Y., Tracey, K. J., Moldawer, L. L., Hesse, D. G., Manogue, K. R., Kenney, J. S., Lee, A. T., Kuo, G. C., Allison, A. C., Lowry, S. F., and Cerami, A. (1989b). Antibodies to cachectin/TNF reduce interleukin-1-beta and interleukin-6 appearance during lethal bacteremia, *J. Exp. Med.*, *170*: 167.

Fraker, D. L., Stovroff, M. C., Merino, M. J., and Norton, J. A. (1988). Tolerance to tumor necrosis factor in rats and the relationship to endotoxin tolerance and and toxicity, *J. Exp. Med.*, *168*: 95.

Fraker, D. L., Merino, M. J., and Norton, J. A. (1989). Reversal of the toxic effects of cachectin by concurrent insulin administration, *Am. J. Physiol.*, *256*: E725.

Franke, F. E. (1944). Action of toxic doxes of the polysaccharide from *Serratia marcescens* (*Bacillus prodigiosus*) in the dog and guinea pig, *J. Natl. Cancer Inst.*, *5*: 185.

Grau, G. E., Fajardo, L. F., Piguet, P. F., Allet, B., Lambert, P. H., and Vassalli, P. (1987). Tumor necrosis factor (cachectin) as an essential mediator in murine cerebral malaria, *Science*, *237*: 1210.

Grunfeld, C., Wilking, H., Neese, R., Gavin, L. A., Moser, A. H., Gulli, R., Serio, M. K., and Feingold, K. R. (1989). Persistance of the hypertriglyceridemic effect of tumor necrosis factor despite development of tachyphylaxis to its anorectic/cachectic effects in rats, *Cancer Res.*, *49*: 2554.

Hegedus, S. I., and Schorr, W. F. (1972). Acquired hypertrichosis lanuginosa and malignancy, *Arch. Dermatol.*, *106*: 84.

Hesse, D. G., Tracey, K. J., Fong, Y., Manogue, K. R., Palladino, Jr., M. A., Cerami, A. Shires, G. T., Lowry, S. F. (1988). Cytokine appearance in human endotoxemia and non-human primate bacteremia. *Surg. Gynecol. Obstet.*, *166*: 147–153.

Hinshaw, L., Olson, P., and Kuo, G. (1989). Efficacy of post-treatment with anti-TNF monoclonal antibody in preventing the pathophysiology and lethality of sepsis in the baboon, *Circ. Shock*, *27*: 362.

Johnson, R. A., Waddelow, T. A., Caro, J., Oliff, A., and Roodman, G. D. (1989). Chronic exposure to tumor necrosis factor in vivo preferentially inhibits erythropoiesis in nude mice, *Blood*, *74*: 130.

Kettelhut, I. C., and Goldberg, A. L. (1988). Tumor necrosis factor can induce fever in rats without activating protein breakdown in muscle or lipolysis in adipose tissue, *J. Clin. Invest.*, *81*: 1384.

Kettelhut, I. D., Fiers, W., and Goldberg, A. L. (1987). The toxic effects of tumor necrosis factor in vivo and their prevention by cyclooxygenase inhibitors, *Proc. Natl. Acad. Sci. USA*, *84*: 4273.

Kilbourn, R. G., Gross, S. S., Jubran, A., Adams, J., Griffith, O. W., Levi, R., and Lodato, R. F. (1990). N^9-Methyl-L-arginie inhibits tumor necrosis factor–induced hypotension: implications for the involvement of nitric oxide, *Proc. Natl. Acad. Sci. USA*, *87*: 3629.

Kirstein, M., Fiers, W., and Baglioni, C. (1986). Growth inhibition and cytotoxicity of tumor necrosis factor in L929 cells is enhanced by high cell density and inhibition of mRNA synthesis, *J. Immunol.*, *137*: 2277.

Lahdevirta, J., Maury, C. P. J., Teppo, A.-M., and Repo, H. (1988). Elevated levels of circulating cachectin/tumor necrosis factor in patients with acquired immunodeficiency syndrome, *Am. J. Med.*, *85*: 289.

Lee, M. D., Zentella, A., Pekala, P. H., and Cerami, A. (1987). Effect of endotoxin-induced monokines on glucose metabolism in the muscle cell line L6, *Proc. Natl. Acad. Sci. USA*, *84*: 2590.

Lieberman, A. P., Pitha, P. M., Shin, H. S., and Shin, M. L. (1989). Production of tumor necrosis factor and other cytokines by astrocytes stimulated with lipopolysaccharide or a neurotropic virus, *Proc. Natl. Acad. Sci. USA*, *86*: 6348.

Mathison, J. C., Wolfson, E., and Ulelvitch, R. J. (1988). Participation of tumor necrosis factor in the mediation of gram-negative bacterial lipopolysaccharide-induced injury in rabbits, *J. Clin. Invest.*, *81*: 1925.

Matsubara, T., and Ziff, M. (1986). Increased superoxide anion release from human endothelial cells in response to cytokines, *J. Immunol.*, *137*: 3295.

Merrill, J. E., Koyanagi, Y., and Chen, I. S. Y. (1989). Interleukin-1 and tumor necrosis factor-alpha can be induced from mononuclear phagocytes by human immunodeficiency virus type 1 binding to the CD4 receptor, *J. Virol.*, *63*: 4404.

Michie, H. R., Manogue, K. R., Spriggs, D. R., Revhaug, A., O'Dwyer, S., Dinarello, C. A., Cerami, A., Wolff, S. M., and Wilmore, D. W. (1988). Detection of circulating tumor necrosis factor after endotoxin administration. *N. Engl. J. Med.*,*318*: 1481.

Michie, H. R., Sherman, M. L., Spriggs, D. R., Rounds, J., Christie, M., and Wilmore, D. W. (1989). Chronic TNF infusion causes anorexia but not accelerated nitrogen loss, *Ann. Surg.*, *209*: 19.

Mintz, M., Rapaport, R., Oleske, J. M., Connor, E. M., Koenigsberger, M. R., Denny, T., and Epstein, L. G. (1989). Elevated serum levels of tumor necrosis factor are associated with progressive encephalopathy in children with acquired immunodeficiency syndrome, *Am. J. Dis. Child.*, *143*: 771.

Mojorad, M., Hamasaki, Y., and Said, S. I. (1983). Platelet-activating factor increases pulmonary microvascular permeability and induces pulmonary edema, *Bull. Eur. Physiopathol. Respir.*, *19*: 253.

Moldawer, L. L., Svaninger, G., Gelin, J., and Lundholm, K. G. (1987). Interleukin 1 and tumor necrosis factor do not regulate protein balance in skeletal muscle, *Am. J. Physiol.*, *253*: C766.

Moldawer, L. L., Marano, M. A., Wei, H., Fong, Y., Silen, M. L., Kuo, G. C., Manogue, K. R., Vlassara, H., Cohen, H., Cerami, A., and Lowry, S. F. (1989). Cachectin/tumor necrosis factor-alpha alters red blood cell kinetics and induces anemia in vivo, *FASEB J.*, *3*: 1637.

Morrison, S. D. (1975). Origins of nutritional imbalance in cancer, *Cancer Res.*, *35*: 3339.

Natanson, C., Eichenholz, P. W., Danner, R. L., Eichacker, P. Q., Hoffman, W. D., Kuo, G. C., Banks, S. M., MacVittie, T. J., and Parrillo, J. E. (1989). Endotoxin and tumor necrosis factor challenges in dogs simulate the cardiovascular profile of human septic shock, *J. Exp. Med.*, *169*: 823.

Nathan, C. F. (1987). Neutrophil activation on biological surfaces: massive secretion of hydrogen peroxide in response to products of macrophages and lymphocytes, *J. Clin. Invest.*, *80*: 1550.

Nawroth, P. P., and Stern, D. M. (1986). Modulation of endothelial cell hemostatic properties by tumor necrosis factor, *J. Exp. Med.*, *163*: 740.

Oliff, A., Defeo Jones, D., Boyer, M., Martinez, D., Kiefer, D., Vuicolo, G., Wolfe, A., and

Socher, S. H. (1987). Tumors secreting human TNF/cachectin induce cachexia in mice, *Cell, 50*: 555.

Pang, X. P., Hershman, J. M., Mirell, C. J., and Pekary, A. E. (1989). Impairment of hypothalamic-pituitary-thyroid function in rats treated with human recombinant tumor necrosis factor-alpha (cachectin), *Endocrinology, 125*: 76.

Peetre, C., Gullberg, U., Nilsson, E., and Olsson, J. (1986). Effects of recombinant tumor necrosis factor on proliferation and differentiation of leukemic and normal hematopoietic cells in vitro, *J. Clin. Invest., 78*: 1694.

Perlmutter, D. H., Dinarello, C. A., Punsal, P. I., and Colten, H. R. (1986). Cachectin/tumor necrosis factor regulates hepatic acute-phase gene expression, *J. Clin. Invest., 78*: 1349.

Plata-Salaman, C. R., Oomura, Y., and Kai, Y. (1988). Tumor necrosis factor and interleukin-1-beta: suppression of food intake by direct action in the central nervous system, *Brain Res., 448*: 106.

Pober, J. S. (1988). TNF as an activator of vascular endothelium, *Ann. Inst. Pasteur, 139*: 317.

Pober, J. S., Bevilacqua, M. P., Mendrick, D. L., Lapierre, L. A., Fiers, W., and Gimbrone, M. A., Jr. (1986a). Two distinct monokines, interleukin 1 and tumor necrosis factor, each independently induce biosynthesis and transient expression of the same antigen on the surface of cultured human vascular endothelial cells, *J. Immunol., 136*: 1680.

Pober, J. S., Gimbrone, M. A., Jr., Lapierre, L. A., Hendrick, D. L., Fiers, W., Rothlein, R., and Sprinter, T. A. (1986b). Overlapping patterns of activation of human endothelial cells by interleukin 1, tumor necrosis factor, and immune interferon, *J. Immunol. 137*: 1893.

Ranges, G. E., Zlotnik, A., Espevik, T., Dinarello, C. A., Cerami, A., and Palladino, M. A., Jr. (1988). Tumor necrosis factor-alpha/cachectin is a growth factor for thymocytes: synergistic interactions with other cytokines, *J. Exp. Med., 167*: 1472.

Rosenstein, M., Ettinghausen, S. E., and Rosenberg, S. A. (Extravasation of intravascular fluid mediated by the systemic administration of recombinant interleukin 2, *J. Immunol., 137*: 1735.

Rothstein, J. L., and Schreiber, H. (1988). Synergy between stumor necrosis factor and bacterial products causes hemorrhagic necrosis and lethal shock in normal mice, *Proc. Natl. Acad. Sci. USA, 85*: 607.

Rouzer, C. A., and Cerami, A. (1980). Hypertriglyceridemia associated with *Trypanosoma brucei* infections in rabbits: role of effective triglyceride removal, *Mol. Biochem. Parasitol.*, 2: 31.

Sato, N., Goto, T., Haranaka, K., Satomi, N., Nariuchi, H., Mano-Hirano, Y., and Sawasaki, Y. (1986). Actions of tumor necrosis factor on cultured vascular endothelial cells: morphologic modulation, growth inhibition, and cytotoxicity, *J. Natl. Cancer Inst., 76*: 1113.

Seckinger, P., Isaaz, S., and Dayer, J. M. (1989). Purification and biologic characterization of a specific tumor necrosis factor alpha inhibitor, *J. Biol. Chem., 264*: 11966.

Sheppard, B. C., Fraker, D. L., and Norton, J. A. (1989). Prevention and treatment of endotoxin and sepsis lethality with recombinant human tumor necrosis factor, *Surgery, 106*: 156.

Sherry, B. A., Gellin, J., Fong, Y., Marano, M., Wei, H., Cerami, A., Lowry, S. F., Lundholm, K. G., and Moldawer, L. L. (1989). Anticachectin/tumor necrosis factor-alpha antibodies attenuate development of cachexia in tumor models, *FASEB J., 3*: 1956.

Silberstein, D. S., and David, J. R. (1986). Tumor necrosis factor enhances eosinophil toxicity to *Schistsoma mansoni* larvae, *Proc. Natl. Acad. Sci. USA*, *82*: 1055.

Socher, S. H., Friedman, A., and Martinez, D. (1988a). Recombinant human tumor necrosis factor induces acute reductions in food intake and body weight in mice, *J. Exp. Med.*, *167*: 1957.

Socher, S. H., Martinez, D. M., Craig, J. B., Kuhn, J. G., and Oliff, A. (1988b). Tumor necrosis factor not detectable in patients with clinical cancer cachexia, *J. Natl. Cancer Inst.*, *80*: 595.

Starnes, H. F., Jr., Warren, R. S., Jeevanandam, M., Gabrilove, J. L., Larchian, W., Oettgen, H. F., and Brennan, M. F. (1988). Tumor necrosis factor and the acute metabolic response to tissue injury in man, *J. Clin. Invest.*, *82*: 1321.

Stolpen, A. H., Guinan, E. C., Fiers, W., and Pober, J. S. (1986). Recombinant tumor necrosis factor and immune interferon act singly and in combination to reorganize human vascular endothelial cell monolayers, *Am. J. Pathol.*, *123*: 16.

Stovroff, M. C., Fraker, D. L., and Norton, J. A. (1989a). Cachectin activity in the serum of cachectic, tumor-bearing rats, *Arch Surg.*, *124*: 94.

Stovroff, M. C., Fraker, D. L., Travis, W. D., and Norton, J. A. (1989b). Altered macrophage activity and tumor necrosis factor: tumor necrosis and host cachexia, *J. Surg. Res.*, *46*: 462.

Sugarman, B. J., Aggarwal, B. B., Hass, P. E., Figari, I. S., Palladino, M. A., Jr., and Shepard, H. M. (1985). Recombinant human tumor necrosis factor-alpha: effects on proliferation of normal and transformed cells in vitro, *Science*, *230*: 943.

Sun, X.-M., and Hsueh, W. (1988). Bowel necrosis induced by tumor necrosis factor in rats is mediated by platelet-activating factor, *J. Clin. Invest.*, *81*: 1328.

Taylor, F. B., Jr., Chang, A., Esmon, C. T., D'Angelo, A. , Vigano-D'Angelo, S., and Blick, K. E. (1987). Protein C prevents the coagulopathic and lethal effects of *Escherichia coli* infusion in the baboonl, *J. Clin. Invest.*, *79*: 918.

Titus, R. G., Sherry, B., and Cerami, A. (1989). Tumor necrosis factor plays a protective role in experimental murine cutaneous Leishmaniasis, *J. Exp. Med.*, *170*: 2097.

Torti, F. M., Dieckmann, B., Beutler, B., Cerami, A., and Ringold, G. M. (1985). A macrophage factor inhibits adipocyte gene expression: an in vitro model of cachexia, *Science*, *229*: 867.

Tracey, K. J., Beutler, B., Lowry, S. F., Merryweather, J., Wolpe, S., Milsark, I. W., Hariri, R. J., Fahey, T. J., III, Zentella, A., Albert, J. D., Shires, G. T., and Cerami, A. (1986a). Shock and tissue injury induced by recombinant human cachectin, *Science*, *234*: 470.

Tracey, K. J., Lowry, S. F., Beutler, B., Cerami, A., Albert, J. D., and Shires, G. T. (1986b). Cachectin/tumor necrosis factor mediates changes of skeletal muscle plasma membrane potential, *J. Exp. Med.*, *164*: 1368.

Tracey, K. J., Fong, Y., Hesse, D. G., Manogue, K. R., Lee, A. T., Kuo, G. C., Lowry, S. F., and Cerami, A. (1987a). Anti-cachectin/TNF monoclonal antibodies prevent septic shock during lethal bacteraemia, *Nature*, *330*: 662.

Tracey, K. J., Lowry, S. F., Fahey, T. J., III, Albert, J. D., Fong, Y., Hesse, D., Beutler, B., Manogue, K. R., Calvano, S., Wei, H., Cerami, A., and Shires, G. T. (1987b). Cachectin/tumor necrosis factor induces lethal shock and stress hormone responses in the dog, *Surg. Gynecol. Obstet.*, *164*: 415.

Tracey, K. J., Wei, H., Manogue, K. R., Fong, Y., Hesse, D. G., Nguyen, H. T., Kuo, G. C.,

Beutler, B., Cotran, R. S., Cerami, A., and Lowry, S. F. (1988). Cachectin/tumor necrosis factor induces cachexia, anemia, and inflammation, *J. Exp. Med.*, *167*: 1211.

Tracey, K. J., Vlassara, H., and Cerami, A. (1989). Cachectin/TNF (tumour necrosis factor), *Lancet*, *1*: 1122.

Tracey, K. J., Morgello, S., Koplin, B., Fahey, III, T. J., Fox, J., Aledo, A., Manogue, K. R., and Cerami, A. (1990). Metabolic effects of cachectin/TNF are modified by its site of production: cachectin/TNF-secreting tumor in skeletal muscle induces chronic cachexia, while implantation in brain induces predominately acute anorexia. *J. Clin. Invest.*, *86*: 2014–2024.

Vlassara, H., Brownlee, M., Manogue, K. R., Dinarello, C. A., and Pasagian, A. (1988). Cachectin/TNF and IL-1 induced by glucose-modified proteins: role in normal tissue remodeling, *Science*, *240*: 1546.

Waage, A., and Espevik, T. (1988). Interleukin 1 potentiates the lethal effect of tumor necrosis factor-alpha/cachectin in mice, *J. Exp. Med.*, *167*: 1987.

Warren, R. S., Donner, D. B., Starnes, H. F., Jr., and Brennan, M. F. (1987a). Modulation of endogenous hormone action by recombinant human tumor necrosis factor, *Proc. Natl. Acad. Sci. USA*, *84*: 8619.

Warren, R. S., Starnes, H. F., Jr., Gabrilove, J. L., Oettgen, H. F., and Brennan, M. F. (1987b). The acute metabolic effects of tumor necrosis factor administration in humans, *Arch. Surg.*, *122*: 1396.

Warren, R. S., Starnes, H. F., Jr., Alcock, N., Calvano, S., and Brennan, M. F. (1988). Hormonal and metabolic response to recombinant human tumor necrosis factor in rat: in vitro and in vivo, *Am. J. Physiol.*, *255*: E206.

Zhang, Y., Lin, J.-X., and Vilček, J. (1988). Synthesis of interleukin 6 (interferon-beta2/B cell stimulatory factor 2) in human fibroblasts is triggered by an increase in intracellular cyclic AMP, *J. Biol. Chem.*, *263*: 6177.

20

Tissue Damage Caused by TNF and Complement

JAY L. ROTHSTEIN
The Wistar Institute, Philadelphia, Pennsylvania

HANS SCHREIBER
The University of Chicago, Chicago, Illinois

I. INTRODUCTION

An enigma of tumor immunology for decades has been that bacteria or their products injected into tumor-bearing individuals can cause spontaneous tumor necrosis and, in some cases, tumor regression (1). Early attempts in determining the mechanism for such a phenomenon led to the discovery that lipopolysaccharides (LPS) produced by bacteria were responsible for the necrosis of tumors (2). Later it was suggested that LPS had direct effects on the tumor tissue (3). However, O'Malley et al. discovered that tumor-bearing mice treated with LPS produce a substance that upon transfer into a nontreated tumor-bearing animal, also induced tumor necrosis (4), indicating that tumor regression was not a direct effect of LPS but rather was mediated by other factors. The serum of LPS-treated mice was also cytotoxic to certain tumor cell lines in vitro. It was, therefore, hypothesized that LPS produced a substance in vivo that was directly toxic to malignant cells of the tumor (4). Efforts to purify this factor were met with much difficulty, as LPS contamination of the preparations may have contributed to the observed responses in vivo. Finally, Carswell et al. conclusively isolated a serum factor from mice treated with LPS that retained the antitumor capability in vivo and the tumor cell cytotoxicity in vitro, while having no detectable endotoxin contamination (5). This observation was confirmed by other investigators and recently the active component, tumor necrosis factor (TNF), was purified to homogeneity and the gene cloned (6). Furthermore, the recombinant TNF exhibits the same properties as the native material (for a review, see Ref. 7). Consistent with the notion that TNF can damage nontumor tissue is the finding that TNF has been associated with tissue damage occurring in animals exposed to infectious agents (8). Indeed, it is known that TNF can be produced by inflammatory cells exposed in vivo or in vitro to bacteria or viruses (9–13). In fact, animals exposed to endotoxin or bacteria show TNF in their serum soon before these animals die of shock (14,15). We were interested in identifying the components that, along with TNF, cause local or systemic toxicity. In addition, we wanted to elucidate a better understanding of how the interaction of these components can lead to such damage. To this end we have found that TNF and bacteria or their products can synergize systemically to cause lethal shock and locally to cause HN. In addition to TNF and a bacterial component, we have identified two other factors required for the induction of HN; one, the anaphylatoxin C5a, and the other radiosensitive non-T-cell leukocytes. The results of these studies will help identify mechanism responsible for protecting the host against malignancy and infection.

II. TUMOR NECROSIS FACTOR (TNF): A CRITICAL MEDIATOR OF TISSUE DAMAGE

A. TNF Effects in Tumors Resistant to TNF In Vitro

The endotoxin LPS is known to induce the release of TNF into the serum, which when transferred passively into a tumor-bearing animal can cause HN of the tumor (5). Even though TNF is cytotoxic to tumor cells and causes HN of tumors (6), damage to these tumors could be due to the direct cytotoxic action of TNF on the tumor cells, or due to direct damage to the normal tissue (e.g., vascular endothelium) surrounding the tumor, or to a combination of the two mechanisms. Indeed, much of the current research concerning the role of TNF in the pathophysiology of damage in malignant and normal tissue has focused on determining how TNF is able to induce many of the deleterious effects of endotoxin, such as lethal shock and local or disseminated HN (8).

To investigate the mechanism of TNF-mediated necrosis in vivo we initially focused on the effects of TNF on tumor tissue. In this regard we used tumor cell lines that have been previously characterized as being either highly sensitive (1591-RE3), moderately sensitive (1591-RES), or resistant (1591-MRV, AG104A) to the in vitro cytotoxic effects of TNF (16). After an initial period of tumor growth (2 to 3 weeks), syngeneic nude mice were then treated intravenously (IV) with increasing doses of TNF. In all cases, tumors responded to TNF with central necrosis (Table 1) even though the tumor cell lines derived from these tumors were markedly different in their sensitivity to TNF in vitro (Fig. 1). It was

Table 1 Sensitivity ot TRNF in Vitro Does Not Correlate to Sensitivity in Vivo

Cell line[a]	TNF concentration (mg/mouse)[b]	Sensitivity to TNF in vitro[c]	Incidence of HN[d]
1591RE-S	1.0	+	2/2
	3.0		1/1
	10.0		1/1
1591RE-3	1.0	+	2/2
	3.0		1/1
	10.0		1/1
1591RE-MRV	1.0	-	2/2
	3.0		1/1
	10.0		1/1
AG104A	5.0	-	4/4

Source: Modified from Rothstein (19).

[a]Treatment of tumors with TNF began 3 weeks after tumor cell challenge (10^7 cells/mouse SC).

[b]1.0 mg of TNF-α is equivalent to 5×10^4 units of activity on actinomycin D-treated L929 cells. Mice were injected once IV with 0.25 mL of TNF in nonpyrogenic saline at the start of the experiment. HN of tumors was recorded 24 h later.

[c]1591RE-S and 1591RE-3 show > 95% and 40% cytotoxicity, respectively, with 2.5×10^6 U/mL (50 μg.mL) of TNF, whereas 1591RE-MRV and AG104A show no greater than 10% cytotoxicity. See Fig. 1 for details. Data are pooled from two independent experiments.

[d]HN of tumors was assessed 24 h after TNF injection and consisted of dark red to black discoloration of the tumor center.. As described earlier (5), the central region of tumors injected with TNF decreased in size as hemorrhage occurred.

possible that TNF caused this damage by causing toxicity to the normal tissue surrounding the tumor. However, injection of large doses of TNF into normal skin did not cause any tissue damage (20). Therefore, TNF is not a bona fide cytotoxin. Evidently, additional factors are required to sensitize tissue in vivo before TNF can have toxic effects.

B. Synergism Between LPS and TNF in Causing Lethal Shock

TNF is known to be induced in vivo by LPS and may be associated with the local or systemic Shwartzman hemorrhagic reaction after repeated injections of LPS (21). TNF has also been associated with the pathological manifestations of endotoxin shock (14). We were, therefore, interested in determining if endotoxin could sensi-

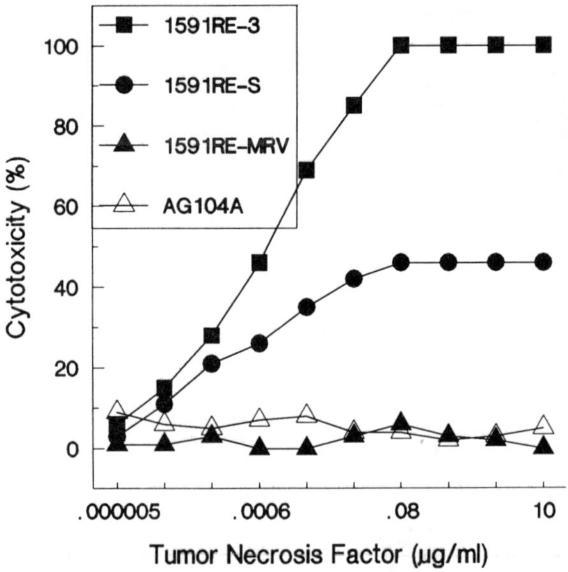

Figure 1 Sensitivity and resistance of selected tumor cell lines to the cytolytic effects of TNF in vitro. Tumor cell susceptibility to TNF was analyzed in a 72-h MTT assay (17); 0% cytotoxicity represents no difference between test wells (with TNF) and control wells (without TNF). Acetinomycin-D-treated, mycoplasma-free L929 cells, used for standardizing the cytotoxic effects (units) of TNF in a 48-h incubation (18), are substantially less susceptible to TNF than the 1591RE-S or 1591RE-3 tumor cells. The SEM for each point indicated was always <10% of the value of each point shown. The data are pooled from two independent experiments. Modified from Rothstein (19).

tize mice to TNF. It is possible that critical factors, in addition to induction of TNF, can be provided by bacteria and bacterial products. Toxicity of TNF in vivo was found only after recombinant preparations became available and had not been observed in previous studies using nonrecombinant sources of TNF (for a review, see Ref. 7). The higher toxicity of recombinant TNF could be due to the use of higher doses, to structural differences between the recombinant and nonrecombinant molecules, or to impurities remaining or introduced into the recombinant preparations during and after purification (7).

Interestingly, we found that an endotoxin-free source of recombinant TNF has a low toxicity in the absence of added endotoxin or other microbial agents as long as tumor-free and pathogen-free animals are used. However, as outlined below, we observed a very strong synergism between TNF and LPS endotoxin or between TNF and other bacteria in causing lethal shock or HN in normal tissues.

When normal pathogen-free C3H/HeN mice were injected IV with human TNF, no lethality was observed except at the highest dose (160 μg per mouse or 8 mg/kg). Even at this dose, only about 10% of the mice died in ≤ 24 h. The symptoms were similar to those observed after injection of high doses of LPS, such as piloerection, lethargy, diarrhea, and fluid exudation around eyes (Table 2, second column). Intravenous injection of 100 μg of LPS alone caused < 10% lethality (Table 2). In contrast, we observed that combined doses of TNF and LPS killed 100% of the mice. Furthermore, doses of LPS as low as 23 ng per mouse caused 50% lethality when applied with a nonlethal dose of TNF. An isobologram of the data (Fig. 2, upper) demonstrated that the combined doses of TNF and endotoxin were markedly synergistic and not merely additive. These data show that small doses of TNF could increase LPS lethality almost a thousandfold. Similar synergism was also observed in BALB/c mice (LPS-sensitive) treated with combinations of TNF and LPS. However, the LPS-resistant strain C3H/HeJ (23) did not develop lethal shock after injection of LPS and TNF (expt. 1, 0/5; expt. 2, 0/5). These findings suggest that the observed toxicity of TNF required LPS or a mediator induced by LPS. In fact, it might be more accurate to say that under these circumstances, TNF is an amplifier of LPS action rather than a mediator of it.

Table 2 LPS Synergizes with TNF in Causing Lethal Shock

	Lethality at dose of LPS (mg)[b]								
Dose of TNF (μg)[a]	0	0.023	0.093	0.38	1.5	6	25	100	400
0.0	0/5	0/2	0/2	0/2	0/5	0/8	0/3	1/17	2/2
0.6	0/5	0/2	0/2	0/2	0/7	0/7	0/7	2/5	2/2
2.5	0/5	0/2	0/2	0/2	1/7	3/7	1/5	4/5	2/2
10.0	0/11	2.6	3.6	3.5	5.7	7.7	2.2	2.2	2.2
40.0	0/18	3/6	4/6	5/5	7/7	7/7	2/2	ND[c]	ND
160.0	2/19	5/5	5/5	2/2	3/3	3/3	1/1	ND	ND

Source: Data from Rothstein and Schreiber (20).
[a]CeH/HeN mice received an intravenous injection of TNF in nonpyrogenic saline at the various doses alone or together with LPS.
[b]Number of deaths/number of mice. Lethality occurred within 2 to 24 h. Data are pooled from two to seven independent experiments, each also containing mice injected with LPS alone and TNF alone as controls. Results are underlined where lethality was observed.
[c]Not done.

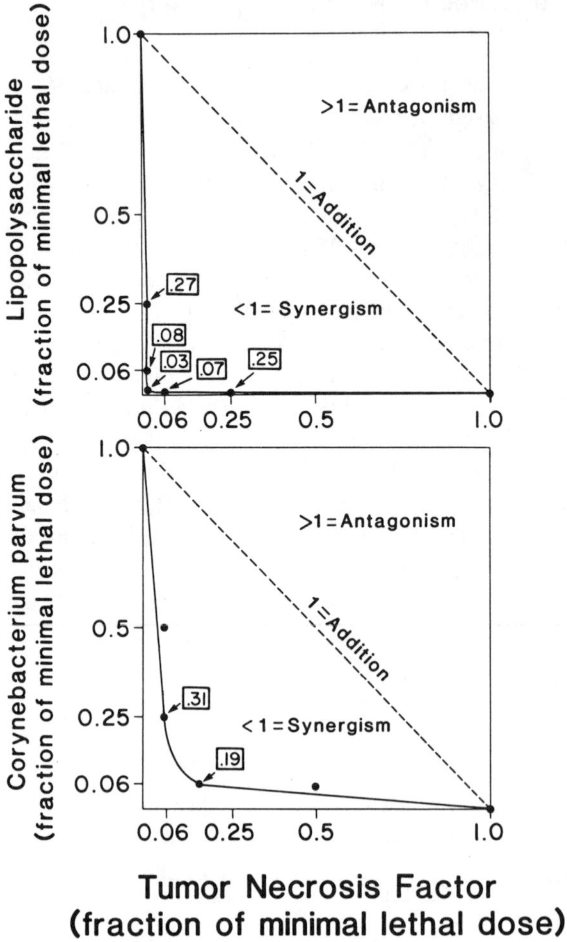

Figure 2 Upper, LPS and TNF, or lower, *C. parvum* and TNF, synergizes in causing lethal shock in mice. The effects are expressed as isobols with solid circles representing doses at which lethality was observed. Doses are plotted as fractions of the lowest (minimal) doses of LPS (100 μg = 1), *C. parvum* (4.8 μg = 1), and TNF (160 μg = 1) that were found to cause any lethality on their own (corner points). At this minimum lethal dose LPS (100 μg) caused 6% lethality, TNF (160 μg) caused 10%, and *C. parvum* (4.8 mg) caused 50% lethality. The two agents show synergism in causing lethal shock when both agents were given together because the sums of the fractions, boxed values smaller than 1, of the minimal lethal doses of these two agents were sufficient to kill the mice. The extremely concave curve in the upper panel is typical for maximum synergism between two agents, in this case LPS and TNF. Lower: *C. parvum* is also synergistic but to a lesser degree. Additive effects would have resulted in a straight line (dashed), with values of the sums equaling 1, and antagonistic effects would have resulted in a convex curve with values of the sums being greater than 1. TNF and LPS toxicity data points are also shown in Table 2. TNF and *C. parvum* toxicity data are derived from two to seven independent experiments each containing control doses of TNF or *C. parvum* alone. Data are from Rothstein and Schreiber (20).

C. Synergism Between LPS and TNF in Causing Hemorrhagic Necrosis

Subcutaneous injection of even high doses of TNF (such as 160 μg) or of LPS (such as 100 μg) alone into normal skin of mice did not cause HN. However, sequential subcutaneous (SC) injection of LPS followed 24 h later by TNF caused a massive HN in 81% of the C3H/HeN mice, of which half eventually died of lethal shock. The importance of this sequence is shown by the finding that simultaneous coinjection of a mixture of 100 μg of LPS and 10 μg of TNF into C3H/HeN mice failed to induce HN at the site of injection. Even though 1 of the 8 mice injected died of shock within 24 h following injection (Table 3) and injection of TNF followed 24 h later by LPS or TNF failed to induce any HN or lethality, it appeared that LPS, but

Table 3 TNF Causes HN in LPS-Prepared Skin: Independence from T-Cell Immunity but Sensitivity to X-Ray

Strain	First injection[a]	Interval (h)	Second injection	Interval (h)	Incidence of necrosis (%)[b]	
C3H/N	LPS + TNF	24			0/8	(0)
Normal	LPS	24	TNF	24	21/26	(81)[c]
	TNF	48			0/5	(0)
	LPS	48			0/5	(0)
	TNF	24	LPS	24	0/5	(0)
650 rad[d]	LPS	24	TNF	24	0/10	(0)
Nude	LPS	24	TNF	24	6/7	(86)[c]
C3H/J	LPS + TNF	24			0/8	(0)
	LPS	24	TNF	24	0/5	(0)
BALB/c	LPS	24	TNF	24	3/4	(75)[c]
	TNF	48			0/5	(0)

Source: Data from Rothstein and Schreiber (20).

[a]Single or mixed reagents were injected subcutaneously in a final volume of 0.25 mL into the lower back skin of mice from which the hair had been removed by a chemical depilator. In all cases the doses of LPS and/or TNF were 100 and 10 μg, respectively.

[b]Number of mice with HN/number of mice. Percentages of mice with HN are given in parentheses. HN was confirmed histologically in 4 mice of the 24 mice tested, showing PML infiltrates and extravasation of blood. In the other instances, the term HN was used to describe a macroscopically visible dark red to black flat discoloration of the skin 0.5 to 2.5 cm in diameter. For each mouse strain, data are pooled from two independent experiments.

[c]Mice were exposed to 650-rad gamma radiation from a ^{137}C source (J. L. Shepard and Associates, San Fernando, CA) 24 h before injections.

[d]The sizes of the HN induced by LPS followed 24 h later by TNF in C3H/HeN, nude, and BALB/cAn mice were similar (1.3 ± 0.1, 1.4 ± 0.2, and 1.4 ± 0.2 cm, respectively).

not TNF, sensitized the SC site for the induction of necrosis. Further, injection of LPS followed by LPS did not cause HN,* suggesting that TNF was indeed needed to elicit the reaction in primed skin. The development of HN required an x-ray-sensitive host component but was independent of a functional T-cell immunity since athymic nude mice developed HN after sequential injections of LPS and TNF (Fig. 3A).

D. Synergism Between TNF and Other Bacteria in Causing Necrosis or Shock

The synergism between TNF and LPS would have much broader implications if TNF also synergized with other groups of bacteria or bacterial products. Mycoplasma (M) organisms do not have a cell wall; they produce lipoglycans, which are similar but not identical to the LPS in the cell wall of gram-negative organisms (24). We therefore injected lysates of either *M. orale*-infected or *M. orale*-noninfected cells together with TNF SC (Table 4). Massive HN of the skin developed at the site of injection of lysates from *M. orale*-infected tumor cells or *M. orale*-infected fibroblasts and TNF, but unlike what was observed after SC injection of LPS and TNF, none of the mice died of the treatment. *M. orale*-infected cell lysates and TNF (Fig. 3B) caused a similar HN in athymic and normal mice, but γ-irradiated mice did not respond, indicating that like TNF- and LPS-induced HN, the induction of HN with mycoplasma-positive cell lysates and TNF was T-cell independent and radiosensitive. Since the LPS-resistant C3H mice responded to mycoplasma and TNF as well as the LPS-sensitive CeH and BALB/cAn mice, it was evident that LPS contamination of the mycoplasma preparations was not the cause of the response. An unrelated (gram-positive) organism, *Corynebacterium parvum*, coinjected SC as a heat-killed bacterial suspension mixed with TNF, also caused massive HN (Fig. 3C) at the site of injection without causing deaths in three strains of mice, including nude mice (Table 4). However, *C. parvum* with TNF injected together IV also synergized in causing lethal shock. The degree of synergism in causing lethality with *C. parvum* and TNF was clearly apparent, albeit less dramatic than that caused by injections of LPS and TNF (Fig. 2, upper and lower).

E. Other Mediators of Tissue Necrosis

As we showed above, the endotoxin-mediated local HN reaction in mice depends on two signals, the LPS as the initiating signal and TNF as the eliciting signal. In the following we have examined whether several other factors could replace the initiating or eliciting signal. Interleukin-1α (IL-1α) has a number of functional

*In rabbits, two successive injections of LPS, first into the skin and second intravenously, are used for the classical local Shwartzman reaction. The result of these injections is a localized HN at the skin site of injection. Mice do not develop HN following this protocol.

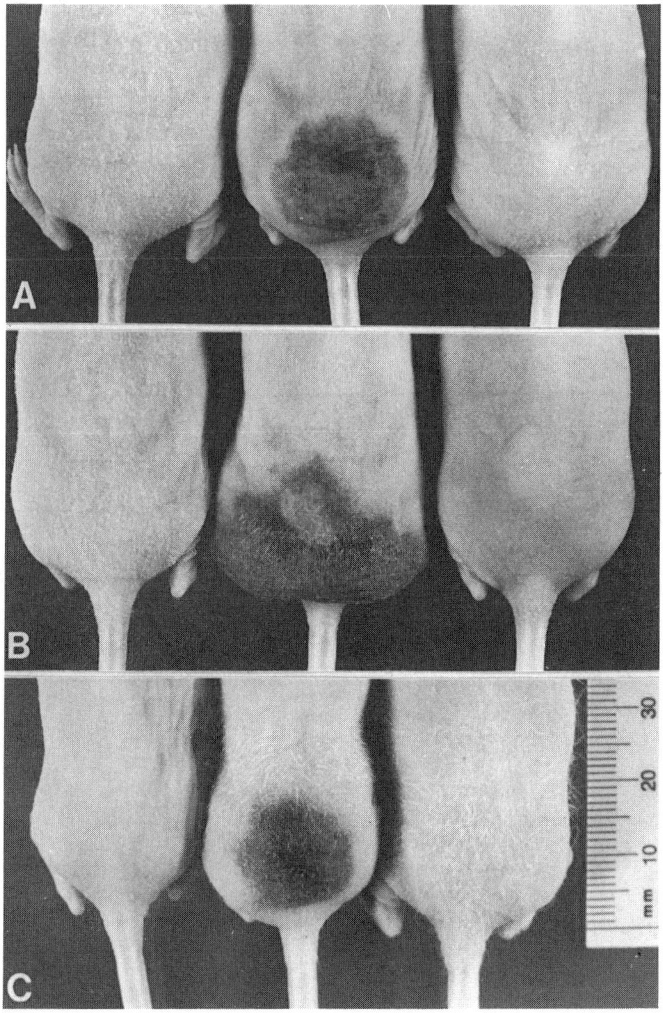

Figure 3 HN induced by TNF and LPS (A). Nude mice were primed with 100 μg of LPS 24 h before start of the experiments and either (right, left) unchallenged or (center) injected with 10 μg of TNF, where HN was detected 24 h later. HN was not seen in mice injected with (left) 10 μg of TNF alone. Center (B) shows HN induced by TNF and *M. orale*-infected lysates. Mice injected with 10 μg of TNF and lysates of 10^7 *M. orale*-infected cells developed HN 24 h later, whereas (left) no necrosis was seen with TNF alone or (right) TNF and lysates from 10^7 *M. orale*-infected cells. Center (C) shows HN induced by *C. parvum* and TNF. Nude mice developed HN 24 h after injection of 300 μg of *C. parvum* and 10 μg of TNF but not with (right) *C. parvum* alone or (left) TNF alone. Data are from Rothstein and Schreiber (20).

TABLE 4 Certain Bacteria Synergize with TNF to Cause HN

Host	Treatment: Bacterium	Treatment: TNF	Incidence of HN necrosis (%)[a]	
C3H/HeN	None	+	0/9	(0)
	M. orale-inf. tumor cells[b]	+	8/9	(89)[c]
	M. orale-inf. tumor cells	–	0/5	(0)
	M. orale-noninf. tumor cells	+	0/7	(0)
	M. orale-noninf. tumor cells	–	0/5	(0)
	M. orale-inf. tumor cells (1 h at 100°C)	+	2/2	(100)[c]
	M. orale-inf. tumor cells (1 h at 100°C)	–	0/2	(0)
	M. orale-inf. fibroblasts	+	9/9	(100)[c]
	M. orale-noninf. fibroblasts	+	0/4	(0)
	C. parvum (killed)	+	13/14	(93)[c]
	C. parvum (killed)	–	0/14	(0)
650 rad	None	+	0/3	(0)
	M. orale-inf. tumor cells	+	0/3	(0)
	C. parvum (killed)	+	1/10	(10)[c]
Athymic	None	–	0/3	(0)
	M. orale-inf. tumor cells	+	2/2	(100)[c]
	M. orale-inf. tumor cells	–	0/4	(0)
	C. parvum (killed)	+	4/4	(100)[c]
	C. parvum (killed)	–	0/5	(0)
C3H/HeJ	None	+	0/7	(0)
	M. orale-inf. tumor cells	+	9/10	(90)[c]
	C. parvum (killed)	+	7/7	(100)[c]
	C. parvum (killed)	–	0/6	(0)
BALB/cAn	None	+	0/5	(0)
	M. orale-inf. tumor cells	+	4/5	(75)[c]
	C. parvum (killed)	+	10/10	(100)[c]
	C. parvum (killed)	–	0/5	(0)
650 rad	None	+	0/5	(0)
	C. parvum (killed)	+	0/5	(0)
Athymic	None	+	0/4	(0)
NCR	*M. orale*-inf. tumor cells	+	3/5	(60)[c]
nudes	*C. parvum* (killed)	+	4/4	(100)[c]

Source: Data from Rothstein and Schreiber (20).

[a]Experiments with more than three mice were pooled from two or more experiments, each containing a negative control (bacterium alone and TNF alone) and a positive control (bacterium and TNF). For other details, see the footnotes of Table 3.

[b]1591-RE and 1316-RE were used as *M. orale*-infected (inf.) tumor cells which induced necrosis in 6/7 and 2/2 mice, respectively. Elsewhere in the table *M. orale*-inf. tumor cells refer to 1591-RE only.

[c]The sizes of the HN induced by *M. orale*-infected lysates and TNF or *C. parvum* and TNF were similar (1.1 cm ± 0.2 SEM, 1.0 ± 0.1, 1.6 ± 0.1, 1.3 ± 0.1, 1.0, 1.3 ± 0.7, 1.9 ± 0.2, 1.6 ± 0.1, 1.4 ± 0.2, 1.6 ± 0.2, 1.5 ± 0.2, 1.1 ± 0.1, 1.3 ± 0.2, respectively, in the sequence mentioned).

[d]The normal fibroblast line, 10T 1/2, and normal heart-lung fibroblasts were used as *M. orale*-inf. fibroblasts which induced necrosis in 4/4 and 4/4 mice, respectively. *M. orale*-noninfected (noninf.) fibroblasts refer to 10T 1/2.

similarities with TNF (for a review, see Ref. 25), and a nonrecombinant course of IL-1α has been implicated in the development of Shwartzman reaction (21). However, Table 5 shows that the recombinant cytokine IL-1α failed to substitute for TNF in synergizing with *C. parvum* to induce HN. Similarly, interferon-γ (IFN-γ) also failed to synergize with *C. parvum* to induce HN. In contrast, LT (26), which demonstrates significant sequence homology to TNF (27), can substitute for TNF in causing HN with *C. parvum*, although in repeated experiments LT was less effective. At present, we do not know whether GM-CSF or G-CSF, which can, like TNF, cause a respiratory burst in polymorphonuclear leukocytes (PML) can replace the TNF signal. IFN-γ is known to synergize with TNF in killing tumor cells in vitro (28–30). However, neither IFN-γ nor IL-1α could replace the bacterial component and synergize with TNF to induce HN, even though IL-1α has been shown to synergize with TNF in inducing lethal shock (31).

Table 5 Neither IL-1α nor IFN-γ Can Substitute for TNF, LT, or *C. parvum* in the Induction of HN

Subcutaneous treatment[a]	Incidence of HN in experiments 1	2	3	4	5	6	7	Incidence of HN (%)[b]
TNF	0/2	0/2	0/2		0/2			0/8 (0)
LT	0/2	0/2						0/4 (0)
IFN-γ	0/2	0/2	0/2			0/2		0/8 (0)
IL-1α						0/2	0/2	0/4 (0)
C. parvum	0/2	0/2	0/2					0/6 (0)
+ TNF	5/5	5/5	2/2	2/2	2/2			16/16 (100)[c]
+ LT	3/5	1/2						4/7 (57)[c]
+ IFN-γ	0/5	0/5	0/2					0/12 (0)
+ IL-1α				0/2	0/2			0/4 (0)
IFN-γ + TNF						0/2	0/2	0/4 (0)
IL-1α + TNF[d]						0/2	0/2	0/4 (0)

Source: Data from Rothstein and Schreiber (20).

[a]C3H/HeN mice were injected SC with *C. parvum* (300 μg) and/or the appropriate recombinant cytokine (each of the latter was used at a dose of 10 μg/mouse). The incidence of HN was determined 24 h later.

[b]Number of mice showing HN/number of mice tested. The percentages are given in parentheses.

[c]The sizes of the HN induced by *C. parvum* and TNF or *C. parvum* and LT were similar (1.7 ± 0.1 and 1.9 ± 0.2 cm, respectively.

[d]IL-1α injected SC (10 μg/mouse) followed 24 h later by TNF (10 μg/mouse) also failed to induce HN (expt. 1: 0/2, expt. 2: 0/2).

Unlike the cytokines tested, the elements that make up the bacterial component are complex. Much is known about the structural backbone of the bacterial cell wall component LPS, which is common to gram-negative bacteria. In fact, a majority of the biological activity of LPS can be associated with the glycolipid backbone moiety commonly referred to as lipid A (32). Lipid A is composed of a phosphorylated glucosamine disaccharide backbone with long chains of fatty acid side groups. Although lipid A is distinct from the parental LPS molecule, Table 6 shows that lipid A was, nonetheless, capable of replacing LPS in the induction of HN with TNF. Furthermore, highly purified lipid A, containing only the diphosphorylated form and without contaminating LPS molecules, or the monophosphorylated derivative of lipid A were equally capable of priming mice for the induction of HN by TNF (Table 6). These data suggest that the bacterial component capable of synergizing with TNF may be a simple compound, such as the lipid A derivative of LPS, which is shared among different gram-negative bacteria. In addition, it is known that tumors produce substances that have structural similarity with the complex oligosaccharides found on the surface of many different bacteria (33). These compounds may all share a similar property enabling both tumors and bacteria to act as priming factors for damage caused by TNF.

III. HUMORAL COMPONENT OF HEMORRHAGIC NECROSIS

A. C5-Deficient Mice Do Not Develop Necrosis

When comparing different mouse strains for possible differences in the HN response to TNF and *C. parvum*, LPS, or *M. orale*-infected cell lysates, we discov-

Table 6 LPS and Nontoxic Derivatives Prime Mice for the Induction of HN by TNF

Priming agent[a]	Incidence of HN (%)[b]	
LPS	8/9	(89)
Lipid A	5/7	(71)
Dilipid A	4/4	(100)
Monolipid A	4/4	(100)

Source: Modified from Rothstein (19).
[a]All agents were SC injected at 100 μg. TNF was injected at the same site 24 h later (10 μg). Di (diphosphoryl), mono (monophosphoryl).
[b]Number of mice (C3H/HeN) responding with HN/total number of mice tested. The diameter of HN lesions were similar (1.2 cm ± 0.3 SEM). Data are pooled from two independent experiments.

ered that certain strains of mice failed to develop HN (Table 7; Fig. 4). Interestingly, these nonresponsive strains are known to have no detectable levels of C5 in the plasma (36,37; for a review, see Ref. 38). In contrast, the C5-sufficient CBA, B10.D2/n, and C3H mouse strains regularly developed HN, as characterized by a round dark red to black flat lesion (Fig. 4) involving the full thickness of the skin, 0.5 to 2.5 cm in diameter (mean diameter, 1.4 cm). HN could be quantified by a ^{51}Cr-labeled blood cell assay previously used to quantify HN induced in tumors by TNF (20). This assay served as a direct measurement of blood cell extravasation. Thus in Fig. 5, C5-sufficient mice show significant extravasation of blood cells as quantified by the retention of ^{51}Cr-labeled blood cells in skin with HN. Consistent with the HN observed macroscopically, Fig. 6 also shows that this effect required injection of *C. parvum* as well as TNF. Injection of *C. parvum* and TNF or *C. parvum* alone into C5-deficient mice showed no difference n retention of ^{51}Cr-labeled blood cells. In addition, these data can be corroborated microscopically by demon-

Table 7 C5-Deficient Mouse Strains Fail to Develop HN When Injected with a Bacterial Agent and TNF

Bacterial agent[a]	Mouse strain	Complement deficiency[b]	Incidence of HN (%)[c]
C. parvum	C3H/HeN	None	13/14 (93)
	C3H/HeJ	None	4/4 (100)
	CBA/J	None	9/10 (90)
	B10.D2/n	C3	14/22 (64)
	DBA/2	C3, C5	0/10 (0)
	B10.D2/o	C3, C5	0/13 (0)
	A\J	C5	0/12 (0)
	AKR	C5	0/7 (0)
LPS	CeH/HeN	None	11/11 (100)
	B10.D2/o	C3, C5	0/10 (0)
M. orale-infected cell lysates	C3H/HeN	None	10/10 (100)
	DBA/2	C3, C5	0/10 (0)

Source: Data from Rothstein et al. (42).

[a]HN was induced by SC coinjection of *C. parvum* and TNF or *M. orale*-infected cell lysates and TNF. Alternatively, HN was induced by SC injection of LPS followed 24 h later by TNF.

[b]Mice deficient in C3 have low, but detectable levels of C3 (34,35). Mice deficient in C5 have no detectable C5 (36,37; for a review, see Ref. 38).

[c]Number of mice responding with HN/ total number of mice tested. HN was assessed 24 h after injection of TNF. The mean diameter of the hemorrhagic lesions of different C5-sufficient mouse strains were similar (1.8 cm ± 0.2 SESM). Data are pooled from two or more independent experiments each containing at least one C5-sufficient and one C5-deficient group of mice.

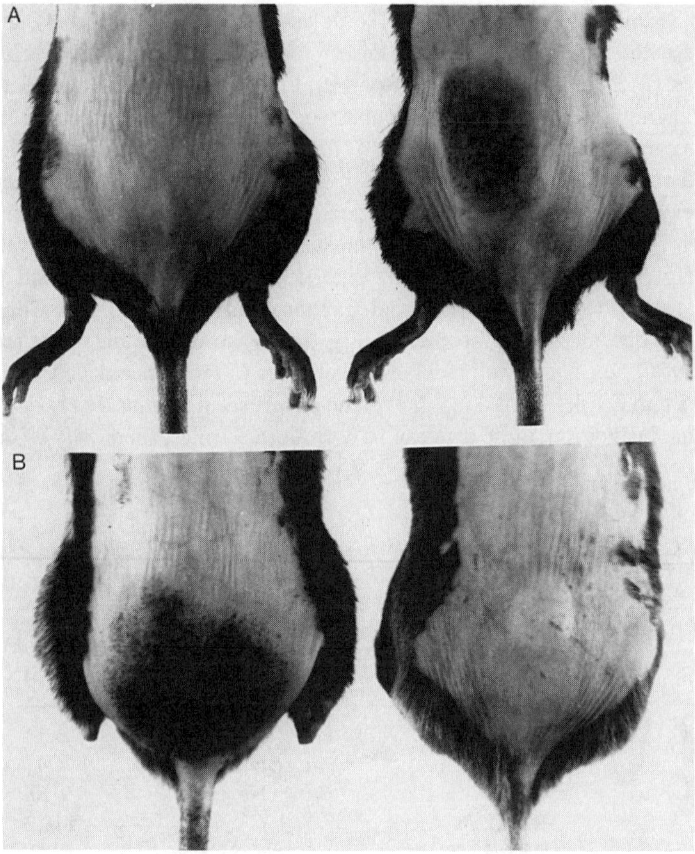

Figure 4 C5-deficient mice fail to develop HN when injected with bacterial agents and TNF. (A) Right: C5-sufficient (B10.D2/n) mice respond with HN 24 h after coinjection of *C. parvum* (400 μg) and TNF (10 μg). Left: C5-deficient (B10.D2/o) mice coinjected with *C. parvum* (400 μg) and TNF (10 mg) fail to respond with macroscopic hemorrhagic lesion. (B) Right: C5-deficient (DBA/2) mice injected with LPS (100 μg) followed 24 h later with TNF (10 μg) do not develop HN. Left: C5-sufficient (C3H/HeN) injected with LPS (100 μg) followed 24 h later by TNF (10 μg) respond with HN. Data are from Rothstein et al. (42).

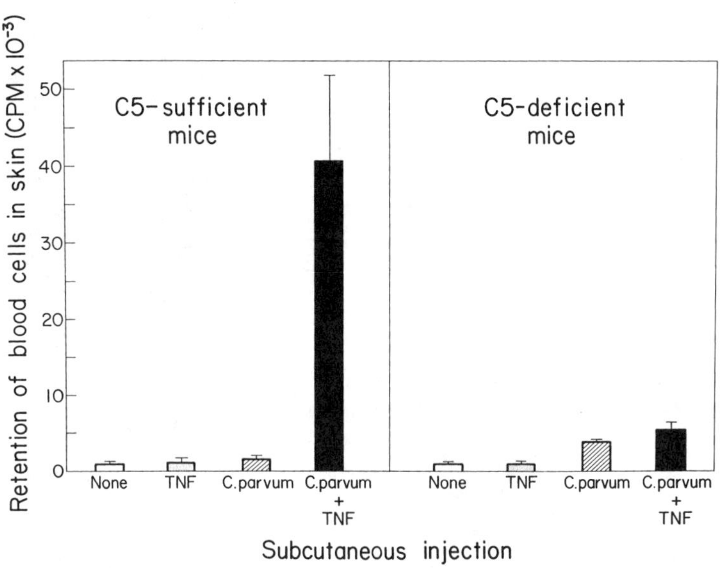

Figure 5 Quantification of the HN developing in C5-sufficient, but not C5-deficient mice after injection of *C. parvum* and TNF. C3H/HeN (C5-sufficient) or B10.D2/o (C5-deficient) mice were injected with either TNF (10 mg) alone, heat-killed *C. parvum* (400 mg) alone, or heat-killed *C. parvum* (400 mg) and TNF (10 μg). 24 h later, retention of [^{51}Cr]blood cells in the skin was quantified by measuring the radioactivity of a 2 $\times$ 2 cm square piece of skin containing the site of injection in the center. For details see the text. Bars represent SEM. Data are pooled from three independent experiments. From Rothstein et al. (42).

strating that the increased retention of ^{51}Cr-labeled blood cells in skin showing HN in C5-sufficient mice is indeed associated with the extravasation of red blood cells (Fig. 6D,E). In contrast, C5-deficient mice show inflammatory infiltrates without extravasation of red cells (Fig. 7).In fact, these inflammatory white blood cell infiltrates may be responsible for the slightly increased retention of ^{51}Cr-labeled blood cells as measured in the skin of C5-deficient mice (Fig. 5). Even though this level is increased significantly ($p < 0.002$) above the level observed in noninjected skin, it is much lower than in mice developing HN. Furthermore, C5-deficient mice lack the potent leukocyte chemoattractant C5a (39), but they nonetheless showed an equal or even greater leukocyte infiltrate when compared to C5-sufficient mice (Fig. 6). Thus the absence of the leukocyte-attractive function of C5a cannot explain the nonresponsiveness in these C5-deficient mice. Interestingly, B10.D2/n mice did not show the same incidence of HN as the other C5-sufficient strains,

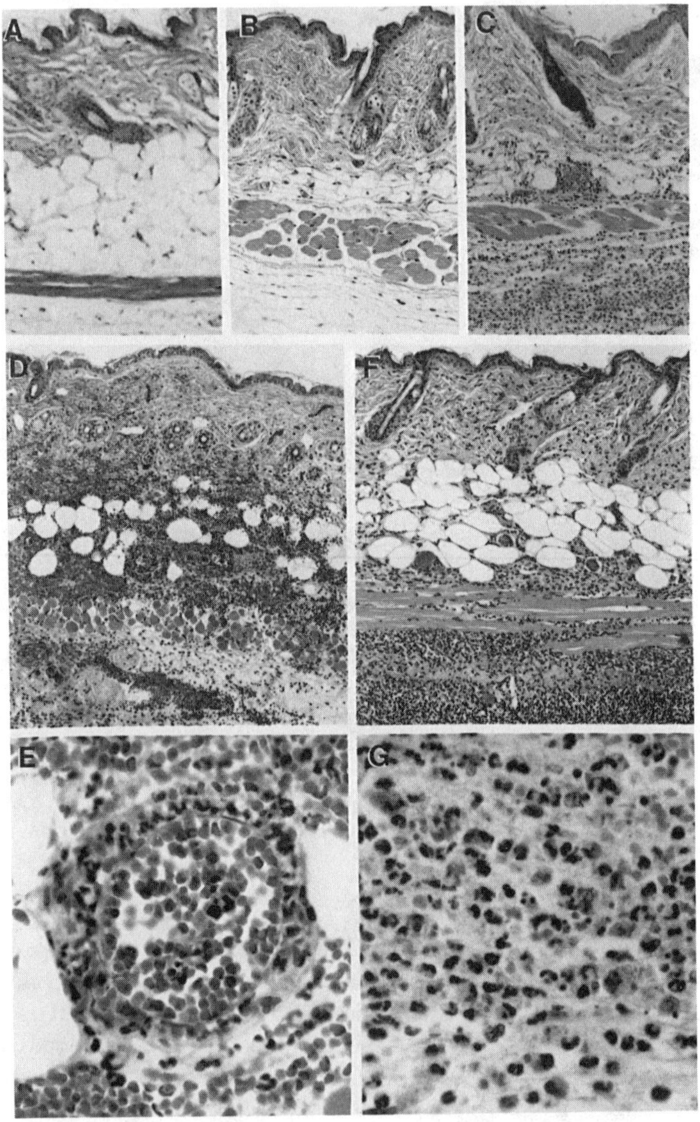

Figure 6 Inflammatory infiltrate without extravasation of red blood cells in skin of C5-deficient mice injected with TNF and *C. parvum*. (A–E) skin sections of C5-sufficient C3H/HeN mice. (A) Noninjected. (B) TNF (10 mg); no infiltrate. (C) *C. parvum* (400 mg); extensive leukocyte infiltrate. (D and E) *C. parvum* (400 μg) and TNF (10 μg); extensive leukocyte infiltrate with extravasation of red blood cells. (F and G) Skin sections of C5-deficient A/J mice injected with *C. parvum* (400 μg) and TNF (10 μg); extensive leukocyte infiltrate but no red cell extravasation (A–D, F, ×99; E and G, ×600). Data are from Rothstein et al. (42).

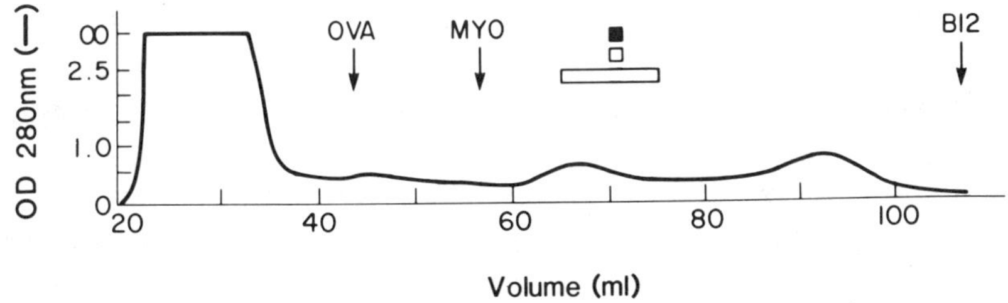

Figure 7 Gel filtration chromatography of acidified zymosan-activated plasma from C5-sufficient mice. Column fractions were collected and monitored for total protein at 280 nm. Elution volumes of low-molecular-weight standards are shown. The molecular weights of ovalbumin (Ova), myoglobin (Myo), and vitamin B12 (B12) are 44,000, 17,000, and 1350, respectively. Closed bar represents protein that eluted at a volume corresponding to an M_r value of 9000 Da enabled C5-deficient mice to develop HN when injected with *C. parvum* and TNF. Open bars represent the relative location of the active single and pooled fractions tested from two independent gel filtrations, thus confirming this M_r. Data taken from Rothstein et al. (42).

which responded 90 to 100% of the time. This difference may be due to the fact that B10.D2/n mice have lower levels of C3 than the other C5-sufficient mouse strains (34), and consequently, the C5 convertase C3a is therefore reduced in B10.D2/n mice.

B. Depletion of Complement Prevents Necrosis

The evidence presented so far is that complement components at or beyond C5 in the complement pathway are necessary, whereas early-acting components of the classical (C1, C2, C4, C3) and the alternative (B, D, P, C3) pathway may contribute but are not sufficient alone to cause HN in animals injected with *C. parvum* and TNF. Depletion of complement components should therefore abrogate the capacity of C5-sufficient mice to respond with HN. Cobra venom factor (CVF) isolated from *Naja naja kaouthia* venom, by generating a C3/C5-convertase, causes the depletion of C3, factor B as well as the terminal (C5–9) components of the complement pathway (40,41). Indeed, C5-sufficient C3H/HeN mice pretreated with two IV injections of purified CVF failed to develop HN 24 h later (42). CVF, however, did not prevent leukocyte attraction since CVF-pretreated mice had an influx of leukocytes equal to the nontreated mice (42). These data therefore demonstrated that the depletion of complement components in C5-sufficient mice prevents the development of HN.

C. C5-Sufficient Plasma Corrects the Defect in C5-Deficient Mice

The data that CVF prevented HN in C5-sufficient mice suggested that C5-deficient mice could be made to respond to TNF and bacteria by providing a source of C5. Indeed, Table 8 shows that plasma injected from C5-sufficient mice was fully capable of supplementing two different C5-deficient mouse strains, B10.D2/o and AKR. Heat inactivation of this plasma at 56°C for 30 min abrogated its capacity to supplement C5-deficient mice, a finding consistent with the notion that complement was indeed the active component. These data show that C5 can sufficiently correct the defect in C5-deficient mice, thus allowing them to respond with HN after coinjection of *C. parvum* and TNF. In addition, these experiments provided a

Table 8 C5-Deficient Mice Supplemented with Plasma from C5-Sufficient Mice Can Respond With HN

C5-deficient responder[a]	Plasma used for supplementation[b]	Retention of blood in skin (CPM ± SEM)[c]	Incidence of HN (%)[d]	
B10.D2/o	Sufficient	22,385 ± 8,552[e]	16/17	(94)
	Deficient	[f]	0/4	(0)
	Sufficient (HI)	5,474 ± 1,375[g]	0/5	(0)
	None	4,105 ± 110	0/5	(0)
AKR	Sufficient		12/14	(86)
	Deficient		0/4	(0)
	Sufficient (HI)		0/3	(0)
	None		9/0	(0)

Source: Data from Rothstein et al. (42).

[a]Mice were coinjected with *C. parvum* and TNF followed by IV injection of plasma 3 h later.

[b]C5-sufficient plasma was collected from C3H/HeN mice. C5-deficient plasma was collected from either AKR, DBA/2, or B10.D2/o mice. C5-sufficient plasma was heat inactivated (HI) by incubation at 56°C for 30 min.

[c]Retention of ^{51}Cr-labeled blood cells in skin of mice isolated 24 h after injection of *C. parvum* and TNF. For details, see Fig. 5.

[d]Number of mice responding with HN/total number of mice tested. HN was observed 24 h after supplementation. The mean diameter (± SEM) of the hemorrhagic lesions were similar between strains (1.8 ± 0.3 cm for B10.D2/0; 1.7 ± 0.3 cm for AKR). Data are pooled from two or more independent experiments.

[e]Mean significantly greater than that of control group ($p < 0.1$) as determined by Student's *t* test.

[f]Not determined.

[g]Mean not significantly different from control group ($p < 0.6$).

useful assay for the identification of the specific complement component needed for HN.

Since many proteins other than C5a are present in zymosan-activated C5-sufficient plasma, we further purified the active component in zymosan-activated plasma that supplemented C5-deficient mice. Zymosan-activated C5-sufficient and C5-deficient plasma was acid precipitated and centrifuged, thus removing unwanted plasma proteins without affecting the acid soluble C5a (43). The supernatant was then size fractionated through a Bio-Gel P60 column and fractions were tested for their capacity to enable C5-deficient mice to respond to TNF and bacteria with HN. While proteins > 60,000 M_r eluting in the void volume had no activity, Fig. 7 and Table 9 show that a pool of fractions corresponding to proteins within the molecular weight range 8000 to 15,000 Da could enable C5-deficient mice to respond with HN after injection of *C. parvum* and TNF. Further analysis of single fractions within this size range revealed that the activity corresponds to a protein with an M_r value of 9000 Da (Fig. 7; Table 9). Similar fractions tested from the zymosan-activated C5-deficient plasma did not supplement treated mice. The molecular weight of this acid-stable protein is consistent with published reports of the molecular ranges from 8000 to 15,000 Da (43,44). These data further implicate C5a in the induction of HN by *C. parvum* and TNF.

Table 9 C5-Deficient Mice Supplemented with a Partially Purified 9000 M_r Protein Respond with HN

Elution volume (mL)	M_r (Da)	Incidence of HN (%)[a]
65–75	11,500–8,000	4/5 (80)
68	10,000	0/4 (0)
71	9,000	2/4 (50)
75	8,000	0/4 (0)
78	7,000	0/4 (0)
78–100	7,000–4,000	0/3 (0)

Source: Data from Rothstein et al. (42).

[a]B10.D2/o mice wre injected with column fractions as described for plasma injections in Table 8. Data are pooled from two independent experiments, each containing as positive control C5-deficient B10.D2/o mice coinjected with *C. parvum* and TNF followed 3 h later by injection with unfractionated C5-sufficient plasma.

D. Plasma Hemolytic Activity Is Not Required for Necrosis

Since C5-deficient mice have a selective genetic defect in their ability to secrete C5 (37,45,46), while having normal levels of all other complement components, two possible pathways involving C5 in the pathological process of HN could be proposed:

1. Locally activated C5 would yield C5b, thus triggering the assembly of the membrane attack complex (C5b-9). This complex, in the presence of leukocytes and TNF, could cause direct vessel damage leading to HN.
2. C5 could be locally activated and the other C5-derived fragment C5a, together with TNF, could interact with infiltrating leukocytes to induce the secretion of hydrolytic enzymes, reactive oxygen intermediates (ROI), and/or vasoactive substances which would ultimately cause vessel damage and HN.

The yeast cell-wall extract zymosan can deplete plasma of many of the hemolytic components of complement while leaving the anaphylatoxins, C3a, and C5a behind (47,48). Table 10 shows that plasma 96% depleted of hemolytic activ-

Table 10 C5-Sufficient Plasma Depleted of Hemolytic Activity Enables C5-Deficient Mice to Respond with HN

Treatment of plasma in vitro[a]	Plasma hemolytic activity (U/mL)[b]	Reduction of plasma C5 activity (%)[c]	Incidence of HN (%)[d]
4°C	165 ± 15	0 ± 0	5/6 (83)
37°C	103 ± 23	51 ± 6	7/8 (88)
37°C + zymosan	<50 ± 0	96 ± 0	9/11 (82)

Source: Rothstein et al. (42).

[a]C5-sufficient plasma was either kept at 4°C, incubated for 2.5 h at 37°C, or incubated at 37°C with 5 mg/mL zymosan for 2.5 h followed by removal of zymosan by centrifugation.

[b]Hemolytic activity of plasma was determined using a standard rabbit erythrocyte hemolysis assay. CH_{50} values of each sample are reported as U/mL ± SEM.

[c]Represents the percent reduction in C5 activity as measured by the capacity of treated plasma to supplement hemolytic activity in C5-deficient plasma. Data are reported as percent reduction in CH_{50} from control ± SEM.

[d]B10.D2/o mice were coinjected with *C. parvum* (400 μg) and TNF (10 μg) 3 h before the start of the experiment and then supplemented with plasma as described in Table 8. HN was assessed 24 h later and reported as the number of mice responding with HN/total number of mice tested. The mean diameter (± SEM) of the hemorrhagic lesions were similar between the groups (1.6 ± 0.1 cm). Data are pooled from three independent experiments.

ity was still completely capable of enabling C5-deficient B10.D2/o mice to respond with HN after injection of *C. parvum* and TNF. These data suggest that the terminal complement components (membrane attack complex) were not needed for HN to occur. The data are consistent, however, with the notion that the missing component required for C5-deficient mice to develop HN is C5a. In fact, C5a should be sufficient to allow these mice to develop HN in response to bacteria and TNF.

IV. LEUKOCYTE INFILTRATION AND TISSUE DAMAGE

TNF is only one of the multiple mediators of inflammation released by inflammatory cells after exposure to bacterial agents, and an interplay of several cells and mediators may be required for effective defense. To dissect these interacting components, it is critical to identify animals that have selective defects in one or the other defense functions. In this regard it is interesting that the LPS-responsive C3H/HeN mice respond with HN to injection of the bacterial endotoxin LPS and TNF, whereas the LPS-nonresponsive C3H/HeJ strain do not. Even though the C3H/HeJ mice respond with HN to injections of *C. parvum* and TNF, they are resistant to the induction of HN by LPS and TNF. However, they do respond microscopically with an influx of leukocytes equal in magnitude to C3H/HeN mice injected with the same agents. In fact, bone marrow-derived leukocytes from C3H/HeN mice can correct the LPS defect in C3H/HeJ mouse strain such that these mice are now sensitive to the lethal effects of LPS (49). Therefore, analogous to the use of the C5 congenic strains in identifying a requirement for C5a in HN (42), the C3H/HeN and C3H/HeJ congenic mouse strains offered insight into the role of the leukocyte component in TNF-mediated HN.

Gamma-irradiation (650 rad), which causes leukopenia, prevented the HN induced by sequential LPS and TNF injections, suggesting the need for a radiosensitive host component in the induction of HN by TNF and bacteria or their products (20). Histological analysis of skin sections from mice treated with either bacterial agents or a combination of bacterial agents and TNF revealed that the infiltration of leukocytes correlated with the onset of HN (20). However, infiltration alone was not the ultimate cause of the damage since skin from LPS-nonresponsive (C3H/HeJ) and C5-deficient mice injected with bacteria and TNF showed significant inflammatory infiltrates, in agreement with an earlier report (50), but did not develop HN. The role of these inflammatory leukocytes in the development of HN is therefore not clearly understood. We were interested in determining whether HN could be dependent on leukocytes.

Coinjection of TNF and *C. parvum* or *M. orale*-infected lysates will lead to HN at the skin site of injection 24 h later (20). In contrast, coinjection of LPS and TNF does not lead to HN, not even in the LPS-responsive C3H/HeN mice. LPS, however, followed 24 h later by TNF injected at the same site will cause HN in C3H/HeN mice (20). Thus the bacterial agents all have in common the capacity to induce

HN when injected with TNF, although the time at which TNF was needed to be injected to cause HN was different for each agent. We suspected that one of the reasons for these differences in kinetics of HN induction might be due to differences among the bacterial agents in conditioning the skin. Since bacterial agents are known to be potent inducers of leukocyte chemotaxis in vivo, differences in chemotactic activity of the agents may be responsible for the observed kinetic differences. Thus serial skin sections were taken from groups of mice injected with bacterial agents to determine the extent of leukocyte infiltration at a given time after injection. Results from a double-blind microscopic analysis revealed that while LPS needed 24 h to accumulate an inflammatory infiltrate, *C. parvum* and *M. orale*-infected cell lysates induced an equally large infiltrate by 3 h (Table 11). In addition, the infiltrate induced by *M. orale*-infected lysates diminished by 12 h, unlike the *C. parvum*-induced infiltrate, which continued to increase through 24 h. These data are consistent with the finding that HN induced by these agents only occurs when TNF is injected at the time of maximum leukocyte accumulation. For example, LPS can induce HN only when TNF is injected 24 h later. In contrast, *C. parvum* can induce HN either when TNF is coinjected or injected 24 h later (but not 48 h later). Finally, *M. orale*-infected cell lysates will induce HN only when simultaneously injected with TNF (by 24 h, TNF injection into *M. orale*-infected cell

Table 11 Time Course of Leukocyte Infiltration into Skin Injected with Bacterial Agents

	Degree of leukocyte infiltration at various times after injection (h)[b]				
Bacterial agent[a]	1	3	9	12	24
LPS	0/1	1	2	3	4
C. parvum	1	4	5	6	5
M. orale lysates	1	4	5	4	3

Source: Data from Rothstein (19).

[a]Bacterial agents were injected SC at start of the experiment, LPS (100 μg), *C. parvum* (400μg), *M. orale*-positive lysates (10^7 cells).

[b]At specified times mice were sacrificed (two per time point) and a 2 × 2 cm square piece of skin was removed with the site of injection in the center. Skin was fixed, sectioned, and stained with hematoxylin and eosin and observed under a light microscope for the degree of leukocyte infiltration in a double-blind fashion. The degree of leukocyte infiltration was quantified as compared to a negative control (normal skin) and scored as positive relative to one another, with 6 designated as the maximum infiltrate observed.

lysate primed skin will no longer induce HN). In all cases the infiltration of leukocytes was associated with the development of HN. Leukocytes can be seen in skin of mice injected with bacteria or clustered around vessels in skin developing HN after injection of bacteria and TNF. These data are consistent with the notion that leukocyte infiltration appears to precede the development of HN. The evidence therefore suggests that leukocytes may be required for, rather than being consequence of, HN.

V. CONCLUDING REMARKS

The studies described here have provided new information concerning the mechanism of tissue damage induced by TNF. Four components were identified that were required for the induction of HN (Fig. 8). Two of these components, TNF and a priming agent such as bacteria or tumors, were applied exogenously, whereas the other two, non-T-cell leukocytes and C5a, were endogenous host components. Under normal pathological conditions, TNF may be supplied endogenously by activated macrophages and/or T cells, which are often found in tumors and at the site of bacterial infections. The omission of any one of these components resulted in the inability to induce local HN. It appears, therefore, that a complex interaction of all four of these components causes HN. Much work has shown that TNF plays an important, if not critical, role in the pathophysiologic events leading to such states as tumor necrosis (2), anorexia (51), cachexia (52), septic shock (8), bone resorp-

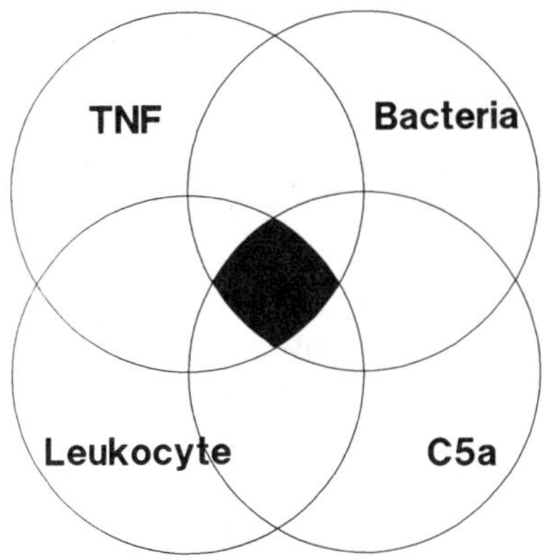

Figure 8 Factors implicated in the induction of HN. Bacteria attract and activate non-T-cell, radiosensitive, bone marrow-derived leukocytes which respond to TNF and C5a, thus leading to the development of HN. Modified from Rothstein (19).

tion (53), allograft rejection (54), and graft-versus-host disease (55). Although TNF does not appear to be associated with tissue damage occurring in the affected host, there are no data to show that TNF is the ultimate mediator in any of these pathological conditions. Indeed, it is known that cachectic cancer patients fail to show detectable levels of TNF in their serum (56) and TNF appears in the serum of patients exposed to infectious agents only transiently and at the onset of acute, rather than chronic, exposure (56,57). Furthermore, antibodies to TNF can prevent the development but not reverse endotoxin-mediated or septic shock in experimental animals (14,15). Although in these situations the actual mechanism of tissue damage is unknown, it would be consistent with the data presented here that additional factors are required for TNF to have these observed effects and that TNF alone cannot cause lethal shock or HN. In fact, our studies show that the capability of TNF to cause HN of tumors was independent of the sensitivity of the tumor cells to be killed by TNF in vitro. In addition, treatment of normal skin with large doses of purified "endotoxin-free" recombinant TNF failed to cause HN.

The Shwartzman reaction (21) is induced by sequential injections of bacterial agents (a SC injection followed 24 h later by an IV injection), resulting in the formation of a localized hemorrhagic skin lesion or, in cases when both injections are IV, systemic toxicity. Historically, the Shwartzman reaction has been studied in rabbits, which by comparison are about 1000 times more sensitive to the effects of endotoxin than are mice (58). It was therefore not surprising that previous attempts to repeat the Shwartzman phenomenon in mice have usually failed (59). Since much of the work concerning TNF-mediated tumor necrosis was studied in mice, we chose to study the effects of endotoxin and TNF using a murine model. Even though we confirmed that the Shwartzman reaction (i.e., after two consecutive injections of a bacterial component) does not occur in mice, we developed a reliable protocol in mice for a strong HN reaction using a bacterial component and TNF. Although we have not used rabbits in our experiments, it is possible that the interactions of TNF, C5a, leukocytes, and bacteria in causing HN in mice provide the basis for the Shwartzman phenomenon described many decades ago (21). One of the enigmas that this phenomenon presents is the lack of specificity (i.e., antigenically different and seemingly unrelated bacterial agents can be used as the two signals for generating the HN phenomenon). An explanation suggested by our work is that the sensitizing agent attracts and activates macrophages and PML, and the eliciting agent causes TNF release from macrophages and C5 activation. The notion that C5a may be generated directly by the eliciting agent is consistent with the fact that a common characteristic of eliciting agents used in the Shwartzman reaction is their capacity to activate complement (60). In this regard it is interesting the C6-deficient rabbits respond with HN after repeated injections of endotoxin, suggesting that C5a is sufficient to cause the localized Shwartzman reaction (61). Alternatively, C5a could be generated locally through the cleavage of C5 by activated macrophages (62). In tumor-bearing mice, where no priming agent is needed for TNF to cause HN, it may be that the tumor alone can provide or elicit signals similar to those given by bacteria. For example, the tumor may directly activate the complement system, thus providing a source of C5a. This is certainly possible since tumors are known to effectively activate the complement system (63–65). In addition, the finding that tumors can induce a considerable macrophage infiltrate (66) is consistent with the need for leukocytes in the induction of HN.

Finally, it is our contention that the observed HN reaction may be a beneficial inflammatory response designed to limit the spread of bacteria from an infected focus and to prevent bacteria and bacterial products to circulate systemically. The first event in this containment reaction would be the attraction of macrophages and PML to the site of infection. At this site the bacterial products, such as LPS, could activate macrophages to produce TNF and C5-cleaving proteolytic enzymes as well as to induce the expression of receptors for C5a and TNF on PML. The PML that bind C5a and TNF would then release hydrolytic enzymes, reactive oxygen intermediates, and/or vasoactive amines that would have direct effects on the vascular endothelium, thus leading to vessel damage and extravasation of blood. The consequence of this local damage would be that the circulation of bacteria or their toxins would be prevented. Septic or endotoxin shock would be the result of the failure of this defense reaction, leading to the circulation of bacterial products which can induce the systemic activation of leukocytes and cause the release of cytokines (including TNF). As we showed, TNF and bacterial products synergize to cause systemic vessel damage, irreversible organ failure, and death. Knowing the precise interacting components and pathways in the development of HN will give us the means to limit the detrimental effects and enhance the beneficial effects of this host protection reaction against foreign invaders.

ACKNOWLEDGMENTS

This work was supported by the National Institutes of Health Grants P01 CA-19266, R37 CA-22677, R01 CA-37156, and T32 AI-07090.

REFERENCES

1. Coley, W. B., Contribution to the knowledge of sarcoma, *Ann. Surg., 14*: 199, 1891.
2. Shear, M. J., and Turner, F. C., Chemical treatment of tumors. V. Isolation of the hemorrhage-producing fraction from *Serratia marcescens* (*Bacillus prodigiosus*) culture filtrate, *J. Natl. Cancer Inst., 4*: 81, 1943.
3. Algire, G. H., Legallaies, F. Y., and Anderson, B. F., Vascular reactions of normal and malignant tissues in vivo. V. The role of hypotension in the action of bacterial polysaccharide on tumors, *J. Natl. Cancer Inst., 12*: 1279, 1952.
4. O'Malley, W. E., Achinstein, B., and Shear, M. J., Action of bacterial polysaccharide on tumors. II. Damage of Sarcoma 37 by serum of mice treated with *Serratia marcescens* polysaccharide, and induced tolerance, *J. Natl. Cancer Inst., 29*: 1169, 1962.

5. Carswell, E. A., Old, L. J., Kassel, R. L., Green, S., Fiore, N., and Williamson, B., An endotoxin-induced serum factor that causes necrosis of tumors, *Proc. Natl. Acad. Sci.* USA, *72*: 36666, 1975.
6. Pennica, D., Nedwin, G. E., Hayflick, J. S., Seeburg, P. H., Derynck, R., Palladino, M. A., Kohr, W. J., Aggarwal, B. B., and Goeddel, D. V., Human tumour necrosis factor: precursor structure, expression and homology to lymphotoxin, *Nature (Lond.), 312*: 724, 1984.
7. Old, L. J., Tumor necrosis factor (TNF), *Science, 230*: 630, 1985.
8. Tracey, K. J., Beutler, B., Lowry, S. F., Merryweather, J., Wolpe, S., Milsark, I. W., Hariri, R. J., Fahey, T. J., Zentella, A. J. D., Albert, J. D., Shires, G. T., and Cerami, A., Shock and tissue injury induced by recombinant human cachectin, *Science, 234*: 470, 1986.
9. Aderka, D., Holtman, H., Toker, L., Hahn, T., and Wallach, D., Tumor necrosis factor induction by Sendai virus, *J. Immunol., 136*: 2938, 1986.
10. Grau, G. E., Fajardo, L. F., Piguet, P. F., Allet, B., Lambert, P. H., and Vassalli, P., Tumor necrosis factor (cachectin) as an essential mediator in murine cerebral malaria, *Science, 236*: 1210, 1987.
11. Clark, I. A., Cowden, W. B., Butcher, G. A., and Hunt, N. H., Possible roles of tumor necrosis factor in the pathology of malaria, *Am. J. Pathol., 129*: 192, 1987.
12. Havell, E. A., Production of Tumor necrosis factor during murine listeriosis, *J. Immunol., 139*: 4225, 1987.
13. Jupin, C., Anderson, S., Damais, C., Alouf, J. E., and Parant, M., Toxic shock syndrome toxin 1 as an inducer of human tumor necrosis factors and γ-interferon, *J. Exp. Med., 167*: 752, 1988.
14. Tracey, K. J., Fong, Y., Hesse, D. G., Manogue, K. R., Lee, A. T., Kuo, G. C., Lowry, S. F., and Cerami, A., Anti-cachectin/TNF monoclonal antibodies prevent septic shock during lethal bacteraemia, *Nature (Lond.), 330*: 662, 1987.
15. Beutler, B., Milsark, I. W., and Cerami, A. C., Passive immunization against cachectin/tumor necrosis factor protects mice from lethal effect of endotoxin, *Science, 229*: 869, 1985.
16. Urban, J. L., Shepard, H. M., Rothstein, J. L., Sugarman, B. J., and Schreiber, H., Tumor necrosis factor: a potent effector molecule for cell killing by activated macrophages, *Proc. Natl. Acad. Sci. USA, 83*: 5233, 1986.
17. Kramer, S. M., and Carver, M. E., Serum-free *in vitro* bioassay for the detection of tumor necrosis factor, *J. Immunol. Methods, 93*: 201, 1986.
18. Mosmann, T., Rapid colorimetric assay for cellular growth and survival: application to proliferation and cytotoxic assays, *J. Immunol. Methods, 65*: 55, 1983.
19. Rothstein, J. L., Tumor necrosis factors and tissue damage, Ph.D. thesis, University of Chicago, 1988.
20. Rothstein, J. L., and Schreiber, H., Synergy between tumor necrosis factor and bacterial products causes hemorrhagic necrosis and lethal shock in normal mice, *Proc. Natl. Acad. Sci. USA, 85*: 607, 1988.
21. Shwartzman, G., Studies on *Bacillus typhosus* toxic substances. I. Phenomenon of local tissue reactivity to *B. typhosus* culture filtrate, *J. Exp. Med., 48*: 247, 1928.
22. Sande, M. A., and Mandell, G. L., Antimicrobial agents, *The Pharmacological Basis of*

Therapeutics (L. S. Goodman, T. W. Rall, and F. Murad, eds.), Macmillan, New York, 1980–1105, 1985.
23. Heppner, G., and Weiss, D. W., High susceptibility of strain A mice to endotoxin and endotoxin-red blood cells cultures, *J. Bacteriol.*, *90*: 696, 1965.
24. Gabridge, M. G., Chandler, D. K. F., and Daniels, M. J., Pathogenicity factors in mycoplasmas and spiroplasmas, *The Mycoplasmas*, Vol. 4 (M. Bazin, ed.), Academic Press, New York, pp. 313–351, 1985.
25. Beutler, B., and Cerami, A., Cachectin and tumor necrosis factor as two sides of the same biologial coin, *Nature (Lond.)*, *320*: 584, 1986.
26. Ruddle, N. H., and Waksman, B. H. Cytotoxicity mediated by soluble antigen and lymphocytes in delayed hypersensitivity. III. Analysis of mechanism. *J. Exp. Med.*, *128*: 1267, 1968.
27. Gray, P. W., Aggarwal, B. B., Benton, C. V., Bringman, T. S. Henzel, W. J., Jarrett, J. A., Leung, D. W., Moffat, B., Ng, P., Scedersky, L. P. Palladino, M. A., and Neddwin, G. E., Cloning and expression of cDNA for human lymphotoxin, a lymphokine with tumor necrosis activity, *Nature (Lond.)*, *312*: 721, 1984.
28. Williams, T. W., and Bellanti, J. A., In Vitro synergism between interferons and human lymphotoxin: enhancement of lymphotoxin-induced target cell killing, *J. Immunol.*, *130*: 518, 1983.
29. Williamson, B. D., Carswell, E. A., Rubin, B. Y., Prendergast, J. S., and Old, L. J., Human tumor necrosis factor produced by B cell lines: synergistic cytotoxic interaction with human interferon, *Proc. Natl. Acad. Sci. USA*, *80*: 5397, 1983.
30. Sugarman, B. J., Aggarwal, B. B., Hass, P. E., Figari, S., Palladino, M. A., and Shepard, H. M., Recombinant human tumor necrosis factor-α: effects on proliferation of normal and transformed cells in vitro, *Science*, *230*: 943, 1985.
31. Waage, A., and Espevik, T., Interleukin 1 potentiates the elthal effect of tumor necrosis factor-α/cachectin in mice, *J. Exp. Med.*, *167*: 1987, 1988.
32. Takayama, K., Qureshi, N., Raetz, C. R. H., Ribi, E., Peterson, J., Cantrell, J. L., Pearson, F. C., Wiggins, J., and Johnson, A. G., Inlfuence of fine structure of lipid A on *Limulus* amebocyte lysate clotting and toxic properties, *Infect. Immun.*, *45*: 350, 1984.
33. Dennis, J. W., Laferte, S., Waghorne, C., Breitman, M. L., and Kerbel, R. S., β1-6 branching of Asn-linked oligosaccharides is directly associated with metastasis, *Nature (Lond.)*, *236*: 582, 1987.
34. Ferreira, A., and Nussenzweig, V., Genetic linkage between serum levels of the third component of complement and the H-2 complex, *J. Exp. Med.*, *141*: 513, 1975.
35. Ferreira, A., and Nussenzweig, V., Control of C3 levels in mice during ontogeny by a gene in the central region of the H-2 complex, *Nature (Lond.)*, *260*: 613, 1976.
36. Cinader, B., Dubiski, S., and Wardlaw, A. C., Distribution, inheritance, and properties of an antigen, MUB1, and its relation to hemolytic complement, *J. Exp. Med.*, *120*: 897, 1964.
37. Erickson, R. P., Tachibana, D. K., Herzenberg, L. A., and Rosenberg, L. T., A single gene controlling hemolytic complement and a serum antigen in the mouse, *J. Immunol.*, 92: 611, 1964.
38. Shreffler, D. C., Variants of complement and other proteins: Mouse, *Inbred and Genetically Deffined Strains of Laboratory Animals*, Part 1, *Mouse and Rat* (P. L. Altman and

D. Dittmer-Katz, eds.), Federation of American Societies for Experimental Biology, Bethesda, Md., pp. 103–104, 2979.

39. Fernandez, H. N., Henson, P. M., Otani, A., and Hugli, T. E., Chemotactic response to human C3a and C5a anaphylatoxins: 1. Evaluation of C3a and C5a leukotaxis in vitro and under simulated in vivo conditions, *J. Immunol., 120*: 109, 1978.
40. Jensen, J., Anaphylatoxin in its relation to the complement system, *Science, 155*: 1122, 1967.
41. Cochrane, C. G., Müller-Eberhard, H. J., and Aikin, B. S., Depletion of plasma complement in vivo by a protein of cobra venom: its effecct on various immunologic reactions, *J. Immunol., 105*: 55, 1970.
42. Rothstein, J. L., Lint, T. F., and Schreiber, H., Tumor necrosis factor/cachectin: induction of hemorrhagic necrosis in normal tissue requires the fifth component of complement (C5), *J. Exp. Med., 168*: 2007, 1988.
43. Wissler, J. H., Chemistry and biology of the anaphylatoxin related serum peptide system. *In* Purification, crystallization and properties of classical anaphylatoxin from rat serum, *Eur. J. Immunol.,* 2: 73, 1972.
44. Fernandez, H. N., and Hugli, T. E., Partial characterization of human C5a anaphylatoxin. I: chemical description of the carbohydrate and polypeptide portions of human C5a, *J. Immunol., 117*: 1688, 1976.
45. Whest, W. H., Wetsel, R., Falus, A., Tack, B., and Strunk, R. C., The fifth component of complement (C5) in the Mouse. Analysis of the molecular basis for deficiency, *J. Exp. Med., 165*: 1442, 1987.
46. Ooi, Y. M., and Colten, H. R., Genetic defect in secretion of complement C5 in mice, *Nature (Lond.), 282*: 207, 1979.
47. Hugli, T. E., and Müller-Eberhard, H. J., Anaphylatoxins: C3a and C5a, *Adv. Immunol., 26*: 1, 1978.
48. Vogt, W., The anaphylatoxin-forming system, *Ergeb. Physiol. Biol. Chem. Exp. Pharmakol., 59*: 160, 1967.
49. Michalek, S. M., Moore, R. N., McGhee, J. R., Rosenstreich, D. L., and Mergenhagen, S. E., The primary role of lymphoreticular cells in the mediation of host responses to bacterial endotoxin, *J. Infect. Dis., 141*: 55, 1980.
50. Moeller, G. R., Terry, L., and Snyderman, R., The inflammatory response and resistance to endotoxin in mice, *J. Immunol., 120*: 116, 1978.
51. Socher, S. H., Friedman, A., and Martinez, D., Recombinant human tumor necrosis factor induces acute reductions in food intake and body weight in mice, *J. Exp. Med., 167*: 1957, 1988.
52. Beutler, B., Mahoney, J., Le Trang, N., Pekala, P., and Cerami, A., Purification of cachectin, a lipoprotein lipase-suppressing hormone secreted by endotoxin-induced RAW 264.7 cells, *J. Exp. Med., 161*: 984, 1985.
53. Bertolini, D. R., Nedwin, G. E., Bringman, T. S., Smith, D. D., and Mundy, G. R., Stimulation of bone resorption and inhibition of bone formation in vitro by human tumour necrosis factors, *Nature (Lond.), 319*: 516, 1986.
54. Maury, C. P. J., and Teppo, A.-M., Raised serum levels of cachectin/tumor necrosis factor α in renal allograft rejection, *J. Exp. Med., 166*: 1132, 1987.
55. Piguet, P.-F., Grau, G. E., Allet, B., and Vassalli, P., Tumor necrosis factor/cachectin is

an effector of skin and gut lesions of the acute phase of graft-vs.-host disease, *J. Exp. Med., 166*: 1280, 1987.

56. Waage, A., Espevik, T., and Lamvik, J., Detection of tumour necrosis factor-like cytotoxicity in serum from patients with septicaemia but not from untreated cancer patients, *Scand. J. Immunol., 24*: 739, 1986.

57. Michie, H. R., Manogue, K. R., Spriggs, D. R., Revhaug, A., O'Dwyer, S., Dinarello, C. A., Cerami, A., Wolff, S. M., and Wilmore, D. W., Detection of circulating tumor necrosis factor after endotoxin administration, *N. Engl. J. Medd., 318*: 1481, 1988.

58. Rothstein, J. L., and Schreiber, H., Relationship of tumour necrosis factor and endotoxin to macrophage cytotoxicity, haemorrhagic necrosis and lethal shock, *Tumour Necrosis Factor and Related Cytotoxins* (G. Bock and J. Marsh, eds.), Wiley, Chichester, England, pp. 124–139, 1987.

59. Kelly, M. G., Smith, N. H., Wodinsky, I., and Rall, D. P., Strain differences in local hemorrhagic response (Shwartzman-like reaction) of mice to a single intradermal injection of bacterial polysaccharides, *J. Exp. Med., 105*: 653, 1957.

60. Fong, J. S. C., Rother, K. O., and Good, R. A., The role of complement in the localized Shwartzman reaction: Studies with congenitally C6-deficient rabbits, *Clin. Exp. Immunol., 16*: 17, 1974.

61. Wilson, G. S., and Miles, A. A., Some non-specific mechanisms in general immunity, *Principles of Bacteriology and Immunity* (R. Knox, M. T. Parker, A. D. Macrae, G. G. Meynell, and E. W. Meynell, eds.), Williams & Wilkins, Baltimore, pp. 1448–1465, 1964.

62. Snyderman, R., Shin, H. S., and Dannenberg, A. M., Macrophage proteinase and inflammation: the production of chemotactic activity from the fifth component of complement by macrophage proteinase, *J. Immunol., 109*: 896, 1972.

63. McConnell, I., Klein, G., Lint, T. F., and Lachmann, P. J., Activation of the alternative complement pathway by human B cell lymphoma lines is associated with Epstein-Barr virus transformation of the cells, *Eur. J. Immunol., 8*: 453, 1978.

64. Dierich, M. P., Schulz, T., Yefenof, and Klein, G., Detection of proteolytic (C3-cleaving) activity on mouse mastocytoma (P815) cells and other mouse cell lines by formation of cell contact with C3-carrying mouse lymphocytes, *eur. J. Immunol., 9*: 928, 1979.

65. Ramos, O. F., Samay, G., Klein, E., Yefenof, E., and Gergely, J., Complement-dependent cellular cytotoxicity: lymphoblastoid lines that activate complement component (C3) and express C3 receptors have increased sensitivity to lymphocyte-mediated lysis in the presence of fresh human serum, *Proc. Natl. Acad. Sci. USA, 82*: 5470, 1985.

66. Evans, R., Macrophages in syngeneic animal tumors, *Transplantation, 14*: 666, 1972.

21

Effects of TNF and Lymphotoxin on Bone Cells

G. R. MUNDY, G. D. ROODMAN, L. F. BONEWALD, T. YONEDA, and M. SABATINI
The University of Texas Health Science Center at San Antonio, San Antonio, Texas

I. INTRODUCTION

As far as is currently known, tumor necrosis factor (TNF) and lymphotoxin (LT) (also known as TNF-α and TNF-β, respectively) have identical effects on bone cells. In vitro, they both stimulate osteoclastic bone resorption. They increase the formation of osteoclasts, enhance the differentiation of committed osteoclast progenitors, and activate performed osteoclastic cells to form lacunae on bone surfaces. They increase osteoblast-like cell replication, and inhibit differentiated function. When injected or infused into intact rodents, these factors induce hypercalcemia. These effects will now be described in detail.

II. OVERVIEW OF NORMAL BONE REMODELING

The integrity of the skeleton is maintained by cellular events that are occurring continuously in localized areas and are responsible for the remodeling of the skeleton. This cellular remodeling process occurs throughout life and is characterized by an orderly sequence of events that begins with the activation of osteoclasts or bone resorbing cells to form resorption lacunae on bone surfaces and concludes with the formation of new bone by osteoblasts or bone-forming cells. Bone remodeling occurs in discrete and localized units or packets throughout the skeleton. Osteoclastic bone resorption and osteoblastic new bone formation are closely associated both chronologically and geographically. Thus it is likely that the bone remodeling sequence is primarily under the control of local factors that are generated in the bone microenvironment. In recent years it has become clear that there are potent local factors produced in the bone microenvironment which can regulate both osteoclast and osteoblast activity. Immune cells (lymphocytes and monocytes) appear to be ideally located as sources for these mediators of osteoclast and osteoblast activity.

The bone loss that occurs with aging is associated with a decrease in both trabecular and cortical bone. This bone loss is due to an imbalance between these coupled processes of osteoblastic bone resorption and osteoblastic bone formation. Osteoporosis occurs when there is a decrease in trabecular and cortical bone mass (predominantly trabecular) such that the structural integrity of the skeleton is compromised and the skeleton is no longer able to provide its support function. As a consequence, the affected bones fracture and compress after trivial trauma. In normal adults, the complex relationship between bone formation and bone resorption changes after the age of 30 (approximately). After this age, bone resorption is always relatively greater than bone formation. In the 10 years following the menopause in females, there is a marked increase in osteoclastic bone resorption due to estrogen deficiency. In older individuals, both men and women, there is a primary decrease in bone formation due to an abnormal decrease in osteoblast vigor. This abnormality may be due either to a decrease in the recruitment of osteoblasts to repair the resorption areas made by osteoclasts or a decrease in the activity of the osteoblasts that have accumulated at the site of resorption and are thus unable to repair it (Darby and Meunier, 1982). Thus both abnormal osteoclast and osteoblast function contribute to the decrease in bone mass that occurs in the elderly.

Advances in the understanding of local bone remodeling have been hampered for a number of years by severe limitations in the technology both in the available culture techniques as well as in the characterization of the peptide factors involved. A major disadvantage is that the peptide factors for many years were poorly defined. However, recent advances in this area have been dramatic, with the biotechnology revolution leading to marked improvements in techniques in protein chemistry and the advent of the recombinant cytokines affecting bone cell function becoming available for testing. In addition, techniques have now been developed for studying bone cell function in patients with bone disease. At the present time we realize that a number of osteotropic cytokines which are produced in the bone microenvironment affect bone cell function. The task confronting workers in this field is to seek out the relative importance of these local regulatory factors which control the bone remodeling sequence.

III. STIMULATION OF OSTEOCLASTIC BONE RESORPTION

TNF and LT were first shown to stimulate osteoclastic bone resorption in organ cultures by Bertolini et al. (1986). These workers found that when added to organ cultures of fetal rat long bones, both cytokines in concentrations of 10^{-9} to 10^{-6} *M* increased the release of previously incorporated ^{45}Ca from organ cultures of these bones after 48 and 120 h or culture. These effects were associated with an increase in the numbers of activated osteoclasts in the bone cultures as determined by histologic assessment. Both cytokines were equipotent. Calcitonin concentrations of 1 to 10 mU/mL inhibited these effects. Tashjian et al. (1987) confirmed these responses in organ cultures of neonatal mouse calvariae and showed that responses to TNF could be inhibited by indomethacin in concentrations of 10^{-5} *M*, indicating that the effects of TNF and LT were related to prostaglandin synthesis in these cultures. This was confirmed by measurement by radioimmunoassay of PGE_1 and PGE_2 in the conditioned media of cultured bones. Gowen et al. (1986) and Gowen and Mundy (1986) found that the effects of TNF on bone resorption in neonatal mouse calvariae was inhibited by interferon-γ in concentrations of 10 to 100 U/mL. Interferon-γ was more effective at inhibiting bone resorption stimulated by TNF and IL-1 than bone resorption stimulated by PTH or 1,25-dihydroxyvitamin D_3 in this system.

The effects of TNF and LT on bone organ cultures can be potentiated by other factors. Stashenko et al. (1987) showed that interleukin-1 (IL-1) had synergistic effects with TNF and LT on bone resorption in fetal rat long bone cultures. The same group also showed that PTH caused synergistic effects when cultured and in addition demonstrated that TGF-α and PTH-rP potentiate the effects of TNF on bone resorption in fetal rat long bone cultures (Sabatini et al., 1987, 1989). The mechanisms responsible for these synergistic effects remain to be demonstrated. In the case of PTH, it is likely that TNF and LT have predominant effects on increasing cell proliferation and increasing the pool of committed osteoclast progenitors (Mundy and Roodman, 1987). PTH has major effects on later stages in osteoclast formation (differentiation and fusion) (Mundy and Roodman, 1987). Thus the combination of these two agents acting at different sites on osteoclast formation may produce a synergistic effect on the generation of osteoclasts.

These organ culture experiments show that TNF and LT stimulate osteoclastic bone resorption but give no indication at what step or steps in the process of osteoclast formation and activation the cytokines act. This issue was examined in a recent study by Pfeilschifter et al. (1989). These workers used a long-term (three-week) human marrow mononuclear cell culture system in which cells with the functional and morphological characteristics of osteoclasts form in vitro in response to specific agents that stimulate proliferation and differentiation. They found that TNF, LT, and IL-1 increase both the proliferation of marrow mononuclear cells and enhance the differentiation of committed progenitors in this system. Increased proliferation was confirmed by autoradiography experiments which showed that osteoclasts treated with these factors showed increased numbers of labeled nuclei. Since the total number of osteoclasts was also increased, these factors must also have stimulated fusion of mononuclear progenitors to form multinucleated osteoclasts. TNF and LT were equipotent in this system, producing effects at concentrations of 10^{-8} to 10^{-10} *M*. These effects of TNF and LT differed from those of TGF-α and the colony-stimulating factors for granulocytes-macrophages and macrophages (CSF-GM and CSF-M) in this system. TGF-α and the CSFs stimulate only the proliferation of the progenitors; they have no effect on fusion or differentiation (Takahashi et al., 1986a; MacDonald et al., 1986). These factors require the addition of 1,25-dihydroxyvitamin D_3 for the formation of osteoclasts. Takahashi et al. (1986b) found that interferon-γ also inhibited the formation of mononuclear cells in this system, consistent with the observations of Gowen et al. (1986) using neonatal mouse calvarial organ cultures.

At least part of the effect of TNF and LT in these systems may be mediated by IL-1 (Roodman et al., 1987). The use of neutralizing antibodies to interleukin-1β inhibits the formation of osteoclasts in response to TNF and LT but not in response to PTH or 1,25-dihydroxyvitamin D. TNF and LT have been shown to induce IL-1 production by mononuclear cells in a number of systems (reviewed in Le and Vilček, 1987).

The effects of TNF and LT on mature osteoclasts were demonstrated by Thomson et al. (1987). These investigators used freshly dispersed mature rat osteoclasts isolated from the endosteal surfaces of tibiae if neonatal rat pups. They showed that TNF and LT increased the capacity of these multinucleated cells to form resorption lacunae on calcified bone matrices. Resorption lacunae were evaluated by scanning electron microscopy. However, the cytokines mediated their effects on the osteoclasts indirectly. Both cytokines stimulated the osteoclasts only when these cells were cultured together with cells of the osteoclast phenotype, either freshly dispersed rat calvarial bone cells or rat osteosarcoma cells with osteoblastic characteristics. The conclusion from these experiments was the TNF and LT caused the osteoblast-like cells to generate a second soluble signal, which in turn activates the osteoclastic cells. A similar population of "helper" or intermediate cells is required by PTH, Il-1, and 1,25-dihydroxyvitamin D in this assay system. The identity of this second signal remains unknown.

The effects of TNF on bone in vivo have been examined by Boyce et al. (1989) and by Johnson et al. (1989). Boyce examined the calvariae of normal mice injected with TNF locally. They found an increase in osteoclast activity on endosteal surfaces and an increase in the whole-blood ionized calcium concentrations in the mice. Johnson et al. (1989) used a different approach. These workers used Chinese hamster ovarian cells, which where transfected with human tumor necrosis factor cDNA in a mammalian expression vector. These cells express appreciable quantities of human TNF. The CHO cells were then inoculated into nude mice and the tumors grew in vivo. Tumor-bearing mice became hypercalcemic and their calvarial bones were examined by quantitative bone histomorphometry. The bones showed increases in osteoclastic bone resorption, with increased numbers of osteoclasts, increased active resorption surfaces, and increased total resorption surfaces (both active and inactive). The most prominent osteoclastic activity was seen along the area of bone adjacent to the surfaces. Mice were also examined that were carrying CHO cells transfected with the empty vector. Tumors grew in these mice just as well, but the mice did not become hypercalcemic and their bones remained normal.

IV. EFFECTS ON OSTEOBLAST ACTIVITY

TNF and LT also stimulate cells with an osteoblast phenotype. Bertolini et al. (1986) showed that TNF and LT caused a decrease in collagenase-digestible protein synthesis in fetal rat calvariae. This effect was seen in concentration of 10^{-7} to 10^{-9} *M*. The effect was relatively specific for collagen synthesis. Noncollagen protein synthesis was not affected. Smith et al. (1987) examined the effects of a group of osteotropic cytokines, including TNF, on cells with the osteoblast phenotype specifically rat osteosarcoma cells. These workers found that TNF and LT, like IL-1, inhibited alkaline phosphatase activity and collagen synthesis in these cells, but stimulated cell proliferation. These effects were seen in concentrations of 10^{-6} to 10^{-10} *M*. Interferon-γ had similar effects on cell proliferation and differentiated function in these cells. Ng et al. (1985) found that the effects of TNF on osteosarcoma cells with the osteoblast phenotype could be seen at much lower concentrations when the cells were co-cultured in the presence of retinoic acid (Ng et al, 1985.).

V. EFFECTS ON CALCIUM HOMEOSTASIS

TNF and LT cause hypercalcemia in normal mice. This has now been shown using a number of different systems and modes of administration. Tashjian et al. (1987) used repeated injections of recombinant human TNF in intact normal mice and found increases in plasma calcium. Sabatini et al. (1988) used Alzet osmotic minipumps and found that after 3 days of continuous infusion, there was a substantial increase in plasma calcium. These workers used recombinant human TNF and found that this was less potent and less powerful than recombinant human IL-1 in the same system, although the responses were similar to those found with parathyroid hormone. Yates (unpublished) used repeated injections of recombinant human TNF and found similar increases in whole-blood ionized calcium after 3 days to those seen with identical doses of IL-1 given in the same manner. As described earlier, Johnson et al. (1989) used Chinese hamster ovarian cells tranfected with human TNF to show that nude mice inoculated with these cells became hypercalcemic. These workers measured circulating human TNF by the L929 (cytotoxicity) biological assay. They found that circulating concentrations of TNF were increased to more than twice the normal range and were associated with substantial increases in the plasma calcium as well as changes in bone histomorphometry showing osteoclastic resorption.

Lymphotoxin has also been shown to cause hypercalcemia. Garrett et al. (1987) infused recombinant human LT into normal mice 72 h using Alzet osmotic minipumps and found that the mice became hypercalcemic. Lymphotoxin was used in doses of 10 to 20 μg/day, similar to those of recombinant human TNF, which cause hypercalcemia in the same system.

VI. ROLE OF TNF AND LT IN PHYSIOLOGIC AND PATHOLOGIC BONE TURNOVER

A. Physiologic Bone Turnover

The potential role of bone resorbing cytokines such as TNF, LT, and IL-1 have been described above under the section on normal bone remodeling. The mechanisms by which the cellular events of the bone remodeling sequence are initiated at specific sites throughout the skeleton remain unknown. However, it is likely that local factors generated in the environment of osteoclasts and on endosteal bone surfaces are important. Cytokines such as IL-1 and TNF are among the most potent osteoclast stimulating factors known. They are clearly candidates for the triggers that initiate remodeling events.

B. Chronic Inflammatory Diseases

Bone resorbing cytokines produced by chronic inflammatory cells are probable stimulants of the local bone resorption that occurs in association with chronic inflammatory diseases. Diseases such as rheumatoid arthritis, periodontal disease, and cholesteatoma are associated with the localized osteolysis that occurs adjacent to collections of the chronic inflammatory cells. In these circumstances it is reasonable to postulate that these collections of activated immune cells comprising lymphocytes and monocytes produce not only peptide cytokines but prostaglandin which could activate adjacent osteoclasts and their progenitors to cause bone resorption.

It was first recognized that activated leukocytes could produce bone resorbing activity by workers at the National Institute of Dental Research (Horton et al., 1972) during studies on the mechanisms responsible for alveolar bone destruction in periodontal disease. When leukocytes were activated by phytohemagglutinin or by dental plaque antigen, they released a number of cytokines, including an activity that caused the release of ^{45}Ca from fetal rat long bones in organ culture. This activity was called *osteoclast activating factor* (OAF). OAF was further characterized and found to have effects similar to PTH (Raisz et al., 1975). For example, it caused not only the release of mineral but also degradation of the bone matrix of the fetal rat long bone cultures. Its effects in this organ culture system are characterized by steep dose-response curves, and it caused rapid increase in osteoclastic bone resorption following either brief or continuous exposure, a phenomenon that Raisz and co-workers have referred to as *induction* (Raisz et al., 1972).

The effects of this activity on bone in vitro were effectively inhibited by phosphate, calcitonin, and cortisol. However, cortisol is more effective at inhibiting OAF than PTH-mediated bone resorption (Mundy et al., 1978). OAF increases osteoclast size in organ cultures and also increased the volume and area of the ruffled borders. The production of OAF required lymphocytes and monocytes to be present (Horton et al., 1974).

Recent information indicates that the biological activity which was present in the activated leukocyte cultures is really due to a network of cytokines, some of which stimulate osteoclastic bone resorption and some of which inhibit it. These cytokines include (in addition to TNF and LT) IL-1, prostaglandins, and differentiation inducing factor (DIF) (Abe et al., 1986, all of which stimulate osteoclastic bone resorption which are produced by immune cells. These include interferon-γ and transforming growth factor β (Gowen and Mundy, 1986; Takahashi et al., 1986a,b; Chenu et al., 1988; Pfeilschifter et al., 1988). Thus the net effects of any crude supernatant media harvested from an activated leukocyte culture will depend on the relative amounts of these cytokines which are present, and the relative excess of the stimulators of bone resorption over the inhibitors.

C. Neoplastic Disease

1. *Myeloma*

The neoplastic disease in which there is best current evidence that an osteotropic cytokine plays a central role in bone destruction is myeloma. Myeloma is a neoplastic disease of plasma cells that is characterized by extensive bone lesions (for a review of bone lesions and hypercalcemia in myeloma, see Mundy and Bertolini, 1986). These lesions may be local and osteolytic or generalized, causing a picture resembling postmenopausal osteoporosis. Eighty percent of patients with myeloma present with the major complaint of bone pain and the extensive bone destruction in this disorder causes serious clinical consequences, such as hypercalcemia, bone pain, and fracture following trivial injury. The cellular mechanisms of bone destruction in myeloma is mediated predominantly by osteoclasts (Mundy et al., 1974a,b; Valentin-Opran et al., 1982). These osteoclasts occur adjacent to myeloma cells, suggesting that they are stimulated by local factors released by the myeloma cells. Osteoblast activity is inhibited and the disorder is characterized by normal serum alkaline phosphatase, indicating that there is an abnormality in the coupling mechanism which normally links bone formation to previous bone resorption. The osteoclasts that are formed in this disorder may be smaller and contain fewer nuclei than the osteoclasts seen in other nonlmyphoid neoplastic disease (C. Marcelli, personal communication).

Myeloma cells produce soluble factors that stimulate osteoclast activity. This was first shown by Mundy et al. (1974a,b) using lymphoid cell lines and cultured myeloma cells. These cells in culture produced bone resorbing activity similar to the bone resorbing activity present in normal activated leukocyte culture supernatants. One of the lymphoid cell lines studied by these workers was derived from a patient with myeloma. The Bence Jones protein in the urine of this patient had the same antigenic determinants as the free light chains of lambda type produced by the cultured tumor cells. This suggests that the cells in culture represented the malignant cells in the patient. The bone resorbing activity produced by these myeloma cell lines and fresh myeloma cells was clearly distinguished from parathyroid hormone, prostaglandins of E series, and 1,25-dihydroxyvitamin D_3 by biological and chemical characteristics.

With more recent knowledge of the cytokines which are present in normal activated leukocyte culture supernatants, Garrett et al. (1987) reexamined the biological activity produced by myeloma cells. These workers looked specifically for IL-1, TNF, and LT. They examined five cell lines from patients with myeloma and one in considerable detail which was obtained from a hypercalcemic patient with extensive bone destruction and hypercalcemic. In all of the cell lines examined, they found culture supernatants contained bone resorbing activity and, in addition, cytotoxic activity. This cytotoxic activity could be neutralized by monoclonal antibodies to LT. Similarly, the bone resorbing activity was neutralized by the antibodies to LT. However, some residual bone resorbing activity remained even after neutralization with LT antibodies. This was in contrast to cytotoxic activity, which was completely neutralized. Il-1 biological activity could not be found in these culture supernatants, nor could expression of IL-1 mRNA. LT and TNF mRNA were expressed in all of the myeloma cell lines. Thus LT was expressed and secreted by the myeloma cells, and TNF was expressed but not secreted. The identity of the residual bone resorbing activity produced by myeloma cell lines that cannot be accounted for by LT, TNF, or IL-1 remains to be determined.

2. *Other Hematologic Disorders*

Cytokines such as LT, TNF, and IL-1 may be important in the bone destruction and hypercalcemia that occurs in other lymphoproliferative disorders. Hypercalcemia and bone destruction are less common in hematologic neoplasms, but occur occasionally in Hodgkin's disease, in T- and B-cell lymphomas, in histiocytic lymphomas, and in Burkitt's lymphoma (Mundy, 1989). There are isolated reports that these neoplasms have been associated with osteotropic factors such as IL-1, the PTH-related protein (PTH-rP), and 1,25-dihydroxyvitamin D_3 (Sato et al., 1988; Motokura et al., 1989; Breslau et al., 1984; Rosenthal et al., 1985; Zaloga et al., 1985; Davies et al., 1985). In one patient with T-cell lymphoma, IL-1α production was convincingly shown by co-purification of bone resorbing activity with IL-1-like activity, inhibition of bone resorbing activity with specific neutralizing antibodies to IL-1α, and demonstration of IL-1-like biological activity in the tumor-conditioned media (Sato et al., 1988). This tumor also produced the PTH-related protein, a tumor factor with sequence homology to PTH at the N-terminus, which also binds to and activates the PTH receptor. Several of these tumors have also been shown convincingly to produce1,25-dihydroxyvitamin D_3 (Breslau et al., 1984; Rosenthal et al., 1985; Zaloga et al., 1985; Davies et al., 1985). The concentrations of this vitamin D metabolite 25-hydroxyvitamin D_3 to 1,25-dihydroxyvitamin D_3 (Fetchick et al., 1986). However, the majority of these lymphomas do not produce 1,25-dihydroxyvitamin D_3. Mundy et al (1978) studied one patient with lymphosarcoma cell leukemia associated with hypercalcemia whose malignant cells produced a macromolecular bone resorbing factor with identical chemical and biological characteristics to the osteoclast activating factor released by normal activated peripheral blood leukocytes. Further characterization of this activity was not possible at the time the study was performed. Since these lymphoproliferative disorders produce a whole range of cytokines, it is likely that IL-1, TNF, and LT will be shown eventually to be produced by at least some of these tumor cells and play a role in the pathophysiology of bone destruction and hypercalcemia.

3. *Solid Tumors*

There is no evidence that spontaneous solid tumors produce TNF or LT, although several solid tumors have now been convincingly shown to produce IL-1 (Sato et al., 1988). This has been demonstrated by inhibition of the bone resorbing activity produced by the tumor cells by neutralizing antibodies to IL-1α and by demonstration of expression of IL-1α mRNA. On the other hand, it is now apparent that the production of TNF by host immune cells in patients with solid tumors can potentially cause a number of paraneoplastic syndromes, including cachexia, anemia, leuko-cytosis, hypertriglyceridemia, and hypercalcemia (Yoneda et al., 1989; Sabatini et al., 1990). The evidence that increased TNF production by host cells can cause hypercalcemia comes from a number of human and animal tumors associated with this syndrome. In one of these tumors, the MH-85 tumor, which was derived from a patient with squamous cell carcinoma of the maxilla, nude mice bearing this tumor develop leukocytosis, cachexia, and hypercalcemia (Yoneda et al., 1989). Circulating concentrations of TNF measured by radioimmunoassay are increased, similar in amount to the circulating TNF concentrations in animals carrying CHO tumors expressing human TNF and causing hypercalcemia and enhanced bone resorption. The cultured MH-85 tumor cells produce no TNF biological activity. On the other hand, conditioned media from these tumors cells stimulates normal host immune cells (peritoneal macrophages, splenic macrophages, peripheral monocytes) to produce TNF biological activity. The hypercalcemia in the tumor-bearing mice is decreased by passive immunization with neutralizing antibodies to TNF administered by intraperitoneal injection. Splenectomy in tumor-bearing mice lowers the plasma calcium, presumably by depleting the animal of host immune cells.

Thus in this tumor it appears likely that the tumor cells are producing a soluble mediator or mediators that provoke normal host immune cells to produce TNF. In turn, TNF is then responsible for hypercalcemia in these animals. The nature of the soluble mediator produced by the tumor cells that provokes TNF production requires further study. However, preliminary purification reveals this activity to be probably comprised of two separate mediators. One of these mediators is neutralized by antibodies to GM-CSF and has GM-CSF biological activity on granulocyte-macrophage colony formation in vitro. Since recombinant human GM-CSF induces TNF production by normal immune cells (Cannistra et al., 1987), it appears likely that this fraction is GM-CSF. The other factor is a separate mediator yet to be characterized.

We have identified several other animal and human tumors in which TNF production by normal host immune cells may be important in the pathophysiology of hypercalcemia. One of these tumors is the A375 human melanoma. This tumor produces large amounts of TGF-α (Sabatini et al., 1990). Tumor-bearing nude mice develop hypercalcemia, cachexia, and hypertriglyceridemia. As with the MH-85 tumor, the tumor cells do not express TNF, but conditioned media harvested from tumor cell cultures stimulates normal host immune cells to produce TNF and IL-1. The major mediator purified from tumor cell-conditioned media, which increases TNF production, can be inhibited by both polyconal and monoclonal antibodies to GM-CSF, suggesting that in this case GM-CSF is primarily responsible for provoking TNF production.

A third tumor that is associated with increased TNF production is the rat Leydig cell tumor (Sabatini, unpublished). This interesting tumor is a widely used model of the humoral hypercalcemia of malignancy which occurs spontaneously in 70% of aged Fischer rats (Jacobs and Huseby, 1967). Tumor-bearing animals develop hypercalcemia and hypophosphatemia. Hypercalcemia is associated with increased osteoclastic bone resorption and increased renal tubular calcium reabsorption (Hirschel-Scholz et al., 1986; Rizzoli et al., 1986). Osteoclastic bone resorption can be demonstrated clearly by quantitative bone histomorphometry (Sica et al., 1983; Martodam et al., 1983). Hypophosphatemia is accompanied by renal phosphate wasting, and tumor-bearing animals also show increased urinary excretion of cAMP (Sica et al., 1983; Troyer et al., 1982). The tumor is nonmetastasizing and hypercalcemia resolves when the tumor is excised (Sica et al., 1983). The tumors produce large amounts of TGF-α and PTH-rP, both of which are associated with increased bone resorption and hypercalcemia (Ibbotson et al., 1983; D'Souza et al., 1984). However, PTH is not expressed by the tumor cells. Circulating concentrations of immunoreactive PTH are not increased and no PTH mRNA can be demonstrated in tumor extracts (Simpson et al., 1983). The tumor cells can readily be grown in culture and produce bone resorbing activity, the majority that can be abrogated by antibodies to epidermal growth factor receptor (Ibbotson et al., 1986).

We found that rats bearing this tumor become extremely cachectic (Sabatini et al., 1990). In addition, they develop hypertriglyceridemia and leukocytosis. The tumor culture media has been examined for TNF biological activity, but none is detectable. However, the tumor-bearing animals have increased circulating concentrations of immunoreactive TNF (approximately 600 pg/mL). This TNF presumably arises from normal host cells, almost certainly cells in the immune system since the tumor-conditioned media stimulate peripheral blood monocytes, splenic cells, and peritoneal macrophages to release TNF. The circulating concentrations of immunoreactive TNF are similar to those found in nude mice bearing Chinese hamster ovarian cell tumors expressing recombinant human TNF and associated with hypercalcemia (Johnson et al., 1989). Production of TNF by host cells occurs in response to a soluble mediator that remains to be identified. Increased TNF production by immune cells is likely working in conjunction with the tumor products TGF-α and PTH-rP in the pathophysiology of hypercalcemia in this model. It is not possible at the present time to assess the relative contributions of each of these factors to the increase in plasma calcium.

In those situations such as the Leydig tumor model, where there is excessive production of TNF in conjunction with TGF-α and PTH-rP, it is likely that the effects of these factors on bone resorption and the development of hypercalcemia are synergistic. PTH-rP at suboptimal doses combined with TGF-α and TNF at doses that alone gave effect in combination were synergistic in resorbing bone in organ cultures (Sabatini et al., 1987). TGF-α TNF, and PTH-rP act at different steps in the formation and activation of osteoclasts (Mundy and Roodman, 1987). Moreover, PTH-rP has the additional effect of enhancing renal tubular calcium reabsorption (Yates et al., 1988). The effects of these factors on osteoclastic bone resorption in organ culture have certainly been shown to be synergistic (Sabatini et al., 1987). In addition, when injected in vivo, the effects of administration of PTH-rP to nude mice appear to be potentiated by TNF injections (Yates, unpublished observations).

Although it is not possible at the present time to determine the exact contribution of TNF to the paraneoplastic syndromes that occur in the rat Leydig tumor, the production of TNF by normal activated immune cells is clearly important. TNF has a wide range of pleiotropic effects, many of which overlap with those of IL-1 (Le and Vilček, 1987). For example, TNF can either inhibit or stimulate the proliferation of tumor cells, it may be the mediator of the tissue effects of endotoxic shock, it inhibits lipoprotein lipase activity *in vitro* and is associated with hypertriglyceridemia in vivo, it stimulates osteoclastic bone resorption both in vitro and in vivo, it inhibits bone formation in vitro, and it causes anemia by inhibition of the proliferation of erythropoietic progenitor cells. It also activates neutrophils, stimulates antibody-dependent cellular cytotoxicity and phagocytosis, and stimulates superoxide anion production. It appears likely, therefore, that many of the clinical features that occur in patients with cancer, such as hypercalcemia, cachexia, and anemia, may at least in part be related to excess production of this mediator by normal host cells.

VII. ROLE OF TNF IN CARTILAGE CELL METABOLISM IN HEALTH AND DISEASE

Less is known about the potential role of cytokines in cartilage degradation than in bone resorption, but the information that is available suggests that factors such as TNF and IL-1 are important. A protein initially called catabolin but later proven to be identical with IL-1 was shown to cause breakdown of cartilage proteoglycans in explants of articular cartilage (Saklatvala et al., 1984). This protein also caused increased bone resorption in organ cultures of murine calvariae and stimulated prostaglandin E_2 and collagenase release by fibroblasts and chondrocytes. The same factor caused a dose-dependent decrease in proteoglycan synthesis in slices of porcine articular cartilage (Tyler, 1985). The proteoglycan molecules that were synthesized appeared to be normal, but were clearly synthesized in reduced number.

Saklatvala (1986) found that human TNF had a similar effect to IL-1 on both proteoglycan synthesis and degradation in articular cartilage. The effects were seen at higher concentrations than those required for IL-1 but were additive with those of IL-1. Neither IL-1 nor TNF caused collagen degradation. Dayer et al. (1985) showed that TNF also had the same effect as IL-1 on collagenase and prostaglandin E_2 production by isolated synovial cells and dermal fibroblasts.

Since both TNF and IL-1 are probably produced in increased amounts in erosive joint disease, particularly when associated with inflammation, these in vitro observations are probably of relevance to the pathophysiology of the progressive erosion of articular cartilage that occurs in these conditions.

ACKNOWLEDGMENTS

Some of the work we have reported here was performed with the help of Grants AR 28149, DE 08569, AR 35188, AR 39357, CA 40035, and DE 08526 from the National Institutes of Health. We are grateful to Thelma Barrios for her expert secretarial assistance.

REFERENCES

Abe, E., Tanaka, H., Ishimi, Y., Chisato, M., Hagashi, T., Nagasawa, H., Tomida, M., Yamaguchi, Y., Hozumi, M., and Suda, T. (1986). Differentiation-inducing factor purified from conditioned media of mitogen-treated spleen cell cultures stimulates bone resorption, *Proc. Natl. Acad. Sci. USA, 83*: 5958.

Bertolini, D. R., Nedwin, G. E., Bringman, T. S., and Mundy, G. R. (1986). Stimulation of bone resorption and inhibition of bone formation in vitro by human tumour necrosis factors, *Nature, 319*: 516.

Boyce, B. F., Aufdemorte, T. B., Garrett, I. R., Yates, A. J. P., and Mundy, G. R. (1989). Effects of interleukin-1 on bone turnover in normal mice, *Endocrinology, 125*: 1141.

Breslau, N. A., McGuire, J. L., Zerwekh, J. E., Frenkel, E. P., and Pak, C. Y. C. (1984). Hypercalcemia associated with increased serum calcitriol levels in three patients with lymphoma, *Ann. Intern. Med., 100*: 1.

Cannistra, S. A., Rambaidi, A., Spriggs, D. R., Herrmann, F., Keefe, D., and Guffin, J. D. (1987). Human granulocyte-macrophage colony-stimulating factor induces expression of tumor necrosis by the U937 cell line and by normal human monocytes, *J. Clin. Invest., 79*: 1720.

Chenu, C., Pfeilschifter, J., Mundy, G. R., and Roodman, G. D. (1988). Transforming growth factor β inhibits formation of osteoclast-like cells in long-term human marrow cultures, *Proc. Natl. Acad. Sci. USA, 85*: 5683.

Darby, A. J., and Meunier, P. J. (1982). Mean wall thickness and formation periods of trabecular bone packets in idiopathic osteoporosis, *Calcif. Tissue Int., 33*: 199.

Davies, M., Hayes, M. E., Mawer, E. B., and Lumb, G. A. (1985). Abnormal vitamin D metabolism in Hodgkin's lymphoma, *Lancet, i*: 1186.

Dayer, J. -M., Beutler, B., and Cerami, A. (1985). Cachectin/tumor necrosis factor stimulates collagenase and prostaglandin E_2 production by human synovial cells and dermal fibroblasts, *J. Exp. Med., 162*: 2163.

Dewhirst, F. E., Ago, J. M., Peros, W. J., and Stashenko, P. (1987). Synergism between parathyroid hormone and interleukin-1 in stimulating bone resorption in organ culture, *J. Bone Miner. Res., 2*: 127.

Fetchick, D. A., Bertolini, D. R., Sarin, P. S., Weintraub, S. E., Mundy, G. R., and Dunn, J. R. (1986). Production of 1,25 dihydroxyvitamin D by human lymphotrophic virus-1 transformed lymphocytes, *J. Clin. Invest., 78*: 592.

Garrett, I. R., Durie, B. G. M., Nedwin, G. E., Gillespie, A., Bringman, T., Sabatini, M., Bertolini, D. R., and Mundy, G. R. (1987). Production of the bone resorbing cytokine lymphotoxin by cultured human myeloma cells, *N. Engl. J. Med., 317*: 526.

Gowen, M., and Mundy, G. R. (1986). Actions of recombinant interleukin-1, interleukin-2 and interferon gamma on bone resorption in vitro, *J. Immunol., 136*: 2478.

Gowen, M., Nedwin, G., and Mundy, G. R. (1986). Preferential inhibition of cytokine stimulated bone resorption by recombinant interferon gamma, *J. Bone Miner. Res., 1*: 469.

Hirschel-Scholz, S., Caverzasio, J., Rizzoli, R., and Bonjour, J. P. (1986). Normalization of hypercalcemia associated with a decrease in renal calcium reabsorption in Leydig cell tumor-bearing rats treated with WR-2721, *J. Clin. Invest., 78*: 319.

Horton, J. E., Raisz, L. G., Simmons, H. A., Oppenheim, J. S., and Mergenhagen, S. E. (1972). Bone resorbing activity in supernant fluid from cultured human peripheral blood leukocytes, *Science, 177*: 793.

Horton, J. E., Oppenheim, J. J>, Mergenhagen, S. E., and Raisz, L. G. (1974). Macrophage-lymphocyte synergy in the production of osteoclast activating factor, *J. Immunol., 113*: 1278.

Ibbotson, K. J., D'Souza, S. M., Ng, K. W., Osborne, C. K., Niall, M., Martin, T. J., and

Mundy, G. R. (1983). Tumor derived growth factor increases bone resorption in a tumor associated with humoral hypercalcemia of malignancy, *Science, 221*: 1292.

Ibbotson, K. J., Harrod, J., Gowen, M., D'Souza, S., Smith, D. D., Winkler, M. E., Derynck, R., and Mundy, G. R. (1986). Human recombinant transforming growth factor alpha stimulates bone resorption and inhibits formation in vitro, *Proc. Natl. Acad. Sci. USA, 83*: 2228.

Jacobs, B. B., and Huseby, R. A. (1967). Neoplasms occurring in aged Fischer rats with special reference to testicular, uterine and thyroid tumors, *J. Natl. Cancer Inst., 39*: 303.

Johnson, R. A., Boyce, B. F., Mundy, G. R., and Roodman, G. D. (1989). Tumors producing human TNF induce hypercalcemia and osteoclastic bone resorption in nude mice, *Endocrinology, 124*: 1424.

Le, J., and Vilček, J. (1987). Biology of disease. Tumor necrosis factor and interleukin 1: cytokines with multiple overlapping biological activities, *Lab. Invest., 56*: 234.

MacDonald, B. R., Mundy, G. R., Clark, S., Wang, E. A., Kuehl, T. J., Stanley, E. R., and Roodman, G. D. (1986). Effects of human recombinant CSF-GM and highly purified CSF-1 on the formation of multinucleated cells with osteoclast characteristics in long term bone marrow cultures, *J. Bone Miner. Res., 1*: 227.

Martodam, R. R., Thornton, K. S., Sica, D. A., D'Souza, S. M., Flora, L., and Mundy, G. R. (1983). The effects of dichloromethylene diphosphonate on hypercalcemia and other parameters of the humoral hypercalcemia of malignancy in the rat Leydig cell tumor, *Calif. Tissue Int., 35*: 512.

Motokura, T., Fukumoto, S., Takahashi, S., Watanabe, T., Matsumoto, T., Igarashi, T., and Ogata, E. (1988). Expression of parathyroid hormone-related protein in a human T cell lymphotrophic virus type I-infected T cell line, *Biochem. Biophys. Res. Commun., 154*: 1182.

Motokura, T., Fukumoto, S., Matsumoto, T., Takahashi, S., Fujita, A., Yamashita, T., Igarashi, T., and Ogata, E. (1989). Parathyroid hormone-related protein in adult T-cell leukemia-lymphoma, *Ann. Intern. Med., 111*: 484.

Mundy, G. R. (1989). Hypercalcemia associated with hematologic malignancies, *Calcium Homeostasis: Hypercalcemia and Hypocalcemia* (M. Dunitz, ed.), Martin Dunitz, London, p. 92.

Mundy, G. R., and Bertolini, D. R. (1986). Bone destruction and hypercalcemia in plasma cell myeloma, *Semin. Oncol., 13*: 291.

Mundy, G. R., and Bonewald, L. F. (1989). Effects of immune cell products on bone, *Macrophage-Derived Cell Regulatory Factors: Cytokines* (C. Sorg, ed.), S. Karger, Basel, p. 38.

Mundy, G. R., and Roodman, G. D. (1987). Osteoclast ontogeny and function, *Bone and Mineral Research V* (W. A. Peck, ed.), Elsevier, Amsterdam, p. 209.

Mundy, G. R., Luben, R. A., Raisz, L. G., Oppenheim, J. J., and Buell, D. N. (1947a). Bone resorbing activity in supernatants from lymphoid cell lines, *N. Engl. J. Med., 290*: 867.

Mundy, G. R., Raisz, L. G., Cooper, R. A., Schechter, G. P., and Salmon S. E. (1974b). Evidence for the secretion of an osteoclast stimulating factor in myeloma, *N. Engl. J. Med., 291*: 1041.

Mundy, G. R., Rick, M. E., Turcotte, R., and Kowalski, M. A. (1978). Pathogenesis of hyperclacemia in lymphosarcoma cell leukemia: role of an osteoclast activating factor-like substance and mechanism of action for glucocorticoid therapy, *Am. J. Med., 65*: 600.

Ng, K. W., Livesey, S. A., Collier, F., Gummer, P. R., and Martin, T. J. (1985). Effect of retinoids on the growth, ultrastructure, and cytoskeletal structures of malignant rat osteoblasts, *Cancer Res., 45*: 5106.

Pfeilschifter, J. P., Seyedin, S., and Mundy, G. R. (1988). Transforming growth factor β inhibits bone resorption in fetal rat long bone cultures, *J. Clin. Invest., 82*: 680.

Pfeilschifter, J., Mundy, G. R., and Roodman, G. D. (1989). Interleukin-1 and tumor necrosis factor stimulate the formation of human osteoclast-like cells in vitro, *J. Bone Miner. Res., 4*: 113.

Raisz, L. G., Trummel, C. L., and Simmons, H. (1972). Induction of bone resorption in tissue culture: prolonged response after brief exposure to parathyroid hormone or 25-hydroxycholecalciferol, *Endocrinology, 90*: 744.

Raisz, L. G., Luben, R. A., and Mundy, G. R. (1975). Effects of osteoclast activating factor from human leukocytes on bone metabolism, *J. Clin. Invest., 56*: 408.

Rizzoli, R., Caverzasio, J., Fleisch, H., Bonjour, J. P. (1986). Parathyroid hormone-like changes in renal calcium and phosphate reabsorption induced by Leydig cell tumor in thyroparathyroidectomized rats, *Endocrinology, 119*: 1004.

Roodman, G. D., Takashashi, N., Bird, A., and Mundy, G. R. (1987). Tumor necrosis factor α (TNF) stimulates formation of osteoclast-like cell (OCL) in long term human marrow cultures by stimulating production of interleukin-1 (IL-1), *Clin. Res., 35*: 515A.

Rosenthal, N., Insogna, K. L., Godsall, J. W., Smaldone, L., Waldron, J. A., and Stewart, A. F. (1985). Elevations in circulating 1,25 dihydroxyvitamin D in three patients with lymphoma-associated hypercalcemia, *J. Clin. Endocrinol. Metab., 60*: 29.

Sabatini, M., Garrett, I. R., and Mundy, G. R. (1987). TNF potentiates the effects of interleukin-1 on bone resorption in vitro, *J. Bone Miner. Res.,* 2(Suppl. 1): 34 (abstr.)

Sabatini, M., Boyce, B., Aufdemorte, T., Bonewald, L., and Mundy, G. (1988). Infusions of recombinant human interleukin-1α, and β cause hypercalcemia in normal mice, *Proc. Natl. Acad. Sci. USA, 85*: 5235.

Sabatini, M., Chavez, J., Mundy, G., and Bonewald, L. (1990). Stimulation of tumor necrosis factor release from monocytic cells by the A375 human melanoma via granulocyte-macrophage colony stimulating factor, *Cancer Res., 50*: 2673–2678 .

Saklatvala, J. (1986). Tumour necrosis factor α stimulates resorption and inhibits synthesis of proteoglycan in cartilage, *Nature, 322*: 547.

Saklatvala, J., Pilsworth, L. M. C., Sarsfield, S. J., Gavrilovic, J., and Heath, J. K. (1984). Pig catabolin is a form of interleukin 1: cartilage and bone resorb, fibroblasts make prostaglandin and collagenase, and thymocyte proliferation is augmented in response to one protein, *Biochem. J., 224*: 461.

Sato, K., Fujii, Y., Kasono, K., Tsushima, T., and Shizume, K. (1988). Production of interleukin-1α and a parathyroid hormone-like factor by a squamous cell carcinoma of the esophagus (EC-GI) derived from a patient with hypercalcemia, *J. Clin. Endocrinol. Metab., 67*: 592.

Sica, D. A., Marodam, R. R., Aronow, J., and Mundy, G. R. (1983). The hypercalcemia rat Leydig cell tumor: a model of the humoral hypercalcemia of malignancy, *Calcif. Tisssue Int., 35*: 287.

Simpson, E., Mundy, G. R., Ibbotson, K., D'Souza, S., Bockman, R, and Jacobs, J. (1983). Absence of parathyroid hormone messenger RNA in non parathyroid tumors associated with hypercalcemia, *N. Engl. J. Med., 309*: 305.

Smith, D., Gowen, M., and Mundy, G. R. (1987). Effects of interferon gamma and other cytokines on collagen synthesis in fetal rat bone cultures, *Endocrinology, 120*: 2494.

Stashenko, P., Dewhirst, F. E., Peros, W. J., Kent, R. L., and Ago, J. M. (1987). Synergistic interactions between interleukin 1, tumor necrosis factor, and lymphotoxin in bone resorption, *J. Immunol., 138*: 1464.

Takahashi, N., MacDonald, B. R., Hon, J., Winkler, M. E., Derynck, R., Mundy, G. R., and Roodman, G. D. (1986a). Recombinant human transforming growth factor α stimulates the formation of osteoclast-like cells in long term human marrow cultures, *J. Clin. Invest., 78*: 894.

Takahashi, N., Mundy, G. R., and Roodman, G. D. (1986b). Recombinant human gamma interferon inhibits formation of human osteoclast like cells, *J. Immunol., 137*: 3541.

Tashjian, A. H., Voelkel, E. F., Lazzaro, M., Goad, D., Bosma, T., and Levine, L. (1987). Tumor necrosis factor α (cachectin) stimulates bone resorption in mouse calvaria via a prostaglandin-mediated mechanism, *Endocrinology, 120*: 2029.

Thomson, B. M., Mundy, G. R., and Chambers, T. J. (1987). Tumor necrosis factors α and β induce osteoblastic cells to stimulate osteoclastic bone resorption, *J. Immunol., 138*: 775.

Troyer, H., Sowers, J. R., and Babich, E. (1982). Leydig cell tumor induced hypercalcemia in the Fischer rat: morphometric and histochemical evidence for a humoral factor that activates osteoclasts, *Am. J. Pathol., 108*: 284.

Tyler, J. A. (1985). Articular cartilage cultured with catabolin (pig interleukin 1) synthesizes a decreased number of normal proteoglycan molecules, *Biochem J., 227: 869.*

Valentin-Opran, A., Charhon, S. A., Meunier, P. J., Edouard, C. M., and Arlot, M. E. (1982). Quantitiative histology of myeloma induced bone changes, *Br. J. Haematol., 52*: 601.

Yates, A. J. P., Gutierrez, G. E., Smolens, P., Travis, P. S., Katz, M. S., Aufdemorte, T. B., Boyce, B. F., Hymer, T. K., Poser, J. W., and Mundy, G. R. (1988). Effects of a synthetic peptide of a parathyroid hormone-related protein on calcium homeostasis, renal tubular calcium reabsorption and bone metabolism, *J. Clin. Invest., 81*: 932.

Yoneda, T., Alsina, M. M., Chavez, J. B., Bonewald, L., and Mundy, G. R. (1989). Hypercalcemia in a human tumor is due to tumor necrosis factor production by host immune cells, *J. Bone Miner. Res., 4*(Suppl. 1): 826 (abstr.)

Zaloga, G. P., Eil, C., and Medbery, C. A. (1985). Humoral hypercalcemia in Hodgkin's disease, *Arch. Intern. med., 145*: 155.

22

Relationship of TNF to Interleukins

RUTH NETA
Armed Forces Radiobiology Research Institute, Bethesda, Maryland

THOMAS J. SAYERS
Program Resources, Inc./DynCorp, Frederick, Maryland

JOOST J. OPPENHEIM
National Cancer Institute, Frederick, Maryland

I. INTRODUCTION

The host response to microbial infection, foreign antigens, and tissue injury is orchestrated by a complex network of endogenous mediators. Prominent among these mediators are cytokines: polypeptide hormones that transmit signals from one cell to another. The cytokines tumor necrosis factor (TNF) and a number of the interleukins have emerged as important mediators of host defense. These cytokines, particularly TNF, IL-1, and IL-6, induce a wide spectrum of biological activities by a variety of cell types in vitro, and have in vivo systemic effects that are often biologically indistinguishable. The apparent redundancy of the activities of these cytokines is perplexing since they are structurally distinct and interact at unrelated cell membrane receptors. In this chapter, in an effort to elucidate the interactions of TNF with these other cytokines, we have therefore compared the production, receptor interactions, intracellular effects, and extracellular in vitro and in vivo effects of TNF with those of interleukins 1, 2, 3, 4, 6, and 8, hematopoietic colony-stimulating factors, as well as transforming growth factor β (TGF-β). This has represented a difficult undertaking since there has been a virtual explosion in the number of studies of the effects of purified recombinant cytokines over the past 5 years. To generate a manageable and useful review we have summarized as much of the available published data as possible in tables and have concentrated on highlighting only the more salient features of the relationships and interactions as well as the unique attributes of these cytokines.

II. INTERACTIONS AND RELATIONSHIPS OF TNF TO IL-1

Despite the many similarities in the biological activities of IL-1 and TNF, the molecular structure and receptors for these cytokines are quite distinct. TNF is now used as a term for two cytokines, TNF-α and TNF-β (or lymphotoxin). Since most of the work in the last few years has been performed using TNF-α, this review will concentrate predominantly on this form of TNF. IL-1 is a term for two polypeptides (IL-1α and IL-1β) that possess a wide spectrum of similar immunologic and nonimmunologic activities. Molecular gene cloning has revealed that IL-1α and IL-1β are products of distinct genes located on chromosome 2 in humans and mouse. IL-1α and IL-1β exhibit about 26% identity at the amino acid level. Neither are glycosylated. Both IL-1α and IL-1β appear to bind to both the p80 and p65 receptors for IL-1.

A. Production of TNF and IL-1

Although IL-1 is produced by almost all cell types and TNF predominantly by leucocytes (Table 1), most studies have been performed on the production of IL-1 and TNF by mononuclear phagocytes. IL-1α, IL-1β, and TNF-α are produced by normal mononuclear cells in response to exogenous stimuli and are often produced simultaneously in response to the same stimuli. Most studies have evaluated the production of these cytokines by human peripheral blood monocytes or murine macrophages in response to potent inducing agents such as bacterial lipopolysaccharide (LPS). Following LPS stimulation, mRNA for TNF and IL-1 is rapidly transcribed (Fenton et al., 1987, 1988; Beutler et al., 1986). However, different intracellular pathways may be involved in LPS induction of IL-1 or TNF gene expression in macrophages since inhibitors of protein kinase C blocked expression of mRNA for both IL-1 and TNF, whereas inhibitors of calmodulin-dependent kinase only blocked the induction of mRNA for IL-1 and did not affect mRNA for TNF-α (Kovacs et al., 1988).

In a recent study, taxol (a plant-derived antitumor drug) was shown to effectively mimic LPS in inducing macrophages to produce TNF-α (Ding et al., 1990b). The best known action of this drug is the stabilization of tubulin polymers. The gene controlling responsiveness to taxol is closely linked to the genes controlling responsiveness to LPS. Thus an intracellular target affected by taxol might be involved in actions of LPS on macrophages and other cells. The effects of taxol on IL-1 production were not reported. The authors concluded that the target for taxol action could be microtubule-associated protein. These findings could lead to new insights into the participation of the cytoskeleton in the response of cells to their environment.

The genes for IL-1 and TNF-α are rapidly transcribed on LPS stimulation and both genes appear to be under the control of short-lived repressor proteins (Collart et al., 1986). Studies on the TNF-α promoter have identified putative κB enhancer motifs which may be important in transcription of the TNF-α gene in response to LPS (Shakov et al., 1990). Elements controlling IL-1 gene expression have not yet been identified. Transcription of of IL-1α appears to be under tighter control than TNF-α in that inhibitors of protein synthesis are sometimes required to observe IL-1α mRNA (Libby et al., 1986a,b).

TNF is initially synthesized as a precursor prohormone of 233 amino acids which possesses a hydrophobic sequence typical of membrane-associated protein. The precursor is cleaved to a mature secreted protein of 157 amino acids (17 kDa) which is secreted (Kriegler et al., 1988). IL-1α and IL-1β are initially synthesized as 33-kDa precursor peptides, and pre IL-1β has little biological activity (Giri et al., 1985). The precursors are cleaved to biologically active forms of IL-1 (17.5 kDa). Since IL-1 possesses no identifiable hydrophobic or transmembrane sequence, the mechanism of secretion is unknown. A membrane form of IL-1 has been hypothesized based mainly on the ability of paraformaldehyde-treated macrophages to replace IL-1 in assays of IL-1 bioactivity (Kurt-Jones et al., 1985, 1986). On using more thorough fixation procedures with glutaraldehyde, no membrane IL-1 can be demonstrated. These inconsistencies have led to the proposal by Suttles et al. (1990) that IL-1 is not found in monocyte membrane fractions but leaks from intracellular pools because of inefficient fixation. Since paraformaldehyde-fixed monocytes were able to kill TNF-sensitive targets, a membrane form of TNF has also been postulated (Decker et al., 1987). Biochemical evidence for a membrane form of TNF has been reported (Kriegler et al., 1988), but Bakouche et al. (1988) reported that membrane-associated TNF did not behave as a typical membrane protein since it could be eluted from human monocytes by either high-salt or low-pH treatment. It was concluded that TNF might be binding back to its own receptor. Using immunofluorescence microscopy, Hofsli et al. (1989) could detect a membrane form of TNF-α, and they argued that this was not TNF-α binding back to its own receptor since the presence of soluble TNF-β did not decrease amounts of membrane TNF-α. TNF-β would be anticipated to block the binding of TNF-α to the common cell surface receptor.

Using sensitive and specific radioimmunoassay techniques to compare levels of secreted and cell-associated IL-1α, IL-1β, and TNF-α from stimulated monocytes, Lonnemann et al. (1989) showed that even by 1 h, secreted TNF-α greatly exceeds cell-associated levels, suggesting that any membrane-bound TNF must be rapidly cleaved to produce the secreted form, and the vast majority of TNF-α protein is in the secreted extracellular form. In contrast, IL-1β was present at roughly equivalent levels as an intracellular and extracellular protein, whereas 90% of the IL-1α re-

Table 1 Induction of IL-1 and/or TNF Production in Different Cell Types

Cell type	Inducing stimulus	Up-regulation of mRNA for: IL-1	TNF
Monocytes/macrophages	LPS	Fenton et al., 1987, 1988	Beutler et al., 1986; Kovacs et al., 1988
	IL-2 + CD3	Numeroff et al., 1988	Steffan et al., 1988; Economou et al., 1989
Mesangial cells	Immune complexes	Werber et al., 1987	
NK cells (LGL)	LPS	Scala et al., 1984a	
	Staph. aureus	Abo et al., 1986	
	PHA or K562 target cells		Degliantoni et al., 1985; Peters et al., 1986
B cells	LPS	Scala et al., 1984b; Matsushima et al., 1985	
	PMA		Yamamoto et al., 1984
T cells	PHA, PMA + ionophore; PMA + CD3		Turner et al., 1987; Cuturi et al., 1987; Steffen et al., 1988; Pawelec et al., 1989
	Allogeneic B cells + antigen	Tartakovsky et al., 1986	

PMN	Zymosan or PMA	Goto et al., 1984; Tiku et al., 1986	
	GM-CSF		Lindemann et al., 1989
Keratinocytes	Constitutive production, UV light	Luger et al., 1981; Kupper et al., 1986a	Oxholm et al., 1988
Smooth muscle	LPS	Libby et al., 1986a	Warner and Libby, 1989
Endothelial cells	LPS	Moissec et al., 1986; Libby et al., 1986b	Libby et al., 1986b
Fibroblasts	TNF or IL-1	Le et al., 1987; Elias et al., 1989	
Astrocytes	LPS	Fontana et al., 1982b; Lieberman et al., 1989	
	New castle disease virus		Lieberman et al., 1989
Microglia	LPS	Giulian et al., 1986	

mained cell associated after 18 h of LPS stimulation. Further study is necessary to elucidate whether IL-1 actually has any intracellular activities in the producing cells.

B. Cell Sources of TNF and IL-1

IL-1 and TNF were initially described as products of mononuclear phagocytes; however, it is now clear that they can both be produced by a wide, range of cell types in response to a variety of stimuli (Table 1). To date, bioassays and immunoassays that measure the release of TNF-α, IL-1α, or IL-1β have been used to quantitate the amount of protein secreted. However, inherent in such methods is the tacit assumption that all cells of a given population secrete equal amounts of a given product. Recent studies suggest that macrophages and monocytes are functionally heterogeneous, with marked differences being observed in the levels of cytokines secreted by different subsets. For example, human alveolar macrophages and peripheral blood monocytes exhibit different profiles of cytokine production on stimulation with LPS. A sensitive and specific ELISA for IL-1β demonstrated that alveolar macrophages and peripheral blood monocytes synthesized equivalent amounts of IL-1β; however, monocytes released three to four times more IL-1β than alveolar macrophages (Wewers and Herzyk, 1989). It was concluded that the limitation in IL-1 release from alveolar macrophages was due to a decrease in processing and release of the IL-1β precursor. In contrast, studies on TNF-α production by alveolar macrophages in response to LPS indicated that these cells secreted six- to eightfold more TNF-α than blood monocytes (Wewers and Herzyk, 1989; Becker et al., 1989). Peripheral blood monocytes themselves produce heterogeneous amounts of IL-1 or TNF-α. When monocytes are fractionated by density gradient centrifugation, denser monocytes consistently produce more IL-1 and TNF on LPS stimulation (Elias et al., 1985). These findings were confirmed by Herrmann et al. (1989b), who additionally noted that TNF-α secretion occurred predominantly in the less dense monocyte fractions. The differences in cytokine secretion by small and large cells could be related to the state of maturation and/or differentiation of individual monocytes. Human blood monocytes that have been differentiated into macrophages after 48 to 96 h in vitro become like tissue macrophages which are characterized by a decreased ability to release IL-1β (Haq and Maca, 1986; Lewis et al., 1989). Cultured monocytes secreted about 80% as much TNF but <10% as much IL-1 as fresh monocytes (Burchett et al., 1988). Furthermore, with increasing duration of in vitro culture macrophages actually produce increasing amounts of an inactive competitive antagonist of IL-1β (Hannum et al., 1990). No such inhibitory analog of TNF has yet been identified. Cytokine production by tissue macrophages (isolated from the peritoneal lavage of women or from the fetal side of the placenta) resembled that of cultured monocytes (Lewis et al., 1989). Heterogeneity of IL-1 and TNF-α production has also been observed during the in vitro differentiation of bone-marrow stem cells (Myers et al., 1989). Although it remains to be demonstrated whether a decrease in IL-1 secretion occurs on differentiation of macrophages in vivo, nonetheless, the differential regulation of IL-1 and TNF-α during phases of monocyte development or differentiation may provide important clues to the regulation of cytokine synthesis and secretion.

Although cells of the macrophage lineage are an important source of IL-1 or TNF, other cells of the lymphoid system can also produce either or both of these cytokines in response to a variety of stimuli in vitro. Purified B cells (Matsushima et al., 1985) produce some extracellular IL-1 activity on stimulation with LPS. This B-lymphocyte-derived IL-1 was biochemically and immunologically similar to monocyte IL-1. Human B lymphoid lines on stimulation with phorbol myristate acetate (PMA) produce large amounts of TNF-β, but TNF-α was not detected (Yamamoto et al., 1984). Interestingly, LPS, which is an extremely good stimulus for IL-1 and TNF production by monocytes, is not always effective in enhancing the production of these cytokines by lymphocytes. In contrast, PMA or phytohemagglutinin (PHA) are good inducers of cytokine production by T and B lymphocytes (Nedwin et al., 1985).

Isolated human T cells as well as T-cell clones have been reported to produce both TNF-α and TNF-β. Optimal stimuli for the production of TNF-α appear to be PHA, PMA, and calcium ionophore or PMA and the antibody OKT3. Murine T-cell clones on stimulation with concanavalin A also produced TNF (Firestein et al., 1989). Certain murine T-cell clones can also produce IL-1α on stimulation with allogeneic B cells; however, the number of clones producing IL-1 is rather limited, and T cells produce IL-1 only after a prolonged period of culture in vitro. The biological importance of T cells as IL-1 producers remains dubious. Highly purified human NK cells or large granular lymphocytes produce IL-1 on stimulation with either LPS or gram-positive bacteria such as *Staphylococcus aureus*. NK cells also produce detectable levels of TNF-*a*; however, in contrast to IL-1 production, LPS does not induce TNF-α production in these cells, whereas PHA- or NK-sensitive targets such as K562 cells do. Consequently, the intracellular pathways utilized by LGL for expression of IL-1 and TNF-α may be quite separate and distinct.

A variety of nonlymphoid cells are also capable of producing IL-1 and/or TNF. Human PMN stimulated with particulate agents such as zymosan or soluble agents such as PMA also release an IL-1-like factor in a dose- and time-dependent manner. PMN have recently been reported to produce mRNA for TNF-α or TNF-β, although no protein was detected (Lindemann et al., 1989).

Keratinocytes were initially identified as cells that could readily produce factors similar or identical to IL-1 (Luger et al., 1981). Interestingly, cultured normal human keratinocytes contain two to four times more IL-1α than IL-1β, in contrast to peripheral blood monocytes, which contain 10 to 20 times more IL-1β than IL-1α mRNA. The reason for this difference in the predominant types of IL-1 produced by monocytes or keratinocytes is unclear. Only keratinocytes that are irradiated with appropriate doses of ultraviolet light (UV-B) produce TNF as well as IL-1.

Human vascular smooth muscle cells can produce both IL-1σ and IL-1β as well as TNF-α in response to stimulation with LPS (Libby et al., 1986a; Warner and Libby, 1989). The mRNAs for IL-1α, IL-1β, and TNF-α are all induced within 4 h, but detection of mRNA for IL-1α or TNF-α usually requires "superinduction" with cycloheximide or anisomycin. Smooth muscle cells were shown to be capable of secreting biologically active IL-1 and TNF-α. Local production of IL-1β could contribute to early responses to injury or infection. Human vascular endothelial cells produce IL-1, in response to LPS (Moissec et al., 1986; Libby et al., 1986b). It should, however, be noted that the minimum levels of LPS required to induce maximal gene expression in vascular endothelial cells were 100-fold higher than those required to stimulate maximal IL-1 production by monocytes. In the case of endothelial cells, although mRNA for TNF-α is upregulated, no TNF-α production has been demonstrated by LPS stimulation of endothelial cell cultures (Libby et al., 1986b). LPS, which is the usual stimulus used to induce high levels of IL-1 by monocytes, did not induce accumulation of IL-1β mRNA in fibroblasts, whereas treatment of the cells with IL-1α or TNF-α did. These cytokines do not induce fibroblasts to produce a significant amount of soluble IL-1β protein (Le et al., 1987; Elias et al., 1989). Furthermore, the 33-kDA IL-1β precursor accumulates, suggesting that fibroblasts either lack the ability to proteolytically process pro-IL-1β or have a defect in IL-1β secretion.

Highly purified cultures of brain astrocytes on stimulation with LPS produce both IL-1 and TNF. In stimulated astrocytes the mRNA for TNF-α was more weakly expressed than mRNA for IL-1α or IL-1β. In contrast, stimulation of astrocytes by the addition of Newcastle disease virus (NDV) resulted in the appearance of abundant TNF mRNA, which appeared within 3 h, reached a maximum by 8 h, and declined by 20 h (Lieberman et al., 1989). The amount of TNF-α released by NDV-stimulated astrocytes was about fourfold greater than that released by LPS-stimulated cells. Neither IL-1α nor IL-1β mRNA were detected in virally stimulated astrocytes. These quantitative differences in cytokine production may reflect the existence in astrocytes of separate pathways for the induction of the genes for TNF-α, IL-1α, and IL-1β. Using newly developed methods to separate astroglia from ameboid microglia, Giulian et al. (1986) demonstrated that microglia produced much higher levels of IL-1 activity than astrocytes on stimulation with LPS. Whether the predominant form of IL-1 released by microglia was IL-1α, IL-1β, or another as yet unidentified member of the IL-1 family is not yet clear.

Although a wide range of cells can produce IL-1 and TNF-α in vitro in response to a variety of stimuli, few studies to date have thoroughly examined which cells predominantly produce the cytokines in vivo, whether these cytokines are produced by cells constitutively or require induction, and the major physiological roles of these proteins.

Using immunohistochemical techniques, both IL-1 and TNF-α have been detected in skin biopies of normal individuals. After UV irradiation of the skin, levels of both cytokines are increased markedly (Oxholm et al., 1988). Mechanical stress, electromagnetic waves or UV, as well as physiological skin flora may play a role as stimuli for induction of these cytokines. On the other hand, production of these cytokines may be linked to epidermal cell differentiation. In recent studies, Tovey et al. (1988) have demonstrated high levels of transcripts for IL-1, TNF-α, and IL-6 in spleen, liver, kidney, and peripheral blood leukocytes of normal individuals. The authors propose that a network of cytokines may act in consort to maintain homeostasis within these tissues. The technique of in situ hybridization has been used to establish the tissue localization of IL-1α and IL-1β in the mouse. These studies suggest that in normal animals many of the IL-1 mRNA-producing cells are tissue macrophages. Organs exposed to environmental antigens and microbial products (lymph nodes, intestine, lung, and uterus) had high frequencies of IL-1 -producing cells. The production of IL-1 mRNA in the thymus and bone marrow suggested that IL-1 may play a role in T-cell differentiation and hemopoiesis (Takacs et al., 1988). The predominance of IL-1 mRNA in cells exposed to environmental stimuli, coupled with the apparent difficulty in detecting mRNA for either IL-1 or TNF in leukocytes isolated under conditions that strictly minimize any stimulation during the isolation procedure, both indicate that the genes for IL-1 and TNF are transcribed only in response to exogenous and endogenous stimuli. Studies on the distribution of cells producing TNF in vivo have not yet been reported.

C. Exogenous Inducers

It has long been recognized that components of bacterial cell walls such as lipopolysaccharide (LPS) or muramyl dipeptide (MDP) are particularly potent inducers of the synthesis and release of both IL-1 and TNF-α by macrophages in vitro. LPS macromolecules are structurally diverse, consisting of a polysaccharide portion and a relatively conserved lipid moiety termed *lipid A*. The lipid A component has been ascribed as accounting for many of the biological properties of LPS. Both IL-1 and TNF-α production in macrophages can be induced by both bacterial and synthetic lipid A, although more lipid A than LPS is usually required to stimulate optimal cytokine production (Loppnow et al., 1986; Kiener et al., 1988; Feist et al., 1989). A monosaccharide precursor of lipid A termed lipid X has little or no effect on TNF production by cultured bone-marrow macrophages or human monocytes (Sayers et al., 1987; Feist et al., 1989) but has been demonstrated to induce increases in both intracellular and extracellular IL-1 (Lasfargues and Chaby, 1988). In addition, a variety of other monosaccharides or disaccharide derivatives preferentially induced either IL-1 or TNF. In an analogous manner, chemical modification of bacterial peptidoglycans such as MDP results in structures that differ in their ability to induce cytokine production (Bahr et al., 1987). Other bacterial components, such as lipoarabinomannan derived from *Mycobacterim tuberculosis*, also enhance TNF-α production by human monocytes (Moreno et al., 1989). It is likely that a number of bacterial constituents may have the ability to trigger monocytes and macrophages directly to release TNF-α and/or IL-1. NK cells can also produce IL-1 in response to gram-positive bacteria (Abo et al., 1986). However, it seems likely that differences in cellular production of IL-1 or TNF in response to modified structures of LPS or MDP may be more quantitative than qualitative. In our view the overall capabilities of the responding cell would be more important than the nature of the exogenous stimulus in determining whether either IL-1 or TNF are produced individually or in combination.

In addition to bacteria, fungi such as *Candida albicans* cause the release of TNF-α from both monocytes and NK cells (Djeu et al., 1988). Whether these cells concomitantly produce IL-1 was not reported. TNF-α has been detected in the sera of patients with acute malaria (Scuderi et al., 1986), and malaria blood-stage parasites have been demonstrated to liberate heat-stable soluble antigens that induce the release of TNF-α by murine macrophages (Taverne et al., 1989). Whether IL-1 was concomitantly induced with TNF-α was not reported. These antigens may be carbohydrate in nature.

Human peripheral blood mononuclear cells (PBMC) preferentially produce TNF-α and TNF-β in response to certain RNA and DNA viruses (Wong and Goeddel, 1986). Aderka et al. (1986) also reported TNF production in response to Sendai virus. Interestingly, Newcastle disease virus can enhance TNF-α production by astrocytes without increasing IL-1 production; consequently, some viruses can preferentially induce TNF without IL-1 in certain cell types. More recent studies have also reported high levels of both TNF-α or IL-1β in sera or culture supernatants of monocytes from AIDS patients (Wright et al., 1988; Enk et al., 1986). However, augmented cytokine production may be a result of HIV infection of cytokine-producing cells or alternatively, an indirect result of the wide variety of opportunistic infections frequently seen in AIDS patients. Infection of the THP-1 monocyte cell line with HIV has shown that HIV-infected cells do not produce detectable amounts of protein or mRNA for TNF-α or IL-1β (Molina et al., 1989). Therefore, HIV infection probably increases both monocyte IL-1β and TNF-α production in an indirect manner. In addition to microbial products, other stimuli, including tobacco glycoprotein (Francus et al., 1989), urate crystals (Di Giovine et al., 1987), and aminated polyglucose (Seljelid et al., 1989) stimulate IL-1 production, and tumor cell membranes (Mannel and Janicke, 1989) can stimulate monocytes to secrete both TNF-α and IL-1. The ability of different cells to produce IL-1 and/or TNF in response to a wide variety of exogenous stimuli is probably a function of the gene repertoire of a given cell type rather than being due to the nature of the stimulant.

Table 2 Induction of mRNA or Protein for Both IL-1 and TNF by Endogenous Mediators

	Induction of mRNA or protein for:	
Endogenous mediator	IL-1	TNF
TNF	Dinarello et al., 1986; Elias et al., 1989; Nawroth et al., 1986	Phillip and Epstein, 1986
OL-1	Dinarello et al., 1987; Warner et al., 1987	Phillip and Epstein, 1986
IFN-γ	Collart et al., 1986	Collart et al., 1986; Gifford et al., 1987
	Hart et al., 1989b	Hart et al., 1989b
IFN-α		Lau and Livesey, 1989
GM-CSF	Lindemann et al., 1988; Sisson and Dinarello, 1988	Lindemann et al., 1988; Sisson and Dinarello, 1988
IL-2	Kasid et al., 1989; Herrmann et al., 1989	Nedwin et al., 1985; Kasid et al., 1989; Herrmann et al., 1989
TGF-β_1	Wahl et al., 1987; Chantry et al., 1989a	Wahl et al., 1987; Chantry et al., 1989a
Immune complexes	Chantry et al., 1989b	Chantry et al., 1989b
Substance P	Cozens and Rowe, 1987; Lotz et al., 1988b	Cozens and Rowe, 1987; Lotz et al., 1988
PAF		Dubois et al., 1989
Leukotriene B_4	Rola-Pleszczynski and Lemaire, 1985	
Endorphins	Apte et al., 1989	

D. Endogenous Inducers

During the course of nonspecific as well as immunologically mediated inflammatory reactions, cytokines and other mediators are produced which in turn regulate each other by competition, interaction, and mutual induction in a series of cascades and circuits with positive and negative feedback effects. Endogenous mediators that induce both IL-1 and TNF are listed in Table 2. IL-1 and TNF participate in self-induction mechanism whereby they induce the production of their respective molecules as well as each other in a variety of cell types. In contrast, IL-6 is not known to be capable of inducing either IL-1 or TNF production.

In addition to cytokines, other endogenous mediators of inflammation can affect IL-1 and TNF-α production. Immune complexes, C5a, and the neuropeptide substance P can induce IL-1 and TNF production in a dose-dependent manner. With increasing C5a concentrations, TNF-α, IL-1α, and IL-1β are all secreted, but TNF-α and IL-1β are secreted in significantly higher concentrations than IL-1α (Okusawa et al., 1988b). The neuropeptide substance P induces production of IL-1 and TNF. Platelet activating factor (PAF) synergizes with MDP in enhancing TNF-α and IL-1 production by alevolar macrophages. The actions of PAF may be mediated by leukotrienes such as LTB4, which are known to enhance IL-1 and TNF synthesis in human monocytes (Rola-Pleszczynski and Lemaire, 1985). Furthermore, addition of LTB4 enhances endotoxin-stimulated IL-1 production by monocytes (Rola-Pleszczynski and Lemaire, 1985). Therefore, in contrast to cyclooxygenase products, lipoxygenase products may play a role in potentiating IL-1 and TNF-α production. Since a wide range of endogenous mediators of inflammation can enhance the concomitant production of both IL-1 and TNF, these cytokines must play a critical and central role in the generation of inflammatory and immune responses.

In conclusion, we consider it likely that during infection TNF and IL-1 are predominantly produced by leukocytes in response to exogenous stimuli, and levels of production are tightly regulated by other endogenous mediators generated during an immune response. However, local production of TNF or IL-1 in nonlymphoid tissues may regulate other aspects of homeostasis unrelated to the immune response. In this regard a recent report on the effects of the hormone estradiol on cytokine production by endometrial cells (Tabibzadeh et al., 1989) is suggestive that IL-1, TNF, and IL-6 have some functions outside the immune system. The detection of high levels of IL-1, TNF-α, and IL-6 transcripts in organs such as spleen, liver, and kidney of normal individuals (Tovey et al., 1988) would tend to reinforce this concept. However, the multiple biological activities ascribed to cytokines such as IL-1 or TNF pose a difficult problem. How can one ligand communicate different signals in different tissues? The most likely answer is that localization of cytokine production is very important and most cells produce just enough of these mediators to affect only those cells in their immediate vicinity. Higher circulating levels may arise only when a coordinated multiorgan response to a particular stimulus is necessary for the benefit of the host. Interestingly, some cytokines can bind to α2-macroglobulin, one of the major serum proteins (James, 1990). This may reveal a new and potentially important mechanism for modulation of cytokine activity in the circulation. Ten years ago, researchers thought of the various body systems as separate entities. However, it now appears that the three major communication systems in the body—the endocrine, nervous, and immune systems—are intimately connected to one another by hormones, neuropeptides, and cytokines. The roles that TNF and IL-1 play in these interactions should become more clear in the next 10 years.

E. Inhibitors

Once the immune system is triggered there is a rapid burst of TNF and IL-1 synthesis followed by a decreased production. The host apparently makes a considerable effort to protect itself from the toxic effects of excessive TNF-α and IL-1 production. Therefore, levels of these cytokines are tightly regulated. Molecules that limit IL-1 and TNF-α gene transcription, bind directly to the cytokine or its receptor, or act at other sites to limit the effects of these cytokines have all been described. Some of these inhibitors are listed in Table 3. Inhibitors such as prostaglandins, corticosteroids, IL-4, IL-6, and TGF-β seem to function predominantly by blocking IL-1 and TNF gene transcription and translation. Inhibitors of the lipoxygenase pathways may inhibit the production of both IL-1 and TNF-α (Dinarello et al., 1984; Schade et al., 1989). In this context a recent report on the effects of dietary supplementation with *n*-3 polyunsaturated fatty acids is of interest. In this study blood leukocytes from volunteers who supplemented their diets with a fish-oil concentrate rich in polyunsaturated fatty acids had a decreased synthesis of IL-1α, IL-1β, and TNF-α in response to LPS in vitro (Endres et al., 1989). The suppression of cytokine production was most evident 10 weeks after cessation of the supplement. The mechanism of suppression of IL-1 and TNF-*a* synthesis remains unknown, but *n*-3 fatty acids induce changes in both cyclooxygenase and lipoxygenase products. One possible mechanism could be a decrease in 5-lipoxygenase metabolites such as LTB4, which may be important in inducing the production of IL-1 and TNF. In contrast, studies in mice have demonstrated enhanced IL-1 and TNF-α production by peritoneal macrophages immediately after cessation of a fish-oil diet, probably due to decreased production of suppressive prostaglandins by macrophages (Lokesh et al., 1990). In clinical studies, dietary supplementation with *n*-3 fatty acids has led to improvement in patients with rheumatoid arthritis and psoriasis.

Proteins that inhibit the biological activities of IL-1 and TNF have been isolated from human urine. One of these proteins, called *uromodulin* (or *Tamm-Horsfall protein*), is an 85-kDa glycoprotein that appears to function by binding to both IL-1 and TNF, thus interfering with the interactions between the cytokines on their receptors (Muchmore and Decker, 1985; Brown et al., 1986). Another more specific IL-1 inhibitor has been purified from the urine of febrile patients (Liao et al., 1984; Balavoine et al., 1986). This inhibitor has an apparent molecular weight of 18 to 25 kDa and is biochemically distinct from uromodulin. Furthermore, it appears to inhibit IL-1 action by binding to the IL-1 receptor and possesses no inhibitory activity against TNF-α (Seckinger et al., 1987). An IL-1 receptor antagonist isolated from human monocytes has recently been purified to homogeneity (Hannum et al., 1990). This inhibitor has similar biochemical properties to the inhibitors isolated from urine. A variety of other IL-1 inhibitors from granulocytes, keratinocytes, submandibular glands, B lymphoblastoid cell lines, and murine retrovirus have

Table 3 Inhibitors of IL-1 and TNF

Mechanism of action	Inhibitor	Inhibition of IL-1	TNF
Transcription and/or translation	Prostaglandins	Kunkel et al., 1986a; Brandwein, 1986	Kunkel et al., 1986b
	Corticosteroids	Synder and Unanue, 1982	Beutler et al., 1986
	IL-4	Hart et al., 1989a; Weiss et al., 1989; Essner et al., 1989	Hart et al., 1989a; Weiss et al., 1989; Essner et al., 1989
	IL-6	Schindler et al., 1990	Schindler et al., 1990; Aderka et al., 1989
	TGF-β	Wahl et al., 1989; Chantry et al., 1989	Espevik et al., 1987
Binding to cytokine	Uromodulin	Muchmore and Decker, 1985; Brown et al., 1986	
	Urine-derived inhibitor		Seckinger et al., 1988; Wallach et al., 1989
Antagonist for receptor binding	Urine-derived inhibitor	Liao et al., 1984; Balavoine et al., 1986; Seckinger et al., 1987	
	Monocyte-derived inhibitor	Hannum et al., 1990; Carter et al., 1990	
Inhibitor of secretion	Plasma α globulins, serine protease inhibitors		Scuderi et al., 1989a, b
Mechanism unknown	α melanocyte stimulating hormone	Cannon et al., 1986; Daynes et al., 1987	

been described, but their relationships to each other and their mechanisms of action are not yet clear. A specific inhibitor of TNF-α has also been isolated from the urine of febrile patients (Seckinger et al., 1988; Wallach et al., 1989). This protein has an apparent molecular weight of 40 to 60 kDa and binds directly to TNF-α. It also binds to TNF-β although it is somewhat less inhibitory, but does not bind to IL-1. In view of the specific nature of inhibitor binding to TNF-α, the inhibitor is proposed to be a shed fragment of the cell surface TNF receptor. These inhibitors may lead to new approaches for the therapy of septic shock and chronic inflammatory diseases.

In addition to specific inhibitors of IL-1 and TNF-α, certain plasma α-globulins (Scuderi et al., 1989) and synthetic serine protease inhibitors (Scuderi, 1989) have been demonstrated to block secretion of TNF-α but not IL-1 by PBMC in response to LPS. Therefore, the processing of IL-1 to the mature extracellular form involves different enzymes. Since α-globulins are a major fraction of circulating plasma proteins, they may function in TNF homeostasis by controlling TNF secretion. The very complex positive and negative regulation of IL-1 and TNF-α probably reflects the many interactions between these cytokines and the microenvironment in which they are produced such that processes like inflammation and repair can be regulated constantly for the benefit of the host.

F. In Vivo Pharmacokinetics

Studies with the intravenous (IV) injection of radiolabeled human IL-1β into mice have shown that there is a rapid initial loss from the circulation 5 to 10 min after injection, followed by a slower loss over the next hour (Newton et al., 1988). Injection by intraperitoneal (IP) or subcutaneous (SC) routes gives an initial peak in circulating IL-1 after 10 min which is sustained over at least the next 7 h (Newton et al., 1988). Injection of radioiodinated murine TNF-α into mice by the IV route similarly showed that TNF-α was rapidly cleared from the plasma with a half-life of 6 to 7 min (Beutler et al., 1985). On administration of human TNF-α to rhesus monkeys, a plasma half-life of 1.2 to 2.1 h was calculated (Greischel and Zahn, 1989). A serum half-life of about 20 min has been estimated for IV injection of TNF-α into cancer patients (Chapman et al., 1987).

Two hours after injection, most tissues examined were found to contain an equal amount of IL-1 on a weight basis with the exception of bone, which contained only half the level found in other tissues, and kidney, which contained four- to eightfold more IL-1. Therefore, it appears that IL-1 may initially distribute with the fluid in the body and then localize more specifically to the tissues (Newton et al., 1988). In contrast, TNF-α rapidly concentrates in the liver, kidney, spleen, and gastrointestinal tract, which all concentrated injected labeled cytokine with respect to plasma levels (Beutler et al., 1985). Whole-brain specimens exhibited the lowest specific activity of any tissue, suggesting that little if any TNF is capable of penetrating the central nervous system. There have been contradictory reports on the ability of IL-1 to cross the blood-brain barrier; one group has demonstrated that IL-1β cannot enter the cerebrospinal fluid from the peripheral circulation (Coceani et al., 1988). However, IL-1α has been reported to cross the rodent blood-brain barrier at an entry rate about 44 times greater than would be predicted by leakage alone (Banks et al., 1989). The major organ of IL-1 clearance appears to be the kidney, since 10 to 20% of the label was found in the urine within hours of injection (Newton et al., 1988). Therefore, although most of the initial decrease in plasma IL-1 occurs due to diffusion into the tissues, the eventual removal probably occurs through the kidneys. No evidence of protein breakdown of IL-1 to lower-molecular-weight forms was observed on administration of radiolabeled human IL-1β to mice. In contrast, nephrectomy significantly reduced but did not eliminate the clearance of recombinant human TNF-α administered to rats (Ferraiolo et al., 1989), so sites other than the kidney may contribute to the elimination of TNF. Indeed, two elimination mechanisms for TNF have been postulated, a nonsaturatable unspecific process (dominant at high doses) dependent on the glomerular filtration of the TNF-α dimer or trimer, and a saturatable process (visible only at low plasma levels) dependent on receptor-mediated internalization of TNF-α. The kidney can rapidly catabolize TNF (Pessina et al., 1987). TNF is rapidly degraded into a low-molecular-weight form after injection, and only degradation products are detected in the urine, supporting the contention that unlike IL-1, TNF can be degraded rapidly.

G. Relationship of Receptors for TNF and IL-1

The findings that TNF and IL-1 have many overlapping effects, yet frequently elicit a synergistic response when administered together suggests that TNF and IL-1 may utilize different means of signaling cells. Indeed, the receptors for TNF-α and TNF-β are distinct from those for IL-1α and IL-1β. At least two distinct receptors have recently been identified for TNF as well as for IL-1. Furthermore, the expression of TNF and IL-1 receptors appears to be independently regulated (Table 4). PMA up-regulates expression of receptors for IL-1 on keratinocytes, whereas PMA diminishes their expression of TNF-receptors (Blanton et al., 1989). TNF receptors are also down-regulated by PKC (Scheurich et al., 1986; Unglaub et al., 1987). This PKC transmodulation of TNF receptors is due to a reduction in binding affinity. Conversely, PKA enhances TNF receptor expression by increasing their synthesis (Scheurich et al., 1989). Less is known concerning the mechanisms regulating IL-1 receptor expression. Both glucocorticoid (GC) hormones and inducers of cAMP up-regulate IL-1 receptor expression (but not affinity) on selected target cells such as B lymphocytes, fibroblasts, and other leukocytes, but not on T cells (Akahoshi et al., 1988). However, GC failed to stimulate a number of receptors for TNF. Consequently, agents that have opposing effects on TNF and IL-1 receptors can potentially favor the actions of one of these cytokines at the expense of the

Table 4 Agents Regulating IL-1 and TNF Receptor Expression

Agent	Target cell(s)	IL-1 receptor	TNF receptor	Reference
PMA	Kerationocytes	↑	↓	Blanton et al., 1989
PKC	Monocyte	?	↓	Scheurich et al., 1989
PKA	Tumor cell lines	?	↑	Scheurich et al., 1989
Microtubule depolymerizers	Endothelial cells, macrophages	?	↓	Ding et al., 1990a
Glucocorticoids	B cells	↑	No effect	Akahoshi et al., 1988
	Fibroblasts	↑	No effect	Akahoshi et al., 1988
PGE_2 and cAMP	B cells	↑	No effect	Akahoshi et al., 1988
	Fibroblasts	↑	No effect	Akahoshi et al., 1988
TGF-β	Bone marrow cells	↓	?	Dubois et al., 1990
	Myelomonocytic lines	↓	?	Dubois et al., 1990
	EL 4 cell lines	↓	?	Dubois et al., 1990
IL-3, G-CSF, GM-CSF	Bone marrow cells	↑	?	Dubois et al., 1990
IFN-γ	Several cell types	?	↑	Aggarwal et al., 1985
IL-2	T lymphocytes	?	↑	Owen-Schaub et al., 1989
PDGF	3T3 fibroblasts	↑	?	Chiou et al., 1989

other. Despite the observations of synergy between IL-1 and TNF, there has been one report that IL-1 reduces the expression of TNF receptors (Holtzmann and Wallach, 1987). Perhaps this down-regulation is a late event that does not interfere with the initial synergy. The effect of TNF on IL-1 receptors has not been reported, but the other cytokines reported to modulate IL-1 and/or TNF receptors are listed on Table 4. A considerable proportion of internalized radiolabeled IL-1 has been observed to localize in the nucleus (Mizel et al., 1987). There are also reports suggesting that both TNF (Smith et al., 1990) and IL-1 (Falk et al., 1990) may also be able to bypass cell membrane receptors and act directly intracellularly. However, the physiological relevance of these effects is unknown.

H. Signal Transduction by TNF and IL-1

Although the information concerning the *initial* postreceptor events is incomplete, the mechanism of action of IL-1 and TNF appear to show some differences as well as similarities (Table 5). TNF and IL-1 both decrease the binding capacity of epidermal growth factor receptors (Bird and Saklatvala, 1989). This is associated with a concommitant increase in the phosphorylation of EGF-R, which occurs independently of protein kinase C. IL-1 selectively induces serine phosphorylation of a cytosolic p65 (Matsushima et al., 1988b). On the other hand, early signal transduction in response to TNF involves rapid phosphorylation of a 26-kDa cytosolic protein at serine residues. Although TNF in some cells activates protein kinase C, the protein kinase responsible for TNF-induced serine phosphorylation remains to be identified (Schutze et al., 1989). Both TNF and IL-1 phosphorylate three distinct 27-kDa cytosolic proteins in fibroblasts (Kaur and Saklatvala, 1989). In addition, TNF-α stimulates the phosphorylation of a mRNA cap-binding protein in a human ME-180 cervical carcinoma cell line. This phosphorylation event may be involved in the signal transduction by TNF-α since the phosphorylation correlated with the cytostatic effects of TNF-α for this cell line (Marino et al., 1989). Shirakawa et al. (1988) report cAMP production in IL-1 responsive cells, which suggests involvement of cAMP-dependent PKA in the signal transduction of IL-1. These investigators further suggest that this signal in turn converts an inactive cytosolic form of NF-κB to a form that translocates to the nucleus and binds DNA (Shirakawa et al., 1989). Although Zhang et al. (1988b) agree that activation of cAMP-dependent protein kinase may contribute to the effects of TNF-α and IL-1 on some cells. However, TNF or IL-1-induced IL-6 gene expression was not as strongly inhabitable by a protein kinase blocker (H-8) as was the action of forskolin on IL-6 gene expression. Consequently, other as yet unidentified mechanisms were felt to mediate the induction of IL-6 gene expression in fibroblasts by TNF and IL-1. Rosoff et al. (1988) have suggested that IL-1 signal transduction involves phospholipid hydrolysis of phosphatidyl choline, yielding increases in cytosolic diacylglycerol levels. Finally, there is evidence suggesting that IL-1 activates G-proteins in EL4

Table 5 Intracellular Effects of TNF and IL-1

	TNF	IL 1
2,5-A synthetase	↑ (Rosenblum and Donato, 1989)	?
EGF receptor kinase	↑ (Rosenblum and Donato, 1989)	?
Phosphorylation of serine residues	↑ (pp. 26–28, Schutze et al., 1989)	↑ (p. 65, Matsushima et al., 1988b)
Diacylglycerol	?	↑ (Rosoff et al., 1988)
Increased cAMP	↑ (Zhang et al., 1988b)	↑ (Shirakawa et al., 1988)
G proteins	↑ (O'Neill et al., (1990)	↑ (Imamura et al., 1988)
Phospholipase A2	↑ (Old, 1990)	?
Phospholipase C	?	↑ (Rosoff et al., 1988)
Cyclooxygenase pathway	↑ (Dayer et al., 1985)	↑ (Rosoff, 1989)
Lipooxygenase pathway	↑ (Kunkel et al., 1989)	↑ (Scales and Kunkel, 1989)
Reactive oxygen intermediates	↑ (Hoffman and Weinberg, 1987)	↑ (No direct effect)
ADP ribosylation	↑ (Agarwal et al., 1988)	?
Manganese superoxide dysmutase	↑ (Wong and Goeddel, 1988) (Visner et al., 1990)	↑ (Masuda et al., 1988) (Visner et al., 1990)
Histidine decarboxylase	↑ (Endo, 1989)	↑ (Endo, 1989)
Ornithine decarboxylase	↑ (Endo, 1989)	↑ (Endo, 1989)
Xanthine oxidase	↑ (Friedl et al., 1989)	No effect

thymoma cell membranes (O'Neill et al., 1990). IL-1 stimulation of a pertussis toxin-sensitive G-protein may lead to the activation of an adenylate cyclase (Chedid et al., 1989). Similarly, TNF induces GTPase activity and GTP in other cell lines (Imamura et al., 1988).

Both TNF and IL-1 frequently both modulate a variety of later intracellular events, such as inducing histidine and ornithine decarboxylase activities (Endo, 1989), enhancing production of MnSOD (Wong and Goeddel, 1988; Masuda et al., 1988), and inhibiting lipoprotein lipase and other intracellular proteins as indicated on Table 5. Differences in the intracellular effects of IL-1 and TNF have been reported less frequently (Table 5). Thus TNF, but not IL-1, is reported to induce xanthine oxidase in endothelial cells (Friedl et al., 1989).

Table 6 Modulation of Oncogenes and Nuclear Factors by TNF and IL-1

	TNF	IL-1
c-fos	↑ (Lin and Vilček, 1987)	↑ (Kovacs et al., 1986)
c-myc	↑ (Lin and Vilček, 1987)	↑ (Kovacs et al., 1986)
c-abl	↑ (Andrews et al., 1989)	↑ (Andrews et al., 1989)
c-jun	↑ (Brenner et al., 1989)	↑ (Muegge et al., 1989)
AP-1	↑ (Brenner et al., 1989)	↑ (Muegge et al., 1989)
NF-κB	↑ (Osborn et al., 1989)	↑ (Shirakawa et al., 1989)

Thus, despite the fact that TNF and IL-1 frequently have the same biological effects on a target cell, the early intracellular events induced by TNF and IL-1 at times appear to differ. The heterogeneity in receptors and signal transduction may account for the synergistic cooperative effects of IL-1 and TNF and may permit each of them to act at relatively low concentrations when in the presence of the other.

I. Regulation of Gene Expression by TNF and IL-1

Both IL-1 and TNF have the capacity to rapidly induce the expression of the same oncogenes and proto-oncogenes (Table 6). Both IL-1 and TNF have been reported to induce oncogenes such as c-fos and c-myb, and to inhibit c-myc. In the case of the two signal models for activation of IL-2 gene expression in T lymphocytes, Muegge et al. (1989) reported that IL-1 enhanced the expression of c-jun mRNA, whereas the antigenic or mitogenic signal enhanced mRNA for c-fos. These two oncogene products then generate an AP-1 transcription factor that mediates the action of IL-1 by binding to an IL-1-responsive element in the promoter region of the IL-2 gene. IL-1 also acts via the PKC pathway and the AP-1 binding site in the promoter region of the amyloid β-protein gene of human endothelial cells (Goldgaber et al., 1989). TNF-α results in prolonged activation of both jun and fos gene expression to generate AP-1, which acts via the AP-1 site in the promoter region to stimulate transcription of the collagenase gene (Brenner et al., 1989). Both TNF-α and IL-1 also activate the nuclear factor (NF) κB transcription factor, which binds the κ immunoglobulin light chain gene enhancer. Osborn et al. (1989) report that TNF and IL-1 by inducing NF-κB in a T-cell line can stimulate HIV gene expression.

In SV40-transformed marrow stromal cell lines, both IL-1α and TNF-α further increased the expression of c-abl transcripts. This data are said to suggest that c-abl may play a role in extracellular matrix expression and the regulation of hematopoiesis by stromal cells (Andrews et al., 1989). IL-1 and TNF also both markedly enhance the expression of reporter genes transcribed from the SV40 early promoter in a T-cell line. These cytokines appear to achieve this effect by activation of preexisting transcription factors (Plaetinck et al., 1989). However, it is not known whether these effects of IL-1 and TNF on oncogenes and proto-oncogenes are exerted by common or distinct intracellular pathways.

IL-1 appears to have a dramatic stimulatory effect on the expression of a number of genes, including those for IL-6, G-CSF, GM-CSF, IL-2, and IL-1 itself by markedly prolonging the half-life of their mRNA from the usual 30 min to greater than 28 h (Bagby, 1989). The mechanism for this posttranscriptional regulation is proposed to involve the induction of ribonuclease inhibitory activities. Although TNF also prolongs the half-life of mRNA for a similar battery of genes, it is reported to be less potent than IL-1. Thus TNF may have a lower capacity to induce gene products than IL-1.

III. INTERACTIONS AND RELATIONSHIPS OF TNF TO IL-6

Although interleukin 6 (IL-6) was identified several years ago, only within the past few years has the multiplicity of biological activities of this molecule been recognized. This recognition has come in large part from the convergence of work from several different laboratories with interests in different fields. These investigators, using very different and seemingly unrelated bioassays, have identified and molecularly cloned the gene encoding a single regulatory protein. This accounts for the various terms used to describe IL-6, such as B-cell stimulating factor 2, interferon β2, 26-kDa protein, myeloma/plastocytoma growth factor, hepatocyte stimulating factor, macrophage granulocyte inducing factor 2, and cytotoxic T-cell differentiating factor.

A. Relation of Cell Sources and Induction of IL-6 to TNF

Like IL-1 and TNF, IL-6 is produced by a wide range of different cell types. IL-6 is induced by a variety of different stimuli and there appear to be distinct differences in the potency of these different stimuli on the various cell types, as listed in Table 12.

In human fibroblasts, IL-6 synthesis can be induced with approximately equal efficacy by two distinct intracellular pathways. One of these pathways is triggered by the activation of protein kinase C (Sehgal et al., 1987), a pathway also thought to be involved in the induction of TNF-α and IL-1. In contrast, the second pathway for IL-6 induction appears to involve increases in intracellular cAMP (Zhang et al., 1988a), which is reported to inhibit TNF-α and IL-1 gene expression. These two pathways appear at least in fibroblasts to act independently, with neither synergistic nor antagonistic interaction. Furthermore, different stimuli may preferentially utilize one or another of these pathways. Activation of protein kinase C may be involved in the induction of IL-6 in fibroblasts in response to diacylglycerols, LPS, IL-1, and TNF. However, IL-1 and TNF may also induce IL-6 production via increases in intracellular cAMP. Activation of G-binding proteins may also be involved in IL-6 induction (Akashi et al., 1990). IL-1, TNF-α, and PDGF are probably the major endogenous stimuli for IL-6 production. IL-6 is unique in that it does not induce IL-1 or TNF-α and therefore does not propagate this cytokine cascade.

Studies on the IL-6 gene indicate that regions −225 to −113 contain the major cis-acting regulatory elements responsible for the activation of the IL-6 promoter by several different cytokines, viruses, and second messenger agonists (Ray et al., 1988). Sequences similar to transcriptional enhancer elements, such as serum responsive element (SRE), consensus sequences for cAMP induction (CRE), activator protein 1 binding (AP-1), NF-κB binding element, and glucocorticoid receptor binding (GRE), have been identified in highly conserved 5′-flanking regions of the IL-6 gene (Tanabe et al., 1988). Recent evidence suggests that NF-κB may be the most important element for IL-6 induction by TNF or IL-1 (e.g., Liberman and Baltimore, MCB 10: 2327, 1990). Future studies are necessary to elucidate similarities and differences in the control of TNF-α and IL-6 gene expression. IL-6 mRNA can be detected within 30 min of stimulating fibroblasts with LPS and reaches maximal levels between 2 and 3 h. The mRNA for IL-6 in common with that of IL-1 and TNF-α can be superinduced in some cells by the addition of cycloheximide (Loppnow and Libby, 1989; Helfgott et al., 1987). A number of apparent molecular weights for IL-6 of 26, 22, and 21 kDa have been reported; however, these differences are probably due to differences in proteolytic processing or glycosylation (Zilberstein et al., 1986). When PBMC were stimulated with LPS, IL-6, like IL-1β and TNF-α, was found mainly in the cell supernatants even within 2 h of stimulation, whereas the majority of IL-1α was cell associated (Schindler et al., 1990). Staining of intracellular TNF-α and IL-6 in monocytes stimulated with LPS has shown that both cytokines accumulate rapidly in the Golgi system (Andersson and Masuda, 1989). Cell fractionation of PBMC indicates that the kinetics of IL-6 production varies between different subsets. The IL-6 mRNA is rapidly induced in monocytes with a peak at 5 h, whereas maximal induction of mRNA in T cells and B cells occurred after 48 h of incubation (Horii et al., 1988). The kinetics of IL-6 production in monocytes and lymphocytes are therefore rather similar to those of TNF-α. IL-1 is not a particularly strong activator of IL-6 production by PBMC, whereas it is extremely potent in inducing IL-6 production in other cells, such as fibroblasts, endothelial cells, and thymocytes. Like TNF, IL-6 is active in the thymocyte co-stimulation assay, which has been used as a bioassay for IL-1. This, together with the fact that TNF and IL-1 induces production of IL-6 by a variety of cells, suggests that some of the pleiotropic effects of TNF and IL-1 are actually mediated by IL-6 or a combination of these cytokines. However, studies of the effects of inhibitors of IL-6, TNF, and IL-1 are needed to define their contributions more precisely.

Corticosteroids such as dexamethasone, which inhibit TNF-α and IL-1 production, also inhibit the accumulation of mRNA for IL-6 in fibroblasts in a dose-dependent manner (Helfgott et al., 1987). However, in contrast to IL-1 and TNF-α, specific serum inhibitors of IL-6 have not been characterized to date.

Injection of LPS, IL-1, and TNF-α into mice results in increases in plasma IL-6 within 3 h. Therefore, IL-1 and TNF can, at least indirectly, exert many of the in vivo activities of IL-6 (Libert et al., 1990).

B. Relationships Between Activities of TNF, IL-1, and IL-6

The available evidence indicates that IL-1 and TNF can be coordinately induced by the same inducers and from the same cell types and tissues. As a result, both are concurrently present in body fluids and tissues. On the other hand, in view of the disparity, in the structures, receptors, and transducing signals of TNF-α and TNF-β, and IL-1α and IL-1β, it was most surprising that their biological effects greatly overlap (Tables 7 and 8). A number of previous reviews have thoroughly discussed the overlapping as well as distinct properties of TNF and IL-1 that are outlined in Table 9 (Le and Vilček, 1987; Dinarello, 1989; Durum and Oppenheim, 1989). Some of the most strikingly divergent activities of IL-1 and TNF are their direct effects on early bone marrow progenitor cells. In culture, IL-1 promotes survival of hematopoietic progenitor cells in the absence of hematopoietic growth factors (Williams and Broxmeyer, 1988). Furthermore, in the presence of CSFs, IL-1 functions as hematopoietin 1, promoting growth and proliferation of early progenitor cells (Mochizuki et al., 1987; Moore and Warren, 1987). In contrast to these stimulatory effects of IL-1, TNF inhibits the development of early progenitor cells in colony assays (Broxmeyer et al., 1986). However, stimulatory effects of TNF on stromal cells of the bone marrow to induce production of CSFs may prevail, leading to a subsequent overall stimulation of hematopoiesis, which may explain the radioprotective properties of TNF. These contrasting properties of TNF may also account for TNF being much less effective as a radioprotector than IL-1 (Neta et al., 1988a).

The overlapping effects of IL-1 and TNF, although at first considered redundant, may be advantageous by providing alternate pathways and may compensate for differences in the production, distribution, and access of these two cytokines in various tissues. Furthermore, the high frequency of synergistic effects of combinations of IL-1 and TNF suggest that presence of both may be necessary to yield maximal biologic effects. Since each of these cytokines stimulates production of the other, it is possible that many of the effects observed following exposure to either IL-1 or TNF can be attributed to their combined action. Our own results sup-

Table 7 Biological Effects Common to TNF and IL-1 In Vitro

Target cell activity	TNF	IL-1	Synergy of TNF and IL-1
Endothelial cells			
Procoagulant activity	Bevilacqua et al., 1986	Bevilacqua et al., 1986	
CSFs	Broudy et al., 1986; Seelentag et al., 1987	Bagby et al., 1986; Seelentag et al., 1987	Seelentag et al., 1987
IL-1	Nawroth et al., 1986		
TNF			
IL-6	Jirik et al., 1989; Shalaby et al., 1989; Mawatari et al., 1989	Jirik et al., 1989; Shalaby et al., 1989	
IL-8	Strieter et al., 1989	Strieter et al., 1989	
MCAF	Sica et al., 1990	Sica et al., 1990	
ELAM, ICAM-1	Pober et al., 1986	Pober et al., 1986	
PDGF	Hajjar et al., 1987		
PGI2	Kawakami et al., 1986	Rossi et al., 1985; Kawakami et al., 1986	
Plasminogen activator inhibitor		Nachman et al., 1986	
PAF	Camussi et al., 1987	Bussolino et al., 1986	
Fibroblasts			
CSFs	Zucali et al., 1988	Zucali et al., 1986; Kushansky et al., 1988	
IL-1	Le et al., 1987		Elias et al., 1989
IL-6	Akashi et al., 1990	Kohase et al., 1986; Van Damme et al., 1987	Elias and Lentz, 1990
IL-8	Larsen et al., 1989a	Larsen et al., 1989a	
MCAF	Larsen et al., 1989b	Larsen et al., 1989b	
ICAM	Rothklein et al., 1988	Dustin et al., 1986;	

		Rothklein et al., 1988	
Mn-SOD	Wong and Goeddel, 1988	Masuda et al., 1988	
c-fos, c-myc	Lin and Vilček, 1987	Lin and Vilček, 1987	
PGE_2	Dayer et al., 1985	Zucali et al., 1986; Raz et al., 1988	Elias et al., 1987
C3 and factor B	Katz and Strunk, 1989	Katz and Strunk, 1989	
Pro-collagen	Postlethwaite et al., 1988		
Collangenase	Dayer et al., 1985	Postlethwaite et al., 1983	
Proliferation	Sugarman et al., 1985	Schmidt et al., 1982	
Hepatocytes			
Acute-phase response proteins	Perlmutter et al., 1986; Darlington et al., 1986	Ramadori et al., 1985; Darlington et al., 1986	
Pancreatic Langerhans cells			
Toxicity			Mandrup-Poulsen et al., 1987
Adipocytes			
Decreasedd lipoprotein lipase	Beutler et al., 1985; Price et al., 1986b	Price et al., 1986a	
Monocytes			
Cytotoxicity	Phillip and Epstein, 1986; Urban et al., 1986	Phillip and Epstein, 1986	
IL-1	Bachwich et al., 1986		
IL-6	Bauer et al., 1988		
IL-8	Matsushima et al., 1988	Matsushima et al., 1988a	
CSFs		Fibbe et al., 1986	
Mn-SOD	Wong and Goeddel, 1988	Masuda et al., 1988	
PGE_2	Bachwich et al., 1986		
PAF	Valone and Epstein, 1988; Camussi et al., 1987	Valone and Epstein, 1988	

Table 7 (continued)

Target cell activity	TNF	IL-1	Synergy of TNF and IL-1
Neutrophils			
Increased LFA	Gamble et al., 1985; Pohlman et al., 1986	Pohlman et al., 1986	
Activation	Shalaby et al., 1985; Klebanoff et al., 1986	Klempner et al., 1978	
PAF	Camussi et al., 1987		
Smooth muscle cells			
Induction of IL-1, PGE_2	Warner and Libby, 1989	Warner et al., 1987; Libby et al., 1988	
Induction of IL-6		Lippnow and Libby, 1990	
Thymocytes			
Co-mitogenic	Ranges et al., 1988	Gery and Waksman, 1972	
T-cell			
Co-mitogenic	Hackett et al., 1988; Yokota et al., 1988	Hackett et al., 1988	
Colony growth	Zucali et al., 1987	Zucali et al., 1987	
Induction of IL-2 receptor	Lowenthal et al., 1989	Falk et al., 1989	
Augment MLR and CTL	Shalaby et al., 1988; Nakano et al., 1989	Plaetinck et al., 1989	
B-cell			
Co-mitogenic	Kehrl et al., 1987; Jelinek and Lipsky, 1987	Jelinek and Lipsky, 1987; Pike and Nossal, 1985; Cavender et al., 1986	
Natural killer cell			
Activation	Ostensen et al., 1987		
Enhanced ADCC	Eisenthal and Rosenberg, 1989	Eisenthal and Rosenberg, 1989	

Astrocytes			
Proliferation	Lachman et al., 1987; Selmaj et al., 1990	Lachman et al., 1987; Giulian and Lachman, 1985	
Chondrocytes			
Degradation of proteoglycan, induction of plasminogen activator, PGE_2	Campbell et al., 1990a, b	Campbell et al., 1988; Campbell et al., 1990a	
Osteoclasts			
Increased proliferation		Dewhirst et al., 1985	
Bone resorption	Bertolini et al., 1986; Saklatvala, 1986		Stashenko et al., 1987
Keratinocytes			
Induction of IL-8	Larsen et al., 1989a	Larsen et al., 1989a	
Synovial cells			
Increased collagenase, PGE_2	Dayer et al., 1985	Mizel et al., 1981	
Enhanced growth	Butler et al., 1988	Butler et al., 1988	
Induction of plasminogen activator	Leizer and Hamilton, 1989	Hamilton, 1987	
Pituitary cells			
Production of ACTH, GH, TSH	Milenkovic et al., 1989	Bernton et al., 1987	
Tumor cells			
Cytostatic	Sugarman et al., 1985 Ruggiero et al., 1987	Onozaki et al., 1985; Ruggiero et al., 1987; Lachman et al., 1986	Ruggiero and Baglioni, 1987
Differentiation	Munker and Koeffler, 1987		Onozaki et al., 1988
Cytotoxicity	Murase et al., 1987 (see reviews for earlier references)		Last-Barney et al., 1988

Table 8 In Vivo Biological Activities Common to TNF and IL-1

Activity	TNF	IL-1	Synergy
Endogenous pyrogen	Dinarello et al., 1986; Dascombe et al., 1989 Kettlehut and Goldberg, 1988	Kampschmidt et al., 1983; Dascombe et al., 1989 Dinarello, 1984	
Slow-wave sleep	Shoham et al., 1987	Krueger et al., 1984	
Renin secretion	Antonipillai et al., 1990	Antonipillai et al., 1990	
Induction of ACTH, corticosteroids	Tracy et al., 1987	Besedovsky et al., 1986; Besedovsky and Del Ray, 1987	
Induction of CRF		Suda et al., 1990	
Hypotension	Okusawa et al., 1988a	Okusawa et al., 1988	Okusawa et al., 1988
Induction of hepatic acute phase proteins	Sipe et al., 1987; Mortensen et al., 1988	Sipe et al., 1987; Mortensen et al., 1988	Mortensen et al., 1988
Decreased cytochrome P450	Ghezzi et al., 1986a	Ghezzi et al., 1986b	
Induction of circulating CSF	Vogel et al., 1987	Vogel et al., 1987	
Induction of circulating IL-6	McIntosh et al., 1989	Neta et al., 1988b	
Neutrophilia	Remick et al., 1986; Ulich et al., 1987	Ulich et al., 1987	Wankowicz et al., 1988; Movat et al., 1987; Sayers et al., 1988
Decreased plasma FE, Zn, increased Cu		Kampschmidt and Pulliam, 1978	
Adjuvant	Jayaraman et al., 1990; Ghiara et al., 1987	Staruch and Wood, 1983; North et al., 1988	

Radioprotection	Neta et al., 1988	Neta et al., 1986, 1988a	Neta et al., 1988a
Protection from lethal hyperoxia			White et al., 1987, 1989
Resistance to bacterial infection	Clark et al., 1987b; Hevell, 1989	Ozaki et al., 1987; Czuprynski et al., 1988; McIntyre et al., 1989	
Antitumor effect	Asher et al., 1987 (see reviews for other references)	Nakamura et al., 1986; North et al., 1988	
Lethality of adrenalectomized mice	Bertini et al., 1988	Bertini et al., 1988	
Weight loss, anorexia	Bodner et al., 1989; Plata-Salaman et al., 1988; McCarthy et al., 1985	Plata-Salaman et al., 1988; McCarthy et al., 1985	Vogel et al., 1988
Lethality (in mice)	Waage and Espevik, 1988		Vogel et al., 1988; Waage and Espevik, 1988
Prevention and therapy of diabetic mice	Jacob et al., 1990	Del Ray and Besedovsky, 1989	
Hypoglycemia	Kettelhut et al., 1987		
Muscle catabolism			Flores et al., 1989
Induction of early endotoxin tolerance			Vogel et al., 1988
Placental injury in rats	Silen et al., 1989	Silen et al., 1989	

port this possibility. Administration to mice of anti-IL-1 receptor antibody significantly reduced TNF-induced radioprotection and the levels of CSF in circulation. Anti-TNF antibody similarly reduced IL-1-induced radioprotection and the titers of IL-1-induced CSF. Thus mutual induction of TNF by IL-1 and IL-1 by TNF and their synergistic interaction may serve to amplify the host's response and would allow for much lower doses of these very potent cytokines to suffice for biological effects.

In addition to IL-1 and TNF, IL-6 has also been implicated as an active participant in host defense, inducing many of the effects originally ascribed to IL-1 and TNF (Kishimoto, 1989), since many of its in vitro and in vivo activities overlap with those of IL-1 and TNF (Tables 10 and 11). It has even been suggested that since both IL-1 and TNF induce IL-6 (Table 12), most of the effects attributed to IL-1 or TNF are actually mediated by IL-6. The available evidence at present indicates that IL-6 frequently acts in combination with IL-1 and/or TNF. Although in a number of experimental models, administration of IL-1, TNF, or IL-6 may lead to an inflammatory response, it is not yet clear how the presence of IL-1, TNF, or IL-6 in the circulation or in tissues affects the disease process. One example is cerebral malaria, where it was noted that antibody to TNF results in reduced TNF in circulation and reduced severity of the disease. As most laboratories do not examine the presence of all three cytokines in body fluids, tissues, or circulation, it remains to be established whether only the selective presence of a given cytokine, IL-1, TNF, or

Table 9 Nonoverlapping Effects of TNF and IL-1

Activity	TNF	IL-1
Hematopoietin 1 (Mochizuki et al., 1987; Moore and Warren, 1987)	-	+
Potentiation of basophil and mast cell histamine release (Massey et al., 1989; Alam et al., 1989)	-	+
Transport across blood brain barrier (Beutler et al., 1985; Banks et al., 1989)	-	+
Production of reactive oxygen intermediate by PMN (Tsujimoto et al., 1986; Nathan, 1987; Georgilis et al., 1987)	+	-
Induction of class 1 MHC (Collins et al., 1986)	+	-
Cytotoxicity for tumor cells (Urban et al., 1986)	+	-
Suppression of hematopoietic progenitor cells (Broxmeyer et al., 1986)	+	-
Vascular leak syndrome (Remick et al., 1987)	+	-

IL-6 can be associated with a specific clinical condition. Another fundamental question that remains to be answered is whether the cytokines detected in the patient's circulation or tissues are identical to these detected under normal conditions. Reports exist indicating that in some situations (e.g., psioriasis), the processing of cytokines may be different in pathological states.

The recently developed antibodies to IL-1 receptor (Chizzoneti et al., 1989; Bomsztyk et al., 1989), or the use of recently identified IL-1 and TNF inhibitors (Wallach et al., 1989; Hannum et al., 1990), may be useful in resolving the present controversies over the contributions of IL-6, TNF, and IL-1 to host defense. Of interest to this interaction are the findings that while IL-1 and TNF both induce IL-6 production (often in synergy), IL-6 can actually suppress IL-1 and TNF production (Aderka et al., 1989; Schindler et al., 1990). Consequently, IL-6 may serve as a feedback inhibitor for its own inducers. Therefore, despite its fever and acute-phase-response-inducing properties, IL-6 may have some anti-inflammatory effects.

To be conclusive, however, studies will need to be conducted using either specific antibody or inhibitors to each of the cytokines to determine their individual contribution.

IV. INTERACTIONS OF TNF AND IL-1 WITH IL-2

Considerable data have been generated documenting mutual interactions of TNF and IL-2 at the level of production (Table 13). We will first review the evidence that IL-2 stimulates mononuclear cells to produce TNF and IL-1. IL-2, together with anti CD3, stimulated purified human T lymphocytes to express mRNA simultaneously for TNF-α and TNF-β (Steffen et al., 1988). These pure T-cell preparations also produced proteins with TNF bioactivity that could be inhibited by anti TNF-α and antilymphotoxin (TNF-β). Furthermore, IL-2 can also activate purified human and murine macrophages to express mRNA for TNF-α and to produce TNF-α (Economou et al., 1989) as well as IL-1 (Numeroff et al., 1988). Both TNF-α and TNF-β have been detected in the supernatants of IL-2-stimulated LAK cells and in the circulation of the majority of patients receiving IL-2/LAK therapy (Gemlo et al., 1988). The toxic effects of immunotherapy with IL-2 and lymphokine-activated killer (LAK) cells has been attributed to the enhanced production of a battery of cytokines, including IL-1 (Herrmann et al., 1989), IFN-γ, TNF-α, and TNF-β (Gemlo et al., 1988). Thus IL-2 is a potent inducer of IL-1 as well as TNF-α and TNF-β production by mononuclear cells in vitro and in vivo.

The fact that TNF, like IL-1, has adjuvant activities and can augment in vivo immune responses is a commonly overlooked activity of TNF. Like human IL-1β, as shown on Table 8, low doses of human TNF-α enhanced murine in vivo antibody responses to a T-cell-dependent antigen (SRBC), but unlike IL-1, TNF-α did not augment the response to a T-cell-independent antigen [type III pneumococcal

Table 10 Overlapping Effects of TNF, IL-1, and IL-6

Activity	TNF	IL-1	IL-6
Increased acute-phase proteins	Andus et al., 1988	Andus et al., 1988; Ramadori et al., 1985	Andus et al., 1988; Geiger et al., 1988
	Mortensen et al., 1988	Mortensen et al., 1988	Gauldie et al., 1987;
Endogenous pyrogen	Dinarello et al., 1986	Dinarello, 1984	Opp et al., 1989
Thymocyte comitogen	Ranges et al., 1988; Vink et al., 1990	Gery and Waksman, 1972; Vink et al., 1990	Lotz et al., 1988a; Vink et al., 1990
T-cell activator (IL-2R)	Lowenthal et al., 1989	Falk et al., 1989	Garman et al., 1987; Lotz et al., 1988; Uyttenhove et al., 1988
CTL differentiation	Shalaby et al., 1988	Plaetinck et al., 1989	Takai et al., 1988; Okada et al., 1988
Stimulation of hypothalamic–pituitary adrenal cascade	Tracy et al., 1987; Milenkovic et al., 1989	Besedovsky et al., 1986; Bernton et al., 1987	Naitoh et al., 1988
Antitumor	Sugerman et al., 1985; Munker and Koeffler, 1987	Nakamura et al., 1986; North et al., 1988	Mule et al., 1990; Morinaga et al., 1989
Myeloid cell differentiation	Onozaki et al., 1988	Onozaki et al., 1988	Shabo et al., 1988;
Adjuvant	Ghiara et al., 1987; Jayaraman et al., 1990	Staruch and Wood, 1983; North et al., 1988	Jayaraman et al., 1990; Takatsuki et al., 1988

Table 11 Presence of TNF, IL-1, and IL-6 in Disease

Disease state	TNF	IL-1	IL-6
Septic shock	Waage et al., 1986; Girardin et al., 1988	Waage et al., 1989a; Girardin et al., 1988	Fong et al., 1989; Waage et al., 1989a
Meningococcal meningitis	Waage et al., 1987		
Infection of CNA	Leist et al., 1988		Houssiau et al., 1988
Malaria	Grau et al., 1987, 1989; Kern et al., 1989; Clark et al., 1987a,b		Kern et al., 1989; Waage et al., 1989
Rheumatoid arthritis	Buchan et al., 1988	Fontana et al., 1982a	Hirano et al., 1988
Scleroderma		Sandborg et al., 1985	
Psoriasis		Camp et al., 1986	Grossman et al., 1989
Experimental allergic encephalitis		Symons et al., 1987	Gijbels et al., 1990
Renal allografts	Maury and Teppo, 1987	Maury and Teppo, 1987	Van Oers et al., 1988
Crohn's disease		Satsangi et al., 1987	
Graft-vs.-host disease	Piquet et al., 1987		
Burn trauma		Kupper et al., 1986	
Pulmonary fibrosis			
Fulminant hepatic failure	Muto et al., 1988	Muto et al., 1988	
Multiple sclerosis	Hoffman et al., 1989; Merrill et al., 1989	Merrill et al., 1989	
Placental injury	Silen et al., 1989	Silen et al., 1989	
Granulomas		Schmidt et al., 1984; Kobayashi et al., 1985	
Multiple myeloma			Kawano et al., 1988
Parasitic infections	Scuderi et al., 1986; Beutler and Cerami, 1987		
Hodgkin's disease		Kortmann et al., 1984	
AIDS	Lahdevirta et al., 1988	Ensoli et al., 1989; Lepe-Zuniga et al., 1987	
Down syndrome		Griffin et al., 1989	
Alzheimer		Griffin et al., 1989	

Table 12 Effect of TNF, IL-1, and Other Stimulatnts on IL-6 Production by Various Cell Types

Cell type	Inducing stumulus	Upregulation of mRNA or protein for IL-6
T cells	PMA + macrophages	Hirano et al., 1985
	Staphylococcal enterotoxin A	Horii et al., 1988
	CD3	Andersson and Masuda, 1989
B cells	*Staphylococcus aureus*	Horii et al., 1988
Thymocytes	IL-1	Helle et al., 1988
	IL-1 + TNF	Bauer et al., 1989
Macrophages/ monocytes	LPS	Nordan and Potter, 1986; Andersson and Masuda, 1989
	HIV	Nakajima et al., 1989
Fibroblasts	IFN-β, PDGF, IL-1, TNF-α, TNF-β, poly I:C, calcium ionophore	Kohase et al., 1986, 1987; Akashi et al., 1990
Endothelial cells	LPS, IL-1, TNF-α	Jirik et al., 1989; Sironi et al., 1989; Loppnow and Libby, 1989
Smooth muscle cells	PDGF, cell division	Loppnow and Libby, 1990
Keratinocytes	IL-1, PMA	Kupper et al., 1988; Kimbauer et al., 1989
Endometrial stromal cells	IL-1, TNF-α, IFN-γ	Tabibzadeh et al., 1989
Astrocytes and microglia	Lymphocytic choriomeningitid virus, IL-1, TNFα, M-CSF	Frei et al., 1989
Synovial cells	IL-1	Symons et al., 1989

polysaccharide (Ghiara et al., 1987)]. However, since Ranges and co-workers (1988) have clearly demonstrated that mouse TNF is a much more potent stimulant of mouse thymocytes than human TNF (Table 7), it appears that the lymphocytic effects of TNF, unlike IL-1, exhibits considerable species specificity. Consequently, it is reasonable to predict that murine TNF in mice will have greater immunostimulatory activity than human TNF. However, the possibility that endogenously produced IL-1 and/or IL-6 mediate some of these effects of TNF cannot be excluded.

The immunostimulatory effects of TNF, like those of IL-1 (Falk et al., 1989), are based in part on both the induction of IL-2 receptor expression (Scheurich et al., 1987) and T-cell proliferation (Hackett et al., 1988) (see Table 7). Using transfection techniques, it has been shown that TNF-α induces at least three nuclear proteins that specifically bind to a κB-like enhancer element present in the promoter region of the gene for the IL-2Rα chain (tac) (Lowenthal et al., 1989). Both TNF-α and IL-1 are comitogenic with PHA or anti-CD3 in stimulating T-lymphocyte proliferation (Hackett et al., 1988). TNF and IL-1 each augment the proliferation of purified T cells even in the presence of optimal stimulatory doses of the other cytokines, suggesting that their actions on T cells probably involve different mechanisms. However, human TNF was less potent than human IL-1 in inducing IL-2 mRNA expression and IL-2 production by human T cells (Hackett et al., 1988). Consequently, IL-1 coinduces a much more prolonged in vitro lymphoproliferative response than TNF. However, the interactions of various cytokines complicates comparisons of efficacy since TNF synergistically amplifies the mitogenic effects of either IL-1 or IL-2 on thymocytes, but it does not augment responses to IL-4 (Ranges et al., 1988).

The foregoing bidirectional interactions of TNF and IL-2 lead to a number of predictable immunological consequences. As shown on Table 7, both monocyte-derived IL-1 and TNF stimulate T-cell colony growth, which can be blocked by anti-IL-1 or anti-TNF, respectively (Zucali et al., 1987). When added together these neutralizing antibodies completely inhibit the stimulatory activity of supernatants from LPS-stimulated monocytes on T-cell colony formation. Therefore, TNF as well as IL-1 contributes to the accessory cell functions of monocytes in the activation of T cells. As shown on Table 7, human recombinant TNF-α and TNF-β augmented lymphoproliferation by responder cells in an MLR (Shalaby et al., 1988). In addition, TNF-α is produced in the course of an MLR, and anti-TNF causes significant reduction of the MLR, implicating TNF-α in allogeneic reactions. Either TNF-α or IL-1 in combination with IL-2 can induce cytolytic activity in a rat and mouse hybrid T-cell line (Plaetinck et al., 1989). Human rTNF-α also augmented the generation of antigen-specific Lyt2^+ CTL from murine spleen cells directed against antigens on syngeneic tumor cells (Nikano et al., 1989). IL-1 (Crump et al., 1989) and TNF-α both can synergize with suboptimal doses of IL-2 in generating human LAK cells (Chouaib et al., 1988). This interaction between TNF and IL-2 was associated with induction of increased numbers of binding sites for IL-2 on LAK cells and was completely inhibited by anti-tac (IL-2Rα) antibodies (Chouaib et al., 1988). Conversely, as shown on Table 4, IL-2 has been documented to induce expression of TNF receptors on normal human T lymphocytes (Owen—Schaub et al., 1989). Consequently, TNF and IL-2 may also regulate each other's activities at the level of receptor expression.

Like IL-1, TNF promotes the in vitro antibody-dependent cellular cytotoxic (ADCC) activity of IL-2-activated murine thymic and spleen cells (Eisenthal and

Rosenberg, 1989). These cytokines augmented the lytic ability of the IL-2-induced ADCC. Both TNF and IL-2 are capable of inducing tumoricidal activity in human peripheral blood monocytes (Philip, 1988). However, whereas monocytes activated by IL-2 can lyse both TNF-sensitive and TNF-insensitive tumor target cells, TNF-activated monocytes kill only TNF-sensitive tumor cells. This was demonstrated by showing that anti-TNF antibodies can completely block the antitumor activities of TNF, but not of IL-2-activated monocytes against TNF-resistant tumor cells. Overall, the observations above indicate that TNF and IL-2 interact on lymphoid as well as monocytic cell types that are engaged in specific as well as nonspecific host defenses.

V. INTERACTIONS OF TNF AND IL-1 WITH IL-4

Based on rather limited available data, as shown on Table 3, IL-4 unexpectedly appears to suppress the production of TNF-α, IL-1, and PGE_2 (Hart et al., 1989a). Preincubation of 90% purified human monocytes with LPS with or without IFN-γ when followed by low doses of human IL-4 results in partial inhibition of the expression of mRNA for TNF-α and IL-1 (Essner et al., 1989) and a reduction in cytokine production to nondetectable levels (Hart et al., 1989a; Weiss et al., 1989). This suppressive effect of IL-4 on monocytes resembles that of glucocorticoids in counteracting the monocyte-activating effect of IFN-γ. Despite reports of stimulating effects of IL-4 on murine monocytes, these findings suggest that IL-4 may have some anti-inflammatory functions in humans.

VI. INTERACTIONS OF TNF AND IL-1 WITH IL-8 AND RELATED CYTOKINES

The observations that TNF and IL-1 have little or no in vitro chemotactic activity for neutrophils, but nevertheless actively recruit neutrophils to accumulate at sites of infection, led to experiments showing that both these cytokines are potent inducers of expression of mRNA for the neutrophil chemoattractant now known as IL-8. As shown on Table 7, IL-8 is produced by a variety of cells in response to IL-1 and TNF such as PBMC (Matsushima et al., 1988), fibroblasts, keratinocytes (Larsen et al., 1989a), and endothelial cells (Strieter et al., 1989). IL-8 is also an in vitro chemoattractant for T lymphocytes and activates neutrophils to release superoxide anions and lysosomal enzymes. Administration of IL-8 induces lymphocytic and neutrophilic infiltration and increases in vascular permeability as reviewed by Matsushima and Oppenheim (1989). However, to what degree the acute inflammatory activities of TNF and IL-1 are mediated by IL-8 remains to be established using specific inhibitors of IL-8.

A number of the other members of this new family of IL-8-related cytokines, including Gro or melanoma growth factor (Golds et al., 1989) and monocyte chemotactic and activating factor (Larsen et al., 1989b), are also induced by both TNF-α and IL-1. On the other hand, there have been no reports that any of the 8- to 10-kDa cytokines in this group have the capacity to induce other cytokines, such as TNF or IL-1. Consequently, these novel cytokines may be more restricted in their activities than TNF and IL-1 and do not appear to perpetuate the cytokine cascade.

VII. TNF INTERACTION WITH HEMATOPOIETIC GROWTH FACTORS; GM-CSF, G-CSF, and CSF-1

TNF effects on hematopoiesis are bimodal. On one hand, TNF inhibits in vitro and in vivo growth and proliferation of normal bone marrow progenitor cells, BFU-E and GM-CFU, as well as proliferation of several leukemic cell lines (Peetre et al., 1986; Broxmeyer et al., 1986). TNF acts as a differentiation factor for the myeloid leukemic cells, suggesting that it may have potential benefit in the treatment of myeloid leukemias. On the other hand, TNF induces the production of CSFs in bone marrow stromal cells, endothelial cells, and fibroblasts. As a result, its net effect on hematopoiesis may be stimulatory. However, continuous administration of TNF, as well as presence of TNF in circulation (e.g., following more than seven repeated injections of IL-1 to primates) were associated with suppressed myelopoiesis (Gasperetto et al., 1989). The suppressive factor was present in the serum and was neutralized by addition of anti-TNF antibody. Exposure of mature monocytes to TNF caused more than 90% down-regulation of CSF-1 receptors. Since TNF is stimulatory to monocytes, the observed down-modulation of CSF-1 receptors may represent a regulatory event of selecting one of several activation pathways.

VIII. RELATIONSHIP OF TNF TO TGF-β

TGF-β was first identified in supernatants of transformed fibroblasts through its ability to induce nonneoplastic cells to express a transformed phenotype and exhibit non-contact-inhibited growth (DeLarco and Todaro, 1978; Roberts et al., 1980). Originally obtained and purified to homogeneity from platelets (Assoian and Sporn, 1986), TGF-β is now known to be produced by many different cells and tissues, including activated macrophages and T and B lymphocytes (Sporn et al., 1986). Like TNF, IL-1, and IL-6, TGF-β has pleiotropic activities, which although in general growth inhibitory, depend greatly on the type of responding cell and the presence of other growth factors.

The growth as well as functional activities of hepatocytes, keratinocytes, T and B lymphocytes, and NK cells are inhibited by TGF-β (Roberts et al., 1985). In direct contrast, TNF has stimulatory effects on these cell types (Table 7). TGF-β may regulate hematopoiesis by suppressing proliferation and development of early hematopoietic progenitor cells (Keller et al., 1988). TNF is also inhibitory to growth of hematopoietic progenitors (BFU-E and GM-CFU) but at a somewhat later stage in lineage progression (Broxmeyer et al., 1986; Peetre et al., 1986). However, unlike TGF-β, TNF can by stimulating stromal cells, produce hematopoietic colony growth factors, thereby having a net stimulatory effect on hematopoiesis.

A number of the inhibitory effects of TGF-β appear to result from its interference with the activities of other cytokines on cells. For example, TGF-β inhibits IL-1 or TNF costimulation of thymocyte proliferation (Ristow, 1986). The finding that TGF-β down-regulates the expression of IL-1 receptors (Dubois et al., 1990) suggests that this could contribute to the inhibitory action of TGB-β on IL-1 effects (Table 4). The effect of TGF-β on receptors for TNF is not yet known.

Examination of the effects of TGF-β and TNF on the generation and action of CTL (induced in MLC) revealed that TGF-β inhibits the generation but not the function of CTL (Ranges et al., 1987). Addition of TNF to MLC reversed the inhibitory effects of TGF-β. Conversely, TGF-β and TNF synergize in their induction of human leukemic cell line differentiation (De Benedetti et al., 1990). Combinations of TGF-β and TNF synergistically inhibited proliferation and induced monocytic differentiation of both HL-60 and U937 cells. Since treatment with TNF induced an increase in TGF-β receptors, it was suggested that the synergy may depend in part on the increased receptor expression.

Although many of the stimulatory effects of TNF on immune and other cell types are antagonized by TGF-β, TGF-β and TNF also have some overlapping biological properties, including stimulation of fibroblast proliferation (giving rise to fibrosis, which is the basis of its wound-healing effects), up-regulation of the epidermal growth factor receptors, and inhibition of myeloblast differentiation (Vilček et al., 1986; Assoian et al., 1984; Palombella et al., 1987; Miller et al., 1988; Massague et al., 1986). Both cytokines also share the capacity to induce angiogenesis. As shown on Table 3, TGF-β regulates IL-1 and TNF at the level of production (Chantry et al., 1989a). Exposure of unstimulated peripheral blood mononuclear cells (PBMC) to TGF-β alone caused an increase in mRNA levels for IL-1α, IL-1β, and TNF-α to levels similar to that seen in LPS-stimulated cells. This increase was shown to be due to increased transcription and not due to message stabilization. The transcribed mRNA, however, was not translated into protein. The mechanism for this inability to translate the transcribed message remains to be elucidated. In contrast to its direct stimulation of mRNA for IL-1 and TNF, TGF-β inhibited LPS induction of IL-1 and TNF, but not induction of these two cytokines with PHA. Because different cell populations are known to respond to the two mitogenic signals, these results suggest that the eventual effects of TGF-β depend on the identity of the responding cell subpopulations as well as presence of other growth factors interacting with these cells and with TGF-β.

SUMMARY AND CONCLUSIONS

It is evident from this review that TNF exhibits complex interactions with other cytokines at the level of production and in its effects. Studies designed to determine the role of TNF in the animal models or cell culture system using pure recombinant molecules have revealed that TNF never operates by itself, but instead operates within a network of cytokines. First, the multitude of exogenous as well as endogenous signals, which induce TNF production, concomitantly also stimulate the production of a battery of other inflammatory cytokines: IL-1, IL-6, IL-8, multiple CSFs, IFN, and TGF-β. Moreover, TNF itself stimulates the production of most of these cytokines. Thus even when pure recombinant TNF is used, it readily generates the production of other interactive cytokines. This apparent redundancy in the production of cytokines with overlapping effects presumably has protective advantage for the host. Furthermore, interaction of these cytokines is more economical and amplifies the responses to subtoxic doses of potentially harmful cytokines.

Cytokine interaction may lead to either synergistic (as for many TNF-IL-1 interactions) or antagonistic effects (TNF and TGF-β, for example). These may depend on (1) the modulation of receptor expression of one cytokine by another (IFN-γ-enhancing receptor expression for TNF, and TGF-β down-regulation of IL-1 receptors), (2) stabilization of the cytokine message by one another (induction of IL-6 by TNF or IL-1), (3) interactions at the level of signal transduction, (4) gene expression, or (5) at the posttranslational level. Thus the receptor repertoire, which is a function of the cell type and stage of development, actually determines the net effects of a particular combination of interactive cytokines. Clearly, the mechanisms of these interactions will need to be elucidated to better understand their biological function and to permit cytokines to be used clinically to the advantage of the host.

Acknowledgement. This project has been funded at least in part with the Federal funds from the Department of Health and Human Services under contract number NO1-CO-74102 with Program Resources, Inc. The content of this publication does not necessarily reflect the views or policies of the Department of Health and Human Services, nor does mention of trade names, commercial products, or organizations imply endorsement by the U. S. Government. By acceptance of this article, the publisher or recipient acknowledges right of the U. S. Government to retain a nonexclusive, royalty-free license in and to any copyright covering the article.

REFERENCES

Abo, T., Sugawara, S., Amenomori, A., Itoh, H., Rikiishi, H., Moro, I., and Kumagai, K. (1986). Selective phagocytosis of gram-positive bacteria and interleukin 1-like factor production by a subpopulation of large granular lymphocytes, *J. Immunol., 136*: 3189-3197.

Aderka, D., Holtmann, H., Toker, L., Hahn, T., and Wallach, D. (1986). Tumor necrosis factor induction by Sendai virus, *J. Immunol., 136*: 2938-2942.

Aderka, D., Le, J., and Vilček, J. (1989). IL-6 inhibits lipopolysaccharide-induced tumor necrosis factor production in cultured monocytes, U937 cells, and in mice, *J. Immunol., 143*: 3517-3523.

Agarwal, S., Drysdale, B.-E., and Shin, H. S. (1988). TNF-mediated cytotoxicity involves ADP ribosylation, *J. Immunol., 140*: 4187–4192.

Aggarwal, B. B., Eessalu, T. E., and Hoss, R P. E. (1985). Characterization of receptors for human TNF and their regulation of IFNγ, *Nature (London), 318*: 665–667.

Akahoshi, T., Oppenheim, J. J., and Matsushima, K. (1988). IL 1 stimulates its own receptor expression on human fibroblasts through the endogenous production of prostaglandin(s), *J. Clin. Invest., 82*: 1219–1224.

Akashi, M., Loussararian, A. H., Adelman, D. C., Saito, M., and Koeffler, H. P. (1990). Role of lymphotoxin in expression of interleukin 6 in human fibroblasts stimulation and regulation, *J. Clin.Invest., 85*: 121–129.

Alam, R., Welter, J. B., Forsythe, P. A., Lett-Brown, M. A., and Grant, J. A. (1989). Comparative effect of recombinant IL 1, -2, -3, -4, and -6, IFN-γ, granulocyte-macrophage colony stimulating factor, tumor necrosis factor α, and histamine-releasing factors on the secretion of histamine from basophils, *J. Immunol., 142*: 3431–3435.

Andersson, V., and Matsuda, T. (1989). Human interleukin 6 and tumor necrosis factor α production studied at the single cell level, *Eur. J. Immunol., 19*: 1157–1160.

Andrews, D. F., Nemunaitis, J. J., and Singer, J. W. (1989). Recombinant TNFα and IL 1α increase expression of c-abl proto-oncogene mRNA in cultured human marrow stromal cells, *Proc. Natl. Acad. Sci. USA, 86*: 6788–6792.

Andus, T., Geiger, T., Hirano, T., Kishimoto, T., and Heinrich, P. C. (1988). Action of recombinant human interleukin 6, interleukin 1β and tumor necrosis factor α on the mRNA induction of acute-phase proteins, *Eur. J. Immunol., 18*: 739–746.

Antonipillai, I., Wang, Y., and Horton, R. (1990). Tumor necrosis factor and interleukin-1 may regulate renin secretion, *Endocrinology, 126*: 273–278.

Apte, R. N., Oppenheim, J. J., and Durum, S. K. (1989). β-Endorphin regulates interleukin 1 production and release by murine bone marrow macrophages, *Int. Immunol., 1*: 456–470.

Asher, A., Mule, J. J., Reichert, C. M., Shiloni, E., and Rosenberg, S. A. (1987). Studies on the antitumor efficacy of systemically administered recombinant tumor necrosis factor against several murine tumors in vivo, *J. Immunol., 138*: 963–974.

Assoian, R. K., and Sporn, M. B. (1986). Type-beta transforming growth factor in human platelets: release during platelet degranulation and action on vascular smooth muscle cells, *J. Cell Biol., 102*: 1217–1223.

Assoian, R. K., Frolik, C. A., Roberts, A. B., Miller, D. M., and Sporn, M. B. (1984). Transforming growth factor β controls receptor levels for epidermal growth factor in NRK fibroblasts, *Cell, 36*: 35–41.

Bachwich, P. R., Chensue, S. W., Larrick, J. W., and Kunkel, S. L. (1986). Tumor necrosis factor stimulates interleukin-1 and prostaglandin E_2 production in resting macrophages, *Biochem. Biophys. Res. Commun., 136*: 94–101.

Bagby, G. C., Jr. (1989). Interleukin 1, stromal cells, granulopoiesis and the inflammatory response, *Biotherapy, 1*: 225–261.

Bagby, G. C., Dinarello, C. A., Wallace, P., Wagner, C., Hefeneider, S., and McCall, E. (1986). Interleukin 1 stimulates granulocyte-macrophage colony-stimulating activity release by vascular endothelial cells, *J. Clin. Invest., 78*: 1316–1323.

Bahr, G. M., Chedid, L. A., and Behbehani, K. (1987). Induction, in vivo and in vitro, of macrophage interleukin-1 by adjuvant-active synthetic muramyl peptides, *Cell. Immunol., 107*: 443–454.

Bakouche, O., Ichinoe, Y., Heicappell, R., Fidler, I. J., and Lachman, L. B. (1988). Plasma membrane-associated tumor necrosis factor: a non-integral membrane protein possibly bound to its own receptor, *J. Immunol., 140*: 1142–1147.

Balavoine, J.-F., de Rochemonteix, B., Williamson, K., Seckinger, P., Cruchard, A., and Dayer, J.-M. (1986). Prostaglandin E_2 and collagenase production by fibroblasts and synovial cells is regulated by urine-derived human interleukin 1 and inhibitor(s), *J. Clin. Invest., 78*: 1120–1124.

Banks, W. A., Kastin, A. J., and Durham, D. A. (1989). Bidirectional transport of interleukin-1α across the blood-brain barrier, *Brain Res. Bull., 23*: 422–437.

Bauer, J., Ganter, U., Geiger, T., Jacobshagen, U., Hirano, T., Matsuda, T., Kishimoto, T., Andus, T., Acs, G., Gorek, W., and Ciliberto, G. (1988). Regulation of interleukin 6 expression in cultured human blood monocytes and monocyte derived macrophages, *Blood, 72*: 1134–1140.

Bauer, J., Bauer, T. M., Kalb, T., Tage, T., Lengyel, G., Hirano, T., Kishimoto, T., Acs, G., Mayer, L., and Gerok, W. (1989). Regulation of IL 6 receptor expression in human monocytes and monocyte-derived macrophages, *J. Exp. Med., 170*: 1537–1549.

Becker, S., Devlin, R. B., and Haskill, J. S. (1989). Differential production of tumor necrosis factor, macrophage colony stimulating factor, and interleukin 1 by human alveolar macrophages, *J. Leukocyte Biol., 45*: 353-361.

Bernton, E. W., Beach, J. E., Holaday, J. W., Smallridge, R. C., and Fein, H. G. (1987). Release of multiple hormones by direct action of interleukin-1 on pituitary cells, *Science, 238*: 519-521.

Bertini, R., Bianchi, M., and Ghizzi, P. (1988). Adrenolectomy sensitizes mice to the lethal effect of interltukin 1 and tumor necrosis factor, *J. Exp. Med., 167*: 1708–1712.

Bertolini, D. R., Nedwin, G. E., Bringman, T. S., Smith, D. D., and Mundy, G. R. (1986). Stimulation of bone resorption and inhibition of bone formation in vitro by human tumor necrosis factor, *Nature, 319*: 516–518.

Besedovsky, H., and Del Ray, A. (1987). Neuroendocrine and metabolic responses induced by interleukin-1, *J. Neurosci. Res., 18*: 172–178.

Besedovsky, H., Del Ray, A., Sorkin, E., and Dinarello, C. A. (1986). Immunoregulatory feedback between interleukin-1 and glucocorticoid hormones, *Science, 233*: 652–654.

Beutler, B., and Cerami, C. (1987). Cachectin–tumor necrosis factor: a cytokine that mediates injury initiated by invasive parasites, *Parasitol. Today, 3*: 345-346.

Beutler, B. A., Milsark, I. W., and Cerami, A. (1985). Cachectin/tumor necrosis factor: production, distribution, and metabolic fate in vivo, *J. Immunol., 135*: 3972–3977.

Beutler, B., Krochin, N., Milsark, I. W., Luedke, C., and Cerami, A. (1986). Control of cachectin (tumor necrosis factor) synthesis: mechanisms of endotoxin resistance, *Science, 232*: 977–980.

Bevilacqua, M. P., Pober, J. S., Majeau, G. R., Fiers, W., Cotran, R. S., and Gimbrone, M. A. (1986). Recombinant tumor necrosis factor induces procoagulant activity in cultured human vascular endothelium: characterization and comparison with the actions of interleukin 1, *Proc. Natl. Acad. Sci. USA, 83*: 4533–4537.

Bird, T. A., and Saklatvala, J. (1989). IL 1 and TNF transmodulate EGF receptors by a protein kinase C independent mechanism, *J. Immunol., 142*: 126–133.

Blanton, R. A., Kupper, T. S., McDougall, J. K., and Dower, S. (1989). Regulation of IL 1 and its receptor in human keratinocytes, *Proc. Natl. Acad. Sci. USA, 86*: 1273–1277.

Bodnar, R. J., Pasternack, G. W., Mann, P. E., Paul, D., Warren, R., and Donner, D. B. (1989). Mediation of anorexia by human recombinant tumor necrosis factor through a peripheral action in the rat, *Cancer Res., 49*: 6280–6284.

Bomsztyk, K., Sims, J. E., Stanton, T. H., Slack, J., McMahan, C. J., Valentine, M. A., and Dower, S. K. (1989). Evidence for different interleukin 1 receptors in murine B- and T-cell lines, *Proc. Natl. Acad. Sci. USA, 86*: 8034–8038.

Brandwein, S. R. (1986). Regulation of interleukin 1 production by mouse peritoneal macrophages, *J. Biol. Chem., 261*: 8624–8632.

Brenner, D. A., O'Hara, M., Angel, P., Chojkier, M., and Karin, M. (1989). Prolonged activation of jun and collagenase genes by TNFα, *Nature, 3377*: 661–663.

Broudy, V. C., Kaushansky, K., Segal, G. M., Harlan, J. M., and Adamson, J. W. (1986). Tumor necrosis factor α stimulates human endothelial cells to produce granulocyte-macrophage colony stimulating factor, *Proc. Natl. Acad. Sci. USA, 83*: 7467–7471.

Brown, K. M., Muchmore, A. V., and Rosenstreich, D. L. (1986). Uromodulin, an immunosuppressive protein derived from pregnancy urine, is an inhibitor of interleukin 1, *Proc. Natl. Acad. Sci. USA, 83*: 9119–9123.

Broxmeyer, H. E., Williams, D. E., Lu, L., Cooper, S., Anderson, S. L., Beyer, G. S., Hoffman, R., and Rubin, B. Y. (1986). The suppressive influence of human tumor necrosis factor on bone marrow hematopoietic progenitor cells from normal donors and patients with leukemia: synergism of tumor necrosis factor and interferon-γ, *J. Immunol., 136*: 4487–4495.

Buchan, G., Barrett, K., Turner, M., Chantry, D., Maini, R. N., and Feldmann, M. (1988). Interleukin-1 and tumor necrosis factor mRNA expression in rheumatoid arthritis: prolonged production of IL-1α, *Clin. Exp. Immunol., 73*: 449–455.

Burchett, S. K., Weaver, W. M., Westfall, J. A., Larsen, A., Kronheim, S., and Wilson, C. B. (1988). Regulation of tumor necrosis factor/cachectin and IL 1 secretion in human mononuclear phagocytes, *J. Immunol., 140*: 3473–3481.

Bussolino, F., Breviaro, F., Tetta, C., Aglietta, M., Mantovani, A., and Dejana, E. (1986). Interleukin 1 stimulates platelet-activating factor production in cultured human endothelial cells, *J. Clin. Invest., 77*: 2027–2033.

Butler, D. M., Michieletto, D. S., and Hamilton, J. A. (1988). Stimulation of human synovial fibroblast DNA synthesis by recombinant human cytokines, *J. Rheumatol., 15*: 1463–1470.

Camp, R. D. R., Finchman, N. J., Cunningham, F. M., Greaves, M. W., Morris, J., and Chu, A. (1986). Psoriatic skin lesions contain biologically active amounts of an interleukin 1-like compound, *J. Immunol., 137*: 3469–3474.

Campbell, I. K., Piccoli, D. S., Butler, D. M., Singleton, D. K., and Hamilton, J. A. (1988). Recombinant human interleukin-1 stimulates human articular cartilage to undergo resorption and human chondrocytes to produce both tissue-and urokinase-type plasminogen activator, *Biochem. Biophys. Acta, 967*: 183–194.

Campbell, I. K., Piccoli, D. S., and Hamilton, J. A. (1990a). Stimulation of human chondrocyte prostaglandin E_2 production by recombinant human interleukin-1 and tumor necrosis factor, *Biochem. Biophys. Acta, 105*: 310–318.

Campbell, I. K., Piccoli, D. S., Roberts, M. J., Muriden, K. D., and Hamilton, J. A. (1990b). The effect of tumor necrosis factor α and β on the resorption of human articular cartilage and on the production of plasminogen activator by human articular chondrocytes, *Arthritis Rheum., 33*: 542–552.

Camussi, G., Bussolino, F., Salvidio, G., and Baglioni, C. (1987). Tumor necrosis factor/cachectin stimulates peritoneal macrophages, polymorphonuclear leukocytes, and vascular endothelial cells to synthesize and release platelet activating factor, *J. Exp. Med., 166*: 1390–1404.

Cannon, J. G., Tatro, J. B., Reichlin, S., and Dinarello, C. A. (1986). α Melanocyte stimulating hormone inhibits immunostimulatory and inflammatory actions of interleukin 1, *J. Immunol., 137*: 2232-2236.

Carter, J. G., Deibel, M. R., Dunn, C. J., Tomich, C.-S. C., Laborde, A. L., Slightom, J. L., Berger, A. E., Bienkowski, M. J., Sun, F. F., McEwan, R. N., Harris, P. K. W., Yem, A. W., Waszak, G. A., Chosay, J. G., Sieu, L. C., Hardee, M. M., Zurcher-Neely, H. A., Reardon, I. M., Heinrikson, R. L., Truesdall, S. E., Shelly, J. A., Eessalu, T. E., Taylor, B. M., and Tracey, D. E. (1990). Purification, cloning, expression and biological characterization of an interleukin-1 receptor antagonist protein, *Nature, 344*: 633–637.

Cavender, D. E., Haskard, D. O., Joseph, B., and Ziff, M. (1986). Interleukin 1 increases the binding of human B and T lymphocytes to endothelial cell monolayers, *J. Immunol., 136*: 203–207.

Chantry, D., Turner, M., Abney, E., and Feldmann, M. (1989a) Modulation of cytokine production by transforming growth factor-β, *J. Immunol., 142*: 4295–4300.

Chantry, D., Winearls, C. G., Maini, R. N., and Feldmann, M. (1989b). Mechanism of immune complex-mediated damage: induction of interleukin 1 by immune complexes and synergy with interferon-γ and tumor necrosis factor-α, *Eur. J. Immunol., 19*: 189–192.

Chapman, P. B., Lester, T. J., Casper, E. S., Gabrilove, J. L., Wong, G. Y., Kempin, S. J., Gold, P. J., Welt, S., Warren, R. S., Stames, H. F., Sherwin, S. A., Old, L. J., and Oettgen, H. F. (1987). Clinical pharmacology of recombinant human tumor necrosis factor in patients with advanced cancer, *J. Clin. Oncol., 5*: 1942–1951.

Chedid, M., Shirakawa, F., Naylor, P., and Mizel, S. B. (1989). Signal transduction pathway for IL 1. Involvement of a pertussis toxin sensitive GTP-binding protein in the activation of adenylate cyclase, *J. Immunol., 142*: 4301–4306.

Chiou, W. J., Bonin, P. D., Harris, P. K. W., Carter, D. B., and Singh, J. P. (1989). PDGF induces IL 1 receptor gene expression in BALB/c 3T3 fibroblasts, *J. Biol. Chem., 264*: 21441-21445.

Chizzonite, R., Truitt, T., Kilian, P. L., Stern, A. S., Nunes, P., Parker, K. P., Kaffka, K. L., Chua, A. O., Lugg, D. K., and Gubler, U. (1989). Two high-affinity interleukin 1 receptors represent separate gene products, *Proc. Natl. Acad. Sci. USA, 86*: 8029–8033.

Chouaib, S., Bertoglio, J., Blay, J.-Y., Marchiol-Fournigault, C., and Fradelizi, D. (1988). Generation of lymphokine-activated killer cells: synergy between tumor necrosis factor and interleukin 2, *Proc. Natl. Acad. Sci. USA, 85*: 6875–6879.

Clark, I. A., Cowden, W. B., Butcher, G. A., and Hunt, N. H. (1987a). Possible roles of tumor necrosis factor in the pathology of malaria, *Am. J. Pathol., 129*: 192–199.

Clark, I. A., Hunt, N. H., Butcher, G. A., and Cowden, W. B. (1987b). Inhibition of murine malaria (*Plasmodium chabaudi*) in vivo by recombinant interferon-γ or tumor necrosis factor, and its enhancement by butylated hydroxyanisole, *J. Immunol., 139*: 3493–3496.

Coceani, F., Lees, J., and Dinarello, C. A. (1988). Occurrence of interleukin 1 in cerebrospinal fluid of the conscious cat, *Brain Res., 446*: 245–250.

Collart, M. A., Belin, D., Vassalli, J.-D., de Kossodo, S., and Vassalli, P. (1986). γ interferon enhances macrophage transcription of the tumor necrosis factor/cachectin, interleukin 1, and urokinase genes, which are controlled by short-lived repressors, *J. Exp. Med., 164*: 2113–2118.

Collins, T., Lapierre, L. A., Fiers, W., Strominger, J. L., and Pober, J. S. (1986). Recombinant human tumor necrosis factor increases mRNA levels and surface expression of HLA-A, B antigens in vascular endothelial cells and dermal fibroblasts in vitro, *Proc. Natl. Acad. Sci. USA, 83*: 446–450.

Cozens, P. J., and Rowe, F. M. (1987). Substance P is a potent inducer of TNF and IL 1 secretion by macrophages: a potential role for TNF in the pathogenesis of asthma, *Immunobiology, 175*: 7.

Crump, W. L., III, Owen-Schaub, L. B., and Grimm, E. A. (1989). Synergy of human recombinant interleukin 1 with interleukin 2 in the generation of lymphokine-activated killer cells, *Cancer Res., 49*: 149–153.

Cuturi, M. C., Murphy, M., Costa-Giomi, M. P., Weinmann, R., Perussia, B., and Trinchieri, G. (1987). Independent regulation of tumor necrosis factor and lymphotoxin production by human peripheral blood lymphocytes, *J. Exp. Med., 165*: 1581–1594.

Czuprynski, C. I., Brown, J. F., Young, K. M., Cooley, A. J., and Kurz, R. S. (1988). Effects of murine recombinant interleukin 1α on the host response to bacterial infection, *J. Immunol., 140*: 962–968.

Darlington, G. J., Wilson, D. R., Lackman, L. B. (1986). Monocyte-conditioned medium, interleukin 1, and tumor necrosis factor stimuate the acute phase response in human hepatomal cells in vitro, *J. Cell Biol., 103*: 787–793.

Dascombe, M. J., Rothwell, N. J., Sagay, B. O., and Stock, M. J. (1989). Pyrogenic and thermogenic effects of interleukin 1β in the rat, *Am. J. Physiol., 256*: E7–E11.

Dayer, J.-M., Beutler, B., and Cerami, A. (1985). Cachectin/tumor necrosis factor stimulated collagenase and prostaglandin E_2 production by human synovial cells and dermal fibroblasts, *J. Exp. Med., 162*: 2163–2168.

Daynes, R. A., Robertson, B. A., Cho, B.-H., Burnham, D. K., and Newton, R. (1987). α-melanocyte-stimulating hormone exhibits target cell selectivity in its capacity to affect interleukin 1-inducible responses in vivo and in vitro, *J. Immunol., 139*: 103–109.

De Benedetti, F., Falk, L. A., Ellingsworth, L. R., Ruscetti, F. W., and Faltynek, C. R. (1990). Synergy between transforming growth factor-β and tumor necrosis factor-α in the induction of monocytic differentiation of human leukemic cell lines, *Blood, 75*: 626–632.

Decker, T., Lohmann-Mattes, M. L., and Gifford, G. E. (1987). Cell-associated tumor necrosis factor (TNF) as a killing mechanism of activated cytotoxic macrophages, *J. Immunol., 138*: 957–962.

Degliantoni, G., Murphy, M., Kobayashi, M., Francis, M. K., Perussia, B., and Trinchieri, G. (1985). Natural killer (NK) cell-derived hematopoietic colony-inhibiting activity and NK cytotoxic factor: relationship with tumor necrosis factor and synergism with immune interferon, *J. Exp. Med., 162*: 1512–1530.

DeLarco, J. E., and Todaro, G. J. (1978). Growth factors from murine sarcoma virus transformed cells, *Proc. Natl. Acad. Sci. USA, 75*: 4001–4005.

Del Rey, A., and Besedovsky, H. (1989). Antidiabetic effects of interleukin 1, *Proc. Natl. Acad. Sci. USA, 86*: 5943–5947.

Dewhirst, F. E., Stashenko, P. P., Mole, J. E., and Tsurumachi, T. (1985). Purification and partial sequence of human osteoclast-activating factor: identity with interleukin 1β, *J. Immunol., 135*: 2562-2568.

Di Giovine, F. S., Malawista, S. E., Nuki, G., and Duff, G. W. (1987). Interleukin 1 (IL 1) as a mediator of crystal arthritis: stimulation of T cell and synovial fibroblast mitogenesis by urate crystal-induced arthritis, *J. Immunol., 138*: 3213-3218.

Dinarello, C. A. (1984). Interleukin-1, *Rev. Infect. Dis., 6*: 51-95.

Dinarello, C. A. (1989). IL 1 and its biologically related cytokines, *Adv. Immunol., 44*: 153-205.

Dinarello, C. A., Bishai, I., Rosenwasser, L. J., and Coceani, F. (1984). The influence of lipoxygenase inhibitors on the in vitro production of human leukocytic pyrogen and lymphocyte activating factor (interleukin 1), *Int. J. Immunopharmacol., 6*: 43-50.

Dinarello, C. A., Cannon, J. G., Wolff, S. M., Berheim, H. A., Beutler, B., Cerami, A., Figari, I. S., Palladino, M. A., Jr., and O'Connor, J. V. (1986). Tumor necrosis factor (cachectin) is an endogenous pyrogen and induces production of interleukin 1, *J. Exp. Med., 163*: 1433-1450.

Dinarello, C. A., Ikejima, T., Warner, S. J. C., Orencole, S. F. Lonnemann, G., Cannon, J. G., and Libby, P. (1987). Interleukin 1 induces interleukin 1. I. Induction of circulating interleukin 1 in rabbit in vivo and in human mononuclear cells in vitro, *J. Immunol., 139*: 1902-1910.

Ding, A. H., Porteu, F., Sanchez, E., and Nathan, C. F. (1990a). Down regulation of TNF receptors on macrophages and endothelial cells by microtubule depolymerizing agents, *J. Exp. Med., 171*: 715-727.

Ding, A. H. Porteu, F., Sanchez, E., and Nathan, C. F. (1990b). Shared actions of endotoxin and taxol on TNF receptors and TNF release, *Science, 248*: 370-372.

Djeu, J. Y., Blanchard, D. K., Richards, A. L., and Friedman, H. (1988). Tumor necrosis factor induction by *Candida albicans* from human natural killer cells and monocytes, *J. Immunol., 141*: 4047-4052.

Dubois, C., Bissonnette, E., and Rola-Pleszczynski, M. (1989). Platelet-activating factor (PAF) enhances tumor necrosis factor production by alveolar macrophages: prevention by PAF antagonists and lipoxygenase inhibitors, *J. Immunol., 143*: 964-970.

Dubois, C. M., Ruscetti, F. W., Palaszynski, E. W., Falk, L. A., Oppenheim, J. J., and Keller, J. R. (1990). Down regulation of IL 1 receptor expression on progenitor cells by TGFβ, *Molecular and Cellular Biology of Cytokines* (J. J. Oppenheim, M. Powanda, M. Kluger, and C. A. Dinarello, eds.), Alan R. Liss/Wiley, New York (137-142).

Durum, S. K., and Oppenheim, J. J. (1989). Macrophage derived mediators: IL 1, TNF, IL 6, IFN and related cytokines, *Fundamental Immunology*, 2nd ed. (W. E. Paul, ed.), Raven Press, New York.

Durum, S. K., Oppenheim, J. J., and Neta, R. (1989). Immunophysiological role of interleukin-1, *Immunophysiology: Role of Cells and Cytokines in Immunity and Inflammation* (J. J. Oppenheim and E. Shevach, eds.), Oxford University Press, Oxford, pp. 210-215.

Dustin, M. L., Rothlein, R., Bhan, A. K., Dinarello, C. A., and Springer, T. A. (1986). Induction of IL 1 and interferon-γ, tissue distribution, biochemistry and function of a natural adherence molecule (ICAM-1), *J. Immunol., 137*: 245-254.

Economou, J. S., McBride, W. H., Essner, R., Rhoades, K., Golub, S., Holmes, E. C., and

Morton, D. L. (1989). Tumor necrosis factor production by IL 2-activated macrophages in vitro and in vivo, *Immunology, 67*: 514-519.

Eisenthal, A., and Rosenberg, S. A. (1989). The effect of various cytokines on the in vitro induction of antibody-dependent cellular cytotoxicity in murine cells, *J. Immunol., 142*: 2307-2313.

Elias, J. A., and Lentz, V. (1990) Interleukin 1 and tumor necrosis factor synergistically stimulate fibroblasts interleukin 6 production by stabilizing interleukin 6 messenger RNA, *J. Immunol., 145*: 161-166.

Ellias, J. A., Chien, P., Gustillo, K. M., and Schreiber, A. D. (1985). Differential interleukin-1 elaboration by density-defined human monocyte subpopulations, *Blood, 66*: 298-301.

Elias, J. A., Gustillo, K., Baeder, W., and Freundlich, B. (1987). Synergistic stimulation of fibroblast prostaglandin production by recombinant interleukin 1 and tumor necrosis factor, *J. Immunol., 138*: 3812-3816.

Elias, J. A., Reynolds, M. M., Kotloff, R. M., and Kern, J. A. (1989). Fibroblast interleukin 1β synergistic stimulation by recombinant interleukin 1 and tumor necrosis factor and post-transcriptional regulation, *Proc. Natl. Acad. Sci. USA, 86*: 6171-6175.

Endo, Y. (1989). Induction of histidine and ornithine decarboxylase activities in mouse tissue by recombinant IL 1 and TNF, *Biochem. Pharmacol., 38*: 1287-1292.

Endres, S., Ghorbani, R., Kelley, V. E., Georgilia, K., Lonnemann, G., van der Meer, J. W. M., Cannon, J. G., Rogers, T. S., Klempner, M. S., Weber, P. C., Schaefer, E. J., Wolff, S. M., and Dinarello, C. A. (1989). The effect of dietary supplementation with *n*-3 poly unsaturated fatty acids on the synthesis of interleukin 1 and tumor necrosis factor by mononuclear cells, *N. Engl. J. Med., 320*: 265-271.

Enk, C., Gerstoft, J., Moller, S., and Remvig, L. (1989). Interleukin 1 activity in the acquired immunodeficiency syndrome, *Scand. J. Immunol., 23*: 491-497.

Ensoli, B., Nakamura, S., Salahuddin, S. Z., Biberfeld, P., Larsson, L., Beaver, B., Wong-Staal, F., and Gallo, R. C. (1989). AIDS-Kaposi's sarcoma-derived cells express cytokines with autocrine and paracine growth effects, *Science, 243*: 223-226.

Espevik, T., Figari, I. S., Shalaby, M. R., Lackides, G. A., Lewis, G. D., Shepard, H. M., and Pallandino, M. A. (1987). Inhibition of cytokine production by cyclosporin A and transforming growth factor β, *J. Exp. Med., 166*: 571-576.

Essner, R., Rhoades, K., McBride, W. H., Morton, D. L., and Economou, J. S. (1989). IL 4 down-regulates IL 1 and TNF gene expression in human monocytes, *J. Immunol., 142*: 3857-3861.

Falk, W., Mannel, D. N., Darjes, H., and Krammer, P. M. (1989). IL 1 induces high affinity IL 2 receptor expression of $CD4^-8^-$ thymocytes, *J. Immunol., 143*: 513-517.

Falk, W., Albrecht, M. P., Stricker, K., Serfling, E., and Krammer, P. H. (1990). Internalization of IL 1 is required for IL 2 gene activation in EL4 thymoma cells, *Molecular and Cellular Biology of Cytokines* (J. J. Oppenheim, M. C. Powanda, M. J. Kluger, and C. A. Dinarello, eds.), Alan R. Liss/Wiley, New York (191-196).

Feist, W., Ulmer, A. J., Musehold, J., Brade, H., Kusumoto, S., and Flad, H.-D. (1989). Induction of tumor necrosis factor-alpha by lipopolysaccharide and defined lipopolysaccharide partial structures, *Immunobiology, 179*: 293-307.

Fenton, M. J., Clark, B. D., Collins, K. L., Webb, A. C., Rich, A., and Auron, P. E. (1987).

Transcriptional regulation of the human pro-interleukin 1β gene, *J. Immunol., 138*: 3972-3979.

Fenton, M. J., Vermeulen, M. W., Clark, B. D., Webb, A. C., and Auron, P. E. 91988). Human pro-IL-1β gene expression in monocytic cells is regulated by two distinct pathways, *J. Immunol., 140*: 2267-2273.

Ferraiolo, B. L., McCabe, J., Hollenbach, S., Hultgren, B., Pitti, R., and Wilking, H. (1989). Pharmacokinetics of recombinant human tumor necrosis factor α in rats: effects of size and number of doses and nephrectomy, *Drug Metab. Dispos., 17*: 369-372.

Fibbe, W. E., Van Damme, J., Billiau, A., Voogt, P. J., Duinkerken, N., Kluck, P. M. C., and Falkenburg, J. H. F. (1986). Interleukin 1 (22 K factor) induces release of granulocyte-macrophage colony stimulating activity from human mononuclear phagocytes, *Blood, 68*: 1316-1321.

Firestein, G. S., Roeder, W. D., Laxer, J. A., Townsend, K. S., Weaver, C. T., Hom, J. T., Linton, J., Torbett, B. E., and Glasebrook, A. L. (1989). A new Murine $CD4^+$ T cell subset with an unrestricted cytokine profile, *J. Immunol., 143*: 518-525.

Flores, E. A., Bistrian, B. R., Pomposelli, J. J., Dinarello, C. A., Blackburn, G. L., and Istfan, N. W. (1989). Infusion of tumor necrosis factor/cachectin promotes muscle catabolism in the rat, *J. Clin. Invest., 83*: 1614-1622.

Fong, Y., Moldawer, L. L., Marano, M., Wey, H., Tatter, S. B., Clarick, R. H., Santhanam, U., Sherris, D., May, L. T., Sehgal, P. B., and Lowry, S. F. (1989). Endotoxemia elicits increased circulating β_2-IFN/IL 6 in man, *J. Immunol., 142*: 2321-2324.

Fontana, A., Hengartner, H., Weber, E., Fehr, K., Grob, P. J., and Cohen, G. (1982a). Interleukin 1 activity in the synovial fluid of patients with rheumatoid arthritis, *Rheumatol. Int., 2*: 49-53.

Fontana, A., Kristensen, F., Dubs, R., Gemsa, D., and Weber, E. (1983b). Production of prostaglandin E and an interleukin-1 like factor by cultured astrocytes and C6 glioma cells, *J. Immunol., 129*: 2413-2419.

Francus, T., Manzo, G., Canki, M., Thompson, L. C., and Szabo, P. (1989). Two peaks of interleukin 1 expression in human leukocytes cultured with tobacco glycoprotein, *J. Exp. Med., 170*: 327-332.

Frei, K., Malipiero, U. V., Leist, T. P., Zinkernagel, R. M., Schwab, M. E., and Fontana, A. (1989). On the cellular source and function of interleukin 6 produced in the central nervous system in viral diseases, *Eur. J. Immunol., 19*: 689-694.

Friedl, H. P., Tiu, G. O., Ryan, U. S., and Ward, P. A. (1989). Mediator-induced activation of xanthine oxidase in endothelial cells, *FASEB J., 3*: 2512-2518.

Gamble, J. R., Harlan, J. M., Klebanoff, S. J., and Vadas, M. A. (1985). Stimulation of the adherence of neutrophils to umbilical vein endothelium by human recombinant tumor necrosis factor, *Proc. Natl. Acad. Sci. USA, 82*: 8667-8671.

Garman, R. D., Jacobs, K. A., Clark, S. C., and Raulet, D. H. (1987). B-cell-stimulatory factor 2 (b2 interferon) functions as a second signal for interleukin 2 production by mature murine T cells, *Proc. Natl. Acad. Sci. USA, 84*: 7629-7633.

Gasperetto, C., Laver, J., Abboud, M., Gillio, A., Smith, C., O'Reilly, R. J., and Moore, M. A. S. (1989). Effects of IL 1 on hematopoietic progenitors: evidence of stimulatory and inhibitatory activities in a primate model, *Blood, 74*: 547-550.

Gauldie, J., Richards, C., Harnish, D., Lansdorp, P., and Baumann, H. (1987). Interferon β_2/B-cell stimulatory factor type 2 shares identity with monocyte-derived hepatocyte-stimulating factor and regulates the major acute phase protein response in liver cells, *Proc. Natl. Acad. Sci. USA, 84*: 7251–7255.

Geiger, T., Andus, T., Klapproth, J., Hirano, T., Kishimoto, T., and Heinrich, P. C. (1988). Induction of rat acute-phase proteins by interleukin 6 in vivo, *Eur. J. Immunol., 18*: 717–721.

Gemlo, B. T., Palladino, M., Jaffe, H., Espevik, T., and Rayner, A. (1988). Circulating cytokines in patients with metastatic cancer treated with recombinant IL 2 and lymphokine activated killer cells, *Cancer Res., 18*: 5864–5867.

Georgilis, K., Schaefer, C., Dinarello, C. A., and Klempner, M. S. (1987). Human recombinant interleukin 1β has no effect on intracellular calcium or on functional responses of human neutrophils, *J. Immunol., 138*: 3403–3407.

Gery, I., and Waksman, B. H. (1972). Potentiation of the T-lymphocyte response to mitogens. II. The cellular source of potentiating mediator(s), *J. Exp. Med., 136*: 143–155.

Ghezzi, P., Saccardo, B., and Bianchi, M. (1986a). Recombinant tumor necrosis factor depresses cytochrome P450-dependent microsomal drug metabolism in mice, *Biochem. Biophys. Res. Commun., 136*: 316–321.

Ghezzi, P., Saccardo, B., Villa, P., Rossi, V., Bianchi, M., and Dinarello, C. A. (1986b). Role of Interleukin-1 in the depression of liver drug metabolism by endotoxin, *Infect. Immun., 54*: 837–840.

Ghiara, P., Boraschi, D., Nencioni, L., Ghezzi, P., and Tagliabue, A. (1987). Enhancement of in vivo immune response by tumor necrosis factor, *J. Immunol., 139*: 3676–3679.

Gifford, G. E., and Lohmann-Matthes, M.-L. (1987). Gamma interferon priming of mouse and human macrophages for induction of tumor necrosis factor production by bacterial lipopolysaccharide, *J. Natl. Cancer Inst., 78*: 121–124.

Gijbels, K., Van Damme, J., Proost, P., Put, W., Carton, H., and Billiau, A. (1990). Interleukin 6 production in the central nervous system during experimental autoimmune encephalomyelitis, *Eur. J. Immunol., 20*: 233–235.

Girardin, E., Grau, G. E., Dayer, J.-M., Roux-Lombard, P., and Lambert, P.-H. (1988). Tumor necrosis factor and interleukin-1 in the serum of children with severe infectious purpura, *N. Engl. J. Med., 319*: 397–400.

Giri, J. G., Lomedico, P. T., amd Mizel, S. B. (1985). Studies on the synthesis and secretion of interleukin 1. I. A 33,00 molecular weight precursor for interleukin 1, *J. Immunol., 134*: 333–349.

Giulian, D., and Lachman, L. B. (1985). Interleukin-1 stimulation of astroglial proliferation after brain injury, *Science, 228*: 497–499.

Giulian, D., Baker, T. J., Shih, L.-C. N., and Lachman, L. B. (1986). Interluekin 1 of the central nervous system is produced by ameboid microglia, *J. Exp. Med., 164*: 594–604.

Goldgaber, D., Harris, H. W., Hla, T., Maciag, T., Donnelly, R. J., Jacobson, J. S., Vitek, M. P., and Gadjusek, D. C. (1989). IL 1 regulates synthesis of amyloid β-protein precursor mRNA in human endothelial cells, *Proc. Natl. Acad. Sci. USA, 86*: 7606–7610.

Golds, E. E., Mason, P., and Hyirkos, P. (1989). Inflammatory cytokines induce synthesis and secretion of GRO protein and neutrophil chemotactic factor but not β2-microglobulin in human synovial cells and fibroblasts, *Biochem. J., 259*: 585–588.

Goto, F., Nakamura, S., Goto, K., and Yoshinaga, M. (1984). Production of a lymphocyte proliferation potentiating factor by purified polymorphonuclear leukocytes from mice and rabbits, *J. Immunol., 53*: 683-692.

Grau, G. E., Fajardo, L. F., Piguet, P. F., Allet, B., Lambert, P. H., and Vassalli, P. (1987). Tumor necrosis factor (cachectin) is an essential mediator in murine cerebral malaria, *Science, 237*: 1210-1212.

Grau, G. E., Taylor, T. E., Molyneux, M. E., Wirima, J. J., Vassalli, P., Hommel, M., and Lambert, P.-H. (1989). Tumor necrosis factor and disease severity in children with falciparum malaria, *N. Engl. J. Med., 320*: 1586-1591.

Greischel, A., and Zahn, G. (1989). Pharmacokinetics of recombinant human tumor necrosis factor alpha in rhesus monkeys after intravenous administration, *J. Pharmacol. Exp. Ther., 251*: 358-361.

Griffin, W. S. T., Stanley, L. C., Ling, C., White, L., MacLeod, V., Perrot, L. J., White, C. L., III, and Araoz, C. (1989). Brain interleukin 1 and S-100 immunoreactivity are elevated in Down syndrome and Alzheimer disease, *Proc. Natl. Acad. Sci. USA, 86*: 7611-7615.

Grossman, R. M., Krueger, J., Yourish, D., Granelli-Piperno, A., Murphy, D. P., May, L. T., Kupper, T. S., Sehgal, P. B., and Gottlieb, A. B. (1989). Interleukin 6 is expressed in high levels in psoriatic skin and stimulates proliferation of cultured human keratinocytes, *Proc. Natl. Acad. Sci. USA, 86*: 6367-6371.

Hackett, R. A., Davis, L. S., and Lipsky, P. E. (1988). Comparative effects of tumor necrosis factor-α and IL 1β on mitogen-induced T cell activation, *J. Immunol., 140*: 2639-2644.

Hajjar, K. A., Hajjar, D. P., Silverstein, R. L., and Nachman, R. L. (1987). Tumor necrosis factor-mediated release of platelet-derived growth factor from cultured endothelial cells, *J. Exp. Med., 166*: 235-245.

Hamilton, J. A. (1987). Interleukin 1β and interleukin 1α stimulate the plasminogen activator activity and prostaglandin E_2 levels of human synovial cells, *Arthritis Theum., 30*: 562-566.

Hannum, C. H., Wilcox, C. J., Arend, W. P., Joslin, F. G., Dripps, D. J., Heimdal, P. L., Armes, L. G., Sommer, A., Eisenberg, S. P., and Thompson, R. C. (1990). Interleukin 1 receptor antagonist activity of a human interleukin 1 inhibitor, *Nature, 343*: 336-340.

Haq, A. U., and Maca, R. D. (1986). Role of IFN-γ and α in IL 1 synthesis and secretion of in vitro differentiated human macrophages: a comparative study, *Immunobiology, 171*: 451-460.

Hart, P. H., Vitti, G. F., Burgess, D. R., Whitty, G. A., Piccoli, D. S., and Hamilton, J. A. (1989a). Potential antiinflammatory effects of interleukin 4: Suppression of human monocyte tumor necrosis factor α, interleukin 1, and prostaglandin E_2, *Proc. Natl. Acad. Sci. USA, 86*: 3803-3807.

Hart, P. H., Whitty, G. A., Piccoli, D. S., and Hamilton, J. A. (1989b). Control by IFNγ and PGE2 of TNFα and IL 1 production by human monocytes, *Immunology, 66*: 376-383.

Havell, E. A. (1989). Evidence that tumor necrosis factor has an important role in antibacterial resistance, *J. Immunol., 143*: 2894-2899.

Helfgott, D. C., May, L. T., Sthoeger, Z., Tamm, I., and Sehgal, P. B. (1987). Bacterial lipopolysaccharide (endotoxin) enhances expression and secretion of β2-interferon by human fibroblasts, *J. Exp. Med., 166*: 1300-1309.

Helle, M., Brakenhoff, J. P. J., de Groot, E. R., and Aarden, L. A. (1988). Interleukin 6 is involved in interleukin 1 induced activities, *Eur. J. Immunol., 18*: 957-959.

Herrmann, F., Gebauer, G., Lindemann, A., Brach, M., and Mertelsmann, R. (1989b). Interleukin 2 and interferon gamma recruit different subsets of human peripheral blood monocytes to secrete interleukin 1 beta and tumor necrosis factor alpha, *Clin. Exp. Immunol., 77*: 97–100.

Herrmann, F., Cannistra, S. A., Lindemann, A., Blohm, D., Rambaldi, A., Mertelsmann, R. H., and Griffin, J. D. (1989a). Functional consequences of monocyte IL 2 receptor expression: induction of IL 1β secretion by IFN-gamma and IL 2[1], *J. Immunol., 142*: 139–143.

Hirano, T., Taga, T., Nakano, N., Yasukawa, K., Kashiwamura, S., Shimizu, K., Nakajima, K., Pyun, K. H., and Kishimoto, T. (1985). Purification to homogeneity and characterization of human B-cell differentiation factor (BCDF or BSF-2), *Proc. Natl. Acad. Sci. USA, 82*: 5490–5494.

Hirano, T., Matsuda, T., Turner, M., Miyasaka, N., Buchan, G., Tang, B., Sato, K., Shimizu, M. Maini, R., Feldman, M., and Kichimoto, T. (1988). Excessive production of interleukin 6/B cell stimulatory factor-2 in rheumatoid arthritis, *Eur. J. Immunol., 18*: 1797–1801.

Hoffman, M., and Weinberg, J. B. (1987). Tumor necrosis factor-α induces increased hydrogen peroxide production and Fc receptor expression, but not increased Ia antigen expression by peritoneal macrophages, *J. Leukocyte Biol., 42*: 704–707.

Hoffman, F. M., Hinton, D. R., Johnson, K., and Merrill, J. E. (1989). Tumor necrosis factor identified in multiple sclerosis brain, *J. Exp. Med., 170*: 607–612.

Hofsli, E., Bakke, O., Nonstad, U., and Espevik, T. (1989). A flow cytometric and immunofluorescence microscopic study of tumor necrosis factor production and localization in human monocytes, *Cell Immunol., 122*: 405–415.

Holtzmann, H., and Wallach, D. (1987). Down regulation of the receptors for tumor necrosis factor by interleukin 1 and 4β-phorbol-12-myristate-13-acetate[1], *J. Immunol., 139*: 1161–1167.

Horii, Y., Muraguchi, A., Suematsu, S., Matsuda, T., Yoshizaki, K., Hirano, T., and Kishimoto, T. (1988). Regulation of BSF-2/IL 6 production by human mononuclear cells. Macrophage-dependent synthesis of BSF-2/IL 6 by T cells, *J. Immunol., 141*: 1529–1535.

Houssiau, F. A., Bukasa, K., Sindic, C. J. M., Van Damme, J., and Van Snick, J. (1988). Elevated levels of the 26K human hybridoma growth factor (interleukin 6) in cerebrospinal fluid of patients with acute infection of the central nervous system, *Clin. Exp. Immunol., 71*: 320–323.

Ikebuchi, K., Wong, G. G., Clark, S. C., Ihle, J. N., Hirai, Y., and Ogawa, M. (1987). Interleukin 6 enhancement of interleukin 3-dependent proliferation of multipotential hemopoietic progenitors, *Proc. Natl. Acad. Sci. USA, 84*: 9035–9039.

Imamura, K., Sherman, M. L., Spriggs, D., and Kufe, D. (1988). Effect of TNF on GTP and GTPase activity in HL60 and L929 cells, *J. Biol. Chem., 263*: 10, 247–253.

Jacob, C. O., Aiso, S., Michie, S. A., McDevitt, H. O., and Acha-Orbea, H. (1990). Prevention of diabetes in nonobese diabetic mice by tumor necrosis factor (TNF): similarities between TNF-α and interleukin 1, *Proc. Natl. Acad. Sci. USA, 87*: 968–972.

James, K. (1990). Interactions between cytokines and α2-macroglobulin, *Immunol. Today, 11*: 163–166.

Jayaraman, S., Martin, C. A., and Dorf, M. E. (1990). Enhancement of in vivo cell-mediated immune responses by three distinct cytokines, *J. Immunol., 144*: 942–951.

Jelinek, D. F., and Lipsky, P. E. (1987). Enhancement of human B-cell proliferation and differentiation by tumor necrosis factor α and interleukin 1, *J. Immunol., 139*: 2970–2976.

Jirik, F. R., Podor, T. J., Hirano, T., Kishimoto, T., Loskutoff, D. J., Carson, D. A., and Lotz, M. (1989). Bacterial lipopolysaccharide and inflammatory mediators augment IL 6 secretion by human endothelial cells, *J. Immunol., 142*: 144–147.

Kampschmidt, R. F., and Pulliam, L. A. (1978). Effect of human monocyte pyrogen on plasma iron, plasma zinc, and blood neutrophils in rabbits and rats, *Proc. Soc. Exp. Biol. Med., 158*: 32–35.

Kampschmidt, R. F., Upchurch, H. F., and Worthington, M. L. (1983). Further comparisons of endogenous pyrogens and leukocytic endogenous mediators, *Infect. Immun., 41*: 6–10.

Kasid, A., Director, E. P., and Rosenberg, S. A. (1989). Induction of endogenous cytokine mRNA in circulating peripheral blood mononuclear cells by IL 2 administration to cancer patients, *J. Immunol., 143*: 736–739.

Katz, Y., and Strunk, R. C. (1989). IL-1 and tumor necrosis factor. Similarities and differences in stimulation of expression of alternative pathway of complement and IFN-β2/IL-6 genes in human fibroblasts, *J. Immunol., 142*: 3862–3867.

Kaur, P., and Saklatvala, J. (1989). IL 1 and TNF increase phosphorylation of fibroblast protein, *FEBS Lett., 241*: 6–10.

Kawakami, M., Ishibashi, S., Ogawa, H., Murase, T., Takaku, F., and Shibata, S. (1986). Cachectin/TNF as well as interleukin 1 increase prostacyclin synthesis in cultured vascular endothelial cells, *Biochem. Biophys. Res. Commun., 141*: 482–487.

Kawano, M., Hirano, T., Matsuda, T., Taga, T., Horii, Y., Iwato, K., Asaoku, H., Tang, B., Tanabe, O., Tanaka, H., Kuramoto, A., and Kishimoto, T. (1988). Autocrine generation and essential requirement of BSF-2/IL-6 for human multiple myelomas, *Nature, 332*: 83–85.

Kehrl, J. H., Miller, A., and Fauci, A. S. (1987). Effect of tumor necrosis factor α on mitogen-activated human B cells, *J. Exp. Med., 166*: 781–791.

Keller, J. R., Mantel, C., Sing, G. K., Ellingsworth, L. R., Ruscetti, S. K., and Ruscetti, F. W. (1988). Transforming growth factor β1 selectively regulates early murine hematopoietic progenitors and inhibits the growth of the IL-3 dependent myeloid leukemia cell lines, *J. Exp. Med., 168*: 737-750.

Kern, P., Hemmer, C. J., Van Damme, J., Gruss, H.-J., and Dietrich, M. (1989). Elevated tumor necrosis factor α and interleukin-6 serum levels as markers for complicated plasmodium falciparum malaria, *Am. J. Med., 87*: 139–143.

Kettelhut, I. C., and Goldberg, A. L. (1988). Tumor necrosis factor can induce fever in rats without activating protein breakdown in muscle or lipolysis in adipose tissue, *J. Clin. Invest., 81*: 1384–1389.

Kettelhut, I. C., Fiers, W., and Goldberg, A. L. (1987). The toxic effects of tumor necrosis factor in vivo and their prevention by cyclooxygenase inhibitors, *Proc. Natl. Acad. Sci. USA, 84*: 4273-4277.

Kiener, P. A., Marek, F., Rodger, G., Lin, P.-F., Warr, G., and Desideno, J. (1988). Induction of tumor necrosis factor, IFNγ and acute lethality in mice by toxic and non-toxic forms of lipid A, *J. Immunol., 141*: 870–874.

Kirnbauer, R., Kock, A., Schwartz, T., Urbanski, A., Krutmann, J., Borth, W., Damm, D.,

Shipley, G., Ansel, J. C., and Luger, T. A. (1989). IFN-β2, B cell differentiation factor 2, or hybridoma growth factor (IL 6) is expressed and released by human epidermal cells and epidermoid carcinoma cell lines, *J. Immunol., 142*: 1922–1928.

Kishimoto, T. (1989). The biology of IL 6, *Blood, 74*: 1–10.

Klebanoff, S. J., Vadas, M. A., Harlan, J. M., Sparks, L. H., Gamble, J. R., Agosti, J. M., and Waltersdorph, A. M. (1986). Stimulation of neutrophils by tumor necrosis factor, *J. Immunol., 136*: 4220–4225.

Klempner, M. S., Dinarello, C. A., and Gallin, J. I. (1978). Human leukocyte pyrogen induces release of specific granule contents from human neutrophils, *J. Clin. Invest., 61*: 1330–1336.

Kobayashi, K., Allred, C., Cohen, S., and Yoshida, T. (1985). Role of interleukin 1 in experimental pulmonary granuloma in mice, *J. Immunol., 134*: 358–364.

Kohase, M., Henriksen-DeStefano, D., May, L. T., Vilcek, J., and Sehgal, P. B. (1986). Induction of β_2-interferon by tumor necrosis factor: a homeostatic mechanism in the control of cell proliferation, *Cell, 45*: 659–666.

Kohase, M., May, L. T., Tamm, I., Vilcek, J., and Sehgal, P. B. (1987). A cytokine network in human diploid fibroblasts: interactions of β-interferons, tumor necrosis factor, platelet-derived growth factor, and interleukin 1, *Mol. Cell. Biol., 7*: 273–280.

Kortmann, C., Burrichter, H., Monner, D., Jahn, G., Diehl, V., and Peter, H. (1984). Interleukin 1-like activity constitutively generated by Hodgkin derived cell lines, *Immunobiology, 166*: 318–333.

Kovacs, E. J., Oppenheim, J. J., and Young, H. A. (1986). Induction of c-fos and c-myc expression in T lymphocytes after treatment with recombinant IL 1α, *J. Immunol., 137*: 3649–3651.

Kovacs, E. J., Radzioch, D., Young, H. A., and Varesio, L. (1988). Differential inhibition of IL 1 and TNF-α mRNA expression by agents which block second messanger pathways in murine macrophages, *J. Immunol., 141*: 3101–3105.

Kriegler, M., Perez, C., Defay, K., Albert, I., and Lu, S. D. (1988). A novel form of TNF/cachectin is a cell surface cytotoxic transmembrane protein: ramifications for the complex physiology of TNF, *Cell, 53*: 45–53.

Krueger, J. M., Walter, J., Dinarello, C. A., Wolff, S. M., and Chedid, L. (1984). Sleep-promoting effects of endogenous pyrogen (interleukin-1), *Am. J. Physiol., 246*: R994–R999.

Kunkel, S. L., Chensue, S. W., and Phan, S. H. (1986a). Prostaglandins as endogenous mediators of interleukin 1 production, *J. Immunol., 136*: 186–192.

Kunkel, S. L., Wiggins, R. C., Chensue, S. W., and Larrick, J. (1986b). Regulation of macrophage tumor necrosis factor production by prostaglandin E_2, *Biophys. Biochem. Res. Commun., 137*: 404–410.

Kunkel, S. L., Remick, D. G., Strieter, R. M., and Larrick, J. W. (1989). Mechanisms that regulate the production and affects of TNFα, *Crit. Rev. Immunol., 9*: 93–117.

Kupper, T. S., Ballard, D. W., Chua, A. O., McGuire, J. S., Flood, P. M., Horowitz, M. C., Langdon, R., Lightfoot, L., and Gubler, U. (1986a). Human keratinocytes contain mRNA indistinguishable from monocyte interleukin 1α and β mRNA: kertinocyte epidermal cell-derived thymocyte activating factor is identical to interleukin 1, *J. Exp. Med., 164*: 2095–2100.

Kupper, T. S., Dietch, E. A., Baker, C. C., and Wong, W. C. (1986b). The human burn wound as a primary source of interleukin 1 activity, *Surgery, 100*: 409-415.

Kupper, T., May, L., Birchall, N., and Sehgal, P. (1988). Keratinocytes produce interleukin 6, a cytokine which can provide a second signal in the activation of T cells, *J. Invest. Dermatol., 90*: 578.

Kurt-Jones, E. A., Beller, D. I., Mizel, S. B., and Unanue, E. R. (1985). Identification of a membrane-associated interleukin 1 in macrophages, *Proc. Natl. Acad. Sci. USA, 82*: 1204-1208.

Kurt-Jones, E. A., Virgin, H. W., and Unanue, E. R. (1986). In vitro and in vivo expression of macrophage membrane IL 1 in response to soluble and particulate stimuli, *J. Immunol., 137*: 10-14.

Kushansky, K., Lin, N., and Adamson, J. W. (1988). Interleukin 1 stimulates fibroblasts to synthesize granulocyte-macrophage and granulocyte colony-stimulating factors, *J. Cllin. Invest., 81*: 92-97.

Lachman, L. B., Dinarello, C. A., Llansa, N. D., and Fidler, I. J. (1986). Natural and recombinant interleukin 1β is cytotoxic for human melanoma cells, *J. Immunol., 136*: 3098-3102.

Lachman, L. B., Brown, D. C., and Dinarello, C. A. (1987). Growth-promoting effect of recombinant interleukin 1 and tumor necrosis factor for a human astrocytoma cell line, *J. Immunol., 138*: 2913-2916.

Lahdevirta, J., Maury, C. P. J., Teppo, A. M., and Repo, H. (1988). Elevated levels of circulating cachectin/tumor necrosis factor in patients with acquired immunodeficiency syndrome, *Am. J. Med., 85*: 289-291.

Larsen, C. G., Anderson, A. O., Oppenheim, J. J., and Matsushima, K. (1989a). Production of IL 8 by human dermal fibroblasts and keratinocytes in response to IL 1 or TNF, *Immunology, 68*: 31-36.

Larsen, C. G., Zachariae, C. O. C., Oppenheim, J. J., and Matsushima, K. (1989b). Production of monocyte chemotactic and activating factor (MCAF) by human dermal fibroblasts in response to IL 1 or TNF, *Biochem. Biophys. Res. Commun., 160*: 1403.

Lasfargues, A., and Chaby, R. (1988). Endotoxin-induced tumor necrosis factor (TNF): selective triggering of TNF and interleukin-1 production by distinct glucosamine-derived lipids, *Cell. Immunol., 115*: 165-178.

Last-Barney, K., Homon, C. A., Faanes, R. B., and Merluzzi, V. J. (1988). Synergistic and overlapping activities of tumor necrosis factor α and IL 1, *J. Immunol., 141*: 527-530.

Lau, A.. S., and Livesey, J. F. (1989). Endotoxin induction of tumor necrosis factor is enhanced by acid-labile interferon-α in acquired immunodeficiency syndrome, *J. Clin. Invest., 84*: 738-743.

Le, J., and Vilček, J. (1987). TNF and IL 1 cytokines with multiple overlapping biological activities, *Lab. Invest., 56*: 234-248.

Le, J., Weinstein, D., Gubler, U., and Vilček, J. (1987). Induction of membrane associated interleukin 1 by tumor necrosis factor in human fibroblasts, *J. Immunol., 138*: 2137-2142.

Leist, T. P., Frei, K., Kam-Hansen, S., Zinkernagel, R. M., and Fontana, A. (1988). Tumor necrosis factor alpha in the cerebrospinal fluid during bacterial, but not viral, meningitis: evaluation in murine model infections and in patients, *J. Exp. Med., 167*: 1743-1748.

Leizer, T., and Hamilton, J. A. (1989). Plasminogen activator and prostaglandin E_2 levels in human synovial fibroblasts, *J. Immunol., 143*: 971-987.

Lepe-Zuniga, J. L., Mansell, P. W. A., and Hersh, E. M. (1987). Idiopathic production of interleukin-1 in acquired immune deficiency syndrome, *J. Clin. Microbiol., 25*: 1695-1700.

Lewis, C. E., McCarthy, S. P., Lorenzen, J., and McGee, J. O. D. (1989). Heterogeneity among human mononuclear phagocytes in their secretion of lyzozyme, interleukin 1 and type-β transforming growth factor: a quantitative analysis at the single-cell level, *Eur. J. Immunol., 19*: 2037-2043.

Liao, Z., Grimshaw, R. S., and Rosenstreich, D. L. (1984). Identification of a specific interleukin 1 inhibitor in the urine of febrile patients, *J. Exp. Med., 159*: 126-136.

Libby, P., Ordovas, J. M., Auger, K. R., Robbins, A. H., Birinyi, L. K., and Dinarello, C. A. (1986a). Endotoxin and tumor necrosis factor induce interleukin 1 gene expression in adult human vascular endothelial cells, *Am. J. Pathol., 124*: 179-185.

Libby, P., Ordovas, J. M., Birinyi, L. K., Auger, K. R., and Dinarello, C. A. Inducible interleukin-1 gene expression in human vascular smooth muscle cells, *J. Clin. Invest., 78*: 1432-1438.

Libby, P., Warner, S. J. C., and Friedman, G. B. (1988). Interleukin-1: a mitogen for human vascular smooth muscle cells that induces the release of inhibitory prostanoids, *J. Clin. Invest., 81*: 487-498.

Liberman, T., and Baltimore, D. (1990). Activation of interleukin 6 gene expression through the NF-κB transcription factor, *Mol. Cell. Biol., 10*: 2327-2334.

Lieberman, A. P., Pitha, P. M., Shin, H. S., and Shin, M. L. (1989). Production of tumor necrosis factor and other cytokines by astrocytes stimulated with lipopolysaccharide or a neurotropic virus, *Proc. Natl. Acad. Sci. USA, 86:* 6348-6352.

Libert, C., Brouckaert, P., Shaw, A., and Fiers, W. (1990). Induction of interleukin 6 by human and murine recombinant interleukin 1 in mice, *Eur. J. Immunol., 20*: 691-694.

Lin, J. X., and Vilček, J. (1987). TNF and IL 1 causes a rapid and transient stimulation of c-fos and c-myc mRNA levels in human fibroblasts, *J. Biol. Chem., 262*: 11908-11911.

Lindemann, A., Riedel, D., Oster, W., Mertelsmann, R., and Herrmann, F. (1988). Recombinant human granulocyte-macrophage colony stimulating factor induces secretion of autoinhibitory monokines by U-937 cells, *Eur. J. Immunol., 18*: 369-374.

Lindemann, A., Riedel, D., Oster, W., Ziegler-Heitbrock, H. W. L., Mertelsmann, R., and Herrmann, F. (1989). Granulocyte-macrophage colony-stimulating factor induces cytokine secretion by human polymorphonuclear leukocytes, *J. Clin. Invest., 83*: 1308-1312.

Lokesh, B. R., Sayers, T. J., and Kinsella, J. E. (1990). Interleukin 1 and tumor necrosis factor synthesis by mouse peritoneal macrophages is enhanced by dietary n-3 polyunsaturated fatty acids, *Immunol. Lett., 23*: 281-286.

Lonnemann, G., Endres, S., Van der Meer, J. W. M., Cannon, J. G., Koch, K. M., and Dinarello, C. A. (1989). Differences in the synthesis and kinetics of release of interleukin 1α, interleukin 1β and tumor necrosis factor from human mononuclear cells, *Eur. J. Immunol., 19*: 1531-1536.

Loppnow, H., and Libby, P. (1989). Adult vascular endothelial cells express the IL 6 gene differentially in response to LPS or IL 1, *Cell. Immunol., 122*: 493-503.

Loppnow, H., and Libby, P. (1990). Proliferating or interleukin 1-activated human vascular smooth muscle cells secrete copious interleukin 6, *J. Clin. Invest., 85*: 731-738.

Loppnow, H., Brade, L., Brade, H., Rietschel, E. T., Kusumoto, S., Shiba, T., and Flad, H. D. (1986). Induction of human interleukin 1 by bacterial and synthetic lipid A, *Eur. J. Immunol., 16*: 1263-1267.

Lotz, M., Jirik, F., Kabouridis, R., Tsukas, C., Hirano, T., Kishimoto, T., and Carson, D. A. (1988a). BSF-2/IL-6 is costimulant for human thymocytes and T lymphocytes, *J. Exp. Med., 167*: 1253-1258.

Lotz, M., Vaugham, J. H., and Carson, D. A. (1988b). Effect of neuropeptides on production of inflammatory cytokines by human monocytes, *Science, 241*: 1218-1221.

Lowenthal, J. W., Ballard, D. W., Bogerd, H., Bohnlein, E., and Greene, W. C. (1989). Tumor necrosis factor-α activation of the IL-2 receptor-α gene involves the induction of kB-specific DNA binding proteins, *J. Immunol., 142*: 3121-3128.

Luger, T. A., Stadler, B. M., Katz, S. I., and Oppenheim, J. J. (1981). Epidermal cell (keratinocyte)-derived thymocyte activating factor (ETAF), *J. Immunol., 127*: 1493-1498.

Mandrup-Poulsen, T., Bendtzen, K., Dinarello, C. A., and Nerup, J. (1987). Human tumor necrosis factor potentiates human interleukin 1-mediated rat pancreatic β-cell cytotoxicity, *J. Immunol., 139*: 4077-4082.

Mannel, D. N., and Janicke, R. (1989). Induction of monokine production by tumor cells, *Lymphokine Res., 8*: 257-261.

Marina, M. W., Pfeffer, L. M., Guidon, P. T., Jr., and Donner, D. B. (1989). TNF induces phosphorylation of a 28-kDa mRNA cap-binding protein in human cervical carcinoma cells, *Proc. Natl. Acad. Sci. USA, 86*: 8417-8421.

Massague, J., Cheiftz, S., Endo, T., and Nadal-Ginard, B. (1986). Type B transforming growth factor is an inhibitor of myogenic differentiation, *Proc. Natl. Acad. Sci. USA, 83*: 8206-8210.

Massey, W. A., Randall, T. C., Kagey-Sobotka, A., Warner, J. A., MacDonald, S. M., Gillis, S., Allison, A. C., and Lichtenstein, L. M. (1989). Recombinant human IL 1 α and Il 1 β potentiate IgE-mediated histamine release from human basophils, *J. Immunol., 143*: 1875-1880.

Masuda, A., Longo, D., Kobayashi, Y., Appella, E., Oppenheim, J. J., and Matsushima, K. (1988). Induction of mitochondrial manganese superoxide dismutase by IL 1, *FASEB J., 1*: 3087-3091.

Matsushima, K., and Oppenheim, J. J. (1989). Interleukin 8 and MCAF: novel inflammatory cytokines inducible by IL 1 and TNF, *Cytokine, 1*: 2-13.

Matsushima, K., Procopio, A., Abe, H., Scala, G., Ortaldo, J. R., and Oppenheim, J. J. (1985). Production of interleukin 1 activity by normal human peripheral blood B lymphocytes, *J. Immunol., 135*: 1132-1136.

Matsushima, K., Morishita, K., Yoshimura, T., Lavu, S., Kobayashi, Y., Lew, W., Appella, E., Kung, H.-F., Leonard, E. J., and Oppenheim, J. J. (1988a). Molecular cloning of a human monocyte-derived neutrophil chemotactic factor (MDNCF) and the induction of MDNCF mRNA by IL 1 and TNF, *J. Exp. Med., 167*: 1883-1893.

Matsushima, K., Shiroo, M., Kung, H., and Copeland, D. T. (1988b). Purification and characterization of a cytosolic 65 kDa phosphoprotein in human leukocytes whose phosphorylation is augmented by stimulation with interleukin 1, *Biochemistry, 27*: 3765–3770.

Maury, C. P., and Teppo, A. M. (1987). Raised serum levels of cachectin/tumor necrosis factor a in renal allograft rejection, *J. Exp. Med., 166*: 1132–1137.

Maury, C. P., and Teppo, A. M. (1988). Serum immunoreactive interleukin 1 in renal transplant recipients, *Transplantation, 45*: 143–147.

Mawatari, M., Kohno, K., Mizoguchi, H., Matsuda, T., Asoh, K.-I., Van Damme, J., Welgus, H. G., and Kuwano, M. (1989). Effects of tumor necrosis factor and epidermal growth factor on cell morphology, cell surface receptors and the production of tissue inhibitor of metalloproteinases and IL 6 in human microvascular endothelial cells, *J. Immunol., 143*: 1619–1627.

McCarthy, D. O., Kluger, M. J., and Vander, A. J. (1985). Suppression of food intake during infection: is interleukin-1 involved? *Am. J. Clin. Nutr., 42*: 1179–1182.

McIntosh, J. K., Jablons, D. M., Mule, J. J., Nordan, R. P., Rudikoff, S., Lotze, M. T., and Rosenberg, S. A. (1989). In vivo induction of IL-6 by administration of exogenous cytokines and detection of de novo serum levels of IL-6 in tumor-bearing mice, *J. Immunol., 143*: 162–167.

McIntyre, K. M., Unowsky, J., DeLorenzo, W., and Benjamin, W. (1989). Enhancement of antibacterial resistance of neutropenic, bone marrow-suppressed mice by interleukin-1α, *Infect. Immun., 57*: 48–54.

Merrill, J. E., Strom, S. R., Ellison, G. W., and Meyers, L. W. (1989). In vivo study of mediators of inflammation in multiple sclerosis, *J. Clin. Invest., 9*: 84–89.

Milenkovic, L., Rettori, V., Snyder, G. D., Beutler, B., and McCann, S. M. (1989). Cachectin alters anterior pituitary hormone release by a direct action in vitro, *Proc. Natl. Acad. Sci. USA, 86*: 2418–2422.

Miller, S. C., Ito, C. H., Blau, H. M., and Torti, F. M. (1988). Tumour necrosis factor inhibits human myogenesis in vitro, *Mol. Cell. Biol., 8*: 2295–2301.

Mizel, S. B., Dayer, J. M., Krane, S. M., and Mergenhagen, S. E. (1981). Stimulation of rheumatoid synovial cell collagenase and prostaglandin production by partially purified lymphocyte activating factor (interleukin-1), *Proc. Natl. Acad. Sci. USA, 78*: 2474–2477.

Mizel, S. B., Kilian, P., Lewis, J., Paganelli, K. A., and Chizzonite, R. A. (1987). The IL 1 receptor dynamics of IL 1 binding and internalization in T cells and fibroblasts, *J. Immunol., 138*: 2906–2912.

Mochizuki, D. Y., Eisenman, J. R., Conlon, P. J., Larsen, A. D., and Tushinski, R. J. (1987). Interleukin 1 regulates hematopoietic activity, a role previously ascribed to hematopoietin 1, *Proc. Natl. Acad. Sci. USA, 84*: 5267-5271.

Moissec, P., Cavender, D., and Ziff, M. (1986). Production of interleukin 1 by human endothelial cells, *J. Immunol., 136*: 2486–2491.

Molina, J.-M., Scadden, D. T., Byrn, R., Dinarello, C. A., and Groopman, J. E. (1989). Production of tumor necrosis factor α and interleukin 1β by monocyte cells infected with human immunodeficiency virus, *J. Clin. Invest., 84*: 733–737.

Moore, M. A. S., and Waren, D. J. (1987). Synergy of interleukin 1 and granulocyte colony stimulating factor: in vivo stimulation of stem cell recovery and hematopoietic regeneration following 5-fluorouracil treatment of mice, *Proc. Natl. Acad. Sci. USA, 84*: 7134–7137.

Moreno, C., Taverne, J., Mehlert, A., Bate, C. A. W., Brealey, R. J., Meager, A., Rook, G. A. W., and Playfair, J. H. L. (1989). Lipoarabinomannan from mycobacterium tuberculosis induces the production of tumor necrosis factor from human and murine macrophages, *Clin. Exp. Immunol., 76*: 240–245.

Morinaga, Y., Suzuki, H., Takatsuki, F., Akiyama, Y., Taniyama, T., Matsushima, K., and Onozaki, K. (1989). Contribution of IL-6 to the antiproliferative effect of IL-1 and tumor necrosis factor on tumor cell lines, *J. Immunol., 143*: 3538–3542.

Mortensen, R. F., Shapiro, J., Lin, B. F., Douches, S. D., and Neta, R. (1988). Interaction of recombinant interleukin-1 (IL-1) and recombinant tumor necrosis factor (TNF) in the induction of mouse acute phase proteins, *J. Immunol., 140*: 2260–2266.

Movat, H. Z., Burrowes, C. E., Cybulsky, M. I., and Dinarello, C. A. (1987). Acute inflammation and Schwartzman-like reaction induced by interleukin-1 and tumor necrosis factor. Synergistic action of the cytokines in the induction of inflammation and microvascular injury, *Am. J. Pathol., 129*: 463–476.

Muchmore, A. V., and Decker, J. M. (1985). Uromodulin: a unique 85-kilodalton immunosuppressive glycoprotein isolated from urine of pregnant women, *Science, 229*: 479–481.

Muegge, K., Williams, T. M., Kant, J., Karin, M., Chin, R., Schmidt, A., Siebenlist, U., Young, H. A., and Durum, S. K. (1989). IL 1 costimulatory activity on the IL 2 promoter via AP-1, *Science, 246*: 249–251.

Mule, J. J., McIntosh, J. K., Jablons, D. M., and Rosenberg, S. A. (1990). Antitumor activity of recombinant interleukin 6 in mice, *J. Exp. Med., 171*: 629–636.

Munker, R., and Koeffler, P. (1987). In vitro action of tumor necrosis factor on myeloid leukemia cells, *Blood, 69*: 1102–1108.

Murase, T., Hotta, T., Saito, H., and Ohno, R. (1987). Effect of recombinant human tumor necrosis factor on the colony growth of human leukemia progenitor cells and normal hematopoietic progenitor cells, *Blood, 69*: 467–472.

Muto, Y., Nouri-Aria, K. T., Meager, A., Alexander, G. J. M., Eddleston, A. L. W. F., and Williams, R. (1988). Enhanced tumor necrosis factor and interleukin-1 in fulminant hepatic failure, *Lancet*, 2(8602): 72–74.

Myers, M. J., Pullen, J. K., Ghildyal, N., Eustis-Turf, E., and Schook, L. B. (1989). Regulation of IL-1 and TNF-α expression during the differentiation of bone-marrow derived macrophage, *J. Immunol., 142*: 153–160.

Nachman, R. L., Hajjar, K. A., Silverstein, R. L., and Dinarello, C. A. (1986). Interleukin 1 induces endothelial cell synthesis of plasminogen activator inhibitor, *J. Exp. Med., 163*: 1595–1600.

Naitoh, Y., Fukata, J., Tominaga, T., Nakai, Y., Tamai, S., Mori, K., and Imura, H. (1988). Interleukin-6 stimulates the secretion of adrenocorticotropic hormone in conscious, freely-moving rats, *Biochem. Biophys. Res. Commun., 155*: 1459–1463.

Nakajima, K., Martinez-Maza, O., Hirano, T., Breen, E. C., Nishanian, P. G., Salazar-Gonzalez, J. R., Fahey, J. L., and Kishimoto, T. (1989). Induction of IL 6 (B cell stimulatory factor 2/IFNβ2) production by HIV, *J. Immunol., 142*: 531–536.

Nakamura, S., Nakata, K., Kashimoti, S., Yoshida, H., and Yamada, M. (1986). Antitumor effect of recombinant human interleukin 1α against murine syngeneic tumors, *Jpn. J. Cancer Res., 77*: 767–773.

Nakano, K., Okugawa, K., Furuichi, H., Matsui, Y., and Sohmura, Y. (1989). Agumentation of the generation of cytotoxic T lymphocytes against syngeneic tumor cells by recombinant human tumor necrosis factor, *Cell. Immunol., 120*: 154–164.

Nathan, C. F. (1987). Neutrophil activation on biological surfaces: massive secretion of hydrogen peroxide in response to products of macrophages and lymphocytes, *J. Clin. Invest., 80*: 1550–1560.

Nawroth, P. P., Bank, I., Handley, D., Cassimens, J., Chess, L., and Stem, D. (1986). Tumor necrosis factor/cachectin interacts with endothelial cell receptors to induce release of interleukin 1, *J. Exp. Med., 163*: 1363–1375.

Nedwin, G. E., Svedersky, L. P., Bringman, T. S., Palladino, M. A., and Goeddel, D. V. (1985). Effect of interleukin 2, interferon-γ, and mitogens on the production of tumor necrosis factors α and β, *J. Immunol., 135*: 2492–2497.

Neta, R., and Oppenheim, J. J. (1988). Cytokines in therapy of radiation injury, *Blood, 72*: 1093–1095.

Neta, R., Douches, S. D., and Oppenheim, J. J. (1986). Interleukin-1 is a radioprotector, *J. Immunol., 136*: 2483–2485.

Neta, R., Sztein, M. B., Oppenheim, J. J., Gillis, S., and Douches, S. D. (1987). In vivo effects of IL-1. I. Bone marow cells are induced to cycle following administration of IL-1, *J. Immunol., 139*: 1861–1866.

Neta, R., Oppenheim, J. J., and Douches, S. D. (1988a). Interdependence of the radioprotective effects of human recombinant IL-1, TNF, G-CSF, and murine recombinant G-CSF, *J. Immunol., 140*: 108–111.

Neta, R., Vogel, S. N., Sipe, J. D., Wong, G. G., and Nordan, R. P. (1988b). Comparison of in vivo effects of human recombinant IL 1 and human recombinant IL 6 in mice, *Lymphokine Res., 7*: 403–412.

Neta, R., Oppenheim, J. J., and Durum, S. (1990). The cytokine concept, *The Role of Lymphokines in Immunity* (S. Cohen, ed.), CRC Press, Boca Raton, Fla., pp. 29–41.

Newton, R. C., Uhl, J., Covington, M., and Back, O. (1988). The distribution and clearance of radiolabelled human interleukin-1 beta in mice, *Lymphokine Res., 7*: 207–216.

Nordan, R. P., and Potter, M. (1986). A macrophage-derived factor required by plasmacytomas for survival and proliferation in vitro, *Science, 233*: 566–569.

North, R. J., Neubauer, R. H., Huang, J. J. H., Newton, R. C., and Loveless, S. E. (1988). Interleukin 1-induced T-cell-mediated regression of immunogenic murine tumors, *J. Exp. Med., 168*: 2031–2043.

Numeroff, R. P., Aaronson, F. R., and Mier, J. W. (1988). IL-2 stimulates the production of IL-1α and IL-1β by human peripheral blood mononuclear cells, *J. Immunol., 141*: 4250–4257.

Okada, M., Kitahara, M., Kishimoto, S., Matsuda, T., Hirano, T., and Kishimoto, T. (1988). BSF-2/IL-6 functions as killer helper factor in the in vitro induction of cytotoxic T cells, *J. Immunol., 141*: 1543–1549.

Okusawa, S., Gelfand, J. A., Ikejima, T., Connoly, R. J., and Dinarello, C. A. (1988a). Interleukin 1 induces a shock-like state in rabbits: synergism with tumor necrosis factor and the effect of cyclooxygenase inhibition, *J. Clin. Invest., 81*: 1162–1172.

Okusawa, S., Yancey, K. B., van der Meer, J. W. N., Endres, S., Lonnemann, G., Hefter, K., Frank, M. M., Burke, J. F., Dinarello, C. A., and Gelfand, J. A. (1988b). C5a stimulates secretion of tumor necrosis factor from human mononuclear cells in vitro, *J. Exp. Med., 168*: 443–448.

Old, L. J. (1990). Tumor necrosis factor, *TNF: Structure, Mechanism of Action, Role in Disease and Therapy* (B. Bonavida and G. Granger, eds.), S. Karger, Basel, pp. 1–30.

O'Neill, L. A. J., Bird, T. A., and Saklatvala, J. (1990). Interleukin 1 increases GTP binding and hydrolysis in membranes of a thymoma cell line (EL4 NOB.1), *The Molecular and Cellular Biology of Cytokines* (J. J. Oppenheim, M. C. Powanda, M. J. Kluger, and C. A. Dinarello, eds.), Alan R. Liss/Wiley, New York (197–202).

Onozaki, K., Matsushima, K., Aggarwal, B. B., and Oppenheim, J. J. (1985). Human interleukin 1 is a cytocidal factor for several tumor cell lines, *J. Immunol., 135*: 3962–3968.

Onozaki, K., Urawa, H., Tamatani, T., Iwamura, Y., Hashimoto, T., Baba, T., Suzuki, H., Yamada, M., Yamamoto, S., Oppenheim, J. J., and Matsushima, K. (1988). Synergistic interactions of interleukin 1, interferon-β, and tumor necrosis factor in terminally differentiating a mouse myeloid leukemic cell line (MI): evidence that interferon-β is an autocrine differentiating factor, *J. Immunol., 140*: 112–119.

Opp, M., Obal, F., Jr., Cady, A. B., Johannssen, L., and Krueger, J. M. (1989). Interleukin-6 is pyrogenic but not somnogenic, *Physiol. Behav., 45*: 1069–1072.

Oppenheim, J. J., Matsushima, K., Yoshimura, T., Leonard, E. J., and Neta, R. (1989a). Relationship between interleukin 1 (IL 1), tumor necrosis factor (TNF) and a neutrophil attracting peptide (NAP-1), *Agents Actions, 26*: 134–140.

Oppenheim, J. J., Neta, R., Tiberghien, P., Gress, R., Kenny, J., and Longo, D. (1989b). Interleukin 1 enhances survival of irradiated mice treated with allogeneic bone marrow cells, *Blood, 74*: 2257–2263.

Osborn, L., Kunkel, S., and Nabel, G. J. (1989). TNFα and IL 1 stimulate the human immunodeficiency virus (HIV) enhancer by activation of the nuclear factor κB, *Proc. Natl. Acad. Sci. USA, 86*: 2336–2340.

Ostensen, M. E., Thiele, D. L., and Lipsky, P. L. (1987). Tumor necrosis factor α enhances cytolytic activity of human natural killer cells, *J. Immunol., 138*: 4185–4191.

Owen-Schaub, L. B., Crump, W. L., Morin, G. I., and Grimm, E. A. (1989). Regulation of lymphocyte TNF receptors by IL 2, *J. Immunol., 143*: 2236–2241.

Oxholm, A., Oxholm, P., Staberg, B., and Bendtzen, K. (1988). Immuno-histological detection of interleukin 1-like molecules and tumor necrosis factor in human epidermis before and after UVB-irradiation in vivo, *Br. J. Dermatol., 118*: 369–376.

Ozaki, Y., Ohashi, T., Minami, A., and Nakamura, S. (1987). Enhanced resistance of mice to bacterial infection induced by recombinant human interleukin 1 α, *Infect. Immun., 55*: 1436–1442.

Palombella, V. J., Yamashiro, D. J., Maxfield, F. R., Decker, S. J., and Vilcek, J. (1987). Tumor necrosis factor increases the number of epidermal growth factor receptors on human fibroblasts, *J. Biol. Chem., 262*: 1950–1954.

Pawelec, G., Sayers, T., and Busch, F. W. (1989). Regulation of normal myelopoiesis and chronic myelogenous leukemia cell proliferation through a non-cytotoxic mechanism by a γ/S T cell clone, *Immunol. Lett., 33*: 199–204.

Peetre, C., Gullberg, U., Nilsson, E., and Olsson, I. (1986). Effects of recombinant tumor necrosis factor on proliferation and differentiation of leukemic and normal hemopoietic cells in vitro, *J. Clin. Invest., 78*: 1694–1700.

Perlmutter, D. H., Dinarello, C. A., Punzal, P. I., and Colten, H. R. Cachectin/tumor necrosis factor regulates hepatic acute-phase gene expression, *J. Clin. Invest., 78*: 1349–1354.

Pessina, G. P., Pacini, A., Bocci, V., Maioli, T., and Naldini, A. (1987). Studies on tumor necrosis factor (TNF): metabolic fate and distribution of human recombinant TNF, *Lymphokine Res.*, *6*: 35–44.

Peters, P. M., Ortaldo, J. R., Shalaby, M. R., Svedersky, L. P., Nedwin, G. E., Bringman, T. S., Haas, P. E., Aggarwal, B. B., Herberman, R. B., Goeddel, D. V., and Palladino, M. A. (1986). Natural killer-sensitive targets stimulate production of TNF-α but not TNF-β lymphocytes, *J. Immunol.*, *137*: 2592–2598.

Philip, R. (1988). Cytolysis of tumor necrosis factor (TNF)-resistant tumor targets: Differential cytotoxicity of monocytes activated by the interferons, IL-2 and TNF, *J. Immunol.*, *140*: 1345–1349.

Phillip, R., and Epstein, L. B. (1986). Tumor necrosis factor as immunomodulator and mediator of monocyte cytotoxicity induced by itself, γ-interferon and interleukin-1, *Nature*, *323*: 86–89.

Piguet, P.-F., Grau, G. E., Allet, B., and Vassali, P. (1987). Tumor necrosis factor/cachectin is an effector of skin and gut lesions of the acute phase of graft-vs.-host disease, *J. Exp. Med.*, *166*: 1280–1289.

Piquet-Pellorce, C., Homo-Delarche, F., and Dy, M. (1989). Interleukin 1 and/or tumor necrosis factor-α synergize with granulocyte-macrophage colony-stimulating factor to enhance histamine synthesis in hematopoietic cells: role of prostaglandin E_2, *Eur. J. Immunol.*, *19*: 1999–2003.

Pike, B. L., and Nossal, G. J. V. (1985). Interleukin 1 can act as a B-cell growth and differentiation factor, *Proc. Natl. Acad. Sci. USA*, *82*: 8153–8157.

Plaetinck, G., Declercq, W., Tavernier, J., Nabholz, M., and Fiers, W. (1987). Recombinant tumor necrosis factor can induce interleukin 2 receptor expression and cytolytic activity in a rat × mouse T cell hybrid, Short Paper, *Eur. J. Immunol.*, *17*: 1835–1838.

Plaetinck, G., Combe, M. C., Corthesy, P., Seckinger, P., and Nabholz, J. (1989). IL 1 and TNF enhance transcription from the SV40 early promoter in a T cell line, *Eur. J. Immunol.*, *19*: 897–904.

Plata-Salaman, C. R., Ooomura, Y., and Kai, Y. (1988). Tumor necrosis factor and interleukin 1 beta: suppression of food intake by direct action in the central nervous system, *Brain Res.*, *448*: 106–114.

Pober, J. S., Gimbrone, M. A., Jr., Lapierre, L. A., Mendrick, D. L., Fiers, W., Rothlein, R., and Springer, T. A. (1986). Overlapping patterns of activation of human endothelial cells by interleukin 1, tumor necrosis factor, and immune interferon, *J. Immunol.*, *137*: 1893–1896.

Pohlman, T. H., Stanness, K. A., Beatty, P. G., Ochs, H. D., and Harlan, J. M. (1986). An endothelial cell surface factor(s) induced in vitro by lipopolysaccharide, interleukin 1, and tumor necrosis factor-α increases neutrophil adherence by a CDw18-dependent mechanism, *J. Immunol.*, *136*: 4548–4553.

Postlethwaite, A. E., Lachman, L. B., Mainardi, C. L., and Kang, A. H. (1983). Interleukin 1 stimulation of collagenase production by cultured fibroblasts, *J. Exp. Med.*, *157*: 801–806.

Postlethwaite, A. E., Raghow, R., Strickling, G. P., Poppleton, H., Seyer, J. M., and Kang, A. H. (1988). Modulation of fibroblast functions of interleukin 1: increased steady-state accumulation of type 1 procollagen messenger RNAs and stimulation of other functions but not chemotaxis by human recombinant interleukin 1α and β, *J. Cell. Biol.*, *106*: 311–318.

Price, S. R., Mizel, S. B., and Pekala, H. (1986a). Regulation of lipoprotein lipase synthesis and 3T3-L1 adipocyte metabolism by recombinant interleukin 1, *Biochem. Biophys. Acta, 889*: 374-381.

Price, S. R., Olivecrona, T., and Pekala, H. (1986b). Regulation of lipoprotein lipase synthesis by recombinant tumor necrosis factor: the primary regulatory role of the hormone in 3T3-L1 adipocytes, *Arch. Biochem. Biophys., 251*: 738-746.

Ramadori, G., Sipe, J. D., Dinarello, C. A. Mizel, S. B., and Colten, H. R. (1985). Pretranslational modulation of acute phase hepatic protein synthesis by murine recombinant interleukin 1 (IL 1) and purified human IL 1, *J. Exp. Med., 162*: 930-942.

Ranges, G. E., Figari, I. S., Espevik, T., and Palladino, M. A., Jr. (1987). Inhibition of cytotoxic T cell development by transforming growth factor β and reversal by recombinant tumor necrosis factor α, *J. Exp. Med., 166*: 991-998.

Ranges, G. E., Zlotnik, A., Espevik, T., Dinarello, C. A., Cerami, A., and Palladino, M. A., Jr. (1988). Tumor necrosis factor α/cachectin is a growth factor for thymocytes, *J. Exp. Med., 167*: 1472-1478.

Ray, A., Tatter, S. B., May, L. T., and Sehgal, P. B. (1988). Activation of the human "β2-interferon/hepatocyte-stimulatory factor/interleukin 6" promoter by cytokines, viruses, and second messenger agonists, *Proc. Natl. Acad. Sci. USA, 85*: 6701-6708.

Raz, A., Wyche, A., Siegel, N., and Needleman, P. (1988). Regulation of fibroblast cyclooxygenase synthesis by interleukin-1, *J. Biol. Chem., 262*: 3022-3029.

Remick, D. G., Larrick, J., and Kunkel, S. L. (1986). Tumor necrosis factor induced alterations in circulating leukocyte populations, *Biochem. Biophys. Res. Commun., 141*: 818-824.

Remick, D. G., Kunkel, R. G., Larrick, J. W., and Kunkel, S. L. (1987). Acute in vivo effects of human recombinant tumor necrosis factor, *Lab. Invest., 56*: 583-590.

Ristow, H. (1986). BSC-1 growth inhibitor/type β transforming growth factor is a strong inhibitor of thymocyte proliferation, *Proc. Natl. Acad. Sci. USA, 85*: 5531-5533.

Roberts, A. B., Lamb, L. C., Newton, D. L., Sporn, M. B., DeLarco, J. E., and Todaro, G. J. (1980). Transforming growth factors: isolation of polypeptides from virally and chemically transformed cells by acid/ethanol extraction, *Proc. Natl. Acad. Sci. USA, 77*: 3494-3498.

Roberts, A. B., Anzano, M. A., Wakefield, L. M., Roche, N. S., Stern, D. R., and Sporn, M. B. (1985). Type β transforming growth factor: a bifunctional regulator of cellular growth, *Proc. Natl. Acad. Sci. USA, 82*: 119-123.

Rola-Pleszczynski, M., and Lamaire, M. (1985). Leukotrenes augment interleukin 1 production by human monocytes, *J. Immunol., 135*: 3958-3961.

Rosenblum, M. G., and Donato, N. J. (1989). TNFα: A multifacted peptide hormone, *Crit. Rev. Immunol., 9*: 21-44.

Rosoff, P. M. (1989). Characterization of the IL 1 stimulated phospholipase C activity in human T lymphocytes, *Lymphokine Res., 8*: 407-413.

Rosoff, P., Savage, N., and Dinarello, C. (1988). Interleukin 1 stimulated diacylglycerol production in T lymphocytes by a novel mechanism, *Cell, 54*: 73-81.

Rossi, V., Breviario, F., Ghezzi, P., Dejana, E., and Mantovani, A. (1985). Prostacyclin synthesis induced in vascular cells by interleukin-1, *Science, 229*: 174-176.

Rothklein, R., Czajkowski, M., O'Neill, M. M., Marlin, S. D., Mainolfi, E., and Merluzzi, V. J. (1988). Induction of intercellular adhesion molecule 1 on primary and continuous cell lines by pro-inflammatory cytokines: regulation by pharmacologic agents and neutralizing antibodies, *J. Immunol., 141*: 1665–1669.

Ruggiero, V., and Baglioni, C. (1987). Synergistic anti-proliferative activity of interleukin 1 and tumor necrosis factor, *J. Immunol., 138*: 661–663.

Ruggiero, V., Latham, K., and Baglioni, C. (1987). Cytostatic and cytotoxic activity of tumor necrosis factor on human cancer cells, *J. Immunol., 138*: 2711–2717.

Saklatvala, J. (1986). Tumor necrosis factor α stimulates resorption and inhibits synthesis of proteoglycan in cartilage, *Nature, 322*: 547–549.

Sandborg, C. I., Berman, M. A., Andrews, B. S., and Friou, G. J. (1985). Interleukin 1 production by mononuclear cells from patients with scleroderma, *Clin. Exp. Immunol., 60*: 294–302.

Satsangi, J., Wolstencroft, R., Cason, J., Aihley, C., Dumonde, D., and Thompson, R. (1987). Interleukin 1 in Crohn's disease, *Clin. Exp. Immunol., 67*: 594–605.

Sayers, T. J., Macher, I., Chung, J., and Kugler, E. (1987). The production of tumor necrosis factor by mouse bone marrow-derived macrophages in response to bacterial lipopolysaccharide and a chemically synthesized monosaccharide precursor, *J. Immunol., 138*: 2935–2940.

Sayers, T. J., Wiltrout, T. A., Bull, C. A., Denn, A. C., III, Pilaro, A. M., and Lokesh, B. (1988). Effect of cytokines on polymorphonuclear neutrophil infiltration in the mouse. Prostaglandin- and leukotriene-independent induction of infiltration by IL-1 and tumor necrosis factor, *J. Immunol., 141*: 1670–1677.

Scala, G., Allavena, P., Djeu, J. Y., Kasahara, T., Ortaldo, J. R., Herberman, R. B., and Oppenheim, J. J. (1984a). Human large granular lymphocytes are potent producers of IL 1, *Nature, 309*: 56–59.

Scala, G. Kuang, Y. D., Hall, R. E., Muchmore, A. V., and Oppenheim, J. J. (1984b). Accessory cell function of human B cells. I. Production of both interleukin 1-like activity and a interleukin 1 inhibitory factor by an EBV-transformed human B cell line, *J. Exp. Med., 159*: 1637–1652.

Scales, W. E., and Kunkel, S. L. (1989). Regulatory interactions between IL 1, TNF and other inflammatory mediators, *Interleukin 1, Inflammation and Disease* (R. Boxford and B. Henderson, eds.), Elsevier, Oxford, pp. 163–172.

Schade, V. F., Burmeister, I., Engel, R., Reinke, M., and Wolter, D. T. (1989). Lipoxygenase inhibitors suppress formation of tumor necrosis factor in vitro and in vivo, *Lympokine Res., 8*: 245–250.

Scheurich, P., Unglaub, B., Maxeiner, B., Thoma, B., Zugmaier, G., and Pfizenmaier, K. (1986). Rapid modulation of TNF membrane receptors by activators of protein kinase C, *Biochem. Biophys. Res. Commun., 141*: 855–859.

Scheurich, P., Thoma, B., Ucer, U., and Pfizenmaier, K. (1987). Immunoregulatory activity of recombinant human TNFα: induction of TNF receptors on human T cells and TNFα mediated enhancement of T cell responses, *J. Immunol., 138*: 1786–1790.

Scheurich, P., Kobrich, G., and Pfizenmaier, K. (1989). Antagonistic control of TNF receptors by protein kinase A and C, *J. Exp. Med., 170*: 947–956.

Schindler, R., Mancilla, J., Endres, S., Ghorbani, R., Clark, S. C., and Dinarello, C. A. (1990). Correlations and interactions in the production of interleukin-6 (IL 6), IL 1 and tumor necrosis factor (TNF) in human blood mononuclear cells: IL-6 suppresses IL 1 and TNF, *Blood, 75*: 40–47.

Schmidt, J. A., Mizel, S. B., Cohen, D., and Green, I. (1982). Interleukin 1, a potential regulator of fibroblast proliferation, *J. Immunol., 128*: 2177–2182.
Schmidt, J. A., Oliver, C. N., Lepe-Zuniga, J. L., Green, I., and Gery, I. (1984). Silica-stimulated monocytes release fibroblast proliferation factors identical to interleukin 1, *J. Clin. Invest., 73*: 1462–1472.
Schutze, S., Scheurich, P., Pfizenmaier, K., and Kronke, M. (1989). Tumor necrosis factor signal transduction tissue-specific serine phosphorylation of 26-kDa cytosolic protein, *J. Biol. Chem., 264*: 3562–3567.
Schwartz, G. N., MacVittie, T. J., Vigneulle, R. M., Patchen, M. L., Douches, S. D., Oppenheim, J. J., and Neta, R. (1987). Enhanced hematopoietic recovery in irradiated mice pretreated with interleukin-1 (IL-1), *Immunopharmacol. Immunotoxicol., 9*: 371–389.
Schwartz, G. N., Patchen, M. L., Neta, R., and MacVittie, T. J. (1990). An increase in the number of spleen colony-forming units (CFU-S) at the time of irradiation is not necessary for the radioprotection of mice pretreated with interleukin-1, *Radiat. Res., 121*: 220–226.
Scuderi, P. (1989a). Suppression of human leukocyte tumor necrosis factor secretion by the serine protease inhibitor *p*-toluenesulphoryl-L-argenine methyl ester (TAME), *J. Immunol., 143*: 168–173.
Scuderi, P., Sterling, K. E., Lam, K. S., Finley, P. R., Ryan, K. J., Ray, C. G., Peterson, E., Slymen, D. J., and Salmon, S. E. (1986). Raised serum levels of tumor necrosis factor in parasitic infections, *Lancet, 2*(8520): 1364–1365.
Scuderi, P., Dorr, R. T., Liddil, J. D., Finley, P. R., Meltzer, P., Raitano, A. B., and Rybski, J. (1989b). Alpha-globulins suppress human leukocyte tumor necrosis factor secretion, *Eur. J. Immunol., 19*: 939–942.
Seckinger, P., Williamson, K., Balavoine, J.-F., Mach, B., Mazzei, G., Shaw, A., and Dayer, J.-M. (1987). A urine inhibitor of interleukin 1 activity affects both interleukin 1α and 1β but not tumor necrosis factor α, *J. Immunol., 139*: 1541–1545.
Seckinger, P., Isaaz, S., and Dayer, J.-M. (1988). A human inhibitor of tumor necrosis factor α, *J. Exp. Med., 167*: 1511–1516.
Seelentag, W. K., Mermond, J.-J., Montesano, R., and Vassalli, P. (1987). Additive effects of interleukin-1 and tumor necrosis factor α on the accumulation of three granulocyte and macrophage colony stimulating factor mRNA in human endothelial cells, *EMBO J., 6*: 2261–2265.
Sehgal, P. B., Walther, Z., and Tamm, I. (1987). Rapid enhancement of B2-interferon/B cell differentiation factor BSF-2 gene expression in human fibroblasts by diacylglycerols and the calcium ionophore A23187, *Proc. Natl. Acad. Sci. USA, 84*: 3663–3667.
Seljelid, R., Figenschau, Y., Bogwald, J., Rasmussen, L. T., and Austgulen, R. (1989). Evidence that tumor necrosis factor induced by aminated β1-3D polyglucose is mediated by a concerted action of local and systemic cytokines, *Scand. J. Immunol., 30*: 687–694.
Selmaj, K. W., Farooq, M., Norton, W. T., Raine, C. S., and Brosnan, C. F. (1990). Proliferation of astrocytes in vitro in response to cytokines: a primary role for tumor necrosis factor, *J. Immunol., 144*: 129–135.
Shabo, Y., Lotem, J., Rubinstein, M., Revel, M., Clark, S. C., Wolf, S. F., Kamen, R., and Sachs, L. (1988). The myeloid blood cell differentiation-inducing protein MGI-2A is interleukin-6, *Blood, 72*: 2070–2073.
Shakhov, A. N., Collart, M. A., Vassalli, P., Nedospasov, S. A., and Jongeeneel, C. V.

(1990). κB-type enhancers are involved in lipopolysaccharide-mediated transcriptional activation of the tumor necrosis factor α gene in primary macrophages, *J. Exp. Med., 171*: 35–47.

Shalaby, M. R., Aggarwal, B. B., Rinderknecht, E., Svedersky, L. P., Finkle, B. S., and Palladino, M. A., Jr. (1985). Activation of human polymorphonuclear neutrophil functions by interferon-γ and tumor necrosis factors, *J. Immunol., 135*: 2069–2073.

Shalaby, M. R., Espevik, T., Rice, G. C., Ammann, A. J., Figari, I. S., Ranges, G. E., and Palladino, M. A., Jr. (1988). The involvement of human tumor necrosis factors-α and -β in the mixed lymphocyte reaction, *J. Immunol., 141*: 499–503.

Shalaby, M. R., Waage, A., and Espevik, T. (1989). Cytokine regulation of interleukin 6 production by human endothelial cells, *Cell. Immunol., 121*: 372–382.

Sherman, M. L., Weber, B. L., Datta, R., and Kufe, D. W. (1990). Transcriptional and posttranscriptional regulation of macrophage-specific colony stimulating factor gene expression by tumor necrosis factor. Involvement of arachidonic acid metabolites, *J. Clin. Invest., 85*: 442–447.

Shirakawa, F., and Mizel, S. (1989). In vitro activation and nuclear translocation of NF-kB catalyzed by cyclic AMP-dependent protein kinase and protein kinase C, *Mol. Cell. Biol., 9*: 2424–2430.

Shirakawa, F., Yamashita, U., Chedid, M., and Mizel, S. (1988). Cyclic AMP-an intracellular second messenger for interleukin 1, *Proc. Natl. Acad. Sci. USA, 85*: 8201–8205.

Shoham, S., Davenne, D., Cady, A. B., Dinarello, C. A., and Krueger, J. M. (1987). Recombinant tumor necrosis factor and interleukin 1 enhance slow-wave sleep, *Am. J. Physiol., 253*: R142–R149.

Sica, A., Wang, J. M., Colotta, F., Dejana, E., Mantovani, A., Oppenheim, J. J., Larsen, C. G., Zachariae, C. O. C., and Matsushima, K. (1990). Monocyte chemotactic and activating factor gene expression induced in endothelial cells by IL-1 and tumor necrosis factor, *J. Immunol., 144*: 3034–3038.

Silen, M. L., Firpo, A., Morgello, S., Lowry, S. F., and Francus, T. (1989). Interleukin-1α and tumor necrosis factor α cause placental injury in the rat, *Am. J. Pathol., 135*: 239–244.

Sipe, J. D., Vogel, S. N., Douches, S. D., and Neta, R. (1987). Tumor necrosis factor/cachectin is a less potent inducer of serum amyloid a synthesis than interleukin-1, *Lymphokine Res., 6*:93–101.

Sironi, M., Breviaro, F., Proserpio, P., Biondi, A., Vecchi, A., Van Damme, J., Dejana, E., and Mantovani, A. (1989). IL 1 stimulates IL 6 production in endothelial cells, *J. Immunol., 142*: 549–553.

Sisson, S. D., and Dinarello, C. A. (1988). Production of interleukin-1α, interleukin-1β and tumor necrosis factor by human mononuclear cells stimulated with granulocyte-macrophage colony-stimulating factor, *Blood, 72*: 1368–1374.

Smith, M. R., Munger, W. E., Kung, H.-F., Takacs, L., and Durum, S. (1990). Direct evidence for an intracellular role for TNFα. Microinjection of TNF kills target cells, *J. Immunol., 144*: 162–169.

Snyder, D. S., and Unanue, E. R. (1982). Corticosteroids inhibit murine macrophage Ia expression and interleukin 1 production, *J. Immunol., 129*: 1803–1805.

Sporn, M. B., Roberts, A. B., Lalage, M. W., and Assoian, R. K. (1986). Transforming growth factor-β: biological function and chemical structure, *Science, 233*: 532–534.

Staruch, M. J., and Wood, D. D. (1983). The adjuvanicity of interleukin 1 in vivo, *J. Immunol., 130*: 2191-2194.

Stashenko, P., Dewhirst, F. E., Peros, W. J., Kent, R. L., and Ago, J. M. (1987). Synergistic interactions between interleukin-1, tumor necrosis factor and lymphotoxin in bone resorption, *J. Immunol., 138*: 1464-1468.

Steffen, M., Ottmann, O. G., and Moore, M. A. S. (1988). Simultaneous production of tumor necrosis factor-α and lymphotoxin by normal T cells after induction with IL-2 and anti-T3, *J. Immunol., 140*: 2621-2624.

Stern, L., and Kunos, G. (1988). Synergistic regulation of pulmonary β-adrenergic receptors by glucocorticoid and interleukin-1, *J. Biol. Chem., 268*: 15876-15879.

Strieter, R. M., Kunkel, S. L., Showelll, H. J., Remick, D. J., Phan, S. H., Ward, P. A., and Marks, R. M. (1989). Endothelial cell gene expression of a neutrophil chemotactic factor by TNF-α, LPS, and IL 1β, *Science, 243*: 1467-1469.

Suda, T., Tozawa, F., Ushiyama, T., Sumitomo, T., Yamada, M., and Demura, H. (1990). Interleukin-1 stimulated corticotropin-releasing factor gene expression in rat hypothalamus, *Endocrinology, 126*: 1223-1228.

Sugarman, B. J., Aggarwal, B. B., Hass, P. E., Figari, I. S., Palladino, M. A., and Shepard, H. M. (1985). Recombinant human tumor necrosis factor α: effects on proliferation of normal and transformed cells in vitro, *Science, 230*: 943-945.

Suttles, J., Carruth, L. M., and Mizel, S. B. (1990). Detection of IL 1α and IL 1β in the supernatants of paraformaldehyde-treated human monocytes. Evidence against a membrane form of IL 1, *J. Immunol., 144*: 170-174.

Symons, J. A., Bundick, R. V., Suckling, A. J., and Rumsby, M. G. (1987). Cerebrospinal fluid interleukin 1 like activity during chronic relapsing experimental allergic encephalomyelitis, *Clin. Exp. Immunol., 68*: 648-654.

Symons, J. A., McDowell, T. L., di Giovine, F. S., Wood, N. C., Capper, S. J., and Duff, G. W. (1989). Interleukin 1 in rheumatoid arthritis: potentiation of immune responses with the joint, *Lymphokine Res., 8*: 365-372.

Tabibzadeh, S. S., Santhanam, U., Sehgal, P. B., and May, L. T. (1989). Cytokine-induced production of IFN-β2/IL 6 by freshly explanted human endometrial cells; modulation by estradiol-17β, *J. Immunol., 142*: 3134-3139.

Takacs, L., Kovacs, E. J., Smith, M. R., Young, H. A., and Durum, S. K. (1988). Detection of IL 1α and IL 1β gene expression by in situ hybridization: tissue localization of IL 1 mRNA in the normal C57BL/6 mouse, *J. Immunol., 141*: 3081-3085.

Takai, Y., Wong, G. G., Clark, S. C., Burakoff, S. J., and Herrmann, S. H. (1988). B cell stimulatory factor-2 is involved in the differentiation of cytotoxic T lymphocytes, *J. Immunol., 140*: 508-512.

Takatsuki, F., Okano, A., Suzuki, C., Chieda, R., Takahara, Y., Hirano, T., Kishimoto, T., Hamuro, J., and Akiyama, Y. (1988). Human recombinant interleukin 6/B cell stimulatory factor 2 (IL-6/BSF-2) augments murine antigen-specific antibody responses in vitro and in vivo, *JH. Immunol., 141*: 3072-3077.

Tanabe, O., Akira, S., Kamiya, T., Wong, G. G., Hirano, T., and Kishimoto, T. (1988). Genomic structure of the murine IL 6 gene: high degree of conservation of potential regulatory sequences between mouse and human, *J. Immunol., 141*: 3875-3881.

Tartakovsky, B., Kovacs, E. J., Takacs, L., and Durum, S. K. (1986). T cell clone producing

IL 1-like activity after stimulation with antigen presenting B cells, *J. Immunol., 137*: 160–166.

Taverne, J., Bate, C. A. W., and Playfair, J. H. L. (1989). Induction of TNF in vitro as a model for the identification of toxic malaria antigens, *Lymphokine Res., 8*: 317–322.

Tiku, K., Tiku, M. L., and Skosey, J. L. (1986). Interleukin 1 production by human polymorphonuclear neutrophils, *J. Immunol., 136*: 3677–3685.

Tovey, M. G., Content, J., Gresser, I., Gugenheim, J., Blanchard, B., Guymarho, J., Poupart, P., Gigon, M., Shaw, A., and Fiers, W. (1988). Genes for IFN-β2 (IL-6), tumor necrosis factor, and IL 1 are expressed at high levels in the organs of normal individuals, *J. Immunol., 141*: 3106–3110.

Tracey, K. J., Lowry, S. F., Fahey, T. S., III, Albert, J. D., Fong, Y., Hesse, D., Beutler, B., Manogue, K. R., Calvano, S., Wei, H., et al. (1987). Cachectin/tumor necrosis factor induces lethal shock and stress hormone responses in the dog, *Surg. Gynecol. Obstet., 164*: 415–422.

Tsujimoto, M., Yokota, S., Vilček, J., and Weissmann, G. (1986). Tumor necrosis factor provokes superoxide anion generation from neutrophils, *Biochem. Biophys. Res. Commun., 137*: 1094–1100.

Turner, M., Londei, M., and Feldmann, M. (1987). Human T cells from auto-immune and normal individuals can produce tumor necrosis factor, *Eur. J. Immunol., 17*: 1807–1814.

Ulich, T. R., del Castillo, J., Keys, M., Granger, G. A., and Ni, R. X. (1987). Kinetics and mechanism of recombinant human interleukin 1 and tumor necrosis factor α induced changes in circulating numbers of neutrophils and lymphocytes, *J. Immunol., 139*: 3406–3415.

Unglaub, R., Maxeiner, B., Thoma, B., Pfizenmaier, K., and Scheurich, P. (1987). Down regulation of tumor necrosis factor sensitivity via modulation of TNF binding capacity by protein kinase C activators, *J. Exp. Med., 166*: 1788–1797.

Urban, J. L., Shepard, H. M., Rothstein, J. L., Sugarman, B. J., and Schreiber, H. (1986). Tumor necrosis factor: a potent effector molecule for tumor cell killing by activated macrophages, *Proc. Natl. Acad. Sci. USA, 83*: 5233–5237.

Uyttenhove, C., Coulie, P. G., and Van Snick, J. (1988). T cell growth and differentiation induced by interleukin-HPI/IL-6, the murine hybridoma/plasmacytoma growth factor, *J. Exp. Med., 167*: 1417–1427.

Valone, F. H., and Epstein, L. B. (1988). Biphasic platelet-activating factor synthesis by human monocytes stimulated with IL-1β, tumor necrosis factor, or IFN-γ, *J. Immunol., 141*: 3945–3950.

Van Damme, J., Obdenakker, G., Simpson, R. J., Rubira, M. R., Cayphas, S., Vink, A., Billiau, A., and Van Snick, J. (1987). Identification of the human 26 K protein (IFN-β2) as a B-cell hybridoma/plasmocytoma growth induced by interleukin 1 and tumor necrosis factor, *J. Exp. Med., 165*: 914–919.

Van Oers, M. H. J., Van der Heyden, A. A. P. A. M., and Aarden, L. A. (1988). Interleukin 6 (IL-6) in serum and urine of renal transplant recipients, *Clin. Exp. Immunol., 71*: 314–319.

Vilček, J., Palombella, V. J., Henriksen-Destefano, D., Swenson, C., Feinman, R., Nirai, M., and Tsujimoto, M. (1986). Fibroblast growth enhancing activity of tumor necrosis factor and its relationship to other polypeptide growth factors, *J. Exp. Med., 163*: 632–643.

Vink, A., Uyttenhov, C., Wauters, P., and Van Snick, J. (1990). Accessory factors involved in murine T cell activation: distinct roles of interleukin 6, interleukin 1 and tumor necrosis factor, *Eur. J. Immunol., 1*: 1-6.

Visner, G. A., Dougall, W. C., Wilson, J. M., Burr, I. A., and Nick, H. S. (1990). Regulation of manganese superoxide dismutase by lipopolysaccharide, interleukin-1, and tumor necrosis factor, *J. Biol. Chem., 265*: 2856-2864.

Vogel, S. N., Douches, S. D., Kaufman, E. N., and Neta, R. (1987). Induction of colony stimulating factor in vivo by recombinant interleukin-1α and recombinant tumor necrosis factor α, *J. Immunol., 138*: 2143-2148.

Vogel, S. N., Kaufman, E. N., Tate, M., and Neta, R. (1988). Recombinant interleukin 1 α and recombinant tumor necrosis factor alpha synergize in vivo to induce early endotoxin tolerance and associated hematopoietic changes, *Infect. Immun., 56*: 2650-2657.

Waage, A., and Espevik, T. (1988). Interleukin 1 potentiates the lethal effect of tumor necrosis factor α/cachectin in mice, *J. Exp. Med., 167*: 1987-1992.

Waage, A., Espevik, T., and Lamvik, J. (1986). Detection of tumor necrosis factor-like cytotoxicity in serum from patients with septicemia but not from untreated cancer patients, *Scand. J. Immunol., 24*: 739-743.

Waage, A., Halstensen, A., and Espevik, T. (1987). Association between tumor necrosis factor in serum and fatal outcome in patients with meningococcal disease, *Lancet, 2*(8529): 355-357.

Waage, A., Brandtzaeg, P., Halstensen, A., Kierulf, P., and Espevik, T. (1989a). The complex pattern of cytokines in serum from patients with meningococcal septic shock, *J. Exp. Med., 169*: 333-338.

Waage, A. Kaufman, C., Espevik, T., and Husby, G. (1989b). Interleukin 6 in synovial fluid from patients with arthritis, *Clin. Immunol. Immunopathol., 50*: 394-398.

Wahl, S. M., Hunt, D. A., Wakefield, L. M., McCartney-Francis, N., Wahl, L. M., Roberts, A. B., and Sporn, M. B. (1987). Transforming growth factor type β induces monocyte chemotaxis and growth factor production, *Proc. Natl. Acad. Sci. USA, 84*: 5788-5792.

Wallach, D., Holtmann, H., Aderka, D., Rubinstein, M., Auni, Y. S., Sharov, I., and Engelman, H. (1989). Mechanism which take part in regulation of the response to tumor necrosis factor, *Lymphokine Res., 8*: 359-363.

Wankowicz, Z., Megyeri, P., and Issekutz, A. (1988). Synergy between tumor necrosis factor α and interleukin 1 in the induction of polymorphonuclear leukocyte migration during inflammation, *J. Leukocyte Biol., 43*: 349-365.

Warner, S. J. C., and Libby, P. (1989). Human vascular smooth muscle cells: target for and source of tumor necrosis factor, *J. Immunol., 142*: 10-109.

Warner, S. J. C., Auger, K. R., and Libby, P. (1987). Human interleukin 1 induces interleukin 1 gene expression in human vascular smooth muscle cells, *J. Exp. Med., 165*: 1316-1331.

Weiss, L., Haeffner-Cavaillon, N., Laude, M., Cavaillon, J.-M., and Kazatchkine, M. D. (1989). Human T cells and interleukin 4 inhibit the release of interleukin 1 induced by lipopolysaccharide in serum-free cultures of autologous monocytes, *Eur. J. Immunol., 19*: 1347-1350.

Werber, H. I., Emancipater, S. N., Tykocinski, M. L., and Sedor, J. R. (1987). The interleukin 1 gene is expressed by rat glomerular mesangial cells and is augmented in immune complex glomerulonephritis, *J. Immunol., 138*: 3207-3212.

Wewers, M. D., and Herzyk, D. J. (1989). Alveolar macrophages differ from blood monocytes in human IL 1β release: quantitation by enzyme-linked immunoassay, *J. Immunol., 143*: 1635-1641.

White, C. W., Ghezzi, P., Dinarello, C. A., Caldwell, S. A., McMurtry, I. F., and Repine, J. E. (1987). Recombinant tumor necrosis factor/cachectin and interleukin 1 pretreatment decreases lung oxidized glutathione accumulation, lung injury and mortality in rats exposed to hyperoxia, *J. Clin. Invest., 79*: 1868-1876.

White, C. W., Ghezzi, P., McMahon, S., Dinarello, C. A., and Repine, J. E. (1989). Cytokines increase rat lung antioxidant enzymes during exposure to hyperoxia, *J. Appl. Physiol., 66*: 1003-1007.

Williams, D. E., and Broxmeyer, H. E. (1988). Interleukin-1 alpha enhances the in vitro survival of purified murine granulocyte-macrophage progenitor cells in the absence of colony-stimulating factors, *Blood, 71*: 1608-1615.

Wong, G. H. W., and Goeddel, D. V. (1986). Tumor necrosis factors α and β inhibit viral replication and synergize with interferons, *Nature, 323*: 819-822.

Wong, G. H. W., and Goeddel, D. V. (1988). Induction of manganous superoxide dismutase by tumor necrosis factor: possible protective mechanism, *Science, 242*: 941-944.

Wright, S. C., Jewett, A., Mitsuyasu, R., and Bonavida, B. (1988). Spontaneous cytotoxicity and tumor necrosis factor production by peripheral blood monocytes from AIDS patients, *J. Immunol., 141*: 99-104.

Yamamoto, R. S., Johnson, D. L., Masunaka, I. K., and Granger, G. A. (1984). Phorbol myristate acetate induction of lymphotoxins from continuous human B lymphoid cell line in vitro, *J. Biol. Response Modif., 3*: 76-87.

Yokota, S., Geppert, T. D., and Lipsky, P. E. (1988). Enhancement of antigen- and mitogen-induced human T lymphocyte proliferation by tumor necrosis factor-α, *J. Immunol., 140*: 531-536.

Zhang, Y., Lin, J.-X., and Vilček, J. (1988a). Synthesis of interleukin G (interferon β2/B cell stimulatory factor 2) in human fibroblasts is triggered by an increase in intracellular cyclic AMP, *J. Biol. Chem., 263*: 6177-6182.

Zhang, Y., Lin, J.-X., Yip, Y. K., and Vilček, J. (1988b). Enhancement of cAMP levels and of protein kinase activity by TNF and IL 1 in human fibroblasts: role in the induction of IL 6, *Proc. Natl. Acad. Sci. USA, 85*: 6802-6805.

Zilberstein, A., Ruggieri, R., Korn, J. H., and Revel, M. (1986). Structure and expression of cDNA and genes for human interferon-β2, a distinct species inducible by growth-stimulatory cytokines, *EMBO J., 5*: 2529-2537.

Zucali, J. R., Dinarello, C. A., Oblon, D. J., Gross, M. A., Anderson, L., and Weiner, R. S. (1986). Interleukin 1 stimulates fibroblasts to produce granulocyte-macrophage colony-stimulating activity and prostaglandin E_2, *J. Clin. Invest., 77*: 1857-1863.

Zucali, J. R., Elfenbein, J., Barth, K. C., and Dinarello, C. A. (1987). Effects of human interleukin 1 and human tumor necrosis factor on human T lymphocyte colony formation, *J. Clin. Invest., 80*: 772-777.

Zucali, J. R., Broxmeyer, H. E., Gross, M. A., and Dinarello, C. A. (1988). Recombinant human tumor necrosis factor α and β stimulate fibroblasts to produce hematopoietic growth factors in vivo, *J. Immunol., 140*: 840-844.

23

Recombinant Human TNF-α: Preclinical Studies and Results from Early Clinical Trials

SAM SAKS
Xoma Corporation, Berkeley, California

MICHAEL ROSENBLUM
University of Texas, M. D. Anderson Cancer Center, Houston, Texas

I. INTRODUCTION

Tumor necrosis factor (TNF) was originally identified as antitumor activity present in the sera of mice primed with Calmette-Guérin bacillus (BCG) and then treated with endotoxin (1). Preparations of these sera were shown to induce hemorrhagic necrosis in the murine methylcholanthrene-induced sarcoma model (Meth A sarcoma). TNF subsequently was further characterized as a protein product of activated macrophages that could cause hemorrhagic necrosis in the Meth A sarcoma model (2). This cytokine has since been shown to have immunomodulatory and metabolic activities as well as antiproliferative effects on tumor cells (2–5). TNF-α is one of two related cytotoxic cytokines, the other being TNF-β (lymphotoxin), a T-cell product that also causes hemorrhagic necrosis in the Meth A model (3,6,7). TNF-α and TNF-β share an amino acid sequence homology of approximately 30% and the same cell surface receptor (7,8).

Demonstration of the in vitro and in vivo antiproliferative and immunomodulatory activities of TNF-α has led to the initiation of clinical trials designed to evaluate its potential as an antineoplastic agent (9). Preclinical and clinical studies were initially limited by the availability of purified TNF from natural sources and by the presence of endotoxin and other biologically active molecules in those preparations. The application of recombinant DNA methodology has resulted in the production of large quantities of highly purified (>99%) recombinant human tumor necrosis factor α for both preclinical and clinical studies. The 157 amino acid sequence of recombinant TNF (rTNF) is identical to the naturally occurring protein (10). There is one disulfide bond between positions 69 and 101. The molecular weight is approximately 17,000 Da with a specific activity of approximately 4×10^7 units per milligram protein in the L-cell cytotoxicity assay with actinomycin D (11,12). The natural product is not glycosylated. In this chapter we review the preclinical and early clinical studies performed with rTNF.

II. PRECLINICAL STUDIES

A. Antiproliferative Effects

rTNF has both in vitro and in vivo antiproliferative activity against a variety of human tumor cells (13,14). Although it has cytotoxic and cytostatic effects on malignant cells, it does not inhibit and, in fact, may stimulate the growth of diploid fibroblast cell lines. A broad range of inhibitory activity has been demonstrated for rTNF in vitro against human colon carcinoma, breast carcinoma, cervical carcinoma, melanoma, myeloma, and myeloid leukemia cell lines (9,15–20). Included among the sensitive cell lines are those known to be resistant to cytotoxic antineoplastic drugs (18,20). The human tumor stem cell assay has shown an equally broad range of antiproliferative activity for rTNF (22). Of further note is that cell lines chronically exposed to vincristine or doxorubicin to induce pleiotropic drug resistance develop increased sensitivity to rTNF (21). This increased sensitivity does not appear to be mediated by the P glycoprotein. Doses of rTNF <2.5 ng can inhibit some lung and colon cancer cell lines. The differentiating activity of rTNF has also been shown to occur with leukemia cell line targets. Synergistic cytotoxic effects of rTNF in combination with other differentiating agents such as retinoic acid have been reported (17,22,24).

The mechanism of TNF cytotoxic effects against human tumor cells is not completely understood. Cell cycle analysis indicates that sensitive tumor cells accumulate in the G2 phase of the cell cycle (27). TNF must first bind to a cell surface receptor and then be internalized to produce cytotoxicity (28). Receptors are necessary for cells to exhibit sensitivity to the inhibitory effects of TNF, although not all cells that have receptors are sensitive. The number of receptors per cell does not appear to correlate with the degree of sensitivity to TNF antiproliferative effects. The cytotoxicity of TNF can be enhanced by inhibitors of protein synthesis such as cycloheximide (31). This suggests that inhibition of protein synthesis may prevent production of intracellular factors which could otherwise counteract the antiproliferative effects of TNF. Moreover, down-regulation of c-*myc* and c-*myb* oncogene expression has been observed in HeLa and leukemia cell lines following exposure to TNF (29,30). It has also been postulated that synergy with actinomycin

D and other alkylating agents many be mediated through the inhibition of the cellular enzyme topoisomerase II (32).

Synergy between TNF and other cytokines has been well documented with respect to antiproliferative effects. Perhaps the most striking and well-studied example is the synergy observed with the combination of TNF and γ-interferon (IFN-γ) (18,33). Cytotoxic synergy has been observed even when tumor cell lines are minimally sensitive to the single agents (18). The mechanism by which this synergy occurs is unknown. Receptors for TNF are increased on the cell surface following exposure to IFN-γ, although the magnitude of the increase is not great enough to account for the degree of synergy. Scheduling may be important since in vitro antitumor effects are greatest when IFN-γ exposure precedes TNF or when cells are exposed to both agents simultaneously. Synergistic antiproliferative effects of TNF and IFN-γ are observed not only on bone marrow precursors from leukemic patients but also on progenitor cells from normal individuals, albeit to a lesser extent (35). Finally, it should be noted that synergistic cytotoxicity has also been reported when TNF is combined with other biologics, such as IL-1 and IL-2 (34,36). Lymphokine-activated killer (LAK) cell generation by IL-2 is enhanced by TNF and TNF has been measured in LAK cell supernatants (37), suggesting that synergistic interactions between these two cytokines may play a role in the antitumor effects observed with interleukin-2 plus LAK cell therapy.

In vivo cytotoxic and cytostatic antitumor activity of rTNF has been documented against syngeneic murine tumors, human tumor xenografts in nude mice, and in fresh human tumors in the subrenal capsule assay of immunologically intact mice. Antitumor activity has been observed following intravenous, subcutaneous, and intraperitoneal administration. Not all cell lines that demonstrate in vitro antiproliferative effects after rTNF treatment are sensitive in vivo and some tumors that display in vivo activity are not sensitive in vitro. The classic Meth A cell line is relatively insensitive to rTNF in vitro, and antiproliferative activity is not observed if it is implanted intraperitoneally in mice (M. Palladino, personal communication). However, the Meth A cell line implanted subcutaneously undergoes hemorrhagic necrosis following rTNF therapy. Increased survival can also be demonstrated in these animals. This suggests that the degree of vascularization of the tumor may determine in vivo sensitivity to rTNF. Moreover, the sensitivity of different murine sarcoma cell lines in vivo has been related to the immunogenicity of the cell line tested (38). It should be noted that rTNF cannot only induce tumor regression and prolong survival but can also produce cures (14,38) and tumor-specific immunity (14). Tumor-specific immunity can be demonstrated by the inability to reestablish tumors from the same cell line in animals that have been cured by rTNF treatment.

Pharmacokinetic and tissue distribution studies of rTNF have been performed in mice (44). These studies have revealed that rTNF is rapidly cleared following intravenous injection with a plasma half-life of approximately 20 min. Tissue distribution studies using labeled human rTNF in mice show a wide distribution with prominent uptake in the liver and kidneys. The observation that labeled material is not found in the brain suggests that rTNF does not cross the intact blood-brain barrier to a significant extent.

B. Immunomodulatory Effects

The immunomodulatory properties of rTNF suggest that indirect host-mediated effects might be as important as direct cytotoxic actions in achieving antitumor effects in vivo. Immunomodulatory effects have been shown to occur with a wide range of effector cells including neutrophils, lymphocytes, and macrophages. For example, rTNF up-regulates constitutively expressed HLA antigens and enhances the ability of IFN-α to induce class I and II HLA antigens on tumor cells (45). Augmentation of antibody-dependent cellular cytotoxicity (ADCC) has also been observed (56).

TNF is a major mediator of macrophage cytotoxicity and the sensitivity of human tumor cell lines to rTNF correlates with their sensitivity to macrophage-mediated cytotoxicity (46). The induction of macrophage cytotoxicity by other cytokines is inhibited by antibodies to TNF (26). Activated macrophages produce TNF in a large quantities accounting for up to 5% of all protein produced (B. Beutler, personal communication). Peroxide generation is increased after exposure to rTNF, as is true for IFN-α. IFN-α treated macrophages increase their production of TNF. Induction of TNF mRNA in macrophage cell lines treated with rTNF suggests that autocrine regulation may occur (47,53).

Neutrophil peroxide generation and phagocytosis of latex beads are both enhanced by rTNF (48,49). Moreover, neutrophil adherence to endothelial surfaces is increased by rTNF (50). This is thought to result from the induction of adherence antigens on both the endothelial and neutrophil cell surface (54). This may be an important component of the mechanism of the hemorrhagic necrosis seen in the Meth A sarcoma and other tumor models (51). rTNF increases the efflux of neutrophils out of blood vessels and is a chemotactic factor for polymorphonuclear leukocytes and monocytes (52). TNF is also an important regulator of T-lymphocyte function. Both the induction of IL-2 receptors on T cells and the mixed lymphocyte reaction (MLR) are stimulated by TNF (56). Receptors for TNF are also increased on activated T cells (55). TNF is a mediator of natural killer (NK) cell activity, although the sensitivity of human cell lines to NK cell-mediated killing does not correlate with sensitivity to TNF (59).

The complex interactions between TNF and other lymphokines and monokines are still being explored. rTNF stimulates IL-1 release by macrophages and endothelial cells (51). T-cell activation by IL-1 is more significant than that induced by rTNF, although rTNF induces greater T-cell cytotoxicity in vitro and in vivo. IFN-γ regulates rTNF receptors and synergizes with rTNF in up-regulating class II expression. rTNF and IFN-γ are present in LAK cell supernatants (37). The recent production of many of these cytokines by recombinant technology will further enhance the understanding of these components of the immune system. Understanding these interactions will facilitate a more rational approach to combination cytokine therapy.

C. Anti-infective Activity

A broad range of anti-infective activities have been identified for TNF. Cytotoxic activity has been observed against the malaria parasite *Plasmodium falciparum* (57) and TNF has been shown to protect against malarial infection in mice (51). Eosinophils can be activated by TNF to kill schistosomes and elevated levels of TNF have been found in patients with parasitic diseases such as leishmaniasis (58).

TNF is produced during septic shock and may play a role in host defense to bacterial infection (59). For example, an endotoxin-resistant strain of mice has been identified that is deficient in TNF production when stimulated with LPS (62). However, disparate hemodynamic effects have been observed when endotoxin treatment has been compared to rTNF treatment in primates (data on file, Genetech, Inc.). Moreover, antibodies to TNF are unable to reverse shock after endotoxin is administered to mice (61). While TNF may play a role in the pathophysiology of endotoxic shock, it is likely that there are several other mediator proteins and/or peptides are involved in this complex biologic event.

Direct antiviral activity, including selective cytotoxicity against virally infected target cells, has been documented for rTNF (62,63). Both RNA and DNA viruses have been shown to be sensitive to rTNF in these studies, including human immunodeficiency virus. The antiviral effects of rTNF can be augmented synergistically by IFN-α (63).

D. Metabolic Effects

Among the best studied metabolic effects of rTNF are its role in lipid and bone metabolism. rTNF inhibits lipoprotein lipase, an activity that can be used to create a sensitive bioassay (64). It has also been demonstrated that treatment of 3T3-L1 cells with rTNF inhibits the production of adipocyte-specific gene products, which are markers of adipocyte differentiation (65). More recently, the effects on 3T3-L1 cells have also been demonstrated following treatment with TNF-β as well as with IFN-γ (66). In addition, inhibition of lipoprotein lipase activity has been observed in cancer patients receiving IFN-α (67). The demonstration that changes in lipid metabolism may be mediated by other cytokines and the inability of highly purified rTNF to cause cachexia in mice treated repeatedly with low doses (51), suggest that TNF is not the sole mediator of cachexia in humans. Moreover, high circulating levels of TNF activity have not been identified in cachectic cancer patients.

With respect to effects on bone metabolism, both TNF-α and TNF-β stimulate bone resorption and inhibit bone formation in vitro (68). This activity is also observed with IL-1, and combinations of rTNF and IL-1 can result in synergistic effects on bone resorption (69). Since these effects on bone metabolism depend on the inhibition of osteoblasts and the stimulation of osteoclasts, the TNFs are thought to be important components of osteoclast activating factor (OAF) activity, which is found in patients with multiple myeloma (70). The TNFs and IL-1 may also be responsible for the bone resorption seen in chronic inflammatory diseases such as rheumatoid arthritis.

III. RESULTS OF EARLY CLINICAL TRIALS

A. Single-Dose Phase I Studies

Single-does phase I studies of rTNF in cancer patients designed to explore the tolerance and pharmacokinetics of rTNF in humans were initiated in 1985 (72,73,75). In two of these trials, patients received escalating single dose of rTNF up to 200 $\mu g/m^2$ by intravenous (IV) bolus and up to 250 $\mu g/m^2$ by intramuscular (IM) or subcutaneous (SQ) injection. Both the starting dose and dose escalation scheme were based on extensive preclinical toxicology studies in rodents and primates that preceded the human trials. The most commonly observed systemic toxicities in humans were fever, chills, fatigue, and headache, which were noted with all routes of administration. Fever and chills were almost universal symptoms and appeared to be dose dependent. Significant hypotension was observed only rarely and was easily corrected with intravenous fluid replacement. No weight loss was observed. Local toxicity (inflammation) at the injection site was observed following subcutaneous and to a lesser extent, intramuscular administration, at doses of 100 $\mu g/m^2$. Biopsy of the injection site in a limited number of patients revealed a mixed cellular infiltrate. The inflammatory reaction consisted of induration and erythema peaking at 1 to 3 days and resolving within 5 to 7 days.

The most frequent laboratory abnormalities observed following the administration of single doses of rTNF included mild to moderate anemia without reticulocytosis, and mild hyperglycemia. Sporadic leukopenia and hepatic transaminase elevations were also noted. No consistent changes in coagulation parameters were observed, including prothrombin, partial thromboplastin and thrombin times, fibrinogen, or fibrin split products. Factor VIII antigen and other acute-phase reactants such as C reactive protein were noted to increase following low doses of rTNF. rTNF did not induce platelet aggregation in vitro (74). Neither renal insufficiency nor electrolyte abnormalities were observed. Finally, an immunoassay for the detection of both neutralizing and nonneutralizing antibodies to rTNF was performed at the end of treatment and up to 28 days after the last injection with negative results.

Table 1 Serum Pharmacokinetic Summary of rTNF after IV Bolus Administration[a]

Dose (μg/m^2)	Number of patients	Half-life (min)	V_d (L)	AUC (ng/mL x min)
25	3	15.9 ± 3.6	66 ± 30	10.5 ± 2.7
35	5	13.9 ± 1	13.3 ± 5	19.7 ± 5.3
50	4	16 ± 2	13.4 ± 1.1	89.6 ± 13.9
60	5	18 ± 0.4	17.7 ± 4	114.6 ± 26.5
100	3	17 ± 2	12 ± 4	224.8 ± 69

[a] Values expressed as means ± SEM. V_d, volume of distribution; AUC, area under the concentration curve.

The therapeutic trials with recombinant human TNF would not be complete without studies of the pharmacokinetic behavior of this agent. A variety of groups (75,83,85) have examined the pharmacokinetics of TNF after IV administration. A phase I clinical trial of rTNF was performed at M. D. Anderson Cancer Center (75). Patients received TNF at dose levels ranging from 1 to 200 μg/m^2 administered as an intravenous bolus or by the intramuscular route. To evaluate pharmacokinetics, venous blood sample were collected before injection and at 20 min, 40 min, and 1, 1.5, 2, 4, 6, 8, 12, 18, and 24 h following IM doses, and at 5, 10, 20, and 40 min, and 1, 1.5, 2, 4, 6, 8, 12, 18, and 24 h after IV doses. Blood samples were centrifuged and the serum was decanted and stored at -20°C until analysis. Serum rTNF liters were measured by ELISA at Genentech, Inc. A solid-phase ELISA was performed using a sandwich technique with two polyclonal antibodies to rTNF, one of which was conjugated to a horseradish peroxidase label. The ELISA assay can detect rTNF reliably at 100 to 2800 pg/mL. In addition, a bioassay (L-M cell cytotoxicity with actinomycin D added) (11) was performed on specimens that were positive in the ELISA.

The mean serum concentrations at each time point for all patients at a given dose were calculated. Individual serum rTNF clearance curves were constructed and nonlinear regression analyses were performed for each patient. Serum concentrations, half-lives, volumes of distribution, and the area under the concentration curve (AUC) were then calculated for each patient individually using standard pharmacokinetic techniques (98).

Table 1 is a summary of the pharmacokinetic parameters calculated from the ELISA-detectable concentrations of rTNF in the serum of patients receiving IV bolus doses of rTNF ranging from 5 to 100 μg/m^2. The dose-corrected area under the curve for rTNF given by IV bolus administration appears to increase with in-

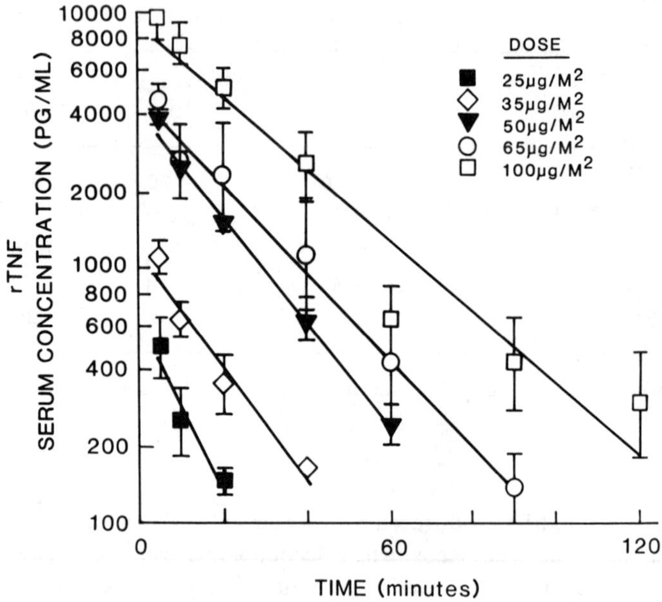

Figure 1 Disappearance from serum of patients after bolus (IV) administration of various doses of recombinant TNF-a. TNF-a concentrations were determined by ELISA assay. Data points shown represent the mean TNF-a concentration determined in several patients. For further details, see Ref. 72. (Reprinted with permission of Cancer Research.)

creasing doses (Fig. 1; Table 1). The apparent volume of distribution (*Vd*) was 66 L at the 25-μg/m^2 dose. The decrease in apparent volume of distribution *Vd* observed with increasing doses of rTNF suggests saturation of clearance mechanisms responsible for extravascular distribution. The saturation of these mechanisms appeared to be maximal at doses of 50 μg/m^2 and above. After IV bolus injection, the clearance of ELISA-detectable material closely fit ($r^2 > 0.95$) an open, one-compartment mathematical model (Fig. 1). Moreover, determinations of rTNF activity in the serum following IV bolus administration using the L-M cell cytotoxicity bioassay correlated with ELISA measurements (data not shown). In contrast to the IV bolus route, IM-administered rTNF was not consistently detected in patients' sera by ELISA until doses reached 150 μg/m^2 or greater. Peak serum levels were usually obtained within 2 h and ELISA-positive material occasionally persisted for 24 h after the injection. None of the patients has circulating antibodies to TNF prior to the study, nor did any patient develop antibodies by the completion of the study.

The clearance of rTNF as measured by ELISA following IV bolus administration was monoexponential, suggesting an open one-compartment mathematical model (Fig. 1). This appears to be similar to the pharmacokinetics of other recombinant lymphokines (99,100). In contrast to the IV route of administration, IM-administered rTNF occasionally resulted in sustained concentrations of rTNF in serum. Because of the small number of measurements for each patient studied, pharmacokinetic calculations were not possible after IM administration.

Pharmacokinetic studies by Creaven et al. (83) have shown that the half-life in plasma was less than 30 min after IV administration. Pharmacokinetic studies by Moritz et al. (101) showed a serum half-life in humans ranging from 11 to 17 min at doses between 0.04 and 0.16 mg/m^2 but found a prolonged clearance with a plasma half-life ranging from 54 to 70 min at the dose range 0.20 to 0.28 mg/m^2. In murine models (102), rTNF was found to have a plasma half-life of approximately 10.5 min. Therefore, the clearance of human TNF in murine models is rapid and monophasic, similar to the clearance of human TNF in humans. rTNF pharmacokinetics appear to be dose dependent with decreasing clearance and increasing half-life as the dose is increased. This observation indicates that extra caution must be applied as the dose of rTNF is escalated.

Although not a principal objective in the single-dose phase I trials of rTNF, all patients were monitored for evidence of antitumor effects. Several patients, including individuals with lymphoma, renal cancer, colon cancer, and myeloma, showed objective evidence of tumor regression, although no complete or partial responses were observed. These observations confirmed that rTNF could be administered to humans safely, in a dose range associated with anticancer effects without the appearance of severe dose-limiting toxicities such as shock or cachexia.

B. Multiple-Dose Phase I Studies

Following the completion of the single-dose phase I trials of rTNF multiple-dose phase I studies were initiated to determine the tolerance and toxicity of repeated administration of rTNF using treatment schedules suitable for evaluation in the phase II setting (76,78–86). These studies explored several different schedules of administration [including continuous (daily), pulse (5 days every 2 to 3 weeks), and intermittent (once or 3 times weekly) schedules] as well as different routes of administration (subcutaneous, intramuscular, and intravenous). Rates of intravenous infusion were also varied from 30 min to 24 h. The patient population studied was limited to patients with advanced, usually heavily pretreated malignancies. A Karnofsky performance score of 60% was necessary for patient enrollment. Preserved hematologic, renal, and hepatic function was also required. Patients with clinically significant cardiac or vascular disease were excluded, as were patients with intracranial metastases.

The principal objective of these multiple-dose phase I trials was to define the maximum tolerated dose (MTD) for phase II testing. To this end, patients were extensively monitored for clinical and laboratory evidence of rTNF-related toxicity. Patients underwent repeated physical examination and monitoring of routine hematology, clinical chemistry, coagulation, and urinalysis parameters. In addition, in some studies, patients were more extensively monitored for evidence of metabolic effects of rTNF therapy, with particular emphasis on lipid and protein metabolism. Limited studies of in vivo immunomodulatory effects of rTNF were also undertaken, including monitoring of changes in immunologic phenotype as determined by cell sorter analysis (77). Although the determination of antitumor effects was not a principal objective of these multiple-dose phase I trials, all patients were evaluated for evidence of anticancer effect so as to obtain some indication as to appropriate targets for phase II trials. Finally, all patients were monitored for the occurrence of antibody to rTNF using an immunoassay capable of detecting both neutralizing and nonneutralizing antibodies.

The spectrum of clinical toxicities associated with multiple-dose administration of rTNF in these phase I trials was similar to that observed following single-dose administration. The most commonly occurring systemic toxicities included fever, chills, fatigue, and headache. The fever and chills appeared to be dose dependent and were occasionally dose limiting. Such symptoms were generally more severe following short intravenous infusions compared with continuous intravenous infusions and intramuscular or subcutaneous injections. The severity of the chills appeared to be disproportionate to the degree of temperature elevation. Both fever and chills were largely controlled by pharmacologic intervention with such agents as acetaminophen, meperidine, and nonsteroidal anti-inflammatory drugs. In contrast to the constitutional toxicity associated with interferon administration, there was little evidence of tolerance; that is, the intensity of the fever and chills decreased only minimally following prolonged courses of rTNF therapy. Constitutional toxicities other than fever and chills were noted less frequently following rTNF treatment. Progressive incapacitating fatigue, as is commonly observed following interferon therapy at high doses, was unusual following treatment with rTNF. Headache was noted sporadically; however, it was severe in a minority of patients requiring narcotic analgesics for relief. Gastrointestinal toxicity such as nausea, vomiting, and diarrhea occurred in a minority of patients. Anorexia was less common than with interferon therapy and there were no observations of severe weight loss in patients receiving rTNF in these multiple-dose phase I trials. It should be noted, however, that the mean duration of therapy with rTNF in these studies was less than 2 months, so that it is possible that more prolonged courses of therapy might be associated with weight loss.

A number of preclinical observations suggested that hypotension might be a dose-limiting toxicity for rTNF in humans, and indeed, this proved to be the case in several of the multiple-dose phase I trials. Effects on blood pressure were clearly dose related, so that precipitous unexpected decreases in blood pressure leading to clinical shock did not occur, at least in the clinical trial experience reported thus far in the United States (77–87). Hypotension associated with rTNF therapy was partially prevented by prehydration with normal saline and/or by hydration during the first 6 h following therapy. The use of pressors to correct rTNF-induced hypotension was required only rarely. As a dose-limiting toxicity, hypotension was most clearly associated with short intravenous infusions (30 min) as opposed to more prolonged infusions and intramuscular or subcutaneous injection. It is of interest that the maximum tolerated dose for once weekly or five-times-weekly treatment schedules was approximately the same, in the range 150 to 225 $\mu g/m^2$ day for one preparation of rTNF (77–83). This suggests that the hypotensive effects of rTNF do not extend beyond a 24-h period. In fact, if repeated doses are administered at least 8-h intervals, the maximum tolerated dose for a single infusion of rTNF is relatively unaffected (83).

As was the case for single-dose phase I trials, dose-limiting local inflammation following intramuscular or subcutaneous injection of rTNF was observed in the multiple-dose phase I studies. In most patients, these effects were limited to erythema and induration at the injection site, which tended to peak approximately 2 to 3 days after injection and to resolve within 7 days. Ulceration at the injection site was observed in an occasional patient, but these lesions healed without scarring. Local inflammation proved to be a dose-limiting toxicity for both subcutaneous and intramuscular injection at doses greater than 75 and 150 $\mu g/m^2$ per day, respectively. Some tolerance to local inflammatory effects of rTNF has been observed in multiple-dose phase I trials involving daily subcutaneous or intermuscular injections.

All patients entered on these multiple-dose phase I trials of rTNF were carefully monitored for clinical toxicities involving vital organs such as the heart, lungs, and central nervous system. Cardiac toxicity appears to be a rare occurrence following rTNF therapy. There have been only rare reports of acute ischemic events and arythymias in association with rTNF therapy, although these may only represent exacerbation of underlying cardiac disease. Following initial observations that patients with extensive underlying pulmonary tumor and/or infection may develop respiratory insufficiency in the setting of rTNF therapy, attempts were made to monitor patients prospectively for pulmonary toxicity using diffusing capacity (DLCO). The results of this prospective monitoring revealed a decrease of approximately 10 to 15% may occur following prolonged therapy at high doses, but this decrease in DLCO is readily reversible following discontinuation of treatment and is not associated with clinical symptomatology (87). In view of these observations, patients with extensive pulmonary tumor and/or infection and evidence of respiratory insufficiency as indicated by spirometry or arterial blood gas measurements should be excluded from clinical trials of rTNF. There have been only rare reports of other pulmonary toxicities, such as acute bronchospasm in association with rTNF therapy. These events have been reversible and have not been associated with the formation of antibody to rTNF. Finally, central nervous system toxicity has been only infrequently observed in multiple-dose phase I trials of rTNF and may be related to route of administration. Patients receiving continuous intravenous infusions and intramuscular injections have rarely experienced transient focal neurological deficits, including aphasia and extremity weakness. These symptoms have occurred in the absence of underlying central nervous system pathology, including metastatic disease as documented by CT scans and electroencephalograms. The etiologic basis for these CNS toxicities remains unknown. Seizures have also occasionally been observed following rTNF therapy, although in the majority of cases, these have been related to the presence of previously unsuspected intracranial metastases.

The most commonly observed laboratory abnormalities following rTNF therapy in multiple-dose phase I trials involve changes in various hematologic and metabolic parameters. With respect to the former, leukopenia, thrombocytopenia, and anemia have all been observed, although they are rarely dose-limiting toxicities. Leukopenia is more common following continuous intravenous infusion, whereas thrombocytopenia appears to be more common following subcutaneous an intramuscular injection, suggesting different mechanisms of action. Thrombocytopenia may be dose limiting when rTNF is administered by subcutaneous or intramuscular injection. Acute granulocytopenia has been observed immediately following short infusions of rTNF (30 min) followed by a rebound above baseline over the next several hours. If intravenous infusions are administered once or three times weekly, cumulative granulocytopenia is quite uncommon. Although 30-min infusions for 5 consecutive days often results in a decrease in granulocytes at the end of the treatment cycle, clinically significant granulocytopenia is rare. Recovery to baseline usually occurs within 72 to 96 h. Transient eosinophilia and monocytosis have also been observed on this schedule, particularly after the second and third day of therapy. However, no significant change in lymphocyte subsets has been noted to date. The kinetics of the leukocyte changes following short intravenous infusions of rTNF on various schedules suggests changes in the compartmentalization and/or bone marrow release of circulating white blood cells as opposed to an effect on myelopoiesis. However, the latter mechanism of action may be important following prolonged exposures to rTNF, such as would occur following continuous intravenous infusion and intramuscular or subcutaneous injection. With respect to the anemia observed following multiple-dose administration of rTNF, the decrease in hemoglobin is generally mild, not associated with reticulocytosis, and rarely requires transfusion. Several of the multiple—dose phase I trials of rTNF have involved extensive monitoring of patients for evidence of rTNF-related metabolic effects. Although mild hyperglycemia and hypertriglyceridemia have been observed, the degree of hypertriglyceridemia may be less than that observed with other cytokines, such as IFN-γ (67).

Hypercholesterolemia has not been seen. There is evidence of increased free fatty acid turnover and negative nitrogen balance, although these observations must be regarded as preliminary (77). rTNF also appears to induce an acute-phase inflammatory response, as evidenced by increases in serum cortisol and factor VIII antigen, as well as decrease in serum zinc (76). Finally, in the majority of multiple-dose phase I trials of rTNF, there has been little evidence of either hepatic or renal toxicity other than sporadic increases in serum transaminases and serum creatinine measurements. However, clinical trials with one preparation of rTNF have identified both hepatic toxicity and renal insufficiency as dose-limiting toxicities (83,84). Whether this is the result of the particular treatment regimen tested or the composition of the product itself is presently unresolved. Electrolyte abnormalities following rTNF therapy have been quite rare. As has been the case in early clinical trials with other recombinant lymphokines, patients treated with rTNF in multiple-dose phase I studies have been monitored for the occurrence of antibody to TNF using an assay capable of detecting both neutralizing and nonneutralizing antibodies. Results have been reported thus far only for the rTNF preparation from one manufacturer (88); antibodies have yet to be detected in more than 150 patients who received repeated doses of rTNF by intravenous infusion and intramuscular or subcutaneous injection.

Early phase II trials have now been completed for both systemic and local routes of administration. Phase I combination therapy trials with rTNF and interferon-γ, interleukin-2, and cytoxic chemotherapy have also been completed. Therapeutic activity has not been seen in single-agent phase II trials of systemic administration in patients with melanoma, renal cancer (89), and Kaposi's sarcoma (90). Hematologic malignancies such as acute myelogenous leukemia did not respond to rTNF therapy in phase II trials. Synergistic toxicity has not been a problem when rTNF has been combined with other lymphokines in phase I trials (91–93), although inhibition of interferon-γ's immunomodulatory activity has been noted (94) for that combination. No evidence of synergistic efficacy is available from these combination trials. It is unclear if lack of efficacy can be attributed to the timing of administration of each agent. Although these phase II results are discouraging, issues of dose intensity, therapeutic regimen, and immunomodulatory effects are still being studied and have led some to the conclusion that TNF is "still a promising agent" (95).

In contrast to trials of systemic administration, efficacy has been observed in trials utilizing local therapy with rTNF (8,97). Perhaps this apparent increased activity is due simply to dose intensity at the tumor site, although other factors, such as time of exposure and immunomodulatory effects, may be playing a role. Certainly, response rates and duration need to be more clearly defined before any final conclusions can be drawn from these studies. One interesting activity observed in intraperitoneal studies is reduction of ascites in patients with peritoneal carcinomatosis without a reduction in tumor (A. Markowitz, personal communication). This observation suggests a possible palliative role for rTNF in patients with intraperitoneal disease, although larger studies are needed to further define the response rates and therapeutic index.

IV. SUMMARY

The application of recombinant DNA technology to the production of tumor necrosis factor has resulted in the availability of large quantities of a highly purified protein product. This product has been evaluated extensively in preclinical studies, which have documented a direct cytostatic and cytotoxic effect on human tumor cells, as well as a variety of immunomodulatory effects on various immune effector cells, including neutrophils, macrophages, and T cells. In addition, a number of anti-infective and metabolic effects have been documented.

In addition to its in vitro effects, rTNF has been shown to have antitumor activity in vivo in preclinical studies involving both transplantable murine tumors and human tumor xenografts. Such observations have led to the evaluation of rTNF as a potential antineoplastic agent in humans. Both single- and multiple-dose phase I studies have confirmed that rTNF can be safely administered to patients with advanced malignancies in a dose range associated with anticancer effect without concomitant serious toxicities such as shock and cachexia. The most commonly observed clinical toxicities include constitutional symptoms, such as fever, chills, headache, and fatigue, and toxicities, which can be at least partially controlled with concomitant administration of nonsteroidal anti-inflammatory drugs, such as acetaminophen and meperidine. Hypotension, which occurs at high doses administered by short intravenous infusion, can usually be prevented by prehydration with intravenous fluids or otherwise controlled by the administration. An intense local inflammatory reaction at the injection site as well as thrombocytopenia appear to be the dose-limiting toxicities after subcutaneous and intramuscular administration. Neurologic toxicity is infrequent, except following continuous intravenous infusion, where it may manifest as transient focal neurologic deficits or seizure. Prolonged administration of rTNF at higher doses may be associated with transient, subclinical decreases in diffusing capacity. Patients with underlying cardiopulmonary disease should be excluded from rTNF therapy in future clinical studies until the end-organ toxicities of this agent are better defined. For at least one preparation of rTNF there appears to be no evidence for the formation of antibodies to rTNF in patients who receive multiple administrations of the agent. Pharmacokinetic studies have shown a relatively rapid clearance following intravenous infusion with a half-life of 15 to 30 min and dose-dependent pharmacokinetics. rTNF can be detected in the serum following intramuscular or subcutaneous injection at only relatively high doses, suggesting a decreased bioavailability with the routes of administration.

Early phase I studies defined tolerable dose ranges for each route of administration and began to explore immunomodulatory and metabolic effects of rTNF. Phase I combination studies and early phase II work has not suggested major therapeutic activity for systemic administration of rTNF. Local therapy studies have shown initial promise but will require further study before conclusions can be drawn about its utility.

REFERENCES

1. Carswell, E. A., Old, L. J., Kassel, R. L., Green, S., Fiore, N., and Williamson, B., An endotoxin-induced serum factor that causes necrosis of tumors, *Proc. Natl. Acad. Sci. USA, 72*(9): 3666–3670, 1975.
2. Hoffmann, M. K., Oettgen, H. F., Old, L. J., Mittler, R. S., and Hammerling, U., Induction and immunological properties of tumor necrosis factor, *J. Reticuloendothel. Soc., 23*(4): 307–319, 1978.
3. Granger, G. A., Orr, S. L., and Xamamoto, R., Lymphotoxins, macrophage cytotoxins and tumor necrosis factor: an interrelated family of antitumor effector molecules, *J. Clin. Immunol., 5*: 217–266, 1985.
4. Talmadge, J. E., Tribble, H. R., Pennington, R. W., Phillips, R. W., and Wiltrout, R. H., Immunomodulatory and immunotherapeutic properties of recombinant gamma interferon and recombinant tumor necrosis factor in mice, *Cancer Res., 47*: 2563–2570, 1987.
5. Beutler, B., Greenwald, D., Hulmes, J. D., Chang, M., Pan, Y. C., Mathison, J., Ulevitch, R., and Cerami, A., Identity of tumor necrosis factor and the macrophage-secreted factor cachectin, *Nature, 316*: 552–554, 1985.
6. Pennica, D., Nedwin, G. E., Hayflick, J. S., Seeburg, P. H., Derynck, R., Palladino, M. A., Kohr, W. J., Aggarwal, B. B., and Goeddel, D. V., Human tumor necrosis factor: precursor structure, expression, and homology to lymphotoxin, *Nature, 312*: 724–729, 1984.
7. Gray, P. W., Aggarwal, B. B., Benton, C. V., Bringman, T. S., and Henzel, W. J., Cloning and expression of CDNA for human lymphotoxin, a lymphokine with tumor necrosis activity, *Nature, 312*: 721–724, 1984.
8. Aggarwal, B. B., Eessalu, T. E., and Hass, P. E., Characterization of receptors for human tumor necrosis factor and their regulation by gamma interferon, *Nature, 318*: 665–667, 1985.
9. Helson, L., Carswell, E. A., and Old, L. J., Effect of tumor necrosis factor on cultured human melanoma cells, *Nature, 258*: 731, 1975.
10. Aggarwal, B., Kohr, W., Hass, P., Moffat, B., Spencer, S. A., Henzel, W. J., Bringman, T. S., Nedwin, G. E., Goeddel, D. V., and Harkins, R. N., Human tumor necrosis factor production, purification and characterization, *J. Biol. Chem., 260*: 2345–2354, 1985.
11. Kramer, S. M., and Carver, M. W., Serum-free in vitro bioassay for the detection of tumor necrosis factor, *J. Immunol. Methods, 92*: 201–206, 1986.
12. Kramer, S. M., Carver, M. E., and Apperson, S. M., Comparison of TNF-α and TNF-β

cytolytic biological activities in a serum-free bioassay, *Lymphokine Res., 5*(Suppl. 1): 139–143, 1986.

13. Sugarman, B. J., Aggarwal, B. B., Hass, P. E., Figari, I. S., Palladino, M. A., and Shepard, H. M., Recombinant human tumor necrosis factor-α: effects on proliferation of normal and transformed cells in vitro, *Science, 230*: 943–945, 1985.
14. Palladin, M. A., Shalaby, M. R., Kramer, S. M., Ferrgiola, B. L., Baughman, R. A., Deleo, A. B., Crase, D., Marafino, B., Aggarwal, R. B., Rigari, I. S., Liggitt, D., and Patton, J. S., Characterization of the antitumor activities of human tumor necrosis factor-alpha and the comparison with other cytokines: induction of tumor specific immunity, *J. Immunol., 138*: 4023–4032, 1987.
15. Ruggiero, V., Latham, K., and Baglioni, C., Cytostatic and cytotoxic activity of tumor necrosis factor on human cancer cells, *J. Immunol., 138*: 2711–2717, 1987.
16. Watanabe, N., Niitsu, Y., Neda, H., Sone, H., Yamaguchi, N., Umersu, T., and Urushizaki, I., Antitumor effects of tumor necrosis factor against various primarily cultured human cancer cells, *Jpn. J. Cancer Res., 76*(11): 1115–1119, 1985.
17. Munker, R., and Koeffler, H. P., In vitro action of tumor necrosis factor on myeloid leukemia cells, *Blood, 69*: 1102, 1987.
18. Schiller, J., Bittner, G., Storer, B., and Willson, J. K., Synergistic antitumor effects of tumor necrosis factor and gamma-interferon on human colon carcinoma cell lines, *Cancer Res., 47*: 2809–2813, 1987.
19. Rosenblum, M. G., Donato, N., Kessler, D., and Gutterman, J., Preliminary characterization of human recombinant tumor necrosis factor antiproliferative effects on human cancer cells in culture, *Proc. Am. Assoc. Cancer Res., 28*: 398, 1987.
20. Salmon, S. E., Soehnlen, B., and Scuderi, P., Natural product-resistant leukemia and myeloma cells exhibit sensitivity to recombinant tumor necrosis factor, *Blood, 66*(5 Suppl. 1): 229, 1985.
21. Soehnlen, B., Liv, R., and Salmon, S. E., Recombinant tumor necrosis factors exhibit antitumor activity against clonogenic human tumor cells and synergism with gamma interferon, *Proc. Am. Assoc. Cancer Res., 26*: 303, 1985.
22. Trinchieri, G., Kobayashi, M., Rosen, M., Ioudon, R., Murphy, M., and Perussia, B., Tumor necrosis factor and lymphotoxin induce differentiation of human myeloid cell lines in synergy with immune interferon, *J. Exp. Med., 164*: 1206–1225, 1986.
23. Ottegen, H. F., et al., Exdotoxin-induced tumor necrosis factor, *Recent Results Cancer Res., 75*: 207–212, 1980.
24. Peetre, C., Gulliberg, V., Nilsson, E., Olsson, I., Effects of recombinant tumor necrosis factor on proliferation and differentiation of leukemic and normal hematopoietic cells in vitro, *J. Clin. Invest., 78*: 1694–1700, 1986.
25. Philip, R., and Epstein, L. B., Tumor necrosis factor as immunomodulator and mediator of monocyte cytotoxcity, *Nature, 323*: 86–89, 1986.
26. Nissen-Meyer, J., Rigmor, A., and Espevik, T., Comparison of recombinant tumor necrosis factor involved in monocyte-mediated cytotoxicity, *Cancer Res., 47*: 2251–2258, 1987.
27. Darzynkiewica, A., Carter, S. P., and Old, L. J., Cell cycle-specific effects of tumor necrosis factor, *Cancer Res., 44*: 83–90, 1984.
28. Kull, F. C., Jacobs, S., and Cuatrecasas, P., Cellular receptor for ^{125}I-labeled tumor

necrosis factor: specific binding, affinity labeling, and relationship to sensitivity, *Proc. Natl. Acad. Sci. USA, 82*: 5756, 1985.

29. Yarden, A. and Kimchi, A., Tumor necrosis factor reduces C-MYC expression and cooperates with interferon-γ in HELA cells, *Science, 234*: 1419–1421, 1986.
30. Schachner, J., Blick, M., Gutterman, J., et al., Suppression of C-MYC and C-MYB expression in leukemic cell line sensitive to recombinant tumor necrosis factor alpha, *Proc. Am. Assoc. Cancer Res., 28*: 400, 1987.
31. Ruff, M. R., and Gifford, G. E., Rabbit tumor necrosis factor: mechanism of action, *Infect. Immun., 31*: 380–385, 1981.
32. Alexander, R. B., Nelson, W. G., and Coltey, D. S., Synergistic enhancement by tumor necrosis factor of in vitro cytotoxicity from chemotherapeutic drugs targeted at topoisomerase II, *Cancer Res., 47*: 2403–2406, 1987.
33. Salmon, S. E., and Young, L., Antitumor effects of tumor necrosis factor is markedly enhanced by gamma interferon, *Proc. Am. Soc. Clin. Oncol., 5*: 222, 1986.
34. Ruggiero, and Baglioni, C., Synergistic anti-proliferative activity of interleukin-1 and tumor necrosis factor, *J. Immunol., 138*(3): 661–663, 1987.
35. Broxmeyer, H. E., Williams, D. E., Lu, L., Cooper, S., Anderson, S. L., Beyer, G. S., Hoffman, R., and Rubin, B. Y., The suppressive influences of human tumor necrosis factors on bone marrow hematopoietic progenitor cells from normal donors and patients with leukemia: synergism of tumor necrosis factor and interferon-gamma, *J. Immunol., 136*: 4487–4495, 1986.
36. Owen-Schaub, L. B., Gutterman, J. U., and Grim, E., Recombinant tumor necrosis factor-alpha is synergistic with interleukin in the generation of human lymphokine activated killing (in press).
37. Gemlo, B. T., Palladino, M. A., Jaffe, H. S., Eessalu, T. E., et al., Circulating cytokine levels in patients with metastic cancer treated with recombinant interleukin-2 and lymphokine activated killer cells (in press).
38. Asher, A., Mule, J. J., Reichert, C. M., Shiloni, E., and Rosenberg, S. A., Studies on the anti-tumor efficacy of systemically administered recombinant tumor necrosis factor against several murine tumors in vivo, *J. Immunol., 138*(3): 963–974, 1987.
39. Kramer, S. M., Aggarwal, B. B., Eessalu, T. E., McCabe, S. M., Ferraiolo, B. L., Figori, S. I., and Palladino, M. A. Characterization of the in vitro and in vivo species preference of human and murine tumor necrosis factor-alpha (in press).
40. Chun, M., and Hoffman, M. K., Combination immunotherapy of cancer in a mouse model: synergism between tumor necrosis factor and other defense systems, *Cancer Res., 47*: 115–118, 1987.
41. Winkelhake, J. L., Stampfl, S., and Zimmerman, R. J., Synergistic effects of combination therapy with human recombinant interleukin-2 and tumor necrosis factor in murine tumor models, *Cancer Res., 47*: 3948–3953, 1987.
42. Rothstein, J. L., and Schreiber, H., Synergy between tumor necrosis factor and bacterial products causes hemorrhagic necrosis and lethal shock, *Immunobiology, 175*: 31, 1987.
43. Creasey, A. A., Reynold, M. T., and Laird, W., Cures and partial regression of murine and human tumors by recombinant human tumor necrosis factor, *Cancer Res., 46*: 5687–5690, 1986.
44. Baughman, R. A., Ferraiolo, B., Vandlen, R., Aggarwal, B., and Moore, S. A., Phar-

macokinetics and tissue distribution of recombinant tumor necrosis factor-alpha in rodents, *Pharm. Res., 3*: 1415, 1986.
45. Pfizenmaier, K., Scheurich, P., Schluter, C., and Krönke, M., Tumor necrosis factor enhances HLA-A, B, C and HLA-DR gene expression in human tumor cells, *J. Immunol., 138*(3): 975–980, 1987.
46. Urban, J. L., Shepard, H. M., Rothstein, J. L., Sugarman, B. J. and Schreiber, H., Tumor necrosis factor: a potent effector molecule for tumor cell killing by activated macrophages, *Proc. Natl. Acad. Sci. USA, 83*: 5233–5237, 1986.
47. Hensel, G., Mannel, D. N., Pfizenmaier, K., Krönke, M., et al., Autocrine stimulation of TNF-alpha mRNA expression in HL-60 cells, *Lymphokine Res., 6*(2): 119–125, 1987.
48. Larrick, J. W., Graham, D., Toy, K., Lin, L. S., Senyk, G., and Fendly, B. M., Recombinant tumor necrosis factor causes activation of human granulocytes, *Blood, 69*: 640–644, 1986.
49. Shalaby, M. R., Aggarwal, B. B., Rinderknecht, E., Suerdsky, L. P., Finkle, R. B., and Palladino, M. A., Activation of human polymorphonuclear neutrohil functions by interferon-gamma and tumor necrosis factors, *J. Immunol., 135*(3): 2069–2073, 1985.
50. Gamble, J. R., Harlan, J. M., Klebanoff, S. J., and Vadas, M. A., Stimulation of the adherence of neutrophils to umbilical vein endothelium by human tumor necrosis factor, *Proc. Natl. Acad. Sci. USA, 82*: 8667–8671, 1985.
51. Old, L. J., Polypeptide mediator network, *Nature, 326*: 330–331, 1987.
52. Ming, W. J., Bersami, L., and Mantovani, A., Tumor necrosis factor is chemotactic for monocytes and polymorphonuclear leukocytes, *J. Immunol., 138*: 1469–1473, 1987.
53. Kohase, M., Henriksen-De Stefano, D., May, L. T., Vilček, J., and Sehgal, P. B. Induction of B_2 interferon by tumor necrosis factor: a homeostatic mechanism in the control of cell proliferation, *Cell, 45*: 659–666, 1986.
54. Klebanoff, S. J., Vadas, M. A., Harlan, J. M., Sparks, L. H., Gambel, J. R., and Agosti, J. M. Stimulation of neutrophils by tumor necrosis factor, *J. Immunol., 136*: 1433–1450, 1986.
55. Scheurich, P., Thoma, B., Ucer, V., and Pfizenmaier, K. Immunoregulatory activity of recombinant human tumor necrosis factor: induction of rTNF receptors on human T-cells and TNF-alpha mediated enhancement of T-cell responses, *J. Immunol., 138*: 975–982, 1987.
56. Shalaby, M. R., Hirabayashi, S. F., Suedersky, L. P., Palladino, M. A. Regulation of immune function in vitro by recombinant tumor necrosis factor and lymphotoxin, *Fed. Proc., 44*: 569, 1985.
57. Haidaris, C. G., Haynes, J. D., Meltzer, M. S., and Allison, A. C. Serum containing tumor necrosis factor is cytotoxic for the human malaria parasite *Plasmodium falciparum, Infect. Immun., 42*(1): 385–393, 1983.
58. Scuderi, P., Lam, K. S., Ryan, K. J., Finley, P. R., Ray, G., Peterson, E., and Salmon, S. Raised serum levels of tumor necrosis factor in parasitic infections, *Lancet, 2:* 1364–1365, 1986.
59. Ostensen, M. E., Thiele, D. L., and Lipsky, P. E. Tumor necrosis factor-α enhances cytolytic activity of human natural killer cells, *J. Immunol., 138*: 4185–4191, 1987.
60. Tracy, K. J., Beutler, B., Lowry, S. R., et al. Shock and tissue injury induced by recombinant human cachectin, *Science, 230*: 630–632, 1986.

61. Beutler, B., Milsark, I., and Cerami, A. Passive immunization of cachectin/tumor necrosis factor protects mice from the lethal effects of endotoxin. *Science, 229*: 869–871, 1985.
62. Mestan, J., Digel, W., Mittnacht, S., Hillen, H., Blohm, D., Moller, A., Jacobsen, H., and Kirschner, H. Antiviral effects of recombinant tumor necrosis factor in vitro, *Nature, 323*: 816–819, 1986.
63. Wong, G. H., and Goeddel, D. V. Tumor necrosis factor α and β inhibit virus replication and synergize with interferons, *nature, 323*: 819–822, 1986.
64. Beutler, B., Milsark, I., and Cerami, A. Cachectin/tumor necrosis factor: production distribution and metabolic fate in vivo *J. Immunol., 135*(6): 3972–3977, 1985.
65. Torti, F. M., Dieckmann, B., Beutler, B., Cerami, A., and Ringold,, G. M. A macrophage factor inhibits adipocyte gene expression: an in vitro model of cachexia, *Science, 229*: 867–869, 1985.
66. Patton, J. S., Shepard, H. M., Wilking, H., Lewis, G., Aggarwal, B. B., Eessulu, T. E., Gavin, L. A., and Grunfled, C. Interferons and tumor necrosis factors have similar catabolic effects on 3T3 L1 cells, *Proc. Natl. Acad. Sci. USA, 83*: 8313–8317, 1986.
67. Kurzrock, R., Rohde, M. F., Quesada, J. R., Gianturco, S. J., Bradley, W. A., Sherwin, S. A., and Gutterman, J. U. Recombinant interferon-gamma induces hypertriglyceridemia and inhibits post-heparin lipase activity in cancer patients, *J. Exp. Med., 164*(4): 1093–1101, 1986.
68. Bertolini, D. R., Nedwin, G. E., Bringman, T. S., Smith, D. D., and Mundy, G. R. Stimulation of bone resorption and inhibition of bone formation in vitro by human tumor necrosis factors, *Nature, 319*: 516–518, 1986.
69. Stashenko, P., Dewhirst, F. E., Peros, W. J., Kent, R. L., and Ago, J. M. Synertistic interactions between interleukin-1 tumor necrosis factor, and lymphotoxin in bone resorption, *J. Immunol., 138*(5): 1464–1468, 1987.
70. Garrett, I. R., Durie, B. G. M., Nedwin, G. E., Gillespie, A., Bringman, T., Sabatini, M., Bertolini, D. R., and Mundy, G. R. Production of lynphotoxin, a bone resorbing cytokine, by cultured human myeloma cells. *N. Engl. J. Med., 317*(a): 526–531, 1987.
71. Prince, W. S., Harder, K. J., Saks, S., Reed, B. R., Chen, A. B., and Jones, A. J. S. ELISA for quantitation of tumor necrosis factor-alpha in serum (in press).
72. Blick, M. B., Sherwin, S. A., Rosenblum, M. G., and Gutterman, J. U. A phase I trial of recombinant tumor necrosis factor (rTNF) in cancer patients, *Proc. Am. Soc. Clin. Oncol., 5*: 53, 1986.
73. Chapman, P. B., Lester, R. J., Casper, E. S., Gabrilove, J. L., Kempin, S., and Welt, S. Phase I study of recombinant tumor necrosis factor (rTNF), *Proc. Am. Soc. Clin. Oncol., 5*: 905, 1986.
74. Kempin, S., Gold, P., Glaser, B., Carroll, W., Lester, T., Chapman, P., Gabrilove, J., Casper, E., and Oettgen, H. Hemostatic alterations in patients receiving recombinant tumor necrosis factor (rTNF), *Blood, 335*(a): 1218, 1986.
75. Blick, M., Sherwin, S. A., Rosenblum, M., and Gutterman, J. Phase I study of recombinant tumor necrosis factor in cancer patients, *Cancer Res., 47*: 2986–2989, 1987.
76. Gabrilove, J. L., Starnes, H. F., Begas, A., Casper, E., Chapman, P., Engert, A., Jacabows, I. A., Gasson, J., Templeton, M. A., Sherwin, S., Brennen, M., and Oettgen, H. F. A phase I study of intravenously administered rTNF-alpha inpatients with advanced cancer, *Proc, Am. Soc. Clin. Oncol., 6*: 973, 1987.

77. Engert, A., Gabrilove, J. L., Welk, K., et al. Cell surface marker analysis on peripheral blood mononuclear cells from patients with advanced malignancy treated with recombinant tumor necrosis factor-alpha (rTNF), *Proc. Am. Assoc. Cancer Res., 28*: 187, 1987.
78. Feinberg, B., Kurzrock, R., Talpaz, M., Blick, M., Saks, S., and Gutterman, J. U. Phase I study of recombinant tumor necrosis factor-alpha in patients, *J. Clin. Oncol., 6*: 1328–1334, 1988.
79. Jakabowski, A., Casper, E., Gabrilove, J., Lester, T., Sherwin, S., Old, L. J., Oettgen, H. Phase I trial of intramuscularly administered tumor necrosis factor in adults with advanced cancer, *Proc. Am. Soc. Clin. Oncol., 6*: 956, 1987.
80. Creagen, E., Kovach, J., Moertel, C., Loprinzi, C., and Sherwin, S. Phase I trial of recombinant human tumor necrosis factor (rTNF), *Proc. Am. Soc. Clin. Oncol., 6*: 976, 1987.
81. Trump, D., Remick, S. C., Albertini, D., Nietsing, L., Tombes, M. B., Brown, R., Rosenzweig, B., Tutsch, K., Grem, J. L., and Wilson, J. A clinical trial of recombinant tumor necrosis factor (rTNF) administered three times weekly, *Proc. Am. Assoc. Cancer Res., 28*: 401, 1987.
82. Mertlesmann, R., Gamm, H., Flener, R., et al. Recombinant human tumor necrosis factor alpha (rhTNF-alpha) in advanced cancer: a phase I clinical trial, *Proc. Am. Assoc. Cancer Res., 28*: 399, 1987.
83. Creaven, P. J., Brenner, D. E., Cowens, J. W., Huben, R. P., and Wolp, R. M. A phase I clinical trial of recombinant human tumor necrosis factor given daily for five days, *Cancer Chemother. Pharmacol., 23*: 186–191, 1989.
84. Sherman, M. L., Spriggs, D. R., Arthur, K. A., Imamura, K., Frei, E., III, and Kufe, D. W. Recombinant human tumor necrosis factor administered as a five-day continuous infusion in cancer patients: phase I toxicity and effect on lipid metabolism, *J. Clin. Oncol.,* 1988 Feb. 6, pp. 344–350.
85. Spriggs, D. R., Sherman, M. L., Michie, H., Arthur, K. A., Imamura, K., and Wilmore, D. Recombinant human tumor necrosis factor administered as a 24 hour intravenous infusion: a phase I and pharmacologic study, *J. Natl. Cancer Inst.*, 1988 Sept. 7, pp. 80, 1039–1044.
86. Krigel, R., Comis, R., Padavic, K., Konrad, M., Bradley, E., and Rudolph, A. Phase I trials of recombinant tumor necrosis factor (rTNF) in patients with advanced malignancy, *Proc. Am. Soc. Clin. Oncol., 6*: 241, 1987.
87. Morice, R., Blick, M. B., Ali, M. K., and Gutterman, J. U. Pulmonary toxicity of recombinant tumor necrosis factor (rTNF), *Proc. Am. Soc. Clin. Oncol., 6*: 29, 1987.
88. Kramer, S. M., Carver, M. E., Prince, W. S., Chen, A. B., and Saks, S. R. Analysis of methods for determining human tumor necrosis factor-alpha neutralizing antibody titers: demonstration of lack of antibody production in treated patient, *Immunobiology, 175*: 97, 1987.
89. Figlin, R., Dekernion, J., Sarna, G., Muldower, N., and Saks, S. Phase II study of recombinant tumor necrosis factor in patients with metastatic renal cell carcinoma and malignant melanoma, *Proc. Am. Soc. Clin. Oncol., 7*: 652, 1988.
90. Aboulafia, D., Miles, S. A., Saks, S. R., and Mitsuyasu, R. T. Intravenous recombinant tumor necrosis factor in the treatment of AIDS-related Kaposi's sarcoma, *J. Acquired Immune Defic. Syndr., 2*: 54–58, 1989.

91. Markowitz, A., Parkinson, D., Miller, L., Levitt, D., Saks, S., and Gutterman, J. Phase I study of recombinant interleukin-2 and recombinant tumor necrosis factor, *Proc. Am. Soc. Clin. Oncol., 8*: 1989.
92. Abbruzzese, J. L., Levin, B., Ajani, J. A., et al. A phase I trial of recombinant tumor necrosis factor in patients with advanced gastrointestinal cancer, *Cancer Res.* (in press).
93. Jakubowski, A., Caper, E., Gabrilove, J., Templeton, M. A., Sherwin, S., and Oettgen, H. F. Phase I trial of intravenous tumor necrosis factor plus interferon gamma in patients with advanced cancer, *Proc. Am. Soc. Clin. Oncol., 7*: 1988.
94. Urba, W., Clark, J. W., Longo, D. L., Smith, J. W., Miller, R., Kopp, W. C., Finch, L., Gordon, K.., Farrell, M., Creekmore, S., Stewart, M., Rosen, N., Sherwin, S., and Steis, R. G. Phase I evaluation of the toxicity and immunomodulatory effects of tumor necrosis factor and interferon-gamma, *Proc. Am. Soc. Clin. Oncol., 7*: 641, 1988.
95. Frei, E., and Spriggs, D. Tumor necrosis factor: still a promising agent, *J. Clin. Oncol., 7*: 291–294, 1989.
96. Zukiwski, A., Wallace, S., Gutterman, J., Saks, S., and Mavligit, G. Hepatic arterial infusion of recombinant tumor necrosis factor in patients with metastatic carcinoma, *Proc. Am. Soc. Clin. Oncol., 8*: 476, 1989.
97. Kahn, J. O., Kaplan, J. D., Volberding, P. A., Ziegler, J. L., Saks, S. R., and Abrams, D. I. Intralesional recombinant tumor necrosis factor alpha for AIDS-associated Kaposi's sarcoma: a randomized double-blind trial, *J. AIDS, 2*: 217–223, 1989.
98. Gibaldi, M., and Perrier, D. *Pharmacokinetics*, Marcel Dekker, New York: 1982.
99. Kurzrock, R., Rosenblum, M. G., Sherwin, S. S., Rios, A. A., Talpaz, M., Quesada, J., and Gutterman, J. U. Pharmacokinetics, single-dose tolerance and biological activity of recombinant γ-interferon in cancer patients, *Cancer Res., 45*: 2866–2872, 1985.
100. Gutterman, J. U., Fein, S., Quesada, J., Horning, S. J., Levine, J. F., Alexanian, R., Bernhardt, L., Kramer, M., Spiegel, H., Colburn, W., Trown, P., Merigan, T., and Dziewanowski, Z. Recombinant leukocyte A interferon: pharmacokinetics, single-dose tolerance, and biologic effects in cancer patients, *Ann. Intern. Med., 95*: 549–556, 1982.
101. Mortiz, T., Niederle, N., Baumann, J., May, D., Kurschel, E., Osieka, R., Kempeni, J., Schlick, E., and Schmidt, C. G. Phase I study of recombinant human tumor necrosis factor alpha in advanced malignant disease, *Cancer Immun. Immunother., 29*(2): 144–150, 1989.
102. Flick, D. A., and Gifford, G. E. Pharmacokinetics of murine tumor necrosis factor, *J. Immunopharmacol., 8*(1): 89–97, 1986.

Index